MENTAL ILLNESS AND SOCIAL POLICY

THE AMERICAN EXPERIENCE

MENTAL ILLNESS AND SOCIAL POLICY

THE AMERICAN EXPERIENCE

Advisory Editor
GERALD N. GROB

Editorial Board
ERIC T. CARLSON
BLANCHE D. COLL
CHARLES E. ROSENBERG

A

TREATISE ON INSANITY

IN ITS

MEDICAL RELATIONS

BY

WILLIAM A. HAMMOND

ARNO PRESS

A NEW YORK TIMES COMPANY

New York • 1973

Reprint Edition 1973 by Arno Press Inc.

MENTAL ILLNESS AND SOCIAL POLICY:
  The American Experience
ISBN for complete set: 0-405-05190-5
See last pages of this volume for titles.

Manufactured in the United States of America

———◆———

Library of Congress Cataloging in Publication Data

Hammond, William Alexander, 1828-1900.
    A treatise on insanity in its medical relations.

    (Mental illness and social policy: the American
experience)
    Reprint of the ed. published by D. Appleton, New
York.
    1. Psychiatry--Early works to 1900. I. Title.
II. Series. [DNLM: WM H227t 1883F]
RC340.H3 1973   157   73-2402
ISBN 0-405-05208-1

A

TREATISE ON INSANITY

IN ITS

MEDICAL RELATIONS.

BY

WILLIAM A. HAMMOND, M. D.,

SURGEON-GENERAL UNITED STATES ARMY (RETIRED LIST); PROFESSOR OF DISEASES OF THE MIND AND
NERVOUS SYSTEM, IN THE NEW YORK POST-GRADUATE MEDICAL SCHOOL; PRESIDENT OF
THE AMERICAN NEUROLOGICAL ASSOCIATION, ETC., ETC.

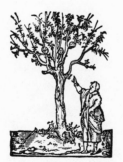

Fructu, non foliis arborem æstima.

NEW YORK:

D. APPLETON AND COMPANY,

1, 3, AND 5 BOND STREET.

1883.

I DEDICATE THIS BOOK

TO

J. S. JEWELL, M. D.,

PROFESSOR OF NERVOUS AND MENTAL DISEASES IN THE CHICAGO MEDICAL COLLEGE,

WHOSE LEARNING

HAS ALWAYS COMMANDED MY HEARTIEST ADMIRATION,

AND WHOSE FRIENDSHIP

IS ONE OF THE GREATEST PLEASURES OF MY LIFE.

PREFACE.

In presenting to the medical profession a new work on the subject of Insanity, it seems proper that I should state the reasons which have induced me to add another volume to the store of medico-psychological literature, and to point out briefly what are, I think, distinctive features of the present production.

I have long been convinced that the term "insanity" has hitherto been applied in altogether too limited and illogical a manner. It has been understood, both in and out of the profession, that a person, in order to be considered the subject of mental aberration, must, at some time or other, present certain marked symptoms, which he cannot avoid exhibiting, and which are sufficient to indicate to the world that he is not in his right mind.

Starting from the points that all normal mental phenomena are the result of the action of a healthy brain, and that all abnormal manifestations of mind are the result of the functionation of a diseased or deranged brain, I do not see why these latter should not be included under the designation of "insanity," as much as the former are embraced under the term "sanity." There can be no middle ground, for the brain is either in a healthy or in an unhealthy condition. If healthy, the product of its action is "sanity;" if unhealthy, "insanity."

Of course, very little of such insanity comes under the signification given to the word by lawyers and the public gen-

erally.   But legal insanity and medical insanity are very
different things, and the two standards can never and ought
never to be the same.   The law establishes an arbitrary and
unscientific line, and declares that every act performed on one
side of this line is the act of a sane mind, while all acts done
on the other side result from insane minds.   This line may be
in one place to-day, and in an entirely different place to-morrow, at the whim or caprice of a Legislature ; it may be established on a certain parallel in one country, and on an entirely
different parallel in another country.   In the State of New
York, for instance, it is drawn at the knowledge of right and
wrong ; and perhaps, all things considered, this is about as
correct a legal line as a due regard for the safety of society
will permit to be made.   But every physician knows that it is
absolutely untenable from his point of view ; that it is not a
medical line, and that there are thousands of lunatics insane
enough to believe themselves to be veritable Julius Cæsars,
and yet sufficiently sane to know that a particular act is contrary to law, and to be fully aware of the nature and consequences of such act.   Hence it follows that, from a medical
stand-point, there is no middle ground between sanity and insanity.   The line of demarkation is sharply drawn, and it is
but a step from one territory to the other.   There is a large
proportion of the population of every civilized community
composed of individuals whose insanity is known only to
themselves, and perhaps to some of those who are in intimate
social relations with them, who have lost none of their rights,
privileges, or responsibilities as citizens, who transact their
business with fidelity and accuracy, and yet who are as truly
insane, though in a less degree, as the most furious maniac
who dashes his head against the stone-walls of his cell.   To
many of these persons life is a burden they would willingly
throw off, if death concerned them alone, for they are painfully conscious of their actual suffering, and morbidly apprehensive in regard to the future.   There are very few people
who have not at some time or other, perhaps for a moment
only, been medically insane.   It is time, therefore, that the

horror of the word should be dissipated, and that the fact should be recognized and acted upon, that a disordered mind is just as surely the result of a disordered brain as dyspepsia is of a deranged stomach; that a scarcely appreciable increase or diminution of the blood-supply to the brain will lead as surely to mental derangement of some kind as an apparently insignificant change of the muscular tissue of the heart to fat, will lead to a derangement of the circulation, and that in the one case there may be a hallucination, a delusion, a morbid impulse, or a paralysis of the will, just as in the other there may be an intermittent pulse, a vertigo, or a fainting-fit. There is no more disgrace to be attached to the one condition than to the other.

To some of the states of mental aberration which are thus, I think, properly to be classed as insanities, I have endeavored to draw attention, to point out their clinical features, and to indicate the treatment proper for them. So far as I know, this is the first systematic attempt in this direction, and some of the forms—though many physicians will recognize them as old acquaintances they have met with in their practice—are now described for the first time.

Again, the alienistic physician, whose practice is not restricted to a lunatic asylum, has peculiar facilities for studying insanity in its first and most curable stages. There are many varieties of mental derangement of which asylum physicians never see the beginning; and there are others, not requiring the restraint of an institution of the kind, which they never see at all. The day has gone by when they were looked upon as the sole exponents of psychological medicine, and in all parts of the civilized world the greatest advances in that division of the healing science and art are made by physicians who are unconnected with asylums.

I have devoted a whole section of this work to the consideration of sleep and some of its derangements, and am indebted to Messrs. J. B. Lippincott & Co., of Philadelphia, the publishers of a little book of mine on the subject,[1] for per-

[1] "On Sleep and its Derangements," Philadelphia, J. B. Lippincott & Co.

1

mission to incorporate some of its chapters into the present volume. I think that a knowledge of the physiology and pathology of this function should form the groundwork of the study of insanity. It is in aberrations of sleep that we often find the first indications of aberrations of mind.

I am also greatly indebted to Dr. R. L. Parsons, late the Medical Superintendent of the New York City Lunatic Asylum, for the use of his voluminous case-books of patients in that institution while it was under his charge. The perusal of these records has been of great assistance to me in my descriptions of several of the forms of insanity.

Again, a word in regard to the classification adopted. In the present state of the patho-anatomy of insanity, a classification, based, as it should be, on the essential morbid conditions giving rise to the symptoms, cannot be made. There are indications, however, that vaso-motor disturbances, by which the amount of intracranial blood is altered either by increase or diminution, are the starting-point at least of almost every known form of mental derangement. In his recent work on Insanity, Luys[1] adopts this view—a view which, I may say, has long been held, though not so thoroughly worked out, by the author of the present volume, and which he has enunciated in several monographs and treatises.[2] It is in this direction that we are to look for the data on which to found a correct system of psychological pathology and a true classification.

In the mean time every author arranges the varieties which he differentiates, to suit himself, and at once with entire consistency proceeds to point out the fallacies and shortcomings of other systems. A classification such as can be made at

[1] "Traité clinique et pratique des maladies mentales," Paris, 1881.

[2] "On Wakefulness," *New York Medical Journal*, 1865.

"Sleep and its Derangements," Philadelphia, 1869.

"On some of the Effects of Excessive Intellectual Exertion," Bellevue and Charity Hospital Reports, New York, 1870.

"A Treatise on the Diseases of the Nervous System," New York, 1871, and subsequent editions to seventh, 1881.

"Cerebral Hyperæmia, the Result of Mental Strain and Emotional Disturbance," New York, 1879.

"On Certain Conditions of Nervous Derangement," New York, 1881.

present can pretend to no more than to arrange the several forms of mental derangement into groups, possessing some one prominent feature in common. Whatever may be the objections to the system I have proposed in this work—and that they are many, no one knows better than I do myself— I hope and believe that it will prove of assistance to the student desirous of investigating the phenomena of insanity. If this expectation is only partially fulfilled, I shall be amply satisfied.

Finally, the objection may be made that, not being the superintendent of a lunatic asylum, I have no business to set up as an authority on insanity, much less to write a book on the subject. To any raising that point I would say that for the last seventeen years I have been a teacher on the subject of " Diseases of the Mind and Nervous System " in four medical colleges of the city of New York, three of them among the largest in the United States, and one the course of instruction in which is given to physicians only. The first professorship of that branch of medical science in this country was held by me; and, furthermore, that, though I cannot claim to have seen so many cases of insanity as the average superintendent of an asylum with its thousand inmates, I do claim that a single case thoroughly studied is worth more as a lesson than a hundred that are simply looked at, and often from afar off. The medical student who dissects one human body is likely to learn more of anatomy than the janitor who sees hundreds of corpses brought to the dissecting-room.

43 West Fifty-fourth Street,
New York, *May 1, 1883.*

CONTENTS.

SECTION I.

GENERAL PRINCIPLES OF THE PHYSIOLOGY AND PATHOLOGY OF THE HUMAN MIND.

SECTION II.

INSTINCT: ITS NATURE AND SEAT.

SECTION III.

SECTION IV.

DESCRIPTION AND TREATMENT OF INSANITY.

A

TREATISE ON INSANITY.

SECTION I.

GENERAL PRINCIPLES OF THE PHYSIOLOGY AND PATHOLOGY OF THE MIND.

CHAPTER I.

NATURE AND SEAT OF THE MIND.

THE brain is the chief organ from which the force called the mind is evolved, and, so far as the present treatise is concerned, may be regarded as the only one. For, though, wherever there is gray nerve-tissue, whether it be in the brain, the spinal cord, or the sympathetic ganglia, nervous force is generated ; and, though all nervous force partakes more or less of the attributes of that which we call mind, its qualities, as exhibited by the force manifested by these latter two organs, are not of such a character, either in health or disease, as to come within the scope of the present treatise. It is with the mind developed by the brain that we have to concern ourselves.

By mind, therefore, I understand a force produced by nervous action, and in man especially by the action of the brain. There are animals without brains, and others again with the cerebral mass so small as to be of much less importance than the spinal cord, and yet in all these there are continual manifestations of the existence of mind. Indeed, in some of them the brain may be removed without, for a time, any considerable impairment of the mental force being produced. As we ascend, however, in the scale of animal life, the brain becomes more and more predominant, until, when we reach the higher orders, at the head of which stands man, it is almost the exclusive seat of the mind.

In former times the dependence of the mind upon the brain was not distinctly and fully recognized. The emotions, for instance, were supposed to have their seat in other organs —some in the heart, others in the liver, the spleen, and the bowels. So firmly was this idea implanted that it even at the present day influences our modes of speech. Thus we say of a man that he has a "good heart," or that his "heart is in the right place"; the boy learns his lessons "by heart," the lover adores his mistress with his "whole heart," and the sinner, when he is converted from his evil ways, undergoes a "change of heart." The influence ascribed to the liver is shown in our words "melancholic" and "choleric," as applied to low-spirited and angry persons; to the spleen in the term "splenetic," as indicating a spiteful individual; and we say of another that he has no "bowels of compassion."

The connection between the mind and the brain is not doubted at the present day, although the character of the relation is still the subject of controversy. On the one hand, it is contended that the brain is only a tool or organ of which the mind makes use in man to manifest itself. According to this view, there is in every human being a mind not dependent upon the nervous system for its existence. On the other hand, it is asserted that the mind is directly the result of nervous action, and especially of the brain, and that if there were no nerve-substance there would be no mind. This view is that which is held by the majority of scientific writers of the present day. The discussion of the question need not, however, concern us here, for, whether the one or the other theory be correct, the brain and nervous system generally must be equally the subject of study in the consideration of either normal or abnormal mental manifestations.

It may, however, be remarked that if the mind is in independent, self-conscious, immaterial personality, using the brain as its instrument for communicating with the external world, it is impossible for us to deny a like principle to the lower animals, differing only in degree as their brains differ from ours. They perceive, experience emotions, have intellects which memorize and exercise judgment, and wills to carry out, in accordance with their powers, the conclusions to which their reasoning leads them.

According to the theological school of philosophers, the mind of an idiot is as good as the mind of Herbert Spencer—

better, perhaps, in a moral point of view. The difference consists, in their opinion, solely in the fact that, whereas Herbert Spencer has a good tool to work with, the idiot has a bad one, and hence the product of his labor is of an inferior quality.

The essential fault of these philosophers is that they confound the mind with the soul. Science has nothing to do with the latter. Its existence is altogether a matter of faith —not of proof—which people believe in or not, according to the education they have received and the subsequent reflection they have bestowed upon the subject. But the mind is found wherever there is gray nerve-matter in action, from the lowest invertebrate animal up to the highest and most intellectual man who walks the earth. With it science may properly concern itself, and with it theologians, as such, have nothing to do.

The several categories of facts which go to establish the connection between the mind and the brain have been well set forth by Mr. Bain,[1] and are in general character similar to those which exist between any other viscus and the product of its action. They are as follows:

1. The action of an organ, even within the limits of health, frequently gives rise to sensations of various kinds, and slight functional derangements are very distinctly felt. Thus the pain of indigestion is referred to the stomach or bowels, as the case may be; disorders of the urinary excretion are manifested by uneasiness in the kidneys; derangements of the secretion of the bile cause pain in the liver; loud noises produce unpleasant feelings in the ears; and excessive or improper use of the eyes causes pain and other abnormalities of these organs. So it is with the brain, and often to a very marked degree. Though ordinarily we are not conscious by any particular sensation that we are using it when we think (and the same is true, *mutatis mutandis*, of the other organs mentioned), yet inordinate mental exertion, or continual disturbance, gives rise to headache, vertigo, and other derangements of sensibility referable to the brain. If the disturbing factor be continued in action, not only are these indications of disorder increased, but the mind shows evidences of derangement, and the organs of the body whose functions are controlled by the brain are likewise affected. As a consequence, insanity and paralysis result, and, upon *post-mortem* exami-

[1] "The Senses and the Intellect," second edition, London, 1864, p. 11.

nation, the brain is found to be the seat of organic disease. There are many persons in whom only very slight mental action invariably produces pain in the head, and others again who are similarly affected by particular kinds of mental exertion, while other kinds, even in excess of proper limits, cause no sensations. Thus some individuals cannot attempt the solution of mathematical problems without suffering from pain in the head, and some experience a like disturbance from the very slight mental effort necessary in adding up a column of figures.

2. Injury or disease of the brain impairs in some way or other the capacity or endurance of the mind. A blow on the head causes confusion of ideas, and, if hard enough, may abolish consciousness or the power of thought altogether. A piece of fractured bone, or a bullet pressing on the brain, likewise destroys the ability to think ; and the same result, or some other indication of mental disturbance, accompanies brain tumors, extravasations of blood within the cranial cavity, congestion, embolism or thrombosis of the cerebral blood-vessels, inflammation, or other disease of the brain. The fact that occasionally, on *post-mortem* examination, severe organic disease of the brain is found to have existed during life without the production of notable symptoms, is no argument against the view here taken. All parts of the brain are not equally concerned in the production of mind, and by far the larger portion—the white substance—is only a medium for the transmission of the nerve-force which has been generated by the gray matter. I think, however, that it may be laid down as a law, admitting of no exception, that injury or disease of the convolutions, or any other portion of the gray tissue, is invariably accompanied by a disturbance of the functions of the brain of a character and extent commensurate with the seat and severity of the lesion. Cases are on record in which the consciousness of the individual has been suspended for several months, from the fact of pressure exerted by depressed bone upon some portion of the cortex, and in which, on the instant that the pressure was removed by surgical interference, consciousness was restored.

3. The action of the brain, like that of any other of the animal organs, results in the disintegration of its substance, and this destruction is in direct proportion to the amount of mental work done. We find, therefore, that the alkaline

phosphates, which are mainly derived from the destructive metamorphosis of the nervous tissue, and which are excreted by the kidneys, are increased in quantity after severe intellectual labor, and are diminished by mental quietude. In a memoir published several years ago, I gave the results of a series of experiments performed upon myself, which show conclusively that increased use of the brain causes increased decay of its tissue, as demonstrated by the largely augmented quantity of phosphates excreted by the urine.[1] As the chemist, by weighing the ashes on the hearth, determines how much wood has been burnt, so the physiologist, by weighing the ashes of the brain—the phosphates—measures the amount of thought which has resulted from the combustion of the encephalon.

4. The size of the brain is well known to bear a direct relation to the intelligence of the individual; and, when all other conditions are alike, it may be said that the largest brain will produce the greatest amount of mental energy. This deduction is based upon the fact that, as a rule, the larger the brain as a whole, the greater is the quantity of gray matter upon which its activity depends. Occasionally there are apparent exceptions to this statement, but there is reason for thinking that they are not so real as they seem. It is entirely consonant with the results of experience to meet with individuals of moderate-sized brains and great intellectual activity in whom the cortical substance is of unusual thickness, and the convolutions of more than ordinary complexity.

At the same time it is a well-known fact that, when the brain is markedly below the average in weight, mental weakness is a necessary concomitant. Thus Dr. Thurnam[2] has shown that the average weight of the brain of Europeans is 49 ounces, while in ten men remarkable for their intellectual development it was 54·7 ounces. Of these, the brain of Cuvier, the celebrated naturalist, weighed 64·5 ounces, Spurzheim's 55·6, and Daniel Webster's 53·5. On the other hand, the brain is small in idiots. In three individuals of very feeble intelligence, whose ages were sixteen, forty, and fifty years, respectively, Tiedemann found the weights of their brains to be 19¾,

---

[1] "Urological Contributions," *American Journal of the Medical Sciences*, April, 1856, p. 330; also, "Physiological Memoirs," Philadelphia, 1863, p. 17.

[2] *Journal of Mental Science*, April, 1866.

25¾, and 22½ ounces. Mr. Gore[1] has reported the case of a woman, forty-two years of age, whose intellect was infantine, who could scarcely say a few words, whose gait was unsteady, and whose chief occupation was carrying and nursing a doll. After death, the weight of her brain was found to be but 10 ounces and 5 grains.

Mr. Marshall[2] has also reported a case of microcephaly existing in the person of a boy twelve years of age, whose brain weighed but 8½ ounces. The convolutions were strongly marked, though few in number and narrow. In a remarkable case which came under my own observation, the individual, a woman twenty-two years of age, was unable to talk, though she could utter a few inarticulate sounds expressive of the more imperious of her wants. The cranium had a circumference of only 14 inches at its largest measurement, and the brain was found to weigh but 23½ ounces. The thickness of the gray matter at no part of the surface exceeded $\frac{1}{25}$ of an inch, and generally was below this point, whereas in the brain of a person of ordinary intelligence it is often more than twice this depth. The convolutions were of very simple structure, and the fissuration comparatively slightly marked. In no adult not an idiot is the cranium less than 17 inches in circumference.

Gratiolet[3] fixes the lowest weight of the human brain in a person of ordinary intelligence at about 31¾ ounces. When the weight is below this, the individual is necessarily an idiot.

Thurnam[4] states that, as the result of his observations, the weight of the female brain is about ten per cent. less than that of the male, and this is about the difference as determined by other observers. Of course this is an average result, for there are many women with larger brains than many men, and of consequently higher mental capacity.

5. Experiments performed upon the nerves and nerve-centres show that from the brain proceeds the force by which muscles are moved ; that it is the chief organ by which sensations are perceived—all the special senses, with the possible

---

[1] " Notes of a Case of Microcephaly," *Anthropological Review*, No. 1, May, 1863, p. 168.

[2] "Brain and Calvarium of a Microcephale, *Anthropological Review*, No. 2, August, 1863, p. 8.

[3] " Anatomie comparée du système nerveux," Paris, 1857, t. ii, p. 318.

[4] *Op. cit.*

exception of touch, having their centres of perception in the brain alone—and that certain portions of the brain are in direct relation with certain faculties of the mind, sensorial operations and muscular actions. Thus, division of a nerve supplying any particular muscle cuts off the connection between the brain and that muscle, and hence the will can no longer act upon it. Division of any nerve of special sense prevents the perception of sensorial impressions. If, for instance, the optic nerve be cut, though the whole optical apparatus of the eye remain unimpaired, the sight is destroyed, for the reason that the communication with the organ of perception is severed. Again, by destroying certain portions of the brain, the power to exercise those sensorial organs which are under the control of the injured regions is lost, faculties of the mind are abolished or impaired, and the ability to move the muscles which derive their innervation from those parts is abolished or diminished. From all of which considerations the connection between the brain and the mind is as clearly made out as any other fact in physiology.[1]

CHAPTER II.

DIVISIONS OF MIND.

The mind, like some other forces, is compound—that is, is made up of several sub-forces. These are: perception, intellect, emotions, and will. All the mental manifestations of which the brain is capable are embraced in one or more of these parts. Either one may be exercised independently of the other, though they are very intimately connected, and in all continuous mental processes are brought more or less into relative and consecutive action. To the consideration of some of the primary facts associated with each of these divisions a brief space may be given.

1. **Perception.**—By perception is to be understood that part

[1] That the spinal cord is likewise the seat of certain elements of mind, or rather is capable of evolving them, can be satisfactorily shown by a parity of reasoning. For the illustrations and arguments relative to this subject, the reader is referred to the author's inaugural address as President of the New York Neurological Society, entitled "The Brain not the Sole Organ of the Mind," *Journal of Nervous and Mental Disease*, January, 1876.

of the mind whose office it is to place the individual in relation with external objects. For the evolution of this force the brain is in intimate relation with certain organs which serve the purpose of receiving the impressions of objects according to their several kinds. These are the organs of the special senses. In order that there may be a perception, there must, therefore, be a special apparatus of an optical, acoustic, olfactory, gustatory, or tactile character, a nerve to transmit to the brain the peculiar impressions made upon the organ, and a ganglionic centre to convert the impression into a perception. The eye, for instance, would be just as capable of receiving images upon the retina if the optic nerve were divided, but the brain would obtain no knowledge of them, and there would, consequently, be no perception. And though the eye and the optic nerve should both be in a normal condition, if the ganglion in connection therewith should be sufficiently diseased, either there would be a perverted perception or none at all. Like reasoning is, of course, applicable to each of the other special senses—hearing, smell, taste, and touch.

But, although no knowledge of external objects can be obtained without the intervention of the special senses, there may be in certain diseased or disordered states of the brain false perceptions which are altogether of esoteric formation. These are called hallucinations, and will engage our attention farther on. For their creation no sense-organ is requisite; indeed, they are quite common in persons who have lost their eyesight or hearing, and who, nevertheless, have frequent hallucinations of either sense. But no hallucination of a sense can exist unless the individual has, at least at some former period, exercised the sense in question.

Perception may exist without there being at the time any superior intellectual act—without any ideation whatever. Thus, if the cerebrum of a pigeon be removed, the animal is still capable of seeing, of hearing, and of exercising the other senses, but it obtains no idea from the impressions which have been made upon the perceptive ganglia. If a candle be moved in front of the eyes, the head is turned in accordance with the motion of the candle, but no alarm is excited, and there is no attempt to escape. If the hand be stretched out as if to seize the bird, it is equally quiet, although previously to the removal of the hemispheres it may have been particularly wild and timid. The discharge of a pistol near its head causes the animal to open its eyes, showing that the sound is heard, but it derives no idea from what would in its normal condition excite the emotion of fear and develop complex muscular actions in its endeavors to get away. If the foot be pinched, an effort is at once made to withdraw the member, and this is repeated as often as the excitation is applied, the animal in the mean time remaining otherwise undisturbed. It is evident, therefore, that no idea is obtained from the impressions which are made on the special sense-organs, and that the memory of them does not exist for a single instant. The mind, with the exception of perception, has been removed with the hemispheres.

In certain abnormal, or *quasi* abnormal, conditions of the system, the several categories of mental faculties, with the exception of perception, appear to be in a state of suspension. Thus, in somnambulism and trance, whether idiopathic or artificially induced, the perceptions often reach a very high degree of acuteness, while the intellect, the emotions, and the will are in abeyance. In the insane a like condition sometimes exists.

Perception is the starting-point of all ideation. An individual born without any of the special senses, or without the essential nervous structures for developing sensorial impressions into perceptions, would be unable to form the simplest possible idea of any object or subject. The avenues of knowledge in such a person would be closed, and—no matter how perfect the rest of the nervous system might be, no matter how complex the cerebral convolutions, or how thick the gray matter of the cortex—there would be no mind. The brain can originate nothing; ideas are not innate; they are derived entirely from without. The brain takes the impressions it receives, converts them into the appropriate perceptions, elaborates these into thousands of varied ideas, develops these primary ideas into thousands of others, and so on, without end; but the beginning is in every case material. The sparks that light up the intellectual, emotional, and volitional fires, come from the things around us; and though the mind of a Socrates might potentially exist in the cerebral cortex of a man without sight, hearing, touch, taste, or smell, it would never kindle into the faintest scintillation, though it endured for an eternity. Such a man would be unable to conceive the

2

idea that one and one make two ; he could never even know
the fact that there is such a number as one, as distinct from
two.   There is no way by which it could be taught to him.

There are reasons for believing that all perceptions are
formed in the optic thalami.   Magendie[1] was the first who
pointed out their relations to sensibility.   He ascertained that
their irritation in animals caused excessive pain, while the
other parts of the brain might be wounded without producing
evidences of suffering.

They have also been regarded as specially the centres for
vision.   Although Todd, Carpenter, and others have considered
the optic thalami as centres for sensorial impressions, Luys,[2]
more than any other physiologist, has developed this idea,
and has adduced arguments in its support which it is difficult
to overlook.   His doctrine is that the optic thalami are reservoirs for all sensorial impressions coming from the periphery
of the nervous system, that with other ganglionic masses they
elaborate these impressions, and that by means of the fibres
of the corona radiata they transmit them to the cortex to be
still further perfectionated by being converted into ideas.   In
his own language : "All sensorial impressions, after having
been received and concentrated in the gray substance of the
optic thalami, are irradiated toward the different regions of
the cortical periphery.   The white central fibres transmit
them, and the gray substance of the convolutions receives and
elaborates them."[3]

Experimental physiology tends to establish this doctrine ;
and, though the position of the optic thalami is such as to
make it a matter of difficulty to act upon them with the same
degree of facility as upon the cortex, the obstacle has been,
in a great measure, overcome by Fournié,[4] and we are thus
placed in possession of data which have a distinct connection
with the point at issue.

Fournié's method consisted in injecting, by means of a
hypodermic syringe, caustic solutions—such as a strong solution of chloride of zinc—into the brain, observing the resulting phenomena, and then, after death, carefully noting the
part of the organ in which the injection had been deposited.

---

[1] " Leçons sur le système nerveux," t. i, p. 103, et seq.
[2] " Recherches sur le système nerveux," Paris, 1865, p. 198, et seq.
[3] Op. cit., p. 346.
[4] " Sur le fonctionnement du cerveau."   Paris, 1873.

Several of his experiments related to the optic thalami, and, without referring to the other results, it may be stated that in every one there was a more or less complete loss of sensation. In one of his cases the needle traversed the cornu ammonis, and the injection was thrown into the centre of the optic thalamus of the left side. As a consequence, there was complete abolition of all sensibility.

As we shall see farther on, there are many facts in morbid anatomy which go to support this view of the relation between the several sensorial organs and the optic thalami.

The accompanying diagram (Fig. 1) exhibits the connec-

Fig. 1.

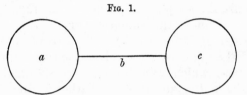

a, organ of sense (eye); *b*, connecting nerve for transmission of impressions; *c*, ganglion for conversion of impressions into perceptions.

tion of an organ of a special sense, as, for instance, the eye, with its perceptive ganglion.

Besides the generally recognized five special senses—*sight, hearing, taste, smell,* and *touch*—there is another, which is known as the muscular sense, the existence of which seems to be well established. By this sense we are enabled to determine, without the assistance of the other senses, the weights of bodies and the exact state of contraction of any particular muscle under the control of the will. It is, probably, also through this sense that the muscular movements are co-ordinated and the requisite degree of contraction initiated and maintained.

But there are others which, though not senses in the strict signification of the word, are, at any rate, sensations, and capable of giving rise to perceptions. They are probably modifications of the sense of touch. They arise through the operations of the various organs of the body, and are intimately associated with imperative needs of the body in its struggle for existence.

These are: *hunger,* the feeling which, starting in the stomach, indicates the necessity for food ; *thirst,* which experienced in the fauces and throat informs us that the organism requires water; the *respiratory sense*, which, when allowed to act to its extreme degree, causes a feeling of suffocation, and which, originating in the lungs, informs us that a due amount of pure air is not being inspired; and the *reproductive* or *genesic sense*, which is intimately concerned with the preservation of the species, but which primarily relates to sexual intercourse and the pleasurable feeling resulting from venereal excitement. The sensation experienced in the bladder when the contained urine is increased beyond a certain quantity, and that felt in the rectum when it is distended with fæces, are still more analogous with touch as it exists in the skin. The pains felt in the different organs and structures of the body when they are the subjects of disease or derangement are also to be embraced under the same category.

All the perceptions are subject to aberrations, either from disorder of the organ which receives them as impressions, the nerve or nerves which transmit the impressions to the brain, or of this latter structure itself. With the first two series of derangements we need not, in the consideration of mental derangement, concern ourselves; the third will be fully brought under notice in a subsequent part of this treatise.

2. **The Intellect.**—In the normal condition of the brain, the excitation of a sense, and the consequent perception, do not stop at the special ganglion of that sense, but are transmitted to a more complex part of the brain, where the perception is resolved into an idea. Thus, the image impressed upon the retina, the perception of which has been formed by a sensory ganglion, ultimately causes the evolution of another force by which all its attributes capable of being represented upon the retina are more or less perfectly appreciated, according to the structural qualities of the ideational centre. To the formation of the idea several important faculties and modes of expression of the intellect contribute.

Thus, if, to employ the example already used, the retina has received the image of a ball, a ganglion converts this into a perception, and a higher one into an idea, and this idea relates to the size, the form, the color, the material, etc., primarily; and the origin, ownership, uses, etc., secondarily. In gaining this conception of the thing, the image of which has been impressed upon the retina, the various faculties of the intellect are brought into action, and the process of thinking is carried on. These faculties, or functions, as generally recognized by metaphysicians, are five in number—*memory, judgment, abstraction, reason,* and *imagination.* Bain[1] reduces them to three—*consciousness of difference, consciousness of agreement,* and *retentiveness.* From a purely philosophical point of view, his classification is more correct than the older one, but, for the purposes of the present inquiry, the latter is to be preferred as being more generally understood, and more in relation with derangements of the intellect.

The region of the brain which is directly concerned with the elaboration of ideas is the cortex. Impressions from the perceptional and emotional centres are transmitted to the ganglionic matter forming the periphery of the brain, and are there converted into ideas. Moreover, it is doubtless this portion in which ideas are stored up for future use, and from which they are brought out when required. The accompanying diagram (Fig. 2) shows the relation which exists.

Fig. 2.

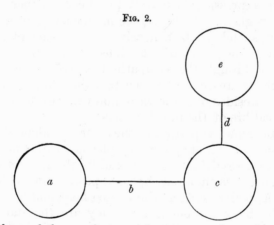

a, the organ of sense ; *b,* the nerve for transmission to *c,* organ of perception ; *d,* the white fibres of the brain transmitting the perception to *e,* the cortex, where it is converted into an idea.

Any one or all of the faculties of the intellect, as above enumerated, may be disordered in insanity.

3. **The Emotions.**—An idea, in its turn, excites another part of the brain to action, and an emotion is produced ; or this last-named force may be evolved under certain circumstances without the intermediation of the idea, but solely from the transmission of a perception to the emotional ganglion.

[1] "The Senses and the Intellect," third edition, New York, 1872, p. 321, *et seq.*

that does not produce at some time or other of its career a
change in the emotional characteristics of the affected individual. Thus, for instance, cerebral hæmorrhages and em-
bolisms are almost invariably accompanied or followed by
marked emotional derangement, and often to the extent of
completely reversing the normal tendencies of the patient.
Referring to this subject in relation to cerebral hæmorrhage,
I have said:[1] "The mental characteristics of the patient will
be found to have undergone a radical change. He is irritable, unreasonable, and fretful. His sense of the proprieties
of life, which may in health have been very delicate, becomes
obtuse, his memory is notably impaired, and his reasoning
powers greatly diminished. The greatest change, however, is
perceived in the emotional faculties. He laughs at the veriest
trifles, and sheds tears profusely at the least circumstance calculated to annoy him. Even for years after, this peculiarity
is noticed." And, again:[2]

"Even after years his emotions are abnormally excitable.
A patient now in the New York State Hospital for Diseases
of the Nervous System informs me that he sheds tears every
time a funeral passes him, and that even hearing of any one's
death, or reading the obituary column in a newspaper, causes
his feelings to get the better of him. In the lightest forms
of the attack this easily aroused emotional disturbance is a
marked feature for years subsequently, if it ever entirely disappears."

In the case of a gentleman, the subject of a very slight
cerebral hæmorrhage, which left scarcely any paralysis after
it, and which the clinical features showed was situated in one
of the ganglia of the left corpus striatum, the grief excited by
the fact that his coffee was cold caused him to shed tears like
a child. This gentleman was normally of great strength of
character, and not given to exhibit his feelings. At the time,
he held one of the highest offices in the Government of the
United States.

A person of my acquaintance had his whole character
changed by a slight attack of cerebral congestion. Naturally
he was of good disposition, amiable in his character, and considerate in his dealings with others; but after a vertiginous
seizure, attended with unconsciousness of but a few moments'

[1] "A Treatise on the Diseases of the Nervous System," seventh edition,
New York, 1881, p. 88.   [2] *Op. cit.*, pp. 92, 93.

duration, his whole mental organization underwent a radical change; he became deceitful, morose, and exceedingly overbearing and tyrannical toward all with whom he came in contact and whom it was safe for him to maltreat. His likes and dislikes were entirely reversed in many important instances.

Bucknill[1] and Tuke refer to the case of a lady whose character had always been distinguished for conscientiousness, whose religious education had been of a sombre kind, and who, suffering from an attack of small-pox, attended with congestion of the brain, recovered with the natural bent of her disposition greatly exaggerated. The irritability of conscience had become an actual disease, destroying her happiness and rendering her incompetent to discharge any of the duties of life.

Intense or long-continued emotional disturbance is among the chief factors in the causation of insanity, as will be fully shown in a subsequent part of this treatise.

McCosh[2] asserts that to the production of an emotion "there is need first of some understanding or apprehension"— that is, of an idea; but I think this is not altogether correct, for it would seem from experience that a simple perception without understanding or apprehension may give rise to marked emotional manifestations. Thus, the feeling of uneasiness in the stomach consequent upon an undigested meal may produce the most profound melancholy; certain indefinable sensations in the generative organs, scarcely perceived, may cause the development of the emotion of love in its most intense form; a gouty pain in the great toe may prompt to the most immeasurable anger. Indeed, emotions may be developed as the direct consequences of disturbances in the viscera, unaccompanied by any sensation whatever, as, for instance, the mental depression, with its accompanying emotional disturbances due to painless liver disorders, and like states developed by morbid conditions of the blood circulating in the brain. In none of these instances is there necessarily the faintest understanding or apprehension. And, as regards the special senses, the fact, that active emotions may be excited through the perceptions they induce without the intervention of the intellect, must, I think, be recognized by all inquirers, although the feeling evolved may not be so

[1] "A Manual of Psychological Medicine," etc., London, 1858, p. 375.
[2] "The Emotions," New York, 1880, p. 1.

strong as when ideation is also brought in as a factor. The sight of a person undergoing bodily pain excites in us a feeling of compassion, provided the sufferer indulges in tears and lamentations, and writhes, let us suppose, under the knife of the surgeon. If, on the contrary, he restrains the manifestations of the pain he is enduring, we look beyond his present condition and contemplate the benefit he is probably to receive from the operation, and the pity we would have felt in the first instance is scarcely, if at all, experienced. Among the insane, the excitation of emotions from illusions and hallucinations, which, as we have seen, are only false perceptions, is common enough.

Many persons are more governed by their emotions than by their intellects in their beliefs and actions. They accept an article of faith because they hear it enunciated amid the surroundings of groined ceilings, stained glass, a dim light, solemn music, and a gorgeous ceremonial, without stopping to submit it to calm investigation when the circumstances are such that the intellect can have full play. Moved by the pity excited at the sight of a weeping wife and children purposely brought into the court-room to influence their judgment, they, as jurymen, acquit a man whom the evidence has clearly shown to be guilty of an atrocious crime. In the one case, the belief will probably be of short duration; in the other, a great wrong is done to society by turning loose upon it a person who will probably do it further injury, and in depriving it of the advantage of example to other would-be offenders against the law. At the same time, the emotions should be allowed their legitimate power in governing our actions, and we can often trust to them as safe guides. With matters of faith or belief, however, they should have nothing to do.

The mechanism of the development of emotions from perceptions and ideas is shown in the accompanying diagram (Fig. 3), in which a is the organ of sense; b, the nerve of transmission; c, the perceptive ganglion; d, the fibres of transmission to e, the ideational ganglion; f, the fibres of transmission to g, the emotional ganglion; and h, fibres of communication between e, the ideational, and g, the emotional ganglia. An emotion, therefore, may be excited in g by a perception coming directly from c, through the fibres f, or indirectly through the fibres d to e, where it is converted into an idea and transmitted to g through the fibres h; or it may be developed from an idea starting from e and reaching g through the fibres h.

Fig. 3.

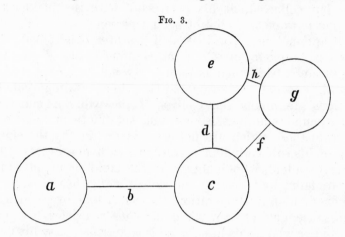

4. **The Will** is that mental force by which the emotions, the thoughts, and the actions are controlled. The product of the force is called a volition.

The influence of the will is greatest in the reverse order in which its subjects are mentioned in the preceding paragraph; that is, it is most powerful over the muscular system of the body, next over the thoughts, the current of which is often regulated and directed by the will, and least of all over the emotions. When we hear of people controlling their feelings, it is not, generally, in reality the feelings which are held in subjection, but merely the manifestation of them. A man, therefore, who possesses the power of preserving his equanimity in the presence of circumstances calculated to rouse the emotions to the highest pitch, is able to abstain from tears or laughter, or the ordinary indications of fear or anger, while the emotion calculated to excite either is experienced to its utmost degree.

A story is told of two officers who were serving together in the Peninsular War, which illustrates this volitional control of the manifestations of a powerful emotion. One of them, whom I will call Captain Smith, was remarkable for his bull-dog bravery, which never failed him, under any circumstances, when mere animal courage was required. The other, Captain Jones, was a good officer, but was thought by some to be deficient in the contempt of danger, which is, after all, the least qualification of a soldier.   The bullets were whistling around, when Captain Smith, riding up to Captain Jones, who stood pale, but collected, at his post, said, with the inexcusable *brusquerie* to be expected of such a person :

"Captain Jones, you look as if you were frightened ! "

"Yes," replied Jones, "I am frightened, and if you were half so much frightened as I am you would run away."

Still, it is not to be doubted that, to a certain extent, the emotions are under the control of the will.   A man may strengthen his emotions, lessen them, subdue them absolutely, or create those which are not natural to him, by the simple force of his will acting in accordance with his desires.   The medical student, whose horror at the sight of blood causes him to faint, by lessening the action of his heart, when he sees his first surgical operation, in a short time overcomes his repugnance, and, after a while, becomes a fearless surgeon. The soldier who in his first battle is so terrified that his urine and fæces escape from him involuntarily, perseveres till he is renowned for his gallantry and daring under the most tremendous fire.

The influence of the will is markedly exhibited in the power to recall or reproduce ideas which have been experienced at some former time.   This power may exist when that of fixing the attention upon subjects is notably diminished. Thus, a person suffers from an attack of cerebral hæmorrhage or other brain disease which lessens the force of the mind. In such a case it often happens that the ability to recall impressions made many years previously remains undiminished, while he finds it impossible to recollect events which occurred only an hour or two ago.   He remembers, with unimpaired vividness, unimportant incidents of his youth, and yet has forgotten the name of the hotel at which he is stopping, or whether or not he ate fish for his dinner.   In the latter circumstances no effort of the will is competent to recall the facts, because he has lost the power of concentrating the attention.   No impression has been formed, and no idea has been evolved.

For the exercise of volition, consciousness is necessary. We are constantly performing acts of which we have at the time no knowledge ; but they are automatic, not voluntary. We will, for example, to go to a friend's house, and we perform the necessary volitional acts initiatory of the proceeding ;

but we do not keep on willing each individual step that we take on our way, and we arrive at the consciousness that we have reached his door, while the will during the journey has either been dormant, or, perhaps, engaged in directing a conversation with a person who has joined us. Such acts are performed by the force evolved from ganglia lower in function than those which produce the will, which simply sets them in operation, and stops them when desirous so to do. Volition is, therefore, an instantaneous and transitory process. Strong determination causes, however, repeated volitional acts of like character. Beattie [1] is, therefore, wrong when he says: "Some acts of the will are transient, others more lasting. When I will to stretch out my hand and snuff the candle, the energy of the will is at an end as soon as the action is over. When I will to read a book or write a letter from beginning to end without stopping, the will is exerted till the reading or the writing be finished. We may will to persist for a course of years in a certain conduct ; to read, for example, so much Greek every day till we learn to read it with ease ; this sort of will is commonly called a resolution."

It requires no profound consideration to perceive the many errors contained in this brief quotation. A resolution to study Greek for a number of years would require thousands of distinct volitional acts for its realization. The idea that while studying each daily lesson the will would be actively engaged in willing the performance of the task is one which our experience emphatically contradicts. After we are conscious of a volition to do a particular thing, the will has nothing further to do with the act.

The will has often been confounded with desire. Thus Hartley [2] says:

"The will appears to be nothing but a desire or aversion sufficiently strong to produce an action that is not automatic, primarily or secondarily. At least, it appears to me that the substitution of these words for the word *will* may be justified by the common usage of language. The will is, therefore, that desire or aversion which is strongest for the present time."

Mr. James Mill [3] apparently holds a like view when he says:

[1] "Elements of Moral Science," vol. i, Edinburgh, 1790, p. 217.
[2] "Observations on Man," etc., 1791, p. 219.
[3] "Analysis of the Human Mind," 1830, p. 279.

"I believe that no case of voluntary action can be mentioned in which it would not be an appropriate expression to call the action desired."

Many other metaphysicians hold a like doctrine—a doctrine which, as Mansel [1] asserts, was overthrown as one of the earliest results of psychological analysis, and which is contrary to the consciousness of every person who has experienced them both, "however much they may have been confounded by the perversity of a few unscrupulous system-makers." Desire and will may, indeed, be the direct opponents of each other. A man may desire his neighbor's watch, but will be very far from making a volitional effort to take it out of his pocket. He often wills in opposition to his desires, and desires in opposition to his will.

Cases in illustration of these points often occur to the physician, although, perhaps, not familiar to the metaphysician. Two instances of the kind are cited by Dr. J. H. Bennet,[2] to whom they were furnished by Sir Robert Christison. In one of them, a gentleman was often unable to do very simple acts which he wished to perform, although his will-power was exerted to its utmost. For instance, in undressing for the night he would be two hours before he could take off his coat, all his mental faculties except the will being perfect. On one occasion, having ordered a glass of water, he was unable to take it off the tray, though desirous of so doing, and the servant was kept standing a half-hour before success attended his efforts. In the other case, if the subject, when walking in the street, came to a break in the line of houses, his will suddenly became inoperative, and he could not, in spite of all his power of volition, proceed another step. An unbuilt-on space in the street was sure to stop him. Crossing a street was also difficult, and on going in or out of a door his movement was always arrested for some minutes.

A similar case has recently come under my own notice. A gentleman from Massachusetts consulted me for what he designated "a paralysis of the will," which was chiefly manifested in undressing himself at night and dressing himself in the morning. It was impossible for him to take off his clothes or to put them on in accordance with the order he wished.

[1] "Metaphysics; or, The Philosophy of Consciousness, Phenomenal or Real," Edinburgh, 1860, p. 171; also, "Encyclopædia Britannica."
[2] "The Mesmeric Mania of 1851," p. 16.

He would begin, for instance, by endeavoring to remove his shoes, but, after vainly trying to bring his will in subjection to his desire, would desist and turn his attention to the task of taking off his coat, with no better success. After an hour or two spent in this way, to no purpose, he would succeed, generally, in getting his clothes off, but quite often he was obliged to summon assistance. In the morning a similar experience was certain to occur. Frequently, as he told me, he would sit for half an hour with his stockings in his hands, unable to determine which one to put on first.

Legrand du Saulle[1] has very thoroughly described such cases under the name of "Folie du doute," and they will subsequently engage our attention more fully.

In certain of the neuroses, notably in hysteria and insanity, this inability to exert the power of the will is a prominent feature. In the latter condition the will is often exercised against the desires and the whole system of thought of the individual, producing what is known as "morbid impulse." In these cases, the will, as it were, breaks loose from the intellect and causes the perpetration of acts of immorality or violence. Even within the limits of mental health some persons are noted for the strength of the will, and others for its feebleness.

The influence of certain narcotics and stimulants in weakening the power of the will is a well-known fact. Among them, opium and alcohol are especially to be noted. The former, in most cases, produces its effect upon the will of the individual without in the slightest degree impairing the intellect. The latter, however, seems to have a more complex action, for it not only diminishes the will-power and places its subject under the control of others, but it prompts to the perpetration of acts of violence, the tendency to which the individual is unable to resist.

The will is also suspended in reverie, in somnambulism, and in the induced condition known as hypnotism. In this last-named state the subject's will is that of some other person; he does as he is told, and his will, and even his perceptions, are under the complete control of the operator. In the normal state of an individual the will has no power over the perceptions. He cannot, for instance, by any effort of his will, alter his perception of color or form, or change the impression

[1] "La folie du doute (avec delire du toucher)," Paris, 1875.

which any one of the sensory organs produces in the perceptional centre.

Like others of the mental faculties, the will-power is greatly developed by education.

While the will is certainly located in the brain, it is by no means certain that in some of the lower animals, at least, it is not also situated in the spinal cord. The acts which are witnessed in the frog after the head has been cut off, and with it, of course, the entire encephalon, are clearly volitional in character, being adapted to the end in view, and such as the animal would perform in its unmutilated state. But, while the brain is the chief, if not the only, seat of the will in man, we have no data by which we are authorized to localize it in any particular part of this organ. Probably each motor and ideational centre is, at the same time, also volitional; but even this is merely an inference.

By certain French physiologists it has been located in the pons Varolii, but without, in my opinion, sufficient warrant from facts.

An idea of the relation of the will to perception and intellect and a volitional act will be obtained from the accompanying diagram (Fig. 4), in which *a* is the organ of sense; *b*, the

FIG. 4.

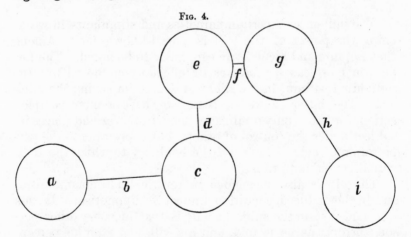

nerve of transmission; *c*, the perceptive ganglion; *d*, fibres of transmission to *e*, ideational ganglion; *f*, communicating fibres with *g*, volitional ganglion; *h*, efferent nerve communicating with *i*, a muscle. An image of a blow about to fall on the finger is formed on the eye, *a*; the image is transmitted by the optic nerve, b, to the perceptive ganglion, c, where it becomes a perception; from c it passes through the white fibres of the brain, d, to e, an ideational centre, where it becomes an idea, being comprehended, and the danger to the finger realized. At once the knowledge excites an impulse either in the ideational centre or in a contiguous one, g, through the intermediation of brain fibres, f; and this impulse—a volition—passes through the nerve h to the muscle i, and the hand is immediately withdrawn.

The mind, therefore, as before stated, is a compound force evolved by the brain—or, rather, a collection of several forces —and its elements are perception, intellect, emotion, and will. The sun, likewise, evolves a compound force, and its elements are light, heat, and actinism. One of these forces—light—is made up of several primary colors; and the intellect of man, one of the mental forces, is composed of faculties. It would be easy to pursue the analogy, but enough has been said to indicate how closely the relationship between brain and mind is that of matter and force.

It is to be regretted that the present state of cerebral anattomy and physiology is such as to prevent our making any precise localizations of the several forces and faculties which go to make up the mind. I have only ventured to do that in a single instance—the optic thalamus as a centre for perception—and even that is questioned by several eminent investigators. The evidence, however, appears to me so explicit on this point that I do not see how it is to be questioned.[1] Much has been done by the labors of Broca, Fritsch and Hitzig, Nothnagel, Meynert, Ferrier, and others, in the direction of the localization of brain functions, but it has been almost entirely confined to the determination of the centres for speech and for motor impulses.

Gall, Spurzheim, Combe, and others, made honest attempts to found the science of phrenology, and, if their localizations of the various faculties of the mind—perceptional, intellect-

---

[1] For the evidence serving to establish the matter in question, reference is made to Magendie, "Leçons sur le système nerveux," t. i, p. 103, et seq.; Luys, "Recherches sur le système nerveux," pp. 198, 344, 346, Paris, 1865; Ritti, "Théorie physiologique de l'hallucination," p. 37, Paris, 1874; Fournié, "Recherches expérimentales sur le fonctionnement du cerveau," Paris, 1873; also, a memoir by the writer, entitled, "Thalamic Epilepsy," in Neurological Contributions, No. 3, p. 1, New York, 1881, in which additional facts are submitted.

ual, emotional, and volitional—had been established, we should have as complete a knowledge of psychological topography as could be desired ; but they built on insufficient data, and, as a consequence, phrenology as a science does not exist at the present time. We know, however, that the gray matter of the brain originates mental operations, and that possibly the gray matter of the spinal cord and of the sympathetic system supplements the process, and, under certain circumstances, especially in the lower animals, may, to a considerable extent, take its place.

We know, also, that the cortical substance of the brain is of far greater importance in the evolution of mind than any other portion of the nervous system, and that it is here that experimentation and other methods of investigation have the greatest prospect of obtaining positive results. It is certainly established that the brain is not a single organ, but consists of a congeries of organs with different functions.

Owing to this fact of our ignorance of the relation existing between the faculties of the mind and the different parts of the brain, and our consequent inability to construct a positive system of cerebral physiology, it is equally beyond our power to propose a classification of the phenomena of insanity based upon morbid anatomy and pathology. We are, therefore, driven to either a psychological or a clinical arrangement, or such a combination of the two as will best serve the purposes of study, till such time as we may become so thoroughly acquainted with the anatomical structure of the brain and its physiology as will admit of a more scientific system.

CHAPTER III.

GENERAL REMARKS ON THE MENTAL AND PHYSICAL CONDITIONS INHERENT IN THE INDIVIDUAL WHICH INFLUENCE THE ACTION OF THE MIND.

IN individuals whose brains are well-formed, free from structural changes, and are nourished with a due supply— neither excessive nor deficient—of healthy blood, the perception, the intellect, the emotions, and the will act in a manner which within certain limits is common to mankind in general. Slight changes in the structure or nutrition of the brain induce corresponding changes in the mind as a whole, or in some one or more of its parts or faculties, while profound alterations are accompanied by more severe and extensive mental disturbances. As no two brains are precisely alike, so no two persons are precisely alike in their mental processes. The argument, therefore, that if the mind resulted from the brain it would be the same in each individual instance, is simply ridiculous, and is made by those who have no conception of the subject of which they write. Thus, M. Simonin,[1] one of the most recent of the antiphysiological psychologists, says:

"If thought is secreted or produced exclusively by a material organ, this secretion ought to have a uniform character, and ought to be always identical with itself, as are other secretions, as the gastric juice secreted by the stomach, the pancreatic juice by the pancreas, etc. How is it, therefore, that this cerebral secretion, which ought always to be identical with itself, as are the secretions of other organic materials, can produce such systems of thought, such calculations, such sublime arrangements, such speculations of the mind as are found in the works of Aristotle, Leibnitz, Lavoisier, Humboldt, Cuvier, Arago, Agassiz, etc. ?"

To this absurd question I would reply by remarking that, if M. Simonin's brain had been exactly like that of Aristotle, his thoughts would also have been exactly like Aristotle's, when evolved by like causes acting under like circumstances. But as M. Simonin's brain is certainly very different from that of the Greek philosopher, so also is the product of his brain different. And I would say, further, that M. Simonin's assumption that the gastric juice and other secretions are alike in all men is as erroneous as are most of the other views contained in his book. No two persons ever lived in whom any one secretion possessed exactly the same composition in each, and hence it is that one man will digest with impunity things which another man's stomach instantly rejects. If M. Simonin has studied cerebral anatomy, and has ever compared two brains—and, being a psychologist whose faith is stronger than his love for facts, he probably disdains any such proofs—he has certainly discovered that there is as much dissimilarity between them as there is between any two peach-trees. How,

[1] " Histoire de la psychologie," etc., Paris, 1879, p. 391.

then, can the product of two such brains—mind—be alike in both?

But mind is not a fluid secretion, to be compared to the gastric juice. It is a force produced by nervous action. As a galvanic battery evolves galvanism, so the brain evolves mind. If the battery is good, the galvanism is good; if the battery is bad, the galvanism is bad. If the gas is good, we get a good light; if the gas is bad, we get a bad light. And, if the brain is good, the mind will certainly be good; and, if the brain is bad, the mind will just as surely be bad. As no two persons ever looked exactly alike, it would be the height of absurdity to expect that any two hearts, or livers, or stomachs, or brains, would be alike.

It would be difficult to find a passage of the same length containing more erroneous statements and false inferences than the following:[1]

"If thought is a pure material secreted by the brain, the product should not be capable of causing a complete disorganization of the human body. Neither the pancreatic juice nor the other visceral secretions ever produce a sudden disorganization. How can the materialistic atheists (*matérialistes-athées*) explain certain facts with which every one is familiar?

"A father, for example, has an only son whom he tenderly loves. This son belongs to an army in the field. The father reads one day that this son has been killed in battle. The intelligence produces in him such a disturbance that he dies suddenly, as if struck by lightning.

"Every sensation, whatever it may be, causes a thought in the brain. The news has caused a thought in the brain of the father, and this thought has instantly deprived him of life. Was this thought pure matter? and why did it cause the father to pass from life to death? How can it be that the brain can secrete such murderous thoughts?"

If M. Simonin is not totally ignorant of all vital phenomena, he must know that, in such a case as the one he supposes, the heart has stopped beating in consequence of the overpowering effect of a strong emotion. I have seen rabbits and birds die in like manner from fear, and M. Simonin denies that they have souls.

And he ought to know that the secretions do, under certain circumstances, become so poisonous as to cause instant death.

[1] *Op. et loc. cit.*

The milk of a nursing mother may, through the influence of great grief, kill the sucking infant with as much suddenness as the father was killed when he heard of his son's death. Thus, Bouchut[1] cites the case of a woman who, much excited by the danger which her husband incurred during a quarrel with a soldier, who was about to use his sword, gave her breast a short time afterward to her child, aged eleven months, and in good health. The infant took a few mouthfuls of her milk, was seized immediately with trembling and panting, and died in a few minutes.

Dr. Carpenter[2] quotes from Mr. Wardrop the case of a mother from whom he had removed a small tumor. All went on well until she fell into a violent passion, and the child, being suckled soon afterward, died in convulsions. Many additional instances might readily be adduced.

It is well known, also, that the saliva of man may, through the power of strong emotions, like anger or terror, become so venomous as to cause death to those on whom it is inoculated.

Finally, it might be suggested to M. Simonin, and those who think with him, that it is no more surprising for death to be caused by a strong emotion originating through the action of the brain than it would be for a like fatal result to come from a murderous soul.

There are differences, therefore, in the minds of men depending upon differences in their brains. These may be inherent in the individual, reaching him through a long line of ancestors, or they may be acquired through the action of extraneous influences upon him ; or, again, they may be such as normally act upon him in the due and regular course of his life. Thus, the brain of a man is different from that of a woman, and there are differences in the resultant mental products. The brain of a child varies in many essential respects from that of an adult, and, as a consequence, the mind is different. Some persons are what is called eccentric, others have peculiar habits and idiosyncrasies, others are geniuses. Temperament, hereditary influence, and constitution, are likewise disturbing factors. So long, however, as the individual peculiarities of mentality are not directly at variance with the average workings of the human mind, or with the person's

[1] " Hygiène de la première enfance," etc., Paris, 1862, p. 177.
[2] " Cyclopædia of Anatomy and Physiology," vol. iv, Part I, art. "Secretion," p. 465.

own methods of normal mind-action, he is sane. If they are at variance, he is insane.

But, within the limits of mental health, marked irregularities are met with in the action of different parts of the mind. Thus, some persons are noted for never perceiving things as the majority of people perceive them. Others are weak in judgment, defective in memory, feeble in powers of application, or vacillating in their opinions; others have the emotional system inordinately or deficiently developed ; others, again, are lacking in volitional power—in the ability to perform certain acts, or to refrain from others, which their reason tells them should be accomplished or omitted, or to follow a definite course of action which they know to be expedient and wise.

In works on insanity, the several influences and conditions to which I refer have not, it appears to me, received due attention.   I propose, therefore, to bring the chief of them to the notice of the reader, premising that no factor which can even in a remote degree influence the mental processes of an individual and no state of being which is liable to develop into insanity are unworthy the consideration of those who propose to study the subject of mental aberration.

CHAPTER IV.

ECCENTRICITY.

PERSONS whose minds deviate in some one or more notable respects from the ordinary standard, but yet whose mental processes are not directly at variance with that standard, are said to be eccentric. Eccentricity is generally inherent in the individual, or is gradually developed in him from the operation of unrecognized causes as he advances in years. If an original condition, it may be shown from a very early period of life, his plays, even, being different from those of other children of his age. Doubtless it then depends upon some peculiarity of brain structure, which, within the limits of the normal range, produces individuality of mental action.

But eccentricity is not always an original condition, for, under certain circumstances, it may be acquired. A person, for instance, meets with some circumstance in his life which tends to weaken his confidence in human nature. He accordingly shuns mankind, by shutting himself up in his own house and refusing to have any intercourse with the inhabitants of the place in which he resides. In carrying out his purpose he proceeds to the most absurd extremes. He speaks to no one he meets, returns no salutations, and his relations with the tradesmen who supply his daily wants are conducted through gratings in the door of his dwelling. He dies, and the will which he leaves behind him is found to devote his entire property for the founding of a hospital for sick and ownerless dogs, "the most faithful creatures I have ever met, and the only ones in which I have any confidence."

Such a man is not insane. There is a rational motive for his conduct—one which many of us have experienced, and which has, perhaps, prompted us to act in a similar manner, if not to the same extent.

Another is engaged in vast mercantile transactions, requiring the most thorough exercise of the best faculties of the mind. He studies the markets of the world, and buys and sells with uniform shrewdness and success. In all the relations of life he conducts himself with the utmost propriety and consideration for the rights and feelings of others. The most complete study of his character and acts fails to show the existence of the slightest defect in his mental processes. He goes to church regularly every Sunday, but has never been regarded as a particularly religious man. Nevertheless, he has one peculiarity. He is a collector of Bibles, and has several thousand, of all sizes and styles, and in many languages. If he hears of a Bible, in any part of the world, different in any respect from those he owns, he at once endeavors to obtain it, no matter how difficult the undertaking, or how much it may cost. Except in the matter of Bibles he is disposed to be somewhat penurious—although his estate is large—and has been known to refuse to have a salad for his dinner on account of the high price of good olive-oil. He makes his will, and dies, and then it is found that his whole property is left in trust to be employed in the maintenance of his library of Bibles, in purchasing others which may become known to the trustees, and in printing one copy, for his library, of the book in any language in which it does not already exist. A letter which is addressed to his trustees informs them that, when he was a boy, a Bible which he had in the breast-pocket of

his coat preserved his life by stopping a bullet which another
boy had accidentally discharged from a pistol, and that he
then had resolved to make the honoring of the Bible the duty
of his whole life.

Neither of these persons can be regarded as insane. Both
were the subjects of acquired eccentricity, which, in all likeli-
hood, would have ensued in some other form, from some other
circumstance acting upon brains naturally predisposed to be
thus affected. The brain is the soil upon which impressions
act differently, according to its character, just as, with the
sower casting his seed-wheat upon different fields, some springs
up into a luxuriant crop, some grows sparsely, and some,
again, takes no root, but rots where it falls. Possibly, if
these individuals had lived a little longer, they might have
passed the border-line which separates mental soundness from
mental unsoundness; but certainly, up to the period of their
deaths, both would have been pronounced sane by all competent laymen and alienists with whom they might have been
brought into contact; and the contest of their wills, by any
heirs-at-law, would assuredly have been a fruitless undertaking.

They chose to have certain ends in view, and to provide
the means for the accomplishment of those ends. There were
no delusions, no emotional disturbance, no hallucinations or
illusions, and the will was normally exercised to the extent
necessary to secure the objects of their lives. At any time
they had it in their power to alter their purposes, and in that
fact we have an essential point of difference between eccentricity and insanity. We may regard their conduct as singular, because they made an unusual disposition of their property; but it was no more irrational than if the one had left his
estate to the "Society for the Prevention of Cruelty to Animals," and the other had devoted his to sending missionaries
to Central Africa.

Two distinct forms of eccentricity are recognizable. In the
one, the individual sets himself up above the level of the rest
of the world, and, marking out for himself a line of conduct,
adheres to it with an astonishing degree of tenacity. For him
the opinions of mankind in general are of no consequence.
He is a law unto himself; what he says and does is said and
done, not for the purpose of attracting attention or for obtaining notoriety, but because it is pleasing to himself. He does

not mean to be singular or original, but he is, nevertheless, both. For every man is singular and original whose conduct, within the limits of reason and intelligence, differs from that of his fellow-men. He endeavors to carry out certain ideas which seem to him to have been overlooked by society to its great disadvantage. Society usually thinks differently; but, if the promulgator is endowed with sufficient force of character, it generally happens that, eventually, either wholly or in part, his views prevail. All great reformers are eccentrics of this kind. They are contending for their doctrines, not for themselves. And they are not apt to become insane, though sometimes they do.

The subjects of the other form occupy a lower level. They affect singularity for the purpose of attracting attention to themselves, and thus obtaining the notoriety which they crave with every breath they inhale. They dress differently from other people, wearing enormous shirt-collars, or peculiar hats, or oddly cut coats of unusual colors, or indulging in some other similar whimsicality of an unimportant character, in the expectation that they will thereby attract the attention or excite the comments of those they meet.

Or they build houses upon an idea perhaps correct enough in itself, as, for instance, the securing of proper ventilation; but in carrying it out they show such defective judgment that the complete integrity of the intellect may, perhaps, be a matter of question. Thus, one gentleman of my acquaintance, believing that fireplaces were the best ventilators, put four of these openings into every room in his house. This, however, was one of the smallest of his eccentricities. He wore a ventilated hat, his clothing was pierced with holes, as were even his shoes; and no one could be in his company five minutes without having his attention directed to these provisions for securing health.

In addition to these advanced notions on the subject of ventilation, he had others equally singular in regard to the arrangement of the furniture in his dwelling and the care that was to be taken of it. Thus, there was one room called the "apostles' room." It contained a table that represented Christ, and twelve chairs, which were placed around it, and typified the twelve apostles; one chair, that stood for Judas Iscariot, was covered with black crape. The floor of this room was very highly polished, and no one was allowed to enter it without slipping their shod feet into cloth slippers that were placed at the door ready for use. He had a library, tolerably large but of little value, and every book in it which contained Judas's name was bound in black, and black lines were drawn around the name wherever it occurred. Such eccentricity as this is not far removed from insanity, and is liable at any time, from some cause a little out of the common way, to pass over the line.

Thus, a lady had since her childhood shown a singularity of conduct as regarded her table furniture, which she would have of no other material than copper. She carried this fancy to such an extent that even the knives and forks were of copper. People laughed at her, and tried to reason her out of her whim, but in vain. She was in her element as soon as attention was directed to her fancy and arguments against it were addressed to her. She liked nothing better than to be afforded a full opportunity to discuss with any one the manifold advantages which copper possessed as a material to be used in the manufacture of every article of table-ware. In no other respect was there any evidence of mental aberration. She was intelligent, by no means excitable, and in the enjoyment of excellent health. She had, moreover, a decided talent for music, and had written several passably good stories for a young ladies' magazine. An uncle had, however, died insane.

A circumstance, trifling in itself, but one, as it afterward resulted, of great importance to her, started in her a new train of thought, and excited emotions which she could not control. She read in a morning paper that a Mr. Koppermann had arrived at one of the hotels, and she announced her determination to call upon him, in order, as she said, to ascertain the origin of his name. Her friends endeavored to dissuade her, but without avail. She went to the hotel, and was told that he had just left for Chicago. Without returning to her home, she bought a railway ticket for Chicago, and actually started on the next train for that city. The telegraph, however, overtook her, and she was brought back from Rochester raving of her love for a man she had never seen, and whose name alone had been associated in her mind with her fancy for copper table furniture. She died of acute mania within a month. In this case erotic tendencies which had never been observed in her before seemed to have been excited by some very indirect and complicated mental process, and these in their turn developed into general derangement of the mind.

In another case, a young man, a clerk in a city bank, had for several years exhibited peculiarities in the keeping of his books. He was exceedingly exact in his accounts, but after the bank was closed always remained several hours, during which he ornamented each page of his day's work with arabesques in different-colored inks. He was very vain of this accomplishment, and was constantly in the habit of calling attention to the manner in which, as he supposed, he had beautified what would otherwise have been positively ugly. His fellow-clerks amused themselves at his expense, but his superior officers, knowing his value, never interfered with him in his amusement. Gradually, however, he conceived the idea that they were displeased with him, and at last the notion became so firmly rooted in his mind that he resigned his position, notwithstanding the protestations of the directors that his idea was erroneous. Delusions of various other kinds supervened, and he passed into a condition of chronic insanity, in which he still remains. In most of the cases occurring under this head the intellectual powers are not of a high order, though there may sometimes be a notable development of some talent, or even a great power for acquiring learning. Painters, sculptors, musicians, mathematicians, poets, and men of letters generally, not infrequently exhibit eccentricities of dress, conduct, manner, or ideas, which not only merely add to their notoriety, but often make them either the laughing-stocks of their fellow-men or objects of fear or disgust to all who are brought into contact with them.

CHAPTER V.

IDIOSYNCRASY.

By idiosyncrasy we understand a peculiarity of constitution by which an individual is affected by external agents in a manner different from mankind in general. Thus, some persons cannot eat strawberries without a kind of urticaria appearing over the body; others are similarly affected by eating the striped bass; others, again, faint at the odor of cer-

tain flowers, or at the sight of blood ; and some are attacked
with cholera-morbus after eating shell-fish—as crabs, lobsters,
clams, or mussels.   Many other instances might be advanced,
some of them of a very curious character.   These several conditions are called idiosyncrasies.

Bégin,[1] who defines idiosyncrasy as the predominance of an
organ, a viscus, or a system of organs, has hardly, I think,
fairly grasped the subject, though his definition has influenced
many French writers on the question.   It is something more
than this—something inherent in the organization of the individual, of which we only see the manifestation when the proper
cause is set in action.   We cannot attempt to explain why
one person should be severely mercurialized by one grain of
blue mass, and another take daily ten times that quantity for
a week without the least sign of the peculiar action of mercury being produced.   We only know that such is the fact ;
and were we to search for the reason, with all the appliances
which modern science could bring to our aid, we should be
entirely unsuccessful.   According to Bégin's idea, we should
expect to see some remarkable development of the absorbent
system in the one case, with slight development in the other ;
but, even were such the case, it would not explain the phenomena, for, when ten grains of the preparation in question
are taken daily, scarcely a day elapses before mercury can be
detected in the secretions, and yet hydrargysm is not produced ; while when one grain is taken, and this condition follows, the most delicate chemical examination fails to discover
mercury in any of the fluids or tissues of the body.

Bégin's definition scarcely separates idiosyncrasy from
temperament, whereas, according to what would appear to be
sound reasoning, based upon an enlarged idea of the physiology of the subject, a very material difference exists.

Idiosyncrasies are often hereditary and often acquired.
Two or more may exist in one person.   Thus, there may be
an idiosyncrasy connected with the digestive system, another
with the circulatory system, another with the nervous system,
and so on.

An idiosyncrasy may be of such a character as altogether
to prevent an individual following a particular occupation.
Thus, a person who faints at the sight of blood cannot be a
surgeon ; another, who is seized with nausea and vomiting

---

[1] "Physiologie pathologique," Paris, 1828, t. i, p. 44.

when in the presence of insane persons, cannot be a superintendent of a lunatic asylum—not, at least, if he ever expects to see his patients. Idiosyncrasies may, however, be overcome, especially those of a mental character.

Millingen[1] cites the case of a man who fell into convulsions whenever he saw a spider. A waxen one was made, which equally terrified him. When he recovered, his error was pointed out to him. The wax figure was put into his hand without causing dread, and shortly the living insect no longer disturbed him.

I knew a gentleman who could not eat soft crabs without experiencing an attack of diarrhœa. As he was exceedingly fond of them, he persevered in eating them, and finally, after a long struggle, succeeded in conquering the trouble.

Individuals with idiosyncrasies soon find out their peculiarities, and are enabled to guard against any injurious result to which they would otherwise be subjected but for the teachings of experience.

Idiosyncrasies may be temporary only—that is, due to an existing condition of the organism, which, though natural or morbid, is of a transitory character. Such, for instance, are those due to dentition, the commencement or the cessation of the menstrual function, pregnancy, etc. These are frequently of a serious character, and require careful watching, especially as they may lead to derangement of the mind. Thus, a lady, Mrs. X, was at one time under my professional care, who, at the beginning of her first pregnancy, acquired an overpowering aversion to a half-breed Indian woman who was employed in the house as a servant. Whenever this woman came near her she was at once seized with violent trembling, which ended in a few minutes with vomiting and great mental and physical prostration, lasting several hours. Her husband would have sent the woman away, but Mrs. X insisted on her remaining, as she was a good servant, in order that she might overcome what she regarded as an unreasonable prejudice. The effort was, however, too much for her, for, upon one occasion when the woman entered Mrs. X's apartment rather unexpectedly, the latter became greatly excited, and, jumping from an open window in her fright, broke her arm, and otherwise injured herself so severely that she was for several weeks confined to her bed. During this period, and for some time afterward,

[1] "Curiosities of Medical Experience," London, 1837, vol. ii, p. 246.

she was almost constantly subject to hallucinations, in which the Indian woman played a prominent part. Even after her recovery the mere thought of the woman would sometimes bring on a paroxysm of trembling, and it was not till after her confinement that the antipathy disappeared.

Millingen [1] remarks that certain antipathies, which in reality are idiosyncrasies, appear to depend upon peculiarities of the senses. Rather, however, they are due to peculiarities of the ideational and emotional centres. The organ of sense, in any one case, shows no evidence of disorder; neither does the perceptive ganglion, which simply takes cognizance of the image brought to it. It is higher up that the idiosyncrasy has its seat. In this way we are to explain the following cases collected by Millingen:

"Amatus Lusitanus relates the case of a monk who fainted when he beheld a rose, and never quitted his cell when that flower was blooming. Scaliger mentions one of his relatives who experienced a similar horror when seeing a lily. Zimmermann tells us of a lady who could not endure the feeling of silk and satin, and shuddered when touching the velvety skin of a peach. Boyle records the case of a man who felt a natural abhorrence to honey; without his knowledge some honey was introduced in a plaster applied to his foot, and the accidents that resulted compelled his attendants to withdraw it. A young man was known to faint whenever he heard the servant sweeping. Hippocrates mentions one Nicanor, who swooned whenever he heard a flute; even Shakespeare has alluded to the effects of the bagpipes. Julia, daughter of Frederick, King of Naples, could not taste meat without serious accidents. Boyle fainted when he heard the splashing of water; Scaliger turned pale at the sight of water-cresses; Erasmus experienced febrile symptoms when smelling fish; the Duke d'Epernon swooned on beholding a leveret, although a hare did not produce the same effect; Tycho Brahe fainted at the sight of a fox; Henry III of France at that of a cat; and Marshal d'Albret at a pig. The horror that whole families entertain of cheese is generally known."

He also cites the case of a clergyman who fainted whenever a certain verse in Jeremiah was read, and of another who experienced an alarming vertigo and dizziness whenever a great height or dizzy precipice was described. In such instances

[1] *Op. cit.*, p. 246.

the power of association of ideas is probably the most influential agent in bringing about the climax. There is an obvious relation between the warnings given by the prophet in the one case, and the well-known sensation produced by looking down from a great height in the other, and the effects which followed.

Our dislikes to certain individuals are often of the nature of idiosyncrasies, which we cannot explain. Martial says:

"Non amo te, Sabidi, nec possum dicere quare;
Hoc tantum possum dicere, non amo te";

or, in our English version:

"I do not like you, Doctor Fell,
The reason why I cannot tell;
But this I know, and that full well—
I do not like you, Doctor Fell."

Some conditions often called idiosyncrasies appear to be, and doubtless are, due to disordered intellect. But they should not be confounded with those which are inherent in the individual and real in character. Thus, they are frequently merely imaginary, there being no foundation for them except in the perverted mind of the subject; at other times they are induced by a morbid attention being directed continually to some one or more organs or functions. The protean forms under which hypochondria appears, and the still more varied manifestations of hysteria, are rather due to the reaction ensuing between mental disorder on the one part, and functional disorder on the other, than to that quasi normal peculiarity of organization recognized as idiosyncrasy.

Thus, upon one occasion I was consulted in the case of a lady who it was said had an idiosyncrasy that prevented her drinking water. Every time she took the smallest quantity of this liquid into her stomach it was at once rejected, with many evident signs of nausea and pain. The patient was strongly hysterical, and I soon made up my mind that either the case was one of simple hysterical vomiting, or that the alleged inability was assumed. The latter turned out to be the truth. I found that she drank in private all the water she wanted, and that what she drank publicly she threw up by tickling the fauces with her finger-nail when no one was looking.

The idiosyncrasies of individuals are not matters for ridicule, however absurd they may appear to be. On the contrary, they deserve, and should receive, the careful consideration of the physician, for much is to be learned from them, both in preventing and treating diseases. In psychiatrical medicine they are especially to be inquired for. It is not safe to disregard them, as they may influence materially the character of mental derangement, and may be brought in as efficient agents in the treatment.

CHAPTER VI.

GENIUS.

THE inherent tendency which some individuals have for original work of a high order, in any department of literature, science, or art, is called genius. Briefly it may be defined to be a power of invention. Great geniuses are rarely met with, but persons born with the capacity for original thought in some new direction, and the energy to make their way to somewhere near the top of the ladder they may attempt to climb, are, fortunately for mankind, by no means rare. There will not probably be more than one Wagner in a generation; but there will be many Verdis, Gounods, Bachs, and Meyerbeers.

The mental operations and results of a great genius are not like those of mankind in general, but the differences are within the normal range, and consist mainly in the fact that they are such as others are not accustomed to, merely because they are new. They are in advance of their time, and hence often induce the belief that their possessor is insane. Most original minds have to encounter this objection at some time or other of their career; and, of course (and logically), the more striking and extravagant are the ideas they enunciate, the more loudly is the allegation of insanity uttered against them. Two or three hundred years ago they were accused of sorcery, witchcraft, or ungodliness, and were in danger of the prison or the stake. Sorcery and witchcraft have disappeared from the indictment, but ungodliness still remains, and lunacy has been added, to stand as prominent charges made against almost every one whose mind is in advance of the ordinary herd—and made, too, by persons of more than average common sense and education. It appears, therefore, that the mere fact of an individual deviating, so far as his mode of thought is concerned, in any notable respect from the path generally followed by mankind, is sufficient to excite the suspicion of insanity. Such deviation is regarded as a reproach, an insult, to the race, which no one has a right to offer. It is never exhibited by persons of mere talent, for talent follows the beaten road, though it follows it well. But genius disdains to be fettered ; it has a contempt for precedent ; it loaths the dull uniformity in which commonplace minds delight, and never rests till it has struck out a road for itself.

If, three hundred years ago, any one had announced that he had discovered a method by which messages could be sent under an ocean three thousand miles wide in a few seconds, and another had claimed that, by a system he had devised, persons a hundred miles apart could converse together as readily as though they stood face to face, they would at first have been objects of derision and pity. If they had persisted, with all the enthusiasm which animates men with genius, in urging the truth of their inventions, and in asking for means to demonstrate them to the world, they would undoubtedly have been imprisoned as agents of the devil and corruptors of morals, or as blasphemers against the immutable laws of the Deity. If a man were in our own time to declare that he had invented a process by which a person could be in two places a hundred miles apart at the same instant, and were to show by his conduct that he had full faith in his assertion, he would certainly be considered a lunatic ; and, if he made himself anyways troublesome to his friends and relations, an insane asylum would ere long receive him within its walls. Nevertheless, to those who know nothing of physics, his claim would be no more preposterous than either of the others, yet both of these have been realized, and their realizers are geniuses. Three hundred years from now those who come after us may be ashamed of their ancestors for doubting that a person can be in two places remote from each other at the same time.

The discrimination of the very highest flights of genius from insanity is a difficult, and at times an impossible, undertaking, for they may exist in one and the same person. If the distinction is to be made, it will be from the careful study of all the characteristics of the alleged genius or lunatic. The latter will generally show signs of mental derangement in

4

more than one direction, and will exhibit that inability to give long-sustained attention to any one subject which is so marked a symptom of insanity. The former will usually be consistent in the one thing which makes him original, whether it be in the work which he does or which he proposes to do. The imagination plays an important part in the mental operations of the man of genius and of the lunatic, but the one makes use of this faculty for the accomplishment of the objects he has in view, while the other becomes its slave, and is led hither and thither by its vagaries.

At the same time, though great genius and insanity are by no means to be regarded as necessarily closely related, there is no doubt that some of those who have made their mark in the world's progress by their transcendent powers of originality and invention have touched closely on the border line, while some again have crossed it. Eccentricity and genius often coexist in the same person, and this fact has served in the minds of some writers as a reason for regarding genius as a morbid mental manifestation. "Genius is a neurosis," says M. Moreau (de Tours),[1] and Dryden has declared that

"Great wit to madness nearly is allied."

No one can read the life of that great genius, Benvenuto Cellini, without reaching the conclusion that in him the two conditions were united. Martin Luther had hallucinations of sight and of hearing ; Pascal constantly saw a yawning precipice at his side ; Napoleon Bonaparte pointed out his star to General Rapp, and declared that it guided him in all his undertakings. Still, we would scarcely say that either of these men was insane ; it is quite certain that all of them were by nature strongly predisposed to insanity, and that the reason why they did not actually pass into that condition was because no sufficiently powerful determining cause was brought into action upon them.

In combating the opinion of M. Moreau (de Tours) that genius is a disease, M. Paul Janet[2] goes to the extreme and asserts that "genius is the human mind in its most healthy and most vigorous state." That this is true of genius as it has existed, and still exists, in some persons, is not to be questioned ; but, with the examples of many others before us, we cannot fail, it appears to us, to arrive at the conclusion that

[1] "Psychologie morbide."

[2] "Le cerveau et la pensée," Paris, 1867, art. "Le génie et la folie," p. 84.

more people of great genius, at one time or other of their lives, exhibit manifestations of insanity than do persons of ordinary mental faculties. And it is not to be doubted that the genius which prompts to exaltation in literature and the fine arts is more apt to be associated with or to end in insanity than that which leads to superiority in any one or more of the sciences. In literature and art the imagination is strained to the utmost if the highest standard of originality and excellence is to be attained, and the imagination is assuredly that faculty of the intellect which is least tolerant of straining. The genius, on the contrary, which is concerned with mathematics, astronomy, or any one of the sciences or mechanical arts, deals with facts instead of fancies ; and there is nothing about facts and their study which in the least predisposes to mental derangement. The great biologists and chemists, for instance, who have become insane, are so few in number that I cannot at this moment recall a single one ; while among great poets, painters, novelists, and musicians, who have either with their genius shown symptoms of insanity, or who toward the close of life passed into fatuity, the names of Tasso, Burns, Swift, Mozart, Hayden, Walter Scott, Blake, and Poe at once come to mind.

The practical lesson to be derived from all this is, that care should be taken that young persons who evince more than ordinary talent for any particular branch of literature, science, or art, should be encouraged to exercise their minds to some extent in other directions. The concentration of the intellect upon a single subject, while yet the individual has scarcely learned how to use his mind, can only be regarded as deplorable.

CHAPTER VII.

HABIT.

WHEN a living being performs an act under the operation of certain impressions which are received, there is a tendency toward the performance of a similar act, if like influences are brought to bear upon the organism. Every time the act is performed, the disposition to repeat it becomes stronger, until at last the tendency is so firmly established that the act is accomplished without the reception of impressions of like character to those which originally gave rise to it, but solely through the force of the newly acquired power. If from any cause the act is impossible of performance, the impulse still exists, and produces more or less unpleasant feeling in the mind, or sensation in the part of the body with which it is in relation.

This disposition to repetition is not limited to physical acts; it prevails in regard to almost every function of the body and mind, and forms often an important element in the production of disease.

Habit, therefore, is periodicity, and may be defined as the disposition which the organism acquires from the frequent reception of certain impressions, the indulgence in certain modes of thought, or the performance of certain acts, to continue in the accustomed course till some more powerful force intervenes.

A person, therefore, who has dined for many years regularly at the same hour, experiences the sensation of hunger when the time for eating arrives; the orator or writer who has long been in the habit of arranging his thoughts in a particular way, or of making use of peculiar modes of expression, follows the familiar methods with such unfailing regularity that, if he has spoken or written much, his style is at once recognized by those who have given it their attention; and the workman, who for years has observed a certain order or sequence in the performance of his duties, continues the system unchanged throughout his whole life.

But all these and other like habits may be broken up. The person who has dined habitually at six o'clock is taken ill, and, attributing his sickness to the fact of eating late in the day, changes his dinner-hour to one nearer noon. The orator or writer, finding that his speeches or essays are not so well received by the public as he would wish, alters his line of thought and characteristic phraseology to others which he thinks will be more effective; and the workman, losing his position, obtains employment in another shop where a change in his methods becomes necessary. Such changes are, however, not accomplished without considerable trouble, and sometimes with great suffering.

An instance cited by Dr. Carpenter [1] will recall many similar ones to the reader.

[1] "Principles of Mental Physiology," etc., London, 1874, p. 354.

" The first child of a young mother was accustomed, before being put into his cradle for his mid-day sleep, to be 'hushed off' in the arms of his mother or his nurse. But, having been told that this was an undesirable practice, his mother, wishing to break him of the habit, one day laid him down awake in his cradle and remained behind the head of it, so as to be out of the infant's sight. He screamed so long and so violently that several times she almost relented, fearing that he would injure himself ; but she had firmness to persevere, and, after a while, the child cried himself to sleep. Next day the screaming fit was much shorter, and on the following day shorter still ; and in a few days the child ceased to cry when laid down, and never did so again."

It is a well-known fact that the impressions or consequences which result from the action of certain agents are less marked as the operation of the cause is repeated. Thus, the system becomes habituated to the action of alcohol, opium, and many other substances, so that while a small quantity will, in the first instance, produce the characteristic result, the dose must be larger each time that it is taken, or be more frequently repeated, in order that a corresponding effect shall be produced.

There are many noxious agents to the action of which the system may become so habituated by frequent repetition or the continuation of their action that no injurious results follow, when, without the protection thus afforded, disease, or even death, would be produced. Persons living in a malarious district, and who are thereby constantly exposed to the deleterious emanations of the locality, are often, in time, so hardened to the influence that it fails to cause its ordinary effects, while, as regards those newly arriving in the region, its power to do harm remains unabated. Acclimation is nothing but the acquisition of immunity from disease by habitual exposure to the morbific elements of some particular place.

In like manner, a perception, an emotion, or a thought, which, when first experienced, caused a good deal of mental and physical disturbance, by repetition loses little by little the energy it once possessed, and scarcely excites a ripple in the usually placid mind or body of the individual.

The influence of habit over the ordinary operations of the economy is constantly seen ; the sensations of hunger and thirst are experienced at stated periods of the day, because, by frequently eating or drinking at those times, the system, as it were, expects a repetition, and hence the regular recurrence of the feelings in question. The action of the same law is seen in the periodical return of the desire to evacuate the bowels at the same hour, when by habit we have become accustomed to the act at that time. So with the desire for sleep, the hour of awaking, and the inexpressible sensations excited by the want of the usual cigar or alcoholic stimulant, with many others which must be familiar to every reader.

The manners and customs of nations are mainly the result of habit, continued through a long succession of generations. It is as difficult to alter them as it is to change a long-established habit of the individual organism.

Some persons are more under the influence of habit than others; they acquire a habit more quickly, and lose it with less facility. So strong are the unpleasant feelings excited by any interruption in the regular course of their habits that they will endure the greatest inconveniences to indulge them. I knew a gentleman whose custom it was to touch a certain tree—on the road from his house to the railway station, a distance of about five miles—as he daily went to his place of business. On one occasion, through absence of mind, he neglected this action, and rode several hundred yards before he discovered his omission. Though feeling annoyed, he continued his journey; but the uncomfortable sensation became too strong for him to endure it any longer, and, after having ridden nearly two miles past the tree, he galloped back, at the risk of missing the train, and touched it as usual.

Many persons, as is well known, have great difficulty in getting to sleep in any other bed than that to which they have become accustomed. No matter how luxurious the bed may be, sleep is effectually banished, often for several hours, and sometimes for the whole night.

In explanation of the essential cause of habit we can bring forward nothing very definite. We know that with inorganic matter a force once acquired will continue indefinitely, if no more powerful force interferes with it. A ball thrown into the air would continue in motion but for the influence exerted by gravity and friction. We can conceive of a similar law being in operation on organized matter. An impression is made upon the brain, and through the nervous system certain thoughts or actions ensue. The impression is not effaced with the accomplishment of the resultant act ; something of it remains to be strengthened, perhaps, by a similar impression made the following day, at the same time, with similar results. The process is in some respects like the registering of impressions to constitute memory, differing mainly in the fact that there is no consciousness of the process, and that there is no voluntary effort made to recall the impressions. This course may continue from day to day until the associated thoughts or actions are produced without the original stimulus, and thus the habit is established.

For instance, a person is induced to smoke a cigar after dinner. The inducement, whatever it may be, constitutes the impression made upon the brain. The persuasion of a friend, the desire to be sociable, or the idea that smoking would be beneficial to the health, prompts to the performance of the act, and the cigar is smoked. It is repeated for the same cause until at last the act of repetition begins to exercise its effect, and the original incentive is lost sight of in the more powerful one which has taken its place. A want has been created. A habit has been fully formed, and it cannot be broken without violence both to mind and body. The oft-repeated impression has left its traces somewhere each time, until at last it assumes a local habitation and becomes permanently fixed in the organism, not to be lost except through some more powerful influence acting in a similar manner to the first.

I have known several instances in which choreic affections have been acquired through a habit of imitating those who were thus disordered in their nervous systems. In one of these a boy mimicked the involuntary facial contortions from which a schoolmate suffered. He kept up the actions at intervals during the morning, and then discovered, to his great dismay, that he had lost the power of control over them, having, in fact, become himself the subject of facial spasms exactly like those of his prototype. Here the original excitation of the will, acting upon a peculiarly sensitive system of motor-cells, impressed them so strongly that, after a few repetitions of the volitional impulse, they were endowed with the power of carrying on the resultant movements through the force evolved by their own action. Several old ladies of strongly benevolent dispositions regarded it as resulting from a special dispensation of Providence.

Stammering, which is a chorea of the muscles of speech, is

also sometimes produced by mimicry of those affected. In one case which came under my observation, the patient, a young man twenty years of age, had suffered for ten years from very severe stammering, which he had contracted by imitating the mode of speech of another boy, who could scarcely articulate a word with facility.

The most striking instance of a disease being continued by habit is furnished by intermittent fever. There can be no doubt that, after the disease has been fairly established through the influence of malaria, the paroxysms occur with more or less regularity after removal to a healthy climate; and this through the force of the habit, which has been induced by the frequent repetition of the attacks. Indeed, so strong is the power of habit over the phenomena which, taken collectively, are known as intermittent fever, that it is quite possible to produce the disease by artificial means.

The very interesting experiment performed by M. Brachet affords us conclusive evidence on this point. This observer took a bath in the Seine every night at twelve o'clock toward the end of October, 1822. The procedure was continued for seven successive nights. After each bath he went to bed, covered himself warmly, in a short time became very hot, and finally broke out in a profuse perspiration. Discontinuing his cold bathing at the expiration of the seven days, M. Brachet was very much surprised to find that, at the hour for taking his bath, he was attacked with shivering, fever, and perspiration in regular order, and not to be distinguished from an ordinary attack of ague. For six successive nights he was thus affected. On the seventh, about midnight, he was summoned to attend a case of labor. The ride heated him, the heat was continued by his standing for some time in front of the fire, and thus the fire was broken up.

There is no doubt that epilepsy is often kept up by habit. Indeed, the occurrence of a single paroxysm from a non-continuing cause, such as an undigested meal, or a splinter under the skin, is sufficient very frequently, in my experience, to cause a predisposition to other attacks, which may last through the whole life of the individual.

Habits may be transmitted by hereditary influence through many successive generations. We are, perhaps, scarcely aware of the fact in all its relations, but a little attention to family histories will bring out many points well calculated to

enlarge our idea of the permanency and immutability characteristic of some mental and physical habits.

Girou de Buzareingues[1] says that he had known a man
who, lying in bed on his back, was in the habit of crossing
his right leg over his left. One of his daughters had the same
habit from birth. She constantly assumed this position in
her cradle, notwithstanding the obstacles which the napkins
offered. And he adds that he knows several girls who resemble their fathers, and who have habits which they have evidently inherited from them, and boys of whom the like is
true as regards their mothers.

Darwin[2] cites a case, on the authority of Mr. F. Galton,
which is still more striking: "A gentleman of considerable
position was found by his wife to have the curious trick,
when he lay fast asleep on his back in bed, of raising his right
arm slowly in front of his face up to his forehead, and then
dropping it with a jerk, so that the wrist fell heavily on the
bridge of the nose. The trick did not occur every night, but
occasionally, and was independent of any ascertained cause.
Sometimes it was repeated incessantly for an hour or more.
The gentleman's nose was prominent, and its bridge often became sore from the blows which it received. At one time an
awkward sore was produced that was long in healing, on account of the recurrence night after night of the blows which
first caused it. His wife had to remove the button from the
wrist of his night-gown, as it made severe scratches, and some
means were attempted of tying his arm.

"Many years after his death his son married a lady who
had never heard of the family incident. She, however, observed precisely the same peculiarity in her husband; but his
nose, from not being particularly prominent, has never as yet
suffered from the blows. The trick does not occur when he is
half asleep, as, for example, when dozing in his arm-chair;
but the moment he is fast asleep it is apt to begin. It is, as
with his father, intermittent, sometimes ceasing for many
nights, and sometimes almost incessant during a part of every
night. It is performed, as it was by his father, with his right
hand.

"One of his children, a girl, has inherited the same trick.
She performs it likewise with the right hand, but in a slightly

---

[1] Cited by Ribot, "L'hérédité," 2ième éd., Paris, 1882, p. 58.
[2] "The Expression of the Emotions," London, 1872, p. 33, note.

modified form ; for, after raising the arm, she does not allow
the wrist to drop upon the bridge of the nose, but the palm
of the half-closed hand falls over and down the nose, striking
it rather rapidly.   It is also very intermittent with this child,
not occurring for periods of some months, but sometimes occurring almost incessantly."

A gentleman informed me that his grandfather had become
accustomed to wake up from sound sleep at twelve o'clock
every night and drink a cup of tea, after which he would lie
down and sleep quietly till morning.   The father of my informant was a posthumous son, and his mother died in childbirth with him.   He was English, and at an early age went
to India with an uncle.   One night, when he was about
twenty years of age, he awoke suddenly with an intense desire for a cup of tea.   He endeavored to overcome the longing, but finally, being unable to sleep, got up, and, proceeding
to an adjoining room, made himself a cup of tea, and then,
going back to bed, soon fell asleep.   He did not mention the
circumstance at that time ; in fact, it made no strong impression on his mind, but the next night the awaking, the desire,
and the tea-making were repeated.   At breakfast the following morning he alluded to the fact that he had twice been
obliged to rise in the middle of the night and make himself a
cup of tea, and laughingly suggested that, perhaps, it would
be as well for him in future to have the materials in his bedroom.   His uncle listened attentively,· and, when the recital
was finished, said : "Yes, have everything ready, for you will
want your tea every night ; your father took it at midnight
for over twenty years, and you are like him in everything."

His uncle was right ; the midnight tea-drinking became a
settled habit.   Several years afterward he returned to England, and there married.   Of this marriage a son—my informant—was born, and six years subsequently the father
died.   The boy was sent to school till he was sixteen years
old, when he was sent to Amsterdam as a clerk in the counting-house of his mother's brother, a banker of that city.

He was kept pretty actively at work, and one night in
particular did not get to bed till after twelve o'clock.   Just
as he was about to lie down the idea struck him that a cup of
tea would be a good thing.   All the servants had retired, so
the only thing to do was to make it himself.   He did so, and
then went to bed.   The next night he again had his tea, and

after that took it regularly, waking from sleep punctually for that purpose at twelve o'clock. Up to that time he had never been a tea-drinker, though he had occasionally tasted it. Writing home to his mother, he informed her that he had taken to the custom of drinking tea, but had acquired the habit of taking it at a very inconvenient hour—twelve o'clock at night. She replied, telling him that he had come honestly by his liking, for his father and grandfather had had exactly the same habit. Previous to the reception of this letter he had never heard of the peculiarity in his father's and grandfather's lives.

Habitual indulgence in some powerful emotion or engrossing train of thought is a very influential cause of insanity.

The proper regulation of the habits conduces more to mental and physical well-being than perhaps any other factor. The ability of an individual to control those habits—which, when indulged in to moderation, are beneficial to the organism, but to excess are injurious—is an indication not only of strong will-power, but is an important influence in preserving the health both of mind and body. All the appetites are more or less under the control of the will, and it is easy in youth or early manhood to bring them into proper subjection, whereas in mature age the matter is much more difficult, and with some persons impossible. As we shall see farther on, there is scarcely a form of mental derangement which may not be incurred by habitual over-indulgence in some one or more of the natural or acquired appetites. As regards purely mental habits, youth is the period during which they may be formed most readily, and with the best prospect of enduring for a lifetime. Then the faculties of the mind are developed with the greatest facility and brought into systematic and habitual action. That, therefore, is the best method of education which most effectually secures these ends.

The matter may be summed up in the following words of Sir Henry Holland:[1] "The formation of new habits, however, is not more important than is the control of those which are casually, and often injuriously, created by the accidents of life, or by individual passions or propensities. These must be governed by the mind, that they do not gain dominion over it. They form an alien power in possession, which it needs strong efforts, both of reason and resolution, to expel. To

[1] "Chapters on Mental Physiology," London, 1852, p. 232.

create and maintain that 'vigor of mind which is able to contest the empire of habit' (Locke) may be rightly asserted as the chief end of all mental discipline."

And the following from Lemoine:[1] "Habit has sometimes been branded with the name of routine, because, as it were, it forms all actions in the same mould, and often usurps the place of reason and the will. But it is not habit which deserves this reproach, and which arrests the progress of science or the perfectionment of life. It is the bad use which is made of it, the idleness of mind and of will, when the agent which has acquired by habit an increase of force and capacity for acting is contented to do with the least effort that which is most easily done, and not to employ this increase of power to perform more difficult acts. If life, science, morality, civilization, progress of all kinds, are stopped at some point of their career, it is not habit which stands in the way; it is some extraneous cause which immobilizes at the same time that it arrests progress. There is nothing in the nature of habit, or in its laws, which can act as a cause of regression, of retardation, or of rest. It is essentially an augmentation of power, and it tends always to the elevation and the improvement of the human race."

In the examination of lunatics, or suspected lunatics, the habits of the individual should form the subject of careful inquiry. Not only is much light thereby thrown upon the mental condition, but important data are supplied toward the formation of a correct prognosis.

CHAPTER VIII.

TEMPERAMENT.

THE subject of temperament, which at one time was an important factor in medical literature, fell a few years ago into unmerited neglect, to be revived quite lately to a position almost equal to that which it occupied among the ancients, and with much clearer ideas of its real value in biological science.

The ancients laid very great stress on the doctrine of the temperaments, and on the influence which these conditions of

-----

[1] " L'habitude et l'instinct; étude de psychologie comparée," Paris, 1875, p. 77.

the system are capable of exercising over diseases. Galen arranged them into four classes, corresponding, as he supposed, to the four different liquids of the body, which, in their turn, represented the four elements—earth, air, fire, and water. The four humors were the bile, the blood, the back bile, and the lymph ; and hence he had the bilious, the sanguineous, the atrabilious, and the lymphatic or phlegmatic temperaments, according to the predominance of one or other of these fluids.

We know, however, that no such connection as that supposed by Galen really exists, yet the names given by him are still those which are in vogue. The individual of sanguine temperament, other things being equal, has no more blood than the one of phlegmatic temperament, nor less lymph ; neither can these fluids be regarded as at all influencing the mental constitution or the physical peculiarities. The same remarks may with truth be applied to the bile, so that there is no necessary or direct connection like that assumed by Galen. But there can be no doubt relative to the existence of certain mental and physical types which present distinct characteristics easily recognizable, so that, from an inspection of the aspect and general bodily construction, we are enabled to define with tolerable certainty the physical peculiarities. These types we call temperaments.

Müller [1] defines temperament as a peculiar permanent condition or mode of mental reaction of the mind and organism. I cannot say that the definition is a very clear or satisfactory one, although perhaps sufficiently so to indicate the idea intended to be expressed.

Temperament is rather the organic constitution dependent upon certain mental or physical peculiarities, innate or acquired. It is the specific difference which gives to persons, or groups of persons, their individuality. We can very readily perceive that it must influence very materially the predisposition to disease. And, in fact, when we come to consider the subject in all its bearings, and with the profundity of which it is worthy, we find it very difficult, if not impossible, to distinguish between temperament and predisposition except by the one feature—that the latter embodies more than the former. And, as we can indicate, with considerable approach to correct-

---

[1] "Elements of Physiology," translated by William Baly, M. D., London, 1842, vol. ii, p. 1406.

ness, the intellectual character of the individual from the color of his hair, eyes, and complexion, the size and shape of his hands and feet, or the peculiarities of his pulse and respiration, so we are enabled, with equal facility, from a similar examination, to designate the diseases to which he is specially liable.

It is not, however, to be asserted that the temperaments are separated from each other by strictly defined lines. If they were, we should probably have more uniformity among authors in their classification. As it is, a very considerable diversity exists, some making but two, and others as high as seven. It is very much with temperaments as it is with the colors of the solar spectrum : they overlap each other, and give rise to certain compound temperaments which possess many of the characteristic marks of distinct conditions, but which may, without much difficulty, be separated into their original constituents.

Cullen was able to see but two temperaments—the sanguineous and the choleric ; all others he regarded as combinations of these two. Bégin,[1] with more propriety, recognizes three—the sanguineous, the lymphatic, and the nervous. I agree with several authors in admitting four—the sanguineous, the lymphatic or phlegmatic, the choleric, and the nervous. This division is that adopted by Devay,[2] and is one which appears to be founded on natural differences. In addition, there is another, which some authors have described as distinct from all others—the insane temperament. This, however, is, I think, only an excessive degree of development of the nervous.

In examining a patient, very little attention is, as a rule, paid to the study of the temperament, although from this source a flood of light can always be obtained to assist in determining the diagnosis, the prognosis, and the treatment, and this is especially true of those diseases of the brain characterized by the existence of mental derangement. In seeking, therefore, to ascertain the particular temperament of an individual, it is necessary to take into consideration, not only his physical peculiarities, but also the mental characteristics he may possess.

And, in making such an investigation, we should, as Royer-

[1] "Physiologie pathologique," Paris, 1828, t. i, p. 56.
[2] "Traité special d'hygiène des familles," etc., Paris, 1858.

Collard [1] declares, bear in mind that a temperament is a more
or less permanent variety of health, and the conditions should
be ascertained, not by examinations made of a single organ
or fluid of the body, but of the blood and the nervous system.
The characteristics of these are to a great extent indicated by
the appearance, the bearing, and the habits of the individual;
but our inquiries may very advantageously extend beyond
these points by employing the several instruments of precision, which, when properly used, are of inestimable value
in such determinations.

The Sanguine Temperament.—This temperament is characterized by great activity of the circulatory and respiratory
apparatus, and by marked vivacity of mind. The pulse is
quick, strong, and bounding; the complexion florid; the hair
red or chestnut color; the eyes blue; the hands and feet
small; the skin thin and fair; the respiration active; the digestion good; the excretion from the skin abundant, while,
owing to this latter cause, the urine is small in quantity and
is high colored. The powers of endurance are very considerable, though not so great as in the choleric temperament, not,
however, so much from any physical defects as from mental
peculiarities. The expression of countenance is cheerful and
hopeful, and activity characterizes all the movements.

In the mental constitution we see the same qualities displayed—modified, of course, by the different material with
which they are associated. There are the same restlessness
and brilliancy, and, while any particular bent is followed, a
good deal of energy is shown. The love of pleasure predominates, but the pleasure must be frequently varied or satiety
is soon produced. Inconstancy is a predominating feature.
Good resolutions are formed but to be broken. Friendships
are readily contracted, to be soon abandoned for others, which,
in their turn, are speedily given up. In love, the individual
of sanguine temperament is fickle and faithless, caring less
for his honor than his pleasure. He engages in great undertakings without counting the cost, and, if unexpected difficulties arise, he soon becomes discouraged, unless he sees
an ultimate advantage to himself from persevering. If success attends his efforts, as it often does, it is more on account
of the rapidity of his actions than the consequence of any

[1] "Des temperaments considérés dans leurs rapports avec la santé." "Memoires de l'academie royale de médecine," t. x, 1843, p. 165.

well-laid plans, or else is the result of that "good luck" of which he is frequently the recipient.

History furnishes many examples of distinguished persons of sanguine temperament. Marc Antony and Plato among the ancients; Charles II, of England, Lorenzo di Medici, the Duke of Richelieu, and Murat, are instances of it. In this country, General Wayne and Henry Clay were good examples of this temperament. Shakespeare, in his inimitable character of Mercutio, has depicted it with masterly power. Poetry, painting, and sculpture have some of their most distinguished cultivators among individuals of the sanguine temperament.

Temperate climates afford the most striking instances of this form of temperament. We see this not only in the mental and physical characteristics of individuals, but in the history of the nations which inhabit countries situated within the temperate zone.

The female sex contains more representatives of it than the male, and youth more than adult age.

The diseases to which persons of the sanguine temperament are peculiarly disposed are those connected with the circulatory system. Thus, they are liable to functional and organic diseases of the heart, aneurisms, and hæmorrhages. Contrary to the generally expressed opinion, I do not believe in any decided proclivity of individuals of this temperament to inflammatory affections. Activity of circulation is not favorable to diseases of this character.

While it cannot be said that the sanguine temperament predisposes to insanity, it modifies the symptoms in accordance with its influence over the mind and body in their normal state. A person of sanguine temperament becoming insane is more apt to be affected with acute mania, or some other form of mental exaltation, in contradistinction to any variety of which mental depression is the characteristic feature. They are not, however, even in their most excited moments, so apt to perpetrate acts of violence as individuals of some of the other temperaments—the choleric, for instance. Being endowed with great vitality, the prognosis is more favorable, other things being equal, in persons of sanguine temperament affected with insanity than in others of different temperaments.

Individuals of the sanguine temperament should abstain

from stimulating articles of food and drink, and should confine themselves to a plain but nutritious diet. They should exercise freely in the open air, avoiding, as far as possible, the direct rays of the summer sun. Overheated and crowded apartments are also injurious. I have seen many cases of acute mania superinduced in persons of sanguine temperament from a disregard of these simple precautions. There is with them generally a predisposition to cerebral hyperæmia, which is very liable to be aggravated into reality, or even intense congestion or inflammation, by any one of the factors cited.

The Lymphatic or Phlegmatic Temperament.—This temperament is the direct opposite of the sanguine in almost every respect. The flesh of persons in whom it exists is flabby and soft; the pulse is infrequent, weak, and languid; the respiration slow; the countenance pale or leaden color; the eyes green or pale gray, and expressionless; the hair very straight, and light-colored. The whole form is rounded, and lacking in that elasticity which characterizes the sanguine temperament.

Mentally, the difference is equally striking. The intellect is slow to act; ideas come with difficulty; but there is by no means necessarily a deficient degree of intelligence, and, though matters may be comprehended and conclusions reached with a tardiness aggravating to those of quicker minds, they are fully as likely to be right in both as those who reason more promptly, and seem to arrive at a judgment with scarcely an effort. Undoubtedly, however, when the lymphatic temperament is excessively developed, there is often a sluggishness of the mental processes almost amounting to stupidity.

The emotions are not easily roused into activity, and are rarely of an ennobling or energetic character. Courage is not a prominent attribute of lymphatic persons, and, though they may not run away at the approach of danger, it is more because they do not at once understand its nature than from any high feeling of pride or honor. The memory is weak, and the power of application, or of concentrating the attention, inconsiderable. There is, therefore, a disinclination to reflective study, or any mental or physical exertion. Men of this temperament have made but little sensation in the world's history. The part they have played has been quiet, unobtrusive, and even insignificant.

5

But it is not to be supposed that this temperament has not its good side. Although prompting to slowness, there is often a perseverance which may compensate for a lack of rapidity. Friendships are not often contracted, but, when once formed, are frequently enduring, in a mild way. Great undertakings are rarely attempted, but those moderate ones which constitute the bulk of the operations of every-day life, and which require neither brilliancy nor energy, are accomplished without bustle or confusion.

As Müller [1] remarks, the subject of the phlegmatic temperament may be a very useful and trustworthy member of society. When rapid action is required, the phlegmatic person is less successful, and others leave him behind ; but, when no haste is desired and delay is admissible, he quietly attains his end while others have committed error upon error, and have been diverted from their course by their passions. The phlegmatic person knows his proper sphere, and does not trespass upon that of others, or come into collision with them. From this conduct, as well as from an orderly and steady course of action, in which he keeps his object in view and avoids self-deception, he derives a contented tone of mind, free alike from turbulent enjoyments and deep suffering. Cold and damp climates are those in which this temperament is generally encountered.

Old age more frequently exhibits it than youth, and it is more often met with in women than in men. It is readily acquired under circumstances favorable to its production. A life in which there is little inducement to either bodily or mental exertion, especially if the surroundings, such as the temperature and humidity of the atmosphere, be propitious, is exceedingly apt to produce it even in persons of directly opposite characteristics.

The varieties of mental derangement which are especially liable to exist in persons of the phlegmatic temperament are a low grade of melancholia—the *melancholie avec stupeur* of the French—and acute dementia. If the subjects of this temperament become affected with acute mania, the mental and bodily excitement does not reach so high a plane as in those of the sanguine temperament. Their delusions are not of so gay a character, and generally relate to plots or designs

[1] "Elements of Physiology," edited by Dr. William Baly, London, 1842, vol. ii, p. 1408.

against them by some real or imaginary persons. Instead, however, of wishing to fight their supposed injurers, as would the man of sanguine temperament, or sitting wringing their hands in anguish, as would he of the choleric temperament, the phlegmatic lunatic takes it all very quietly, and will talk of the malicious attempts which have been made upon his life without evincing the slightest anger or sorrow, and with even a pleasant smile on his countenance.

Persons in whom the lymphatic temperament is strongly marked endure heat well, but cold badly. They should avoid excess at table, but may, with advantage, indulge to moderation in wines or malt liquors. Animal food should constitute a large proportion of their diet.

The Choleric or Bilious Temperament.—The physical and mental characteristics of this temperament are exceedingly well marked. The complexion is dark, or sallow; the hair black, or a dark brown; the eyes black, or hazel; the skin dry and not over-soft, except sometimes in women; the flesh hard and firm; the pulse hard, strong, and frequent; the respiration deep and strong, and the whole form thin, tough, and capable of enduring great fatigue without deleterious consequences.

Mentally, the man of choleric temperament is characterized by firmness, decision, and determination. His mind is quick to form a judgment, his will active and powerful in the accomplishment of his purposes, and his perseverance carries him over all difficulties. His emotions are vivid, but, when it suits his designs, he keeps them under due control. He is irritable, sensitive, and often vindictive, cruel, and unscrupulous. Bold in the conception of a project, constant and indefatigable in its execution, it is among men of this temperament that we find those who in different ages have governed the destinies of the world; full of courage, boldness, and activity, all have signalized themselves by great virtues or great crimes, and have been the terror or admiration of the universe. Such were Alexander, Cæsar, Brutus, Mahomet, Charles XII, the Czar Peter, Cromwell, Sixtus V, and Cardinal Richelieu.

"As love is in the sanguine, so ambition is in the bilious, the governing passion. Observe a man who, born of an obscure family, long vegetates in the lower ranks. Great shocks agitate and overthrow empires; at first a secondary actor in those great revolutions which are to change his destiny, the ambitious man hides his designs from all, and by degrees raises himself to the sovereign power, employing to preserve it the same address with which he raised himself to it.   This is, in a few words, the history of Cromwell and of all usurpers.

"To attain to results of such importance, the profoundest dissimulation and the most obstinate constancy are equally necessary ; these are, further, the most eminent qualities of the bilious.   No one ever combined them in higher perfection than that famous pope who, slowly travelling on toward the pontificate, went, for twenty years, stooping and talking forever of his approaching death, and who, at once proudly rearing himself, cries out : ' I am pope ! ' petrifying with astonishment and mortification those whom his artifice had deceived into his party.

"Such, too, was Cardinal Richelieu, who raised himself to a rank so near to the highest, and was able to maintain himself in it ; feared by the king, whose authority he established ; hated by the great, whose power he destroyed ; haughty and implacable toward his enemies, ambitious of every sort of glory." [1]

Among men of science and letters who have possessed the choleric temperament are Dante, Newton, Spinoza, Galileo, Milton, Pascal, Tasso, Rousseau, Goethe, and Calvin.   In this country the most distinguished representatives of the choleric temperament have been Mr. Calhoun, Mr. Webster, Mr. Lincoln, Generals Grant, Sherman, Sheridan, and Lee, and Mr. Jefferson Davis.

Individuals of the choleric temperament are, perhaps, more subject to insanity than those of any other, unless it be the nervous, next to be described.   The variety to which they are especially liable is melancholia in all its forms, and it sometimes assumes with them the most terrible of all the phases of mental derangement—the suicidal and homicidal. The delusions which are most frequently met with in them are those which relate to injuries done them by others, or horrible crimes which they have themselves perpetrated.   Often they refer to religious subjects, and to the state of eternal damnation into which their souls are to be plunged on account of the enormity of their sins.   The idea that they have

[1] Richerand's "Elements of Physiology," edited by Chapman, Philadelphia, 1818, p. 583.

committed the "unpardonable sin" is a very common delusion with this class of lunatics, and they will often walk the
floor for days and nights at a time, wringing their hands,
moaning, and sobbing, at the thought ever present of the
awful punishment in store for them in the world to come.   I
know of no one point in the whole range of theology which
has inflicted more injury upon the human mind, and caused
more distress, than the doctrine that there is a mysterious sin
which any one may ignorantly commit, and never escape the
eternal wrath of an offended God.   The miserable sufferers
themselves never know what it is, or, if they imagine they
do, are afraid to reveal their knowledge.   One poor girl,
whose anguish of mind was pitiable to witness, informed me,
in answer to my inquiries, that it was "too horrible to mention."

The choleric temperament is more frequently encountered
in the inhabitants of the warmer portions of the temperate
zone than in other localities, and it is more common among
men than among women.

Individuals of the choleric temperament should be spar-
ing in the use of alcoholic liquors and of stimulating articles
of food ; they should exercise freely, be especially careful to
maintain the digestive organs in a healthy condition, and,
above all things, keep the emotions in subjection to the intellect.   A neglect of this last injunction may of itself induce
serious bodily or mental disease.

The Nervous Temperament.—In this temperament the manifestations of nervous energy are markedly prominent, and
give peculiar impress to the whole body and mind.   The
countenance is usually pale, and the features thin and sharp ;
the pulse is quick, small, and frequent, though not weak ;
the respiration active ; the chest and muscular system are
generally not largely developed ; the skin is dry and rough ;
and the digestive functions are performed irregularly.   The
urine is usually copious, and of pale color.

In consequence of the comparative weakness of the muscles, persons of this temperament easily become fatigued ;
though, owing to the activity of the nervous system, they
quickly rally.

Prompt to form opinions and to arrive at conclusions, the
subjects of the nervous temperament are not remarkable for
stability of purpose.   Their intellectual operations are rapid

and brilliant, but, at the same time, not often persistent. Variety is constantly sought for; and the mental efforts, like the physical, are, as it were, spasmodic, full of energy while they last, but soon yielding to others.

Women were formerly much more frequently the subjects of this temperament than men, but, owing to the constant effort to get rich manifested by the male sex in recent times, and the consequent extreme development of the emotional system, and of certain faculties of the intellect, it is now far more common with them. Indeed, I am not sure but that in civilized communities, especially in the large cities of the United States, it has not become the predominating temperament. The man who day after day is kept upon a mental rack by that most harassing of all the emotions—anxiety—will inevitably undergo such psychical and bodily changes as will change him from any other original temperament to the one under notice. Of all the temperaments, it is particularly easy to be acquired. It is the outcome of civilization and refinement, and, probably, but for these agencies, would never have arisen. Among barbarous nations it is almost unknown, and savages never exhibit it; but it is common enough in London, Paris, and New York, and in men who, if they had lived a hundred years ago, would have been as phlegmatic as the most typical Dutchman.

Voltaire and Frederick the Great, of Prussia, are notable examples of the nervous temperament. John Randolph, perhaps, affords the most remarkable example of it among distinguished Americans.

The diseases which are most apt to occur among individuals of the nervous temperament are those which concern the nervous system. Thus, we have the various forms of neuralgia, certain affections of the spinal cord, hysteria in all its protean varieties, chorea, catalepsy, ecstasy, and insanity of all types. In fact, the nervous temperament itself is, if strongly developed, almost a pathological condition. The sensibility is so acute, the capability for receiving mental impressions so decided, and the system is so readily thrown into disorder from slight causes, that the temperament in question may often be considered as the first manifestation of disease. Indeed, it frequently lapses almost insensibly into the condition which Whytt[1] described many years ago, and which has re-

[1] " Observations on the Nature, Causes, and Cure of those Disorders which

cently been very fully considered under the name of "Nervo-sisme" by Bouchut.[1]

Persons of the nervous temperament are very subject to diseases which exist only in their imagination, or which, being slight, are exaggerated by the constant habit of introspection in which they indulge. They are thus very frequently rendered insensible by the morbid attention they give to symptoms which are of no consequence, and which are often by no means abnormal.

The peculiar exaggeration of the nervous temperament to which I have alluded as the insane temperament, is really a morbid condition, and will be more appropriately considered farther on.

As has been said, it rarely happens that the temperaments are so clearly marked that any individual can be said to possess the traits of one without being endowed with some of the attributes of another. Thus, there are the sanguineo-lymphatic, the sanguineo-choleric, the sanguineo-nervous, and so on. Each of these conjoins in itself the manifestations of the temperaments of which it is composed, in an equal or nearly equal degree, or the traits of one may very decidedly predominate, in which case it is named accordingly.

In addition, there are certain conditions which are degenerations of the temperaments. Thus, there are the plethoric state, formed on the sanguineous, in which there is an abnormal development of the circulatory system ; the obese, on the lymphatic, leading to the excessive formation of adipose tissue ; and the melancholic, on the choleric, in which there are extreme activity of the liver and a consequent tendency to disease of the abdominal viscera. These may properly be considered as positive diseases, and, as such, calling for medical intervention.

have been commonly called Nervous, Hypochondriac, or Hysteric," third edition, Edinburgh, 1767.

[1] "De l'état nerveux, aigu et chronique, ou nervosisme," Paris, 1860.

CHAPTER IX.

CONSTITUTION.

By constitution we understand the general condition of the system which results from the permanent state of the organs of the body, and the consequent degree of perfection of their action. A person may, therefore, have either a good or a bad constitution, according as the several organs of the body are of normal or abnormal structure, without or with a tendency to derangement from slight causes, and working properly and in harmony with each other, or acting imperfectly and without co-ordination of functions. In the first case, the vitality of the body, the capability of resisting morbific influences, and of recuperation, are greater than in the last; the functions are performed with energy, the tissues are healthy, and, as a consequence, disorder and disease are not so liable to occur.

On the contrary, persons with weak constitutions are prone to disease upon slight exposure to the operation of causes capable of inducing pathological disturbance. The circulation is weak and languid, and in the extremities, consequently, the temperature is not kept up to the normal standard. Cold hands and feet, even in warm weather, are therefore a subject of constant complaint. Such individuals suffer severely from attacks of disease which persons of strong constitution would endure with scarcely a feeling of discomfort, and recuperate slowly, and often with frequent relapses. Moreover, they are attacked when the others escape.

It is very much the same with a man as with an artificial machine. If the latter is well made, of good material, the several parts strongly put together, and working in harmony with each other, it will resist hard usage better, and do more work, than will the machine which is made of bad materials, in which the different parts are not well proportioned, and which are constructed without a due regard to the work they have to perform.

Constitution differs from temperament, with which it has sometimes been confounded, in this, that while the latter refers to specific and well-defined differences, due to the particular manner in which certain vital processes react on the mind, the former is more general, and relates to the original structure and integrity of the organs and tissues of the body. An individual may possess any temperament conjoined with a good, bad, or indifferent constitution. Constitutions differ from each other only in degree of perfection, while the differences between temperaments are peculiar and radical.

A weak constitution is, to a certain extent, capable of being strengthened by proper hygienic measures. A child born in poverty, and reared under circumstances unfavorable to the full development of the organs of the body, such as insufficient food, clothing, light, and fresh air, may, if the conditions are changed at a sufficiently early period, develop into an adult of good constitution. Even at a late period of life much may be done by the employment of sanitary means to strengthen a constitution originally weak.

The evidences of a feeble constitution are generally sufficiently clear to even superficial observation. The heart, the lungs, and the nervous system are found to be endowed with less than the normal amount of power, and, consequently, the functions appertaining to these organs are imperfectly performed. The chest is narrow and flat, the muscles flabby and weak, and the whole system is wanting in tone.

The factor of constitution is equally powerful with the mind as with the body. Persons whose physical organization is below the normal standard are incapable of long-sustained or intense intellectual action, although the quality of mind produced, dependent as it is on the cerebral structure, may be good. The reason of this is that, if, for instance, the individual has naturally a weak digestive system, one liable to get out of order from those slight exciting causes which no one can altogether avoid, he is incapable of supplying the brain with the nutritive material which it requires to compensate for the waste caused by its action. Hence, the organ easily gets fatigued. Besides, earnest and well-directed brain-work is impossible if the individual is constantly disturbed by uneasy or painful sensations in his abdomen, or in any other part of his body. The attention which is necessary for thought is diverted from the subject under consideration to the place where the pain is felt, and hence the process of reasoning is weak, or is altogether interrupted. *Mens sana in corpore sano* is almost a necessary relation.

A naturally strong constitution may be weakened by excesses or a neglect of the rules of health. The intemperate use of alcohol, inordinate sexual indulgence, long-continued exposure to the action of causes capable of depressing the vital powers, and frequent attacks of disease, will break down the strongest constitution. This is especially seen in the military service. Men originally well constituted and robust, subjected, often without the least attention being paid to their sanitary requirements, to the hardships incident to army life —exposure to all kinds of weather, loss of sleep, want of sufficiently nutritious food and of warm clothing, the absence of proper shelter—fall from the normal standard of health, and remain broken down for the rest of their lives. Tissues which were in the first place capable of performing their office in the economy lose this power in a measurable degree, and the whole organism becomes enfeebled and more susceptible to morbific influences.

And what is true of the body is equally so of the mind. A person with a brain originally well constituted may, by its injudicious use, not only lessen its mental power, but may make it the seat of such organic disease as will reduce him to a state of imbecility. I have seen many individuals who, by working their brain to an extent beyond that which the organ was capable of legitimately accomplishing, could not concentrate the mind for five minutes on the simplest matters without causing headache and mental confusion.

Persons of strong constitutions are not so liable to insanity in any form as those of weak ones. The protective and resisting power of the former is exerted as well upon the brain as upon the other organs of the body. Should such an individual, however, become insane, the probability of recovery is much greater than in another of feeble organization.

It is in early childhood that most can be done to modify original defects of constitution. Weak and sickly children require the utmost care relative to their food, clothing, and physical and mental exercise. A strong meat diet, or, at least, an abundance of milk, eggs, or other animal food, is absolutely necessary when it is desirable to improve the tone of the system. Much injury is often done to children by confining them, as is often done, to a vegetable diet and milk and water. Such children generally remain weak and puny, and, if they live, become adults of feeble constitution. Many, too, are stunted in mind by overtasking their as yet undeveloped brains. The process of hardening, as it is called, whether applied to mind or body, is one which, if injudiciously used without reference to the physical or mental powers of the child, is fraught with danger to the subject upon whom it is tried.

CHAPTER X.

HEREDITARY TENDENCY.

THE hereditary transmission of peculiarities of form, mental character, manner, idiosyncrasies, habits, and proclivity to disease, is no longer a matter of doubt with those best qualified to form an opinion on the subject. In fact, to this tendency of like to beget like we owe the perpetuation of the different species of animals and plants, as well as the great number of varieties produced by the will of man, or by combinations of circumstances.

We see on every side numerous instances of the existence of the law to which reference is made. The different varieties of the dog, of the ox, and other domestic animals, the several kinds of roses, apples, strawberries, and other plants, are all the results of hereditary transmission.

Resemblances in features to parents are extremely common in the progeny. A child looks like its father, its mother, or, perhaps, some collateral relation. The hereditary upper lip of the members of the house of Hapsburg is an example of this fact, and others must be familiar to most persons. In the lower animals the same law applies with equal, if not greater, force. A whole litter of pups, for instance, will be marked like the father or mother, or, perhaps, some like one, and the remainder like the other.

Certain qualities can also be transmitted. Thus, the setter and pointer possess their peculiar accomplishments by hereditary descent from ancestors which were taught to indicate the presence of game by the actions they employ. I knew a lady who could always tell twenty-four hours in advance that rain or snow was at hand. She felt a cold sensation in both ears. Her mother had the same faculty, as has also her daughter. I have already given instances of the hereditary transmission of habits, but the following, which has recently come to my knowledge, will not be out of place:

A lady informed me that her grandmother, who had some

affection of the right eye that rendered the accession of light
to it unpleasant, always worked at her embroidery or sewing
with that eye closed. Her daughter had no ocular disorder,
but, in doing any kind of needle-work, always shut the right
eye. Her daughter, my informant, has a similar habit, which
she acquired when quite young, although constant efforts were
made to break her of the "trick." She came to me for advice
relative to her little girl, eight years old, who, when given
some sewing to do a few days previously, had at once closed
the right eye on beginning her task. Here we have a habit
descending through four generations. Instances like this
almost lead us to the belief that it would be entirely practicable to form a variety of the human race the women of
which would always sew with the right eye closed.

Certain natural deformities or organic deviations are likewise sometimes indubitably transmitted to the progeny. It
is, therefore, by no means rare to find that the immediate ancestors of individuals with superfluous fingers or toes, club-
feet, or hare-lip, were similarly affected.

Accidental anomalies or mutilations are also the subjects of
hereditary transmission. Thus, Grognier[1] states that he has
observed that the colts whose ancestors had for many ascending generations been branded on a particular part of the body
were born with marks corresponding in situation and appearance to those made by the hot iron. According to Blumenbach,[2] a man had the little finger of his right hand badly injured, so that it became crooked. He subsequently had several sons, each of whom had the little finger of the right hand
twisted like that of their father.

Among the Esquimaux and Kamtchatkans it is the custom
to cut off the tails of the dogs used in drawing the sledges. It
is frequently the case that the puppies come into the world
without a tail, or with the appendage very much abbreviated.[3]
Other instances of the same kind are cited by Lucas.

But the most important part of the subject of hereditary
influence which we have at present to consider is in relation
to the transmission of diseases or predispositions to disease.

---

[1] Cited by Lucas, "Traité philosophique et physiologique de l'hérédité naturelle," Paris, 1850, t. ii, p. 492.

[2] Blumenbach, cited from Treviranus by Lucas, op. cit., p. 493.

[3] Langsdorff, cited by Lucas, op. cit., p. 493 ; also Quatrefages, cited by Ribot,
"L'hérédité psychologique," Paris, 1882, p. 9.

Like the transmission of the physical and mental qualities, the transfer of pathological tendencies from parents to offspring must be accepted as a fact amply capable of demonstration, but not susceptible of explanation. When we say that the seminal fluid, being derived from the blood, must possess the abnormal impress of the blood, we assert a proposition just as difficult of demonstration, and in no way an elucidation of the question. Besides, admitting that the seminal fluid of a phthisical person may contain, in an inappreciable form, the germs of tubercles, we could not explain why the offspring of such a person should remain all their lives free from phthisis, and the next generation exhibit unequivocal evidence of the presence of tubercular deposits in the lungs. That the tendency to certain diseases is derived from the seminal fluid of the male, and in an equal or perhaps greater degree from the ovaries of the female, does not admit of a reasonable doubt; but that there are other agencies at work capable of influencing the child while yet unborn is quite as certain. And this fact demands that a distinction shall be made between those diseases or other peculiarities which are connate and those which are purely hereditary. By a connate disease we understand one which the child possesses when born, not necessarily the result of any similar taint or impression received from the system, either of the father or mother, but due to accidents or mental influences operating through the mother. For instance, a child may be born idiotic, not because either of the parents or other ancestors were similarly affected, but through the influence of some severe mental or physical shock received by the mother during her pregnancy. Another may be epileptic—when neither parent has ever been subject to epilepsy or any other disease of the nervous system —if one or other is intoxicated at the time of the intercourse resulting in conception.

Such cases are, of course, not due to hereditary transmission, for a disease cannot be communicated hereditarily which has not affected either of the parents or any other ancestor.

Many interesting cases showing the influence of the maternal mind over the offspring before birth are cited by M. de Frarieré [1] and the elder Séguin. [2] There is no doubt that idiocy,

---

[1] "Éducation antérieure. Influences maternelles pendant la gestation," Paris, 1862.

[2] "Idiocy and its Treatment by the Physiological Method," New York, 1866.

and other forms of disorder of the mind, may be induced in the unborn infant by strong emotional or other mental disturbance in the mother.

A singular fact connected with the transmission of diseases, and also of deformities or resemblances, is that a whole generation, or one or more members of it, are passed over, the disease or other peculiarity appearing in the next; or a child, instead of resembling either of his parents, has the appearance or peculiarities of one of his grandparents. This is called atavism. Its existence was known to the ancients. Aristotle, Galen, Pliny, and Plutarch refer to it, and the latter gives the case of a Greek woman who, having given birth to a black child, was tried for adultery, when it was discovered that she was the fourth generation of an Ethiopian.

A distinction must be made between those diseases which, though hereditary, are congenital, and those which appear after a lapse of time, often considerable. Thus, for example, cataract, deafness, and several kinds of deformities, belong to the first-named class, but the great majority belong to the second, and arise as a consequence of the predisposition which has been transmitted. They are, thus, of very great importance to the physician, because, as the tendency only is conveyed, and this may not be very strong, it is altogether possible frequently to prevent the predisposition being developed into positive disease.

Thus, Voltaire [1] says:

"I have almost with my own eyes seen a suicide whose case deserves the attention of physicians. A man of serious turn of mind, of mature age, and of irreproachable conduct, free from strong passions and above want, killed himself on the 17th of October, 1769, and left a written explanation of his act, addressed to the council of the city in which he was born. This it was thought best not to publish, for fear of encouraging others to quit a life of which so much evil is spoken. In all this there was nothing astonishing; such cases are met with every day. But the sequel is more remarkable. His father and his brother had each committed suicide at the same age as himself. What hidden disposition of the organs, what sympathy, what combination of physical laws, caused the father and his two children to perish by their own hands, by the same method, and at the same age? Was

[1] "Dictionnaire philosophique," art. "Caton du suicide."

it a disease which had long previously been developed in their family, as parents and children are often seen to die of the small-pox, of pneumonia, or of some other disease? Three or four generations become blind, or deaf, or gouty, or scrofulous, at a certain age." Many similar cases have been cited by writers on the subject. The following is within my own knowledge:

A gentleman, well to do in the world, but with a slight hereditary tendency to insanity, killed himself in the thirty-fifth year of his age by cutting his throat while in a warm bath. No cause could be assigned for the act. He had two sons and a daughter—all under age at the time of his death. The family separated, the daughter marrying. On arriving at the age of thirty-five, the eldest son cut his throat while in a warm bath, but was rescued ere life was extinct. At about the same age the second son succeeded in killing himself in the same way. The daughter, in her thirty-fourth year, was found dead in a bath-tub with her throat cut. Her son, at the age of twenty-seven, attempted to kill himself by cutting his throat while in a bath at his hotel in Paris, but did not succeed. Subsequently, at the age of thirty, he made a similar unsuccessful attempt, but was again saved. A year afterward he was found in his bath by his servant with his throat cut from ear to ear.

A very striking physiological fact is not without influence upon the laws of hereditary transmission. It is well known that the children of a woman by her second husband may resemble physically and mentally her first husband, provided she has had children by the latter. The blood of the *foetus in utero* circulates through the system of the mother. This blood has the impress of the father derived through the seminal fluid. It must, therefore, in a greater or less degree, exert an influence upon the organism of the mother. Perhaps this is in accordance with Darwin's provisional theory of pangenesis; but, whether or not, the fact exists. Now the husband, dying, and the mother marrying again and having children, is the medium for transmitting to this second set of offspring the peculiarities of mind and person which she has received from her first husband through his children before they were born. In this way the diseases of a man may be transmitted to children which are not his. In the lower animals, instances of this species of transmission are far from being rare. A bitch will have a litter one half of which will resemble in their markings their progenitor, and the other half a dog by which she has previously had offspring. In the horse the like fact has been noticed, and it doubtless prevails to some extent throughout the entire vertebrate class of animals. Breeders of domestic animals are fully aware of its existence, and are careful that the females used for raising fine stock are not approached by males of bad qualities.

That insanity is often transmitted by hereditary influence is a fact scarcely requiring discussion, but for the circumstance that it has been recently denied by certain medical witnesses in a criminal trial that such was ever its origin. Nevertheless, these gentlemen were by no means the first to advance the hypothesis that insanity is limited in its influence to the individual in whom it first appears, and that it never has heredity for its cause. Its author is Heinroth.[1] He says:

"Insanity is the loss of moral liberty; it never depends on a physical cause; it is not a disease of the body, but of the mind; it is a sin. It is not, and it cannot be, hereditary, for the thinking ego, the soul, is not hereditary. The only things transmitted by generation are temperament and constitution, against which he who has insane ancestors should protect himself if he would escape lunacy. The man who has, during his whole life, before his eyes and in his heart, the image of God, has no fear of ever losing his reason. It is as clear as the light of day that the torments of those wretches called bewitched and possessed are the consequences of the development of remorse of conscience. Man has not only received reason; he has, besides, a certain moral power which cannot be conquered by any physical power, and which never succumbs except under the weight of its own sins."

Commenting on this extraordinary system of mental pathology, M. Lelut[2] says:

"This passage from M. Heinroth contains as many errors as it does phrases. To say that a man who has all his life kept the image of God in his heart will never become insane, is to refuse to recognize the innumerable cases of insanity de-

---

[1] See the German translation of Esquirol's works by Hille, of Dresden, with notes by Heinroth, Leipsic, 1837, cited by Lélut, "Du traitement moral de la folie," Paris, 1840, p. 146; and also by Lemoine, "L'aliéné devant la philosophie, la morale et la société," Paris, 1865, p. 55; also by Ribot, *op. cit.*, p. 140; also by Lucas, *op. cit.*, t. ii, p. 756.   [2] *Op. cit.*, p. 147.

veloped by superstition and an ascetic life; to impute the torments of the bewitched and the possessed of the devil to
remorse of conscience, is to calumniate those unfortunate persons who often have only exaggerated their sins, or have
even accused themselves of crimes they never committed; to
affirm that man has a moral power which cannot be overcome
by any physical force, is to ignore the influence of wounds of
the head, the ingestion of certain poisonous substances, inflammation of the meninges, etc., in the production of insanity. To refuse to admit that insanity may be transmitted by
the process of generation is to refuse to accept the evidence
of that which we see every day."

Lucas[1] asserts that Rush expresses a doubt in regard to
the hereditary transmission of insanity, and the witnesses in
question may have entertained a like opinion relative to his
views. But this is an error, for the great American physician
is emphatic enough when he declares his opinion in the affirmative, and adduces numerous examples in its support. He
says:[2]

"A peculiar and hereditary sameness of organization of
the nerves, brain, and blood-vessels, on which I said formerly
the predisposition to madness depended, sometimes pervades
whole families, and renders them liable to this disease from a
transient or feeble operation of its causes."

He then states that application was made on one day for
the admission of three members of the same family into the
Pennsylvania Hospital, and that he had attended two ladies,
one of whom was the fourth, and the other the ninth, of their
respective families who had been affected with insanity in
two generations. Moreover, he declares that, when there is a
hereditary predisposition to mental aberration, it is induced
by feebler exciting causes than when no such tendency exists.
And, again, that it generally attacks in those stages of life in
which it has appeared in the patient's ancestors, and that
children born previously to the attack of madness in their
parents are less liable to inherit it than those who are born
subsequently.

Without entering at this time into the full consideration
of the question, I will adduce the authority of a few of the

---

[1] *Op. cit.*, t. ii, p. 756.
[2] "Medical Inquiries and Observations upon the Diseases of the Mind,"
fourth edition, Philadelphia, 1830, p. 46.

most eminent writers on mental derangement, premising that, with the exception of Heinroth, already cited, and the modified view of Lordat,[1] I would not know where to find a single negative opinion from any writer on psychological medicine who had received a medical education. Esquirol[2] says:

"Hereditary influence is the most ordinary predisposing cause of insanity, especially with the rich. . . . Insanity is more frequently transmitted by the mothers than by the fathers."

Burrows[3] states that:

"There certainly is no physical error in accounting insanity hereditary. Had the knowledge of this fact merely led to a closer inquiry respecting those with whom a connubial union is contemplated, it would be a commendable foresight, often conducing to the preservation of domestic bliss now too frequently interrupted by the development of this dreadful affliction in the object perhaps of our tenderest affections."

Griesinger[4] says:

"Statistical investigations strengthen very remarkably the opinion generally held by physicians and the laity, that in the greater number of cases of insanity an hereditary predisposition lies at the bottom of the malady ; and I believe that we might, without hesitation, affirm that there is really no circumstance more powerful than this."

Leidesdorf,[5] in speaking of the hereditary character of many cases of insanity, says:

"All alienists have established the importance of this cause, to which an average of one quarter of the cases of insanity is due, though individual statements on this point differ greatly. Marcé goes so far as to assert that in nine tenths of all the cases of insanity hereditary antecedents will be found."

Luys,[6] under the heading of "hereditary cerebral states," says:

[1] "Les lois de l'hérédité physiologique sont-elles les mêmes chez les bêtes et chez l'homme?." Montpellier, 1842, p. 19.

[2] "Des maladies mentales," Paris, 1838, t. i, p. 33.

[3] "An Inquiry into Certain Errors relative to Insanity, and their Consequences, Moral and Physical," London, 1820, p. 9.

[4] "Mental Pathology and Therapeutics," Sydenham Society Translation, p. 150.

[5] "Lehrbuch der psychischen Krankheiten," Erlangen, 1865, p. 128.

[6] "Traité clinique et pratique des maladies mentales," Paris, 1881, p. 214.

"Heredity governs all the phenomena of mental pathology with the same results and the same energy as we see it control moral and physical resemblances in the offspring.

"The individual who comes into the world is not an isolated being separated from his kindred. He is one link in a long chain which is unrolled by time, and of which the first links are lost in the past. He is bound to those who follow him and to the atavic influences which he possesses; he serves for their temporary resting-place, and he transmits them to his descendants. If he comes from a race well-endowed and well-formed, he possesses the characters of organization which his ancestors have given him. He is ready for the combat of life, and to pursue his way by his own virtues and energies.

"But inversely, if he springs from a stock which is already marked with a hereditary blemish, and in which the development of the nervous system is incomplete, he comes into existence with a badly balanced organization; and his natural defects, existing as germs, and in a measure latent, are ready to be developed when some accidental cause arises to start them into activity."

One other authority, and I am done with this question for the present. All admit the ability and knowledge with which the late Dr. Ray discussed all points connected with insanity. Relative to heredity, he says: [1]

"The course of our inquiry, then, leads us to this conclusion—that in the production of insanity there is generally the concurrence of two classes of agencies, one consisting in some congenital imperfection of the brain, and the other in accidental outward events. I do not say that mental disease is never produced by the latter class of cases exclusively. The present limited state of our knowledge forbids so sweeping a conclusion. Cases sometimes occur where the closest investigation discloses, apparently, no cause of cerebral disorder within the patient himself. There is good reason to believe that the number of such cases would be lessened by a deeper insight into the inner life, and a minuter knowledge of those organic movements which lead to disease. We know that, even in those cases in which, to all appearance, the casual incident was most competent of itself to produce the disease, the constitutional infirmity may be often discovered. Drunkenness,

[1] "Contributions to Mental Pathology," Boston, 1873, p. 45.

epilepsy, blows on the head, sunstroke, would seem capable, if anything outward could, of producing insanity ; but, as a matter of fact, we find not unfrequently behind these casual events, firmly seated in the inmost constitution of the brain, the hereditary infirmity.   Can we believe that it took no part in the morbid process ? "

If it be alleged that the disease insanity is not transmitted, but only the tendency to the disease, the same might be alleged of every other morbid condition regarded as hereditary, except those existing at the time of birth, in the parents and offspring.

Phthisis, gout, progressive muscular atrophy, and other indubitable hereditary affections, would from that point of view be non-hereditary.   Besides, how would it be known, in the young infant, whether insanity existed at birth or not? Where there is so little mind as the new-born child possesses, the manifestations of insanity must be so slight as to escape our observation.   Not including cases of idiocy, there is, however, abundant evidence to show that children do occasionally exhibit some of the most intense phases of insanity at very early periods of their lives.   Romberg [1] has seen the case of a child, six years of age, in which there was a blind impulse to destroy everything upon which it could lay its hands.   It rushed through the street with a knife in its hand, and was restrained with difficulty.   Griesinger [2] states that children of three to four years of age often have attacks of crying, of wild restlessness, striking, biting, and endeavoring to destroy, which last only for a time, and which ought to be regarded as true mania.

Dr. Rush [3] saw a case of insanity in a boy of seven years of age, and subsequently one in a child two years, that had been affected with cholera infantum, and another in a child of the same age, that was "affected with internal dropsy of the brain."   "They both discovered the countenance of madness, and they both attempted to bite, first their mothers and afterward their own flesh."

Insanity, as a rule, makes its appearance, when hereditary, at the period of life in which the mind is most active ; and often the inherent condition is so strong that it develops into more intense forms of mental derangement upon exceedingly

[1] "Deutsche Klinik," 1851, p. 178.
[2] *Op. cit.*, p. 142.   [3] *Op. cit.*, p. 55.

slight cause, or even, so far as can be perceived, spontaneously. It cannot, in such cases, be prevented by any means we may employ.

It is a peculiarity of nervous affections that they are not necessarily transmitted to descendants in the same form in which they appear in the ancestors. Thus, the latter may have epilepsy and the progeny neuralgia, migraine, or some variety of mental alienation, or the reverse may occur. Neither when insanity itself is clearly due to hereditary influence is it always the case that a like type of disease is transmitted. The ancestors, for instance, may have had general paralysis, and the descendants will exhibit the several forms of mania or melancholia.

A discussion of the subject of hereditary influence would manifestly be incomplete without reference to that of consanguinity, in regard to which there is, I think, a good deal of misunderstanding.

In the early history of mankind, marriages among blood relations were common. The Persians, Tartars, Scythians, Medes, Phœnicians, Egyptians, and Peruvians, not only married their sisters, but their daughters and their mothers. Instances of such marriages among members of the royal families of antiquity are well known.

The laws of the ancient Germans allowed consanguineous marriages, as did also those of the Arabs up to the period of Mahomet,[1] and the Jews, notwithstanding the prohibitions of Moses, continued them up to the present day. All civilized nations allow them within certain degrees. In the State of New York, for instance, first cousins may marry, as may also uncle and niece, or aunt and nephew. The State of Kentucky, however, prohibits the marriage of first cousins, and of all nearer degrees of relationship.

The dangers of consanguineous marriages have been pointed out by many authors.

M. Rilliet[2] contends that all such marriages are in themselves pernicious, and tend with great certainty to a lowering of the vital force. The effects he divides into two categories:

1. Those which relate to the parents, under which head are:

[1] "La consanguinité et les effets de l'hérédité," par V. La Perre Roo, Paris, 1881, p. 4.

[2] "Lettre sur l'influence de la consanguinité sur les produits du marriage," *Bulletin de l'Academie de Médecine*, t. xxi, p. 746.

a. Failure of conception.

b. Retardation of conception.

c. Imperfect conception.

2. Those which relate to the progeny :

a. Imperfections of various kinds.

b. Monstrosities.

c. Imperfect physical and mental organization.

d. Tendency to diseases of the nervous system, such as epilepsy, imbecility, idiocy, deaf-mutism, paralysis, and various cerebral affections.

e. Tendency to strumous diseases.

f. Tendency to die young.

g. Tendency to succumb to diseases which others would easily resist.

It is easy to see that Rilliet has made several tendencies out of one. Thus, the categories under *b* and *c* are manifestly included in *a*, and those under *f* and *g* in *d* and *e*.

After a full consideration of all that Rilliet has to advance, I feel bound to agree in the main with De Roo [1] in the opinion that common-sense teaches us that all these ills do not proceed from consanguineous marriages, and that it would be very difficult for Rilliet to prove the half of what he has advanced.

Among the opponents of such marriages are Devay,[2] Helliot,[3] and Boudin,[4] in France ; Mitchell,[5] in Great Britain ; and Bemis,[6] in the United States. It was mainly through the exertions of the latter that the State of Kentucky enacted a law prohibiting the marriage of blood relations nearer than second cousins.

It is undoubtedly true that consanguineous marriages often result in the birth of children who are malformed, idiotic, deaf-mutes, or who become in after years the subjects of epilepsy, insanity, and other affections of the nervous system.

On the other hand, it is undoubtedly true that many such marriages take place, the results of which are as perfect in

[1] *Op. cit.*, p. 9.

[2] "Du danger des marriages consanguines," Paris, 1862.

[3] "Contribution à l'étude de la consanguinité," Paris, 1875.

[4] "Dangers des unions consanguines," etc., Paris, 1862.

[5] "On the Influence of Blood Relationships in Marriage," *Memoirs of the Anthropological Society of London*, vol. ii, 1866.

[6] "On the Evil Effects of Marriages of Consanguinity," *North American Medico-Chirurgical Review*, vol. i, 1857, p. 97.

every respect as could be desired. Dr. Bourgeois[1] wrote the history of his own family, which was the issue of a union in the third degree of consanguinity. During the ensuing one hundred and sixty years there were ninety-one marriages, of which sixteen were consanguineous. Of these latter, all were productive, and there was not a single case of malformation or other physical or mental disease in the offspring.

Huth[2] cites from Dr. Thibault the case of a slave-dealer who died in the year 1849, at Widah, Dahomey, leaving behind him four hundred disconsolate widows, and about one hundred children. By order of the king, the whole of this family was interned in a particular part of the country, where reigned the most complete promiscuity. In 1863 there were children of the third generation, and Dr. Thibault, who verified the fact himself, asserts that at that time, although all these people were born from all degrees of incestuous unions, there was not a single case of deaf-mutism, blindness, cretinism, or any congenital malformation. Huth cites many other instances of isolated communities intermarrying continually without detriment to the offspring.

The truth appears to be found in the fact that consanguineous marriages are not. in themselves productive of evil results, either to the parents or offspring; and that the ill consequences are to be ascribed to the operation of the law of hereditary influence, which, of course, is doubled so far as the progeny is concerned. If it is absolutely certain that a family is free from all taint of any kind whatever, there is no physiological reason why a man should not marry any female relative, however near; but, as that can never be positively assumed, it is better to prohibit such marriages down to, or even including, second cousins. There are few persons who cannot call to mind one or more consanguineous marriages which have resulted in idiocy, epilepsy, insanity, or other mental or nervous diseases in the children. I am quite sure that there is a greater tendency to the production of such affections than of any other, many striking examples of the fact having come under my observation.

[1] Cited by Ribot, " De l'hérédité," Paris, 1882.
[2] " The Marriage of Near Kin," etc. London, 1875, p. 161.

CHAPTER XI.

A G E.

TIME, which exercises its influence even upon inorganic bodies, is immeasurably more powerful in its relations with organized beings. They spring into existence, increase, decay, and die according to the laws of their being. 'In some the cycle is completed in a few days, or even hours, in others, in a few years, and in others, again, not until centuries have elapsed.

This is equally true of animals and vegetables. The moth of the silk-worm and certain cryptogamic plants measure the period of their existence by hours, while the crocodile, the elephant, and the oak count hundreds of years of life.

King David fixed the length of human life at seventy years, with eighty as an exceptional limit. Flourens[1] believes, with Buffon, the natural life of man to be one hundred years, and adduces many ingenious arguments in support of his opinion. Instances are not wanting in which even this limit has been greatly exceeded. Thomas Parr, for instance, is said to have lived to the age of one hundred and fifty-two years, and then to have died from indigestion caused by over-eating at a feast given to him by Charles I. Harvey made a *post-mortem* examination of his body, and found all his viscera in normal condition. The cartilages of his ribs were not ossified.

Mr. E. Ray Lankester[2] cites instances in which one hundred and nine and a hundred and eleven years have been reached, but doubts if there is any authenticated instance of more than one hundred and twenty years having been attained. He cites statistics which go to show that in civilized communities the average duration of life is greater in females than in males.

During life the fluids and tissues of the body are constantly undergoing change. New matter is deposited, and the old is renewed with ceaseless activity. The body may be regarded as a complex machine, in which the law that force is only generated by decomposition is fully carried out. Every motion of the body, every pulsation of the heart, every

---

[1] "De la longévité humaine et de la quantité de vie sur la globe," Paris, 1856.
[2] "On Comparative Longevity in Man and the Lower Animals," London, 1870.

thought which emanates from the brain, is accompanied by the destruction of a certain amount of tissue. So long as food is supplied in abundance, and the assimilative functions are not disordered, reparation proceeds as rapidly as decay, and life is the result; but, should nutrition be arrested by any cause for any considerable period, new matter ceases to be formed, and the organs, worn out, act no longer, and death ensues.

The animal body differs from any inorganic machine in the fact that it possesses the power of self-repair. In the steam-engine, for instance, the fuel which serves for the production of steam, and subsequently for the creation of force, can do nothing toward the repair of the parts which have become worn out by use. Day by day, through constant attrition and other causes, the engine becomes less perfect, and must be put in order by the workman. In the animal body, however, the material which serves for the production of force is the body itself, the substances taken as food being first assimilated, and converted into brain-substance, muscle-substance, heart-substance, etc.

The body is therefore undergoing continual change. The hair of to-day is not the hair of yesterday; the muscle which extends the arm is not identically the same muscle after as before the action; old material has been removed and new has been deposited to an equal extent; and, though the weight and form, the chemical constitution, and histological characters are preserved, the identity has been lost. If, however, a muscle be detached from the recently dead body of an animal, accurately weighed, made to contract many times by a current of electricity, and then weighed again, it will be perceived to have lost appreciably a portion of its substance.

So long as the processes of waste and repair exactly counterbalance each other, life continues. If it were possible so to adjust them to each other that neither would be in excess, there is no physiological reason why life, if protected against accidents, should not continue indefinitely. But this is not, with our present knowledge, possible; decomposition eventually predominates, and death from old age results.

The life of man has been variously divided by different authors into artificial stages or periods, the limits of which are by no means accurately fixed. A natural division, which is based upon the physiological course of life, is not only more convenient, but is more correct. In accordance with this principle, therefore, I would divide the life of man into three periods : 1. *The period of increase,* in which the formation of tissues predominates over decay ; this stage extends from birth to about the twenty-fifth year, varying according to individual and sexual peculiarities ; 2. *The period of matur-ity,* in which the two processes counterbalance each other, extending from the twenty-fifth year, or thereabouts, to the thirty-fifth year ; 3. *The period of decay,* in which the tis-sues are not regenerated as rapidly and perfectly as they are broken down and excreted from the system, and reaching from the thirty-fifth year to the extreme limit of human life.[1] Each of these stages is marked by strong peculiarities both of organization and action, and they exhibit immunities to some diseases and susceptibilities to others, which are only to be accounted for by a reference to the physiological condition by which each stage is characterized.

The Period of Increase.—The average height of the human subject at birth is between eighteen and nineteen inches, and the weight about seven pounds. The bones are not yet com-pletely ossified, the muscles are soft, the skin thin and highly vascular, and the circulatory and nervous apparatus devel-oped to a much greater extent comparatively than at any other period of life.

A great tendency exists during the first five years of the period of increase to diseases of the nervous system, and this is at its maximum during the first dentition. Convulsions due to irritation, and inflammation of the brain and its membranes are accordingly of common occurrence. As we have seen, insanity may exist at this time, and this either from heredi-tary transmission or arising from some accidental cause. In addition to the facts cited in the immediately preceding chap-ter, the following are worthy of notice :

Guislain[2] states that he possesses in his notes several re-markable examples of infants who have become maniacs before the age of puberty. He has seen subjects only three or four years old, who up to that age had shown much intelligence and even a precocious development of the mental faculties,

---

[1] This division, which is as old as Aristotle, is preferable to any which has been since devised.

[2] " Leçons orales sur les phrenopathies, ou traité théorique et pratique des maladies mentales," Paris, 1880, t. i, p. 447.

experience suddenly an entire change of character, becoming at first morose and then excited, violent, and exhibiting in their countenances the signs of intellectual derangement. This condition has lasted several months, and has then disappeared, to be replaced by an apparently normal state. Moreover, such instances have occurred in several infants of the same family, in which, nevertheless, insanity was not hereditary.

Morel[1] cites from his own experience the case of a girl ten and a half years old who, on being frightened, fell into convulsions, and immediately lost the faculty of speech. Her mental state was characterized by exacerbations of such a nature that it was necessary to confine her in an asylum, in which she was a constant source of trouble. She seemed never to be happy unless she was destroying everything which came into her hands, and tormenting the adult lunatics.

In another case, which also came under his notice, the subject, a boy five years of age, was suddenly frightened, lost the power of speech, and for three years that he was in an asylum exhibited constant turbulence and frequent maniacal exacerbations.

Dr. Chatelain[2] reports a remarkable case of acute mania occurring in an infant four years and nine months old, who was frightened by a fire-engine. At first she had hallucinations of hearing and of sight, then, as the violence of the disease increased, she was constantly in motion, gesticulated violently, grew angry, struck at persons, wept, and wished to kill her relations. Finally, after several weeks, she became better, and probably entirely recovered.

Several cases of insanity in youths of either sex have come under my observation, but only one in which the subject was of very tender age. This was a boy about six or seven years old, whom I saw in consultation with Dr. E. M. Hunt, of Metuchen, New Jersey. Frequently during the day he would experience attacks of acute maniacal excitement, during which he would bite, kick, and strike at all who came near him, and destroy everything within his power or reach. While the paroxysm was on him he was in constant motion, running and dancing around the room, climbing over the tables and chairs, gesticulating violently, and shouting or talking incoherently

---

[1] "Traité des maladies mentales," Paris, 1860, p. 101.
[2] *Journal de Médicine Mentale*, t. x, p. 322.

at the top of his voice. There was some evidence to show that when an infant in arms he had received a fall, striking his head. The place was pointed out differently by his mother and grandmother, but, acting upon what I conceived was the better evidence, I determined to trephine him. The operation was performed with Dr. Hunt's assistance, the cranium being perforated at the right parietal eminence. No injury of the bone was found, but recovery took place immediately, and the patient is now, as I believe, a healthy and sane young man. It is a notable fact that insanity in young persons is very apt to take the form of mania with destructive tendencies. The patients exhibit strong propensities to kill or torture animals, and to inflict wanton cruelties on their companions.

Strange as it may seem, suicide is by no means an unknown act with very young children. With youths, as we are constantly being informed by the newspapers of the day, it is more common. M. Durand-Fardel[1] found that of 25,760 suicides occurring in France in the ten years from 1835 to 1844, 192 were in persons under sixteen years of age. Of these latter 1 was under five years, 2 between eight and nine years, 2 between nine and ten years, and 6 between eleven and twelve years of age.

Referring to these statistics, Brierre de Boismont[2] says:

"We can understand suicide by infants when we read in the confessions of Saint Augustine that a child at the breast, when its nurse suckled another baby, went into a violent fit of anger at the sight, and almost had convulsions."

According to the census ot 1880 there were in the United States, during the preceding ten years, 2 suicides by children between five and ten years of age; 12 between ten and fifteen years; 66 between fifteen and twenty years; and 136 between twenty and twenty-five years.

Montaigne[3] states that in his time there were many examples of children committing suicide in order to escape from some slight inconvenience.

And this is one of the chief characteristics of suicide when perpetrated by children—that it is generally for some notion

---

[1] "Études sur le suicide chez les enfants," *Annales médico-psychologiques*, Janvier, 1855.

[2] "Du suicide et de la folie suicide," Paris, 1856, p. 68.

[3] "Essais," liv. i, chap. xv, p. 293, édition de Lefèvre.

which to the adult mind appears to be altogether inadequate, often ridiculously so.

Esquirol[1] cites the case of a boy thirteen years old, who, for some trifling cause, hanged himself, leaving a statement in writing that he left his soul to Rousseau and his body to the earth; and from Falret another, also a boy, twelve years of age, who hanged himself because a composition which he hoped would obtain the first place was only twelfth. The following cases are reported by Dr. Forbes Winslow.[2]

Harriet Cooper, aged ten years and two months, upon being reproved for a trifling fault, went upstairs and hanged herself with a pair of cotton braces. Another, named Green, aged eleven, drowned herself from the fear of correction for a trifling fault. And he cites from Casper the statement of Dr. Schlegel that in Berlin between the years 1812 and 1821 no less than thirty-one children of twelve years of age and under committed suicide either because they were tired of existence or had suffered some trifling chastisement.

Collineau[3] refers to the case of a boy ten or twelve years of age, who, on being sent back to college before his holiday was over, hanged himself, as he said in writing, *to make his parents angry.*

Another, ten years old, on being reprimanded by her mother, answered: " If you torment me in this way, you will some day find me hanging to the bed-post "; another of nine years actually threw herself out of the window to avoid a scolding for having broken a goblet; and still another of only five years hanged himself to escape from the bad treatment of his mother.

Cases like these might be cited by the dozen. The daily press makes them familiar to us all; only to-day (August 10th) the New York morning papers report the case of a boy aged fourteen, who, having broken a pane of glass in the shop in which he was employed, was told that he would have to replace it. Afterward he was sent out with a clock which had been repaired, and on which he was to collect a dollar. Then he hired a rowboat, went out on Jamaica Bay, and, anchoring at about three hundred yards from the shore, shot

---

[1] *Op. cit.,* t. i, p. 289.

[2] " The Anatomy of Suicide," London, 1840, p. 269.

[3] " Du suicide chez les enfants," *Journal de Médicine Mentale,* t. viii, 1868, p. 417.

himself with a toy pistol. His dead body was found at the bottom of the boat.

A short time ago a case went the rounds of the press of a boy of ten years who had hanged himself because as he said he was "tired of so much dressing and undressing." Surely there must be an innate abnormal brain-formation in such children, one that if they had lived to attain maturity would have caused infinite trouble to themselves and those around them.

As the age of the individual advances, the body becomes more fully developed and is enabled better to resist disease. By the time puberty is attained, which in the United States is about the sixteenth year for boys and the fifteenth for girls, the tissues have acquired considerable solidity, the bones have become harder, though the epiphyses are not yet consolidated with the shafts, and the circulatory, respiratory, and digestive organs have, in a measure, lost the excessive sensibility by which they were characterized in infancy.

The genital organs, which have hitherto exercised but little influence over the general system, now become capable of performing their functions. In the male the secretion of semen takes place, and in the female menstruation begins. The larynx, which in the infant is small and round, now becomes lengthened, and in the male especially the voice assumes a more grave tone.

The intellectual faculties have not been behindhand. The brain, though relatively smaller, has undergone consolidation and hardening of its substance, and has, in conjunction with the other organs of the system, lost to a material extent the peculiar sensibility to external impressions which belonged to it in early infancy, gaining in strength, in force, and in capacity for improvement.

The relation between the formative and destructive processes is more evenly balanced, and the body has nearly attained the period when growth ceases. This point is in males about the twenty-fifth year, and in females about a year earlier.

Insanity in some one of its several forms, though not especially common about the age of puberty, is nevertheless not infrequently encountered. Its more usual variety is mania, but it is sometimes met with as an affection mainly of the emotions, or as characterized by blind and unreasoning impulses to acts of deceit or violence. Fixed delusions are not a prominent feature, but, as Blandford[1] states, there are perverted feelings, hatred of relations, wanton and indecent behavior, cruelty and destructiveness, and hallucinations of the senses.

Several cases of insanity occurring in young persons have come under my observation, and all were, with one exception, of the types above described, presenting very much the general appearance of reasoning mania, to which attention will subsequently be fully directed. In one of these instances the patient, a young lady about fifteen years of age, had been for some two or more months affected with an impulse to torture and kill every animal which came under her notice. How it originated she could not precisely say, but was disposed to think that the first time she felt it was when witnessing a cat playing with and finally killing a mouse. At once she procured several traps, all so constructed that the animals were captured alive. Then she would put some into a washbasin, and, gradually turning on the hot water, would watch their struggles with the greatest pleasure till they were finally scalded to death. Others she placed in the trap on the top of a hot stove, enjoying their struggles in their frantic efforts to escape. And others again were deliberately cut to pieces with scissors. Upon one occasion she threw a whole litter of kittens into a bucket of boiling water. When the larger animals were not available, she spent her time in catching and killing flies. She confessed to me that her great desire was to steal a baby and skin it alive, but that she was afraid to make the attempt lest she should be arrested and hanged for it. She was at the same time a teacher in a Sunday-school, and she declared that it was with the utmost difficulty she could refrain from enticing one of the younger pupils into a cornfield near which they passed on their way home from church and killing her. She had even gone so far as to put a piece of twine into her pocket, with which she designed strangling her victim, but the fear of the law had always prevented her.

There were periods of remission in which she was a prey to the deepest feelings of remorse, and it was in one of these that she was brought to me by her father, a worthy gentleman, who had endeavored to conceal his daughter's misfortune and to cure her by moral suasion. Not finding this suc-

[1] "Insanity and its Treatment," Edinburgh, 1871, p. 125.

cessful, he had called together a few friends, and together they had prayed for her recovery, also without favorable result.

She reasoned with entire calmness about her misfortune, and with tears in her eyes and much lamentation regretted her inability to control the impulse which moved her, and which she was sure came from the devil. I attributed it, however, to another cause, and, by regulating her menstrual function, succeeded in a short time in restoring her to health. Such cases, however, more properly belong to the following chapter, on sex. Others of similar character will engage our attention in subsequent parts of this treatise.

I am inclined to think that this disturbance of the moral and emotional faculties without marked aberration of the intellect, when occurring in young persons, is more common in girls than in boys.

Later on, during the period from fifteen years of age to twenty-five, the tendency to insanity is still greater, the emotional system is more fully developed, and in both sexes love begins to play an important part in the promotion of mental disorders. The struggle for existence and position has begun, and the individual is sometimes slowly, sometimes rapidly, but always surely, taught that there are trouble and sorrow and exertion before him. To some this knowledge is more than the mind can bear. There are very few at this age and at this day who, according to my experience, injure themselves by intellectual exertion. Occasionally, however, the mind is overtasked, and a *quasi* insane condition is produced, which, if not promptly relieved, terminates in mental alienation. The struggle for position is by no means confined to adults. It exists with the boys and girls in our schools, counting-houses, and even in our workshops. Not long ago a young man, not over sixteen years of age, was brought to me in a high state of acute mania, induced by his efforts to excel in the work of copying letters; and I was shortly afterward consulted in the case of another of like age, who had become melancholic and subject to the delusion that he had committed the "unpardonable sin," the consequence of excessive application to his trade as a violin-maker. This is the exceptional case to the rule of moral perversion only, to which allusion has just been made.

The Period of Maturity.—Some authors consider that physiologically there are but two periods in the life of man, that of increase and that of decline. Strictly speaking, this view may be the correct one, but there is a time when if there is any increase in development it is scarcely perceptible, and if any decline this is so gradually effected that it is inappreciable by any means at our disposal.

This period may very properly therefore be regarded as that at which the formation and destruction of tissues are so nearly balanced that the body may be regarded as fully mature. Tissue is not, as in the preceding stage, deposited faster than it is removed, but the wants of the system are exactly compensated by the deposit of new material to take the place of that removed as effete.

At the beginning of this period, which ordinarily extends from the twenty-fifth to the thirty-fifth year of life, the epiphyses of the bones become firmly incorporated with the shafts, the flesh becomes hard and firm, and the physical strength is at its maximum.

The mental faculties, though more strongly developed than in the former period, are not yet in their prime. This is a curious circumstance, and one which is at variance with our preconceived opinions. Some faculties of the intellect and some of the emotions are, perhaps, equal in force and activity to their development at any other period of life, but, as a whole, the mind is not possessed of the capacity, the strength, the endurance, or the power of concentration, which it has during the next period, when the physical powers have begun to decline.

A little reflection reveals to us the reasons for this, which are two in number:

1. The brain does not attain to its maximum degree of development at the same time as do the other viscera and the osseous and muscular system. So far as size is concerned, it probably does not, as the Brothers Wenzel contended, reach its maximum at the seventh year, but, as Dr. Boyd[1] has shown, it is very nearly as large at this period as it ever will be, and by the twentieth year it has attained to its full size. But, after this point is arrived at, it continues to gain in firmness of structure owing to the gradual loss of a portion of its water, and thus there is a comparative augmentation of brain-tissue, an increase of weight, going on far into the period of decline.

---

[1] Quoted by Thurnam, *op. cit.*

7

2. As the mind feeds on the impressions which reach the brain through the special senses, it has not had time by the end of the period of maturity, which is at the thirty-fifth year, to acquire all the information necessary for it to reach its greatest stage of development, which is during the next period.

It is during the period of maturity that insanity is most common. Wealth and station have generally not yet been fully reached even by those most favorably situated for getting them, while, on the other hand, the contest has terminated disastrously for many who entered upon it with high hopes and expectations. These circumstances cannot fail to increase the wear and tear of brain, and, consequently, to augment the number of cases of mental alienation over those of either the preceding or the following period.

Moreover, it is during this period that the cares of life are greatest in both sexes, through the necessity which exists for providing for a family not yet able to provide for itself. This alone is often a cause of insanity.

The Period of Decline.—The period of decline is marked by as many striking characteristics as those which belong to the period of increase. After the body has remained at nearly a fixed point of development for a few years, varying from five to ten, a disposition is manifested to degeneration. The process of decay becomes more powerful than that concerned in the regeneration of tissues, and, in consequence, the body not only loses weight from the atrophy of its parts, but the functions are less perfectly performed. Thus, the action of the heart becomes weaker and less frequent, the respiration slower, the digestion feebler, the muscles thinner and more rigid, the skin shrunken, the joints stiff, the teeth fall out, the hair becomes gray, the arteries ossified, and the entire form loses its elasticity and becomes less erect than in adult age. The whole tendency of the body is toward consolidation. The generative function is greatly weakened or altogether lost in both sexes, and in the female the menses cease to flow.

The organs of special sense, toward the latter portion of the period, also become involved in the process of degeneration. The eyes lose their brightness, and the sight grows dim and presbyopic. The hearing diminishes in acuteness, the taste is blunted, and the sense of smell is almost, if not altogether, lost at a comparatively early period.

In these changes the mind also participates, but not in an equal ratio to the changes going on in other parts of the body. Indeed there is, during the first ten or fifteen years of this period, an increase in the strength and powers of endurance of the mind, and quite often this process continues for several additional years. The judgment, owing to the experience which the individual has obtained in the affairs of life, becomes riper and more unerring; there is a greater power of determining the value of facts, and a less disposition to be governed by the emotions.

But after a time the intellect becomes less absorptive of perceptions and less creative of ideas. The power of mental concentration is markedly diminished. The memory fails, especially in regard to recent occurrences. The imagination loses the vividness and extensive range of youth and maturity, and the judgment becomes feeble and vacillating. The individual begins to rely on others for advice as to his affairs, and little by little he parts with his own will, even in matters of the smallest importance. The emotions no longer sway the whole being as they once did, and some of them are utterly extinguished. Often, however, a maudlin or fretful condition is developed, which ends with its own expression of tears or sniffles, never prompting to volitional impulses or producing more than a momentary disturbance.

To all this, however, there are sometimes notable exceptions, but yet not enough to invalidate the law that the period in question is one of decline in fact as well as in name.

If the alterations are gradual and uniform throughout the system, death from old age is the consequence; but it rarely happens that derangement of some one important function does not produce this result before the general breaking-up of the vital principle occurs.

During the first ten or fifteen years the decay of the organism is so slowly effected that very little inconvenience results, and occasionally, as has been intimated, we meet with individuals who are able to withstand, to a very advanced period of existence, the tendency to degeneration. But it is nevertheless advancing, imperceptibly it may be, but surely, to the extinction of the principle of life.

Such is a brief outline of some of the conditions which attend the period of decline. The diseases to which it is especially liable are those which are connected with the most important organs of the body—apoplexy, paralysis, and mental affections being chief among them.

Owing to the failure of the nutritive processes of the brain, the power of this organ is so greatly diminished that what is known as senile dementia is a not infrequently engendered pathological state during the latter portion of the period of decline. This condition, which is the result of pathological changes in the brain, rarely makes its appearance before the sixtieth year, and generally not till much later. Willie[1] has shown that there is a positive shrinking of the brain in size and weight, to which, doubtless, the failure of mental power is directly due.

General paralysis, though met with in both the other periods, is far more frequent after the age of thirty-five, when the system has reached its acme, than at any other part of life, or, in fact, than both the others combined.

The cessation of the menstrual flow in women, occurring as it does during this period, is a prolific cause of mental alienation.

But the individual who has attained to an advanced age without suffering from any form of insanity is generally safe for the rest of his existence. Acute mania is rarely met with in these persons, and melancholia, though more common, is nevertheless comparatively infrequent. It is not, indeed, to be expected that, with the exception of senile dementia, old age, when the intellect is dulled and the passions burned out, can afford many examples of active mental alienation. I have, however, witnessed a few cases of what Morel calls senile insanity (*folie senile*) occurring in very old men and women. In some of its features it is not unlike general paralysis ; but it has altogether a different course and character of termination.   There are the same mental exaltation and weakness of the muscular system, conjoined with a peevishness and disregard for the rights and feelings of others which tend to render the subjects a nuisance to those about them, at the very time that they should be exhibiting the calmness and dignity of a majestic old age.   It generally ends either in an attack of acute menengitis or of cerebral hæmorrhage, which quickly carries off the patient.

[1] "Des psychoses de la sénilité," *Allgemeine Zeitschrift für Psychiatrie*, 1873.

CHAPTER XII.

SEX.

AT birth, and for some years afterward, the differences which exist between the sexes are scarcely noticeable, except so far as different conformation of the generative apparatus is concerned. After puberty other evidences of distinct organization appear, and the several peculiarities which mark the sexes become manifest. In the male the voice becomes rough, the penis and testicles enlarge, spermatozoids appear in the seminal liquor, the chest becomes broader and deeper, and hair makes its appearance on the face, the axillæ, and pubes.

In the female the pelvis enlarges, as do also all the organs of generation ; the function of generation, which consists in the periodical discharge of an ovum, accompanied by a flow of blood from the uterus, begins, and hair grows upon the axillæ and pubes. In a short time each sex has fully assumed all the characteristics, both mental and physical, which belong to it, so that an observer is enabled by a casual inspection to determine at once the sex of the individual. In early childhood these differences are so slight that, without an examination of the genital organs, it is often impossible to make the discrimination in question.

Besides these influences there are others of a more general character. The male is stronger and more coarsely and compactly built ; his features are more marked and prominent ; his muscles are more developed ; his bones are larger ; his whole frame taller and broader. In addition, his nervous system, though capable of greater endurance, is not so sensitive to delicate impressions. On the other hand, the female is more slightly and finely organized. Her skin is softer, her features smaller, her muscular system less powerfully developed, her circulation less active, and her figure shorter and more slender.

The capacity of the skull is greater in the male than in the female, and it is remarkable, as Vogt[1] has shown, that the difference in favor of the male increases as the race becomes more civilized. Thus, in savage nations, as the negroes of Africa, the male and female skulls are much more alike in capacity than they are in Europeans. Thus Huschke,[2] of

[1] " Lectures on Man," " Anthropological Society Publication," p. 90.
[2] " Schädel, Hirn und Seele," Jena, 1854.

21 male Germans, found the average cranial capacity to be 1,538·76 cubic centimetres, while of 18 female Germans it was only 1,265·23 cubic centimetres, a difference of 273·53 cubic centimetres. Barnard Davis,[1] of 12 male Australian skulls, found the average capacity to be 1,316·85 cubic centimetres, while of three Australian women it was 1,273·08 cubic centimetres, a difference of only 43·77 cubic centimetres. The largest number of measurements is given by Mantegazza.[2] Of 191 male skulls he found the average capacity to be 1,451 cubic centimetres, and of 101 female skulls the average capacity was 1,338 cubic centimetres, a difference of 113 cubic centimetres in favor of the male skull.

On this point there is no difference among anthropologists, and it may be considered as a settled question that the cranial capacity of the human male is greater than that of the female.

It would naturally follow that, where there is a relatively larger cranium, there would be a relatively larger brain, and this is exactly the case when the male brain is compared with that of the female. The difference has been variously given by authors, according to the nationality of the subjects, but the average, as established by Welcker's[3] observations, appears to be about as correct as such determinations can be made. He found the average male brain to weigh 1,390 grammes, or a little over 49 ounces, and the average female brain 1,250 grammes, or a little over 44 ounces, a difference of about 5 ounces. The proportion existing between the two is, therefore, as 100 : 90. This accords with the observations of Thurnam,[4] to which reference was made in the first chapter of this work.

But, relatively to the weight of the body in the two sexes, the difference is not so great. The body of the female is shorter and weighs less than that of the male. Thurnam determined the average stature of women to be 8 per cent. less than that of men, so that, relatively to her stature, the brain of a woman is but 2 per cent. less than the brain of man.

[1] "Crania Britannica," cited in *Révue d'anthropologie*, Paris, 1873, t. ii, No. 3, p. 482.

[2] "Dei caratteri seperali dei cranio umano," *Archivio per l'Antropologia*, t. ii, 1872, p. 11, *et seq.*

[3] "Untersuchungen über Bau und Wachsthum menschlichen Schädels," Leipzig, 1862.

[4] "On the Weight of the Human Brain and on the Circumstances affecting it," *Journal of Mental Science*, April, 1866.

Quain,[1] summing up the results arrived at by Clendenning, Tiedemann, and Reid, states that, "In a series of 81 males the average proportion between the weight of the brain (encephalon) and that of the body at the age of 20 years and upward was found to be 1 to 36·5; and, in a series of 82 females, to be as 1 to 36·46." According to these figures the proportionate weight of the brain to the body does not differ materially in the two sexes, but what difference there is is in favor of woman. The particular point, however, is not of much importance psychologically, however interesting it may be as a matter of anatomy. If the intelligence depended on the weight of the brain relative to the weight of the body, we could increase or diminish the power of the mind by systems of dietetics. It has not been observed that very thin men are remarkable for their mental vigor, or that very fat ones are on the verge of imbecility.

Some years ago I performed a series of experiments relative to the comparative specific gravities of the male and female brains, which lead, I think, to important results. It is not necessary to go into all the details of them as they relate to the several parts of the encephalon. I will state them so far only as they refer to the gray and white matter of the cerebrum. Twenty brains of each sex were examined, and the results are as follows:

MEN.—*Gray substance.*—Maximum, 1·0372; minimum, 1·0314; mean, 1·0350. *White substance.*—Maximum, 1·0472; minimum, 1·0341; mean, 1·0427.

WOMEN.—*Gray substance.*—Maximum, 1·0325; minimum, 1·0291; mean, 1·0317. *White substance.*—Maximum, 1·0386; minimum, 1·0311; mean, 1·0379.

It is thus seen that both the gray substance and the white are specifically heavier in the male than in the female brain.

Relative to the proportionate development of the different parts of the brain in males and females, Schwalbe[2] has collected the data of most importance.

Huschke regarded it as an essential point of difference between the male and the female brain that, in the latter, the distance of the upper end of the fissure of Rolando from the apex of the frontal lobe, compared with the distance of the same point from the apex of the occipital lobe, is much less

---

[1] "Anatomy of the Human Body," vol. ii, p. 580.

[2] "Lehrbuch der Neurologie," Erlangen, 1880, p. 574, *et seq.*

than in man. Thus, if the entire length of the hemisphere be = 100, there will be found in woman 31·3 in front of the upper end of the fissure of Rolando, while in man there will be 43·9. Huschke concludes from this that in man the frontal lobe is more developed than it is in woman, and that the same is also true of the frontal convolutions. This preponderance of the frontal convolutions in man, Schwalbe continues, has likewise been pointed out by R. Wagner as a characteristic sex differentiation. At all events, it appears to be established by Huschke's investigations that, in the female, the parietal predominates over the frontal lobe. Finally, his statement that, in woman, the fissure of Rolando and also the central convolutions are more perpendicular than in man, as a consequence of the influence exerted by the conformation of the cranium, is generally recognized as correct. Rüdinger asserts that a typical point of difference between the male and the female brain can often be found in the seventh or eighth month of fœtal life, in that the former has the frontal lobe better developed than the latter, and that there is an earlier development of secondary fissures in it and the parietal lobe.

These differences of structure would appear to indicate differences in mind, and that such differences do exist no one who has studied, even cursorily, the course of mental development in the male and female of the human species can doubt. It is not necessary that one should be superior to the other, but that they should be different is an essential deduction from a consideration of the anatomical features of the organ as it exists in man and woman. There are some things in which man excels, there are others in which woman is his superior. To enter fully into the discussion of the subject now is not my purpose. I will only remark that the system which seems to be coming into vogue, of giving a girl exactly the same kind of education as a boy, is, to my mind, supremely absurd. The two sexes may move along paths which approach parallelism at some points of their course, but they can never travel exactly the same road till they have brains presenting exactly the same anatomical configuration and structure.

The beginning of menstruation and its cessation constitute critical periods in the life of the female, and exert a great influence upon her health and mortality.

The first discharge is accompanied, ordinarily, by a variety of abnormal circumstances, such as headache, fever, nervous derangement, pain in the loins and uterus, etc., and even the subsequent returns are often thus attended.

The function of those who are healthy in this respect continues about thirty years, when it becomes more or less irregular, and finally ceases altogether. In some women it is very irregularly performed from the first, and this derangement, when it exists, is a fruitful source of the great variety of nervous and debilitated conditions from which so many women of modern society suffer. Perhaps it is not saying too much to express the opinion, which my experience assures me is well founded, that there is scarcely a woman belonging to the upper classes of society who is not more or less irregular in her menstrual discharges, and this, too, from causes which are the result entirely of an artificial and abnormal mode of existence. Exposure to cold and damp when thinly clothed or shod, late hours in exciting society, the reading of modern works of fiction, which too frequently excite unduly and unhealthily the feelings of a sensitive girl, the avoidance of the duties and obligations of maternity, the cramming of the mind at school with subjects such as civil engineering, differential and integral calculus, and other mathematical studies, which it grasps with difficulty, influence materially the nervous system primarily, and secondarily the generative organs. These, again, react upon the brain, the spinal cord, and the sympathetic ganglia, and hysteria, hypochondria, and other forms of *quasi* insanity are produced, to say nothing of neuralgia, spinal irritation, epilepsy, chorea, nervous dyspepsia, and a dozen other diseases as bad or worse.

As already intimated under another head, the *period of the beginning of menstruation* sometimes leads to very decided conditions of mental derangement. In the preceding chapter I have cited a case in point from my own experience, and one or two additional instances can scarcely fail to be instructive to the student of mental pathology.

A girl aged sixteen, who had never menstruated, but who had suffered no special bodily inconvenience from the circumstance beyond severe periodical headaches, was brought to me to be treated for what was regarded by her friends as insanity, and which was only manifested by an overpowering impulse to set fire to houses. She had made seven distinct attempts, all, however, on the dwellings of members of her own family, and hence, as none were successful, she had hitherto escaped exposure. When questioning her, and examining her thoroughly in other respects, I could discover no defects in her reasoning processes, and no delusions. She was fully aware of her tendency, and regretted, so far at least as words and manner could go, her inability to control herself.

The impulse only came over her once a month, in conjunction with her headache. Scarcely felt as more than a slight impression at first, it grew by degrees, till it finally became so powerful that, as she expressed it, she felt as though she would go wild if she longer resisted. She compared the mental condition to the sensation (*anxietas tibiarum*) sometimes experienced in the legs when they have been kept long in one position, and which causes persons to feel as though, come what may, they must move them. Immediately on setting fire to a building the impulse disappeared, and did not return for a month. Latterly, she had been so closely watched that she had not been able to indulge in her proclivity, which passed off in a few hours, though not without a considerable degree of excitement, almost maniacal, being produced.

In another case, the patient, a girl of fifteen, had made an attempt to kill her brother, an infant, by strangling it as it lay asleep in the cradle. She had been placed in charge of the child while her mother went out on some errand. While sitting watching it, and, as she asserted vehemently, not at all weary of her task, the idea suddenly came into her mind to strangle the child. She accordingly took off one of her garters for the purpose, and placed it around the neck of the sleeping infant, but without drawing it tight. For a little while this appeared to satisfy her, and she got a book and sat down to read. But again the idea occurred to her, and this time stronger than before. She dropped her book, and, going down on her knees, prayed to be delivered from the instigation of the devil, but still the idea increased. Finally, she went to the door to call some one to her assistance, but, before she could open it, the impulse became so overwhelming that she rushed back to the cradle and buckled the garter as tight as she could around the throat of the sleeping child. Then she rushed out of the house, crying, "I have killed my brother! I have killed my brother!" The first person she met was her father, coming home to his midday meal. He, not fully comprehending, but inferring that something terrible had happened, hurried back with her, and arrived not an instant too soon to tear off the band and save the child's life.

Previous to this occurrence the girl had evinced no evidence of mental derangement. She had regularly attended a public school, and had stood well in her classes. She had begun to menstruate at fourteen, but the function had been only twice performed when it stopped. I could discover no sign of insanity, or of even the least abnormality in the action of the mind. She begged, however, that she and the child might not, in future, be compelled to remain in the same house, as she was afraid she would strangle it yet, if she had the opportunity.

I may add that both these cases recovered under treatment.

Several other cases which have come under my care or observation will receive consideration under their proper headings, when the subject of insanity comes to be fully discussed.

The chief feature of the mental derangement occurring at the beginning of menstruation is the impulsive or instinctive character of the manifestations. As I have said[1] on a former occasion, with reference to women generally, and especially with regard to the case of Constance Kant, who was accused of, and who confessed to, the murder of her infant brother:

"Their likes and dislikes are conceived upon the most trivial, and often most erroneous, grounds; they are subject to very whimsical and really ungovernable fancies; their nervous systems are disordered, and thoughts may be conceived and acts committed which, at a subsequent period, would fill their minds with horror. Numerous instances of the kind have come under my observation, and physicians generally will, doubtless, recognize the truth of what I say. Though, in the great majority of young girls who are brought up under proper influences, these psychological evidences of the great change the organism is undergoing rarely make themselves manifest to any but those with whom they are thrown into intimate relations, this is, unfortunately for human nature, not always the case. A slight derangement in the physiological processes which are going on may produce simply an appetite for chalk or slate-pencils; a transient vertigo may cause a radical and permanent change of charac-

[1] " The Medico-Legal Value of Confession as an Evidence of Guilt," " Journal of Psychological Medicine," vol. v., 1871, p. 357.

ter ; an almost unnoticed congestion of the brain may prompt
to the commission of a horrid crime.   Even an adult man is
never the same after as before an attack of cerebral congestion
or hæmorrhage.   From having been kind, considerate, and
gentlemanly, he may become changed to a being of morose
and brutal instincts, which it is impossible for him to restrain
within bounds.   With how much greater force would these
or similar influences act upon the impressionable nervous
organism of a girl when at the most susceptible and critical
stage of her existence ! ''

Delasiauve,[1] among others, has called attention to the abnormal mental condition in which women are sometimes
thrown at each menstrual period.   He has noticed the exaggerated desires, the eccentric appetites, the inexplicable aver-
sions, and especially the instinctive perversions, which impel
them to the perpetration of criminal acts.

Occasionally, women or girls under such circumstances
falsely accuse themselves of all kinds of horrible crimes and
disgusting obscenities.   Doubtless this is sometimes the result of the morbid desire for notoriety, at any cost, with which
they are afflicted, but there is no doubt that they are not infrequently sincere, actually believing that they are the guilty
monsters they represent themselves to be.   During the middle ages it was by no means an uncommon thing for young
girls just beginning menstruation to allege that they had had
sexual intercourse with the devil and other demons, that they
participated in the orgies of the '' Sabbath,'' or that some
monk or priest had, through the power of Satan, bewitched
and seduced them.   Epidemics of alleged '' possession '' and
sorcery, clearly due to menstrual derangements, swept through
the countries of Europe, and led, by the false accusations and
confessions of the affected nuns, to the sacrifice of many innocent persons.[2]

But occasionally the form of insanity developed is of a
much more active character.   Marc[3] cites the case of a girl

---

[1] '' Folie occasionné par la menstruation,'' *Journal de médecine mentale*, t. iv,
1864, p. 241.

[2] For a more complete consideration of this and analogous subjects, the reader
is referred to the author's work, '' On Certain Conditions of Nervous Derangement,'' New York, 1881.

[3] '' De la folie considerée dans ses rapports avec les questions médico-judiciaires,'' Paris, 1840, t. i, p. 317.

who, at each menstrual period, was attacked with furious mania, during which, with a knife in her hand, she attacked those who displeased her or went in the slightest degree in opposition to her wishes.

In an instance that came under my own care, the patient, a young lady, at the beginning of one of her earliest menstrual periods, without any preliminary indications, rushed from the house and ran down the street screaming at the top of her voice, and imploring those she met to save her. As it afterward appeared, she had suddenly, while sitting in the drawing-room talking with her mother, been seized with the delusion that a large negro man was entering the house through the window, and that he was pointing a pistol at her. At each period for several months she had a similar delusion, but eventually she was cured.

Sometimes the only mental faculties which are disordered in their action are the perceptions, causing the production of illusions and hallucinations. Thus, one young lady, who was under my care, always at her menstrual periods had visions of heads and hands floating about in the air near her. They were scarcely ever absent during the whole duration of the discharge. Another saw friends who had long been dead, and who came and sat beside her and talked with her ; and a third had constant hallucinations of hearing voices whispering to her, and telling her to do all kinds of ridiculous acts.

At times, but in my experience not often, there is manifested a very high degree of exaltation of the sexual instincts, and even a depravation of them, constituting the form of insanity known as nymphomania. During the paroxysms of this disease the patient exhibits the most shameless demeanor, indulging in the most obscene gestures and language, conjoined sometimes with maniacal excitement, much agitation, tearing off the clothing, and violence toward herself or others—and all this although her education and associations may have been of the most refined character.

But the period of the beginning of menstruation, if a fruitful source of mental and nervous disorders, is almost equally often a curative agent of like affections. Epilepsy is frequently spontaneously arrested at the inception of the menstrual function, and so also are the several forms of insanity which may have begun in earlier life. Thus, a very distressing but interesting case of acute mania, occurring in a young lady twelve years of age, was suddenly cured on the appearance of the catamenia, at the age of fourteen. In another case, which also came under my observation, the patient, a girl of about eleven years old, was affected with religious melancholy, which disappeared between the second and third menstrual periods, at the age of thirteen ; and in a third instance—the one to which reference has been made in the last chapter—menstruation had been delayed, but, on its being brought on by treatment directed to that end, the mental disorder, quickly yielded. Many like instances are on record, but the following are so striking that I cite them for the instruction they are capable of affording :

Buisson[1] reports the cases of two girls, aged, respectively, twelve and thirteen years, who imagined themselves bewitched by eating potatoes given to them by an old woman to whom they had refused alms. They were taken with vomiting, convulsions, and maniacal fury, during which they lost the faculty of speech, and committed a thousand extravagant acts. After a strong purgative, exhibited probably for the purpose of relieving the bowels of any undigested substances, the delirium increased, but, the menses also appearing, they soon became calm, and remained entirely cured.

And this from Girard : [2]

A thread-winder, aged twelve, of a nervo-sanguineous temperament, suffered from pain in the stomach and bowels, cramps, difficulty of breathing, and the *globus hystericus*. The morbid condition lasted for two years, at which time the following symptoms were noticed : constipation, pain on pressure over the abdomen, irregular distribution of heat, frequency of pulse, and general hyperæsthesia. She then entered the Hôtel Dieu, at Lyons. On the second day she was delirious, had hallucinations of sight and smell, and pains in the thighs and lumbar region. The following day there was a slight menstrual flow. Immediately all the symptoms began to disappear, and, in less than three weeks from her entrance into the hospital, she was discharged cured.

The period of the *cessation of the menstrual discharge* is also one which exercises great influence over the health of the individual, and especially so far as the mind is concerned. It is often the determining agent when hereditary or other pre-

---

[1] Quoted by Berthier in "Des névroses menstruelles," Paris, 1874, p. 220.
[2] Quoted by Berthier, *op. cit.*, p. 225.

disposition exists to mental disease, and, even when there is no such tendency, acts as its own immediate cause.

Most authors upon the subject of insanity have noticed the relation between the menopause and the initiation of symptoms of mental derangement. Generally the melancholic type prevails, and a tendency to suicide is not uncommon; but quite often there are various forms of emotional disturbance or of perversion of the appetite, which are sources of great distress to friends and relatives.

Semelaigne[1] has noticed a fact in this connection to which my attention has also been drawn, and that is, the development of the desire for spirituous liquors as a beverage, producing, in some cases, a veritable form of insanity. As he says, the nervous perversions caused by menstruation are principally occasioned by the cessation of that function, which provokes, with many women, an irresistible temporary or permanent propensity to drink alcoholic liquors to excess. In the beginning, the unhappy subjects take their potations in secret, but, little by little, they lose all sense of shame, and do not hesitate to exhibit in public the spectacle of their deplorable infirmity. Neither rank nor education is any obstacle to the indulgence of this appetite. To procure their favorite liquor there is no deceit they will not practice, or watchfulness they will not evade. If the accustomed stimulus cannot be had, they will resort to the use of anything else that contains alcohol. I have known women, under these circumstances, to drink cologne-water, bay-rum, all kinds of medicinal tinctures, and, in one case, the alcohol that was used to preserve morbid anatomical specimens.

In recent years the appetite for opium, in some one or more of its forms, and chloral, has become developed to a great extent, and I have seen enough of it to know that it, too, is more prone to be exhibited in women at about the period of the cessation of the menstrual flow than at any other time. While not so deleterious, either to body or mind, as the morbid appetite for alcohol, either of these substances, or, indeed, any narcotic, sedative, or stimulant, if used to excess, and as a means of procuring pleasant thoughts, or banishing unpleasant ones, is certain, eventually, to lead to great mental and bodily disorder.

[1] " Du diagnostic de la dipsomanie," *Journal de médicine mentale*, t. i, 1861, p. 212.

Abnormal, erotic, or nymphomaniacal tendencies are some-times excited by the cessation of the menstrual flow, and con-stitute some of the most distressing cases the physician is called upon to treat. In a case of the kind which I saw sev-eral years since, the patient, a married woman, aged forty-six, in whom there was no discoverable hereditary influence toward insanity, at the time that her catamenia were beginning to become irregular was seized with libidinous desires, altogether abnormal in character. Previously she had never exhibited any marked sexual proclivity, and intercourse rarely gave her any pleasure, but now she was continually making indecent propositions to men whom she met, even in the most public places, and in the presence of her own husband. She remained in about the same condition for two years, and then, the menses ceasing altogether, she recovered her health.

Another, a single lady, was, at the period of the meno-pause, affected with hallucinations of sight, of the most ob-scene character, and which haunted her night and day.

Todd cites the case of a Madame X., the mother of ten chil-dren, all of whom she had herself suckled, who began at forty-five to suspect the faithfulness of her husband. Later, she accused him of attempting to murder herself and her chil-dren. A slight improvement in her condition was obtained by sequestration, but eventually the symptoms returned with nymphomaniacal manifestations.

In insane women it is not an uncommon circumstance for sexual aberrations to occur on the supervention of the meno-pause.

In man the accession of puberty is not so efficient an agent in the production of mental disturbance as it is in woman, though occasionally it appears to be the cause of either well-marked lunacy, or of such a perversion of the moral nature as constitutes a condition of *quasi* insanity. There being no physical sign appearing suddenly, like menstruation, it is difficult to associate puberty and mental derangement in boys as cause and effect. Still we do see cases in which, apparently, such a relation exists. We have some right to form such an inference if no other cause can be properly alleged. In the case of a young man, aged fifteen, recently under my charge, I could find no other probable factor than puberty, for the maniacal perversion of the mental faculties which existed. There were hallucinations of sight and hearing, and the fixed

delusion that he was a person whom he designated Sir Peter
Trimble, and who, he claimed, was the greatest traveller the
world had ever known. He would sit by the hour, imagine
himself to be in Central Africa, at the north pole, in China,
Brazil, and other places, real and hypothetical, and carry on
conversations with the natives whom he saw and heard. This
he kept up day after day with wonderful versatility, rarely
visiting the same place twice, or, if he did, evidently encountering different adventures from those which had befallen him
on his first visit. There was one exception to this, however.
Every day he paid a visit to an immense city, as he described
it, which he called Sarominden, and which he said was in the
middle of the wilderness in which the Jews, under Moses and
Joshua, passed forty years. There were no sexual aberrations
of any kind, as I fully satisfied myself, but there were swollen
and painful testicles at times. Evidently, sexual intercourse
would have cured this boy, but I could not find it in my heart
to say so to his father, though, possibly, in time I would have
been less scrupulous, had not Nature stepped in to his relief,
and, by repeated nocturnal emissions, restored the proper degree of equilibrium between his testicles and his brain.

But the insanity of this period in boys is more apt, according to my experience, to present the form of "reasoning
mania." The subject becomes vicious and troublesome, but
is always ready with specious excuses for his conduct. He
commits various petty crimes, and is, perhaps, turned out of
school or his workshop for theft or malicious lying. He runs
away from home to go to sea, or to become a train-robber, or
to fight Indians. Again, he has the "delirium of persecution." People watch him, he declares, as he walks the streets,
and whisper about him, evidently forming combinations to
ruin or murder him. The neighbors, especially those opposite
his residence, are the objects of his continual suspicion. If a
blind is closed, it is in order to watch him through the slats;
if any one leaves the house, it is to tell a confederate of his
movements, and so on, without the slightest regard to probability, or even of possibility.

In another case under my charge, the patient, a young man
of about sixteen years of age, conceived the idea that every
woman who saw him at once fell violently in love with him.
As a consequence, he made himself extremely obnoxious to
many persons, and was continually getting into trouble with

8

the male friends and relatives of his supposed *inamoratas*. Not even several severe beatings which he received were sufficient to cure him of his delusions, and eventually it was found necessary to place him in a private lunatic asylum. He escaped from this place without difficulty, and was next heard of in Cincinnati, where he figured before a police-court for addressing ladies in the street. He was brought home, and, after a year or two, during which he was taken to Europe, entirely recovered, and is now in good health.

Under the head of "Hebephrenia" the insanity of pubescence will be more fully considered.

Gall contended that there was a periodical manifestation in men analogous to that existing in females, though, of course, different from it, and Lévy[1] holds a similar opinion. The latter states that "young and robust persons do not notice this tendency unless their attention is specially directed to it, but men feebly constituted, or endowed with a great degree of irritability, or who have reached the period of their decline, perceive the alteration which their health monthly undergoes : their countenance becomes dull, their perspiration assumes a strange odor, their digestion is more laborious, and sometimes the urine deposits a heavy sediment. The feeling of discomfort is general and inexpressible, and the mind participates in it, for it is more difficult to maintain a train of ideas ; a tendency to melancholy, or perhaps an unusual degree of irascibility, is joined to the indolence of the intellectual faculties. These modifications persist some days, and disappear of themselves.

I have certainly noticed in some of my friends this tendency to some monthly periodical abnormal manifestation. This may be in the form of a headache, or a nasal hæmorrhage, or a diarrhœa, or an abundant discharge of uric acid, or some other unusual occurrence. I think this is much more common than is ordinarily supposed, and that careful examination or inquiry will generally, if not invariably, establish the existence of a periodicity of the character referred to.

The profound changes induced in the female organism by the condition of *pregnancy* could scarcely leave the mind untouched, and we find, in fact, that mental disturbance going far beyond the eccentric "longings" of women in this state is not an infrequent occurrence. This may exhibit itself mainly

[1] " Traité d'hygiène," t. i, p. 122.

as regards the emotions, the subjects becoming irascible, suspicious, jealous, or the victims of profound melancholy ; or the intellect may be involved, and delusions become characteristic features of the disorder. Again, they may manifest the most unreasonable hatred of certain persons, and may make serious attempts to injure or destroy them.

As Morel[1] declares, it is a matter of importance to ascertain whether the mental alienation exhibited during pregnancy is the result of the woman's condition, or whether pregnancy has occurred in a subject already insane. This is an important point in the formation of a prognosis, for, in the former case, the disease will probably disappear with the birth of the child, while in the latter no such favorable termination is to be expected. "In thirty-eight women," he states, "that I have had occasion to treat, and in whom pregnancy was complicated with mental alienation, twelve, at least, were degenerated beings—imbeciles, idiots, or epileptics—in whom pregnancy was only an accident that could not have any influence over the course of an irremediable state. The majority of these unfortunate women were delivered, some without manifesting the slightest interest, and others without possessing the least knowledge of their situation.

"With seventeen other women the insanity which declared itself during the course of the pregnancy was not an isolated phenomenon. It was sometimes due to hereditary transmission, sometimes to neuropathic conditions pre-existent to the pregnancy, and which constituted mental states of a disquieting character. It was observed that, in those with a predisposition to melancholy, there was, in every case, a great irritability of disposition, combined with all the attributes of the nervous temperament, and a tendency to the perpetration of eccentric or unusual acts ; in other cases the hysterical element predominated. In three instances the pregnancy had been advised as a cure for a hysterical neurosis, but without the favorable result that had been expected. It is also to be noted that the greater number of these women were not primiparæ. Some had been pregnant two or three times, and, after each labor, a greater disposition to contract a mental disease had been observed."

Insanity in pregnant women is most apt to make its appearance during the fourth month of gestation.

---

[1] "Traité des maladies mentales," Paris, 1860, p. 202.

As stated by Morel, in the passage quoted, pregnancy is sometimes recommended as a cure for a pre-existing mental derangement. Esquirol[1] states that, though pregnancy, child-birth, and lactation, are means which Nature sometimes adopts for curing insanity, yet such a favorable termination is rare. Though he has often seen childbirth render a maniac more calm, and though, in the case of a lady who, at each of five pregnancies, became insane, to be cured at each delivery, he nevertheless regards such cases as quite exceptional ; and that he has often seen insanity not only persist but become aggravated by these conditions.

Dagonet[2] confirms this opinion, and cites the case of a young girl, the subject of nymphomania, whose condition was rendered much worse by pregnancy and childbirth.

I have never known marriage entered upon for the purpose of curing insanity, but I have repeatedly had it suggested to me for my opinion, and I have always advised against such a course.

During or soon after *childbirth*, in the period intervening before the re-establishment of the menstrual discharge, the mother is liable to a peculiar form of insanity, known as puerperal mania. This, as a distinct type of mental alienation, will engage our attention further on.

The period of *lactation* is also of considerable influence in causing insanity, especially with those who do not suckle their children. The form of insanity is generally similar to that which follows childbirth, and by many authors is regarded as essentially the same condition.

Marcé states that the sex of the child borne by the mother, or nursed by her, is sometimes a determining cause of insanity, women, he says, becoming the subjects of mental alienation after having given birth to male infants, while with every female child they have remained exempt. As he further says, these facts, at first sight, seem inexplicable, till we recall to mind the circumstances that the male child is larger, and, consequently, is born with more difficulty than the female, and that it sucks the breast with more vigor, and hence makes greater demands upon the mother for sustenance. I have not noticed any difference in this respect, nor do I

---

[1] " Des maladies mentales," Paris, 1838, t. i, p. 193.

[2] " Nouveau traité elementaire et pratique des maladies mentales," Paris, 1876, p. 498.

think it has been observed to exist among the women of this country.

Notwithstanding all these factors, which are only effective with the female sex, there are others acting with so much greater force on males as to cause insanity to be much more common in them than in females. The cares incident to providing for a family, the anxieties and wear and tear of mind connected with business and other affairs of the world, and, above all, excessive indulgence in the use of alcoholic liquors and of the sexual organs, and many other influences that will be more specifically considered under another head, are so many powerful agents acting with far greater force on men than on women, and hence aiding in making them more liable to insanity.

Another series of causes tending to make mental alienation more common in men than in women are those which arise from exposure to inclement weather, the direct rays of the sun, noxious vapors and emanations, and to various accidents and injuries, producing wounds of the head.

CHAPTER XIII.

RACE.

THE several races of men are distinguished by great differences—so great, indeed, that they can scarcely be regarded as due to any other cause than a diversity of origin. Climate, hunger, destitution, disease, exposure, degradation, vicious habits and appetites, will, in the course of time, produce many alterations in the form and aspect of organic beings, but they cannot so alter original types as to cause a race, whether of plants or of animals, to lose its identity. Thus, the several varieties of the cabbage are all derived from a wild plant, scarcely edible, growing on the sea-coast rocks of Great Britain. The many kinds of apples all come from a common stock —the crab-apple. The peach, the most luscious of our fruits, has its origin in the bitter-almond of Persia. Yet, however much these plants, and many others that might be mentioned, may have varied from the parent growth, they all evince a tendency to return to the original form when separated from the influences which have given rise to the deviation.

So with the various alterations which animals have undergone through the action of a changed mode of life, or a different climate, continuing through many generations. Restore them to their former conditions of existence, and in a short time the original type is reached. Take, for example, the sheep. The fleece of this animal consists of two kinds of wool intermingled; one is formed of coarse, stiff hairs, the other of short, fine, curly wool. In the merino-sheep this latter is greatly in excess, and hence the value set on fabrics made of it; but, if the animal is removed to a colder region than is natural to it, the coarse, straight hair takes the place of the softer variety, and the value of the whole growth is lost. Replace the merino-sheep in its native climate, and the soft wool soon again becomes predominant.

The turkey, which is found wild in this country, is of a brownish-black color; by the mere act of domestication it becomes wholly changed in its markings, and is frequently met with entirely white. If, however, it is allowed to run wild again in its native forests, the original uniformity of hue is soon resumed.

Other animals, under like circumstances, become changed in the form of their ears, the shape of their skulls, or the character of their horns; but these variations, like the others mentioned, have nothing of permanence about them. They merely exist while the conditions which gave rise to them are in force.

Now, with the several races of mankind the case is altogether different. There are, it is true, certain changes wrought in the physical appearance of man through unfavorable climate and the degenerating influences mentioned. And there are other alterations produced by the action of agents capable of developing his mental and physical organization; but these are quite as transitory in their character as those which ensue in the lower forms of organic beings, to some of which I have just referred, and cannot be held to account for the marked peculiarities which distinguish what are known as the races of men any more than they will explain the differences which exist between the lion and the tiger, the horse and the ass, or the Polar bear and his grizzly representative in the Rocky Mountains.

Place the Caucasian in the tropics of South America, Asia, or Africa, and though his skin may become darker and his hair blacker and coarser, he is, nevertheless, though he remains there for thousands of years, in no danger of being taken for an individual of any other race.

The negro, for nearly four hundred years, has inhabited America. During all that period, his mode of life and the climate to which he has been exposed are altogether different from those natural to him. He has been subjected to humanizing and civilizing influences, his animal wants have been supplied, and yet, except in cases of a mixing of the blood, he presents the same aspects as his progenitors, whose representatives are figured on the monuments of ancient Egypt erected three thousand years ago. Certainly within the historic period there has been no change in the characteristics of the white, yellow, brown, and black races of mankind.

Even in peculiarities which scarcely rise to the height of being racial we observe a permanence which seems to endure under all conditions. For example, the Jews, for nearly two thousand years, have been subjected to varieties of climate, and manners and customs as different from each other as can be found anywhere on the face of the globe, and yet a member of the nation can be as well recognized under the black skin and hair of the African Jew as under the fair skin and red hair of his co-religionist of Norway and Sweden. Before the war, I never met but one Jew in the ranks of the regular army. He had a fair, freckly skin, and hair the color of a carrot. He came from Scotland, and he called himself Ferguson; but he was circumcised, and was as veritable an Israelite in figure, and in the shape of his eyes, nose, and mouth, as any who ever walked the streets of Jerusalem.

There are great differences to be observed in the cranial capacities and cerebral development of the several races of mankind. The late Dr. Morton, of Philadelphia, was among the first to study this subject. His method of determining the capacity of the skull was to fill it with small shot, and then, by measuring these in a graduated vessel, ascertain the cubical contents. He found that the mean cranial capacity in Americans of European descent was 92 cubic inches, in the American Indians 79 cubic inches, and in the negroes 83 cubic inches.

The form of the skull is also a matter of racial difference.

In the negro, for instance, it is long and narrow, constituting the form called *dolichokephalic;* in the Tartar it is broad and short—*brachykephalic;* and in the white or European *mesokephalic*—that is, a mean between the two others.

As regards the weight of the brain in the several races, Thurnam [1] has collected some interesting statistics, by which it appears that the average for male Europeans is about 49 ounces, and for negroes 44·3 ounces, or 1,390 and 1,255 grammes, respectively, while, according to Dr. Clapham, [2] the average brain weight of eleven Chinese males was 50·45 ounces, or about 1,430 grammes. These results are so different from what might have been expected that we may reasonably suppose a source of error to have existed. The subjects were coolies, and they died during the typhoon in Hong-Kong in September, 1874.

As regards the liability to mental derangement, there are very few data at our command, and those we have are complicated by other circumstances than race, which tend to render them of little value. Thus, when it is asserted, and apparently with truth, that negroes are less prone to insanity than the whites, we do not know how much of this immunity is the result of the racial factor, and how much is due to the differences in the mode of life, the degree of activity of the mind, etc., which exist; and the like is true of the American Indian. Place either one of them, in his youth, in New York, let him adopt the manners and customs of the average resident of that city, overwork his mind at school, use alcohol to excess, plunge into the pursuits of money-making with his whole heart and mind, deprive him of a large part of his natural rest—sleep—and prevent him from exercising his body to the extent it requires, and the probability is that he will be as likely to become insane as any white man similarly situated. It is certainly true that barbarous nations do not exhibit so strong a tendency to mental alienation as do those that are civilized, but this is simply because they are barbarous, and not because they belong to different races. As nations advance in civilization, the tendency to all kinds of diseases of the mind is increased, because it is just the very causes which make civilization, and the vices which necessarily ac-

[1] *Op. cit., loc. cit.*

[2] "Journal of the Anthropological Institute of Great Britain and Ireland," vol. vii, p. 90.

company it, that are the most potential agents in producing insanity.

It is a matter of certain knowledge that, since the abolition of slavery, and the consequent elevation of the American negroes in the social scale, the number of cases of insanity among them has greatly increased. In his former condition the negro had no responsibilities and but little care; there was no opportunity for the exhibition of much emotion, and he therefore showed very little. In their original condition in Africa they evinced still less, and probably there, were even less disposed to mental derangement than in America as slaves. Travellers report that the Congo women have so little maternal instinct that their living babies may be pounded in a mortar to appease some evil spirit, while they look on with indifference. In the old days of slavery the parting of families, sold to different masters, rarely caused any marked emotional disturbance.

But long association with whites, and, above all, the abolition of slavery, by which act they were raised to a position of political equality with their former masters, has changed all this. The negro now has responsibilities; he has a wife and children whom he can call his own, and whom he is bound to support. He votes, goes to school, attends church as a critic —selecting his own religion—keeps a shop, or studies some profession. All this is beginning to tell upon his mind. With its development—and he appears to have capacity for considerable mental improvement—the liability to insanity has increased, until now special lunatic asylums are being established for his accommodation, and they are being filled as rapidly as they can be opened.

SECTION II.

INSTINCT; ITS NATURE AND SEAT.

CHAPTER I.

THE NATURE OF INSTINCT.

A WORK on insanity would manifestly be incomplete without some reference to a principle of life present in all organic beings, from the highest to the lowest, from the most insignificant plant to man himself, and which, in all, determines, to a greater or less extent, the character of the acts by which existence is rendered possible. When we bear in mind the fact that, in man, a very considerable proportion of cases of mental derangement have their origin in aberrations of some one or other of the instincts, the propriety of its consideration becomes still more apparent.

A great deal of confusion has existed among physiologists and psychologists relative to the differences between instinct and reason, and undoubtedly there are many difficulties in the way of distinguishing, with perfect accuracy, the manifestations belonging to each. No inconsiderable amount of the obscurity has arisen from the loose manner in which words have been employed and meanings ascribed to them. I shall endeavor, therefore, to give a clear idea of what instinct is, and to separate it, by well-defined limits, from mind, before proceeding to the consideration of its aberrations. In doing this I shall be obliged to quote the views of several eminent authorities, in order to show how various are the opinions held relative to this primal organic force, often more powerful than mind itself.

Montaigne[1] appears to see no difference between the purely

[1] "The Essays of Michael Seigneur de Montaigne," Cotton's translation, p. 283. (Apology for Raimonde de Sebonde.)

instinctive operations of the lower animals and those intellectual acts performed by man.

"As to the rest," he says, "what is there in us that we do not see in the operations of animals? Is there a polity better ordered, the offices better distributed and more inviolably observed and maintained, than that of bees? Can we imagine that such, and so regular, a distribution of employment can be carried on without consideration and prudence?

"The swallows that we see at the return of spring, searching all the corners of our houses for the most commodious places wherein to build their nests, do they seek without judgment, and, among a thousand, choose out the most proper for their purpose without discrimination? In that elegant and admirable contexture of their building, can birds rather make choice of a square figure than a round, of an obtuse than of a right angle, without knowing their properties and effects? Do they bring water and then clay without knowing that the hardness of the latter grows softer by being wet? Do they mat their palace with moss or down without foreseeing that their tender young will lie more safe and easy? Do they secure themselves from the wet and rainy winds, and place their lodgings toward the east, without knowing the different qualities of those winds, and considering that one is more comfortable than the other? Why does the spider make her web straighter in one place and slacker in another? Why now make one sort of knot and then another if she has not deliberation, thought, and conclusion? We sufficiently discern, in most of their works, how much animals excel us, and how unable our art is to imitate them. We, nevertheless, in our more gross performances, employ all our faculties, and apply the utmost power of our souls. Why do we not conclude the same of them? Why should we attribute to, I know not what, natural and servile inclination, the works that excel all we can do by nature and art?"

There is not one of Montaigne's very apposite questions that should not be answered in a way directly the opposite of that to which he evidently inclines. All the acts he cites so eloquently are very different from those reasonable operations which the lower animals do perform, and which theological philosophers regard as instinctive. His error is in a direction the reverse of theirs. He would make all the acts of animals intellectual, while they would give this influence to none.

Pascal[1] had a more correct idea of the difference between instinctive and intellectual acts. "The effects of reasoning," he says, "are continually increasing, while instinct remains always the same. The cells in the honeycomb of the bee were as accurately made a thousand years ago as they are to-day, and each insect formed its hexagon as exactly the first time it made one as the last. Nature, having no other object than to maintain animals in a certain state of perfection, has inspired them with the necessary and never-variable science, so that they shall not perish, and it does not permit them to add to it lest they should pass the limits which have been prescribed."

While sufficiently indicating the general nature of instinctive acts, Pascal has committed the error of regarding instinct as unalterable.

Descartes[2] looked upon all the lower animals as being more or less perfect automata. Beasts, he says, do many things better than we can do them, and, as they invariably fail in doing others, it shows that they do not act from knowledge, but only by the disposition of their organs. He lays very great stress on the assumed fact that none of the lower animals talk—an assertion which has never yet been demonstrated—and from this draws the conclusion that they are devoid of reason. But, with more extensive knowledge of the structure and faculties of the brain, we know that the ability to recollect words, or to articulate them, may be altogether abolished in man without essentially impairing his reasoning power in other directions. Admitting, therefore, that beasts have no faculty of articulate speech, the fact may depend upon a lack of development in the speech tract in the brain, and is no argument against their possession of reason.

Further, he declares that there are in man two principles which govern our actions: the one entirely mechanical and corporeal, which depends solely on the force of the animal spirits and the configuration of the parts, and that may be called the corporeal soul; and the other incorporeal, which feels and reasons. In animals, all movements can be explained by referring them to this one principle, the first-named or corporeal soul. The other, the thinking soul, he denies to them altogether; and instinct is nothing more than the orderly working of the organs, such as takes place in any machine.

[1] " De l'autorité en matière de philosophie," t. ii, p. 270, édition Havet.
[2] " Discours de la méthode," V⁰ partie, Œuvres comp. de Cousin, t. i, p. 186.

He overlooks the fact, however, that, without a force to start the machine and to keep it in action, its parts, though they be absolutely perfect in construction, will remain motionless.

Dr. Reid[1] defines instinct as "a natural, blind impulse to certain actions, without having any end in view, without deliberation, and very often without any conception of what we do."

As an example of instinctive motions, he says: "Thus, a man breathes while he is alive by the alternate contraction and relaxation of certain muscles, by which the chest, and, of consequence, the lungs, are contracted and dilated. There is no reason to think that an infant new-born knows that breathing is necessary to life in its new state, that he knows how it must be performed, or even that he has any thought or conception of that operation; yet he breathes as soon as he is born, with perfect regularity, as if he had been taught, and got the habit by long practice."

Dr. Reid's definition of instinct is essentially correct; but the example he gives is altogether irrelevant, showing, therefore, that he had no clear conception of what he was defining. He has regarded as instinctive an action which is altogether reflex in character. The new-born child does not breathe because of "a natural, blind impulse" to do so, but because the placental connection with its mother, by which its blood was oxygenated, having been severed, and the stimulus of atmospheric air having been applied to its skin, an impression is conveyed to the nerve-centres, is reflected to the respiratory muscles, and breathing takes place. Both the above causes are necessary for the excitation of the respiratory act, for the child does not breathe till pulsation has ceased in the cord, even though it be entirely expelled from the uterus, nor will efforts at respiration be made if access of air be prevented.

We frequently see the reflex character of the respiratory movements demonstrated upon persons who have fainted, or who are in stupor or convulsions, and in whom the actions in question have been temporarily suspended. A little water thrown on the face, a current of air brought to bear upon it, or even a feather brushed across the cheeks, will often procure a deep inspiration of air.

[1] "Essays on the Power of the Human Mind," Edinburgh, 1803, vol. iii, p. 126.

Of other examples adduced by the same author, many are fully as inapplicable as the preceding.

The elder Darwin [1] makes no very clear distinction between instinctive and rational actions, except, perhaps, that they differ in degree. He cites many examples of what are ordinarily considered as belonging to the first-named class, but appears to regard them as being the result of intellection. In the conclusion of his remarks upon the subject he says:

"There is a criterion by which we may distinguish our voluntary acts or thoughts from those that are excited by our sensations. The former are always employed about the *means* to acquire pleasurable objects, or to avoid painful ones, while the latter are employed about the possession of those that are already in our power."

According to the same author, many acts which are ordinarily regarded as instinctive are the results of experience acquired during fœtal existence. Thus, he observes that the fœtus learns to perform certain movements which are excited by a feeling of irksomeness at being kept too long in one position, and that sucking and swallowing are also acquired *in utero*. If, however, all such actions are to be regarded as instinctive, the fact that they have been performed does not afford any explanation of their origin. It merely places the beginning a few months further back, without at all accounting for the cause of their initiation. Indeed, the theory rather obscurely enunciated by Darwin, that instinctive actions are the consequence of sensitive impressions, does not distinguish them from those other actions which are clearly the results of reason and will, through the perceptions. Darwin quotes the following account of an experiment of Galen's:

"On dissecting a goat great with young, I found a brisk embryo, and, having detached it from the matrix, and snatching it away before it saw its dam, I brought it into a certain room where there were many vessels, some filled with wine, others with oil, some with honey, others with milk, or some other liquid, and in others were grains and fruits. We first observed the young animal get upon its feet and walk ; then it shook itself, and afterward scratched its side with one of its feet ; then we saw it smelling to every one of these things that

---

[1] "Zoonomia, or, The Laws of Organic Life," American edition, vol. i, Philadelphia, 1812, art. "Instinct," p. 101, *et seq.*

were set in the room, and, when it had smelt to them all, it drank up the milk."

This passage has been cited by many authors, as affording a beautiful example of instinct, whereas, I think, a little reflection will satisfy the majority of thinking persons that the action described was purely rational and volitional, and one which evinced a great deal of discrimination on the part of the prematurely born kid. It took that food which gave the most pleasurable sensation to its sense of smell. It deliberately made a choice—the result of comparison and judgment. There was nothing instinctive, nothing blind or impulsive. If the kid had not smelt the other substances, but had drunk the first one it touched, the action might have been due to a force which it could not resist, and which might then have been regarded as instinctive.

Broussais[1] falls into the error of regarding all instinctive acts as being due to impressions made upon the senses, and likewise fails to distinguish between such actions and those of a reflex character. The want of health, hunger, thirst, etc., are, therefore, in his opinion, the excitants of motives—respiration, eating, drinking—which are instinctive. But, in fact, such functions are no more kept in operation by instinct than are any other acts which an individual is in the habit of doing, or which he deems it necessary or proper to perform. As well might it be said that, if a person imperatively requires a certain book from a shelf in his library, he is actuated by instinct if he rises from his chair and gets it.

Hartley[2] is more correct than the authors cited when he says that instinctive actions are not the results of external impressions. This germ of lucidity is, however, so mixed up with mystical and confused ideas relative to his theory of vibrations that it is difficult to arrive at a clear conception of his entire meaning.

Sir T. C. Morgan,[3] on the contrary, regards instincts as being due to sensational impressions. He says:

"Those impressions which excite a certain degree of pleasure or pain, or which experience has associated with those affections, stimulate the cerebral system to volition, an action

[1] "A Treatise on Physiology applied to Pathology" (American translation), Philadelphia, 1826, p. 77, et seq.

[2] "Observations on Man," etc., London, 1792, p. 243.

[3] "Sketches of the Philosophy of Life," London, 1818, p. 292.

which influences the muscles and determines their contractions
in a definite and congruous series.

"The actions thus produced may proceed immediately
from the impression, and in close connection with it. They
are then termed *instinctive*. They may result, also, from the
associations which the impression excites, and be governed by
a consciousness of the end to be produced, and then they are
called voluntary.

Cabanis [1] considers the subject of instinct with more philosophical knowledge than any writer of or before his day. As
his views have been received with much attention, and have
exerted a greater or less governing power over all subsequent
inquiries in the same direction, I shall discuss them at some
length.

Philosophers are divided in regard to the following two
points. Some think with Condillac that all the acts of animals are due to reason, and are, consequently, the results of
experience. Others contend that many of their actions are in
no way connected with reason, and that, while all of these
have their source in physical sensibility, they are performed
without any other agency of the will than that which relates
to its action as the director of their execution. These actions
are designated *instinctive*.

Some physiologists contend that sensibility is the only
source of all organic power. Others, among whom Haller is
first, maintain that there is another property, distinct from,
and even independent of, sensibility, which they call irritability. As Cabanis says, however, the dispute is mainly one
of words.

Within the womb of the mother animals do not, properly
speaking, experience any sensation. As soon as they are
born, however—when they respire, when the action of the
external air impresses more energy on their organs, and more
activity, more regularity, on their movements—it is not a
simple change of habits which they experience, but a veritable
new life which begins. From that moment appetites spring
up which they are compelled to gratify by an irresistible internal force. So apt, for instance, is the infant at sucking,
that Hippocrates concluded it was impossible the knowledge
could be acquired so soon after birth, and contended that the

[1] "Rapports du physique et du moral de l'homme," Paris, 1824, t. i, p. 77, *et
seq.*

fœtus learned the necessary movements by sucking the liquor amnii in the mother's womb. This point I have already considered when Darwin's views were under notice. In addition to what was then said, it may be observed that the fœtus certainly does not learn to breathe in its mother's womb, and that the necessary muscular actions toward this object are fully as complex as those concerned in sucking.

Many quadrupeds are born with their eyes shut. Such can only find the nipples of their mother through the senses of smell and touch. These faculties they exercise with great sureness, and kittens will frequently, when half-born, stretch out their necks in search of the source of their future nourishment.

These actions, and many others which could be mentioned, result from internal impressions received by the young of animals during gestation. They are not set in operation by sensations; on the contrary, the animal is prompted by the internal power to employ its senses in order to accomplish its objects. This force, therefore, stands in lieu of the will. In the case of Galen's goat, already quoted, it was instinct which impelled the animal to use its senses. It was not instinct, but reason, which made it select the milk. Instinct is not, therefore, the result of experience, or of reason, or of any choice founded on sensations.

The line, therefore, between rational and instinctive actions can be closely drawn. The former, as Locke and his disciples have proved, are formed from distinct impressions which come to our minds from exterior objects through the medium of our senses. The latter arise from within, as the offspring of a force entirely independent of, and even above, the will. The etymology of the word "instinct" shows conclusively which meaning should properly be attached to it. It is formed from the two Greek radicals, εν, *in;* and στιζειν, *to prick.* According to its derivation, instinct is the product of excitations the stimulus to which is applied from the interior—that is to say, the result of impressions received from within.

Thus, in animals generally, and in man especially, there are two well-defined kinds of impressions, which are the sources, the one of their conscious, the other of their unconscious, determinations; and these two kinds are found, but in different relations to each other, in all species.

From the foregoing brief account and running commentary

on Cabanis's views, it will be seen that he was fully aware of the true source of instinctive actions, and that he clearly distinguished between them and those which result from mental processes.

A writer,[1] whose name is not given, but who has evidently reflected a good deal upon the subject of instinct, and others of an analogous character, makes the great mistake of ascribing instinctive actions to external stimuli. Thus, he says: "We confess, however, that we do not see why the term *instinctive* should not be applied to *all* the actions which are performed *in direct respondence* to an external stimulus." And again:[2]

"We have employed the term instinctive here and elsewhere to denote much more than is included under it by many writers. Some have restricted it to one class of excited actions, some to another; but we think that it may be applied with the greatest propriety to designate all those changes in the muscular system which are immediately excited by impressions from without, which are not respondent upon the exercise of the will, though more or less capable of being controlled by it, and which, if acting alone, deprive the being of the character of a free agent."

This writer, though recognizing what are really instinctive actions, includes among them all reflex, and even voluntary, actions, going further in this respect than any other author whose views have come under my notice. In a subsequent article he reiterates the opinion that the actions in question are all performed in obedience to external stimuli.

Dr. Alison[3] is more exact when he says: "The most correct expression of the difference between an action prompted by instinct and one prompted by reason is, that in the first case the will acts in obedience to an impulse which is directly consequent upon certain sensations or emotions felt or remembered; in the last it acts in obedience to an impulse which results from acts of reasoning and imagination. In a subsequent paragraph, however, Dr. Alison seems disposed to include such purely reflex operations as breathing, winking, coughing, sneezing, vomiting, etc., among instinctive actions.

---

[1] "British and Foreign Medico-Chirurgical Review," vol. v, 1838, p. 491.
[2] *Op. cit.*, p. 505.
[3] "Cyclopædia of Anatomy and Physiology," vol. iii, p. 3, art. "Instinct."

Collineau,[1] in an exceedingly philosophical treatise on the mind, applies the word instinct to all interior sensitive movements, intellectual, affective, and mental, be they voluntary or involuntary, which are exercised without knowledge of the nature or cause, by the being acting immediately, by virtue of organization and inherent disposition.

In psychology, instinct begins everything. It is manifested with the first organic movements. It is, in some respects, an intelligence communicated with life, and which is developed, more or less, according to circumstances, habitudes, and the degree of organization.

Instinct in man is arrested or weakened as soon as we have the intimate feeling or conscience of our intellectual acts, for this intimate feeling, this conscience, is the line of demarcation which is to stand between instinctive actions and those due to intelligence. This line does not actually exist in nature ; it is only a conception of the mind ; in reality, there is always instinct where there is intelligence, even when this latter is greatly in the ascendency, and although reason, for the time being, causes instinct to disappear, it does not accomplish its destruction.

Before the intelligence of a being is brought into active existence there is a force which excites movements, which directs or limits them. It is an attribute of the sensibility already developed ; it is a providential cause which precedes knowledge and reason, but which retains the first place with animals not endowed with the organ of thought, and with those intelligent beings whose intellectual functions are not yet fully developed or sufficiently exercised.

Instinctive dispositions extend to the moral life, and place bounds to an intelligence which cannot be passed without time and labor. Thus it is that nations, like individuals, have their infancy, their middle age, and their decline ; that certain ideas, tastes, and proclivities are suitable to certain sexes, ages, constitutions, peoples, and climates. Instinct is the insensible and often unsuspected link which, by all points, in all times, and in every case, attaches individual life to general life. It is thus that absolute liberty, in regard to which there has been so much dispute, becomes impossible, for man, like the lower animals, enjoys free-will only within the instinctive

[1] "Analyse physiologique de l'entendement humaine," etc., Paris, 1847, p. 37.

limits which are placed to his intelligence, to his affections, and to the agents of his mind.

So far as individuals are concerned, instinct is not infallible ; but, if we regard it as it is manifested in masses and species, we see that it never fails and never deceives.   Its existence is inseparably attached to the organic life of the being.   It controls and determines, with admirable certainty, all actions, even those which require the co-ordination of a large number of organs.   Take, for instance, the numerous and complex acts performed by certain animals at the instant of their birth, as well as by man at all periods of his life.   We can, indeed, say with truth that nature thinks and acts for us in an infinitude of ways that long observation and all the efforts of reason would fail in making us comprehend.

Instinct is, then, innate ; it is present at all epochs of existence, at all moments, while the ideas which come to us acquired by the senses, and which are formed by the intelligence, increase, and are rendered more perfect by exercise and by the various uses to which they are subjected by life.

I have only given a very general idea of M. Collineau's views, and have omitted from his argument much that is interesting.   I do not know where there is a more lucid explanation of the psychology of instinct than is to be found in his admirable volume.   His conclusions in regard to the nature of this faculty are briefly as follows.   He divides all manifestations of instinct into two classes.

1. All spontaneous movements which, in beings endowed with organization and animal life, are constantly in force, according to the species, and more or less directly with a common aim of preservation, reproduction, or propagation.

2. All acts which begin, and can even sometimes be finished, independently of sensation, of comparison, of judgment, of ideas, and of reflection—that is to say, without the aid of the reason or the will, without imitation, without the knowledge of means by which they might be accomplished, or of the results to which they might lead.   The word *instinct* is the indication of the unknown cause, and of the sum total of acts of this nature.

Voisin,[1] though giving no precise definition of insanity, sets out with the observation that he will consider in his treatise the fundamental and primitive forces of our cerebral

[1] " Analyse de l'entendement humaine," etc., Paris, 1858, p. 53, *et seq.*

constitution. He then treats of the "instinct of generation," the "social instinct," the "instinct of self-defence," the "instinct of destruction," etc., showing that, in his opinion, these are primary faculties not acquired by sensation or experience, but originating with the life of the individual, and developing therewith.

Leuret and Gratiolet,[1] in treating of the instincts, enunciate views of which the following is an abstract :

When we voluntarily perform—that is to say, with the knowledge of our will—certain acts, the nature or value of which our intelligence has not estimated, and which it has not prepared, these acts are not attributed to the mind, but to the instinct. We do not apply the term instinct to that general and indefinite tendency by which a simple impulsion, awakening a homogeneous feeling, produces a correlative act. *That* is an automatic reaction, and is not instinct. To fly from a sorrow that threatens us, to combat a harm that has attacked us, to pursue an object that arouses in us pleasing emotions, is to act *automatically*, it is true, but not instinctively. Instinct is not at all a reaction produced in connection with exterior impressions. It is an *innate* tendency, which is due from the first moment of life to the arrangement of the organic mechanism, and to harmonious influences preordained with the world. For instance, let us suppose a clock wound up, and let us suppose the loom of a weaver. As soon as the pendulum of the one is set in motion the hands mark the hour ; and as soon as the hand of the workman raises the lever of the other the fabric begins to be made. Let us further suppose these machines to be gifted with a certain degree of consciousness and personality, the instinct of the clock will be to mark the hour, and that of the loom to weave tissues.

Thus, between inanimate and animate machines there is but one point of difference—the one acts and is ignorant of what it does, the other is restrained by an overpowering principle of which it is conscious. Therefore, when an animal wishes to act, its will is directed toward the organs by which action is possible. No man has the instinct to fly ; no bird has the instinct to grasp things with its wings. The natural will never, therefore, exceeds the limits of possible action. Thus, instincts differ according to species and individuals—

[1] "Anatomie comparée du système nerveux consideré dans ses rapports avec l'intelligence," Paris, 1839–'57, t. ii, p. 632.

that is to say, according to organization. The little duck
which the hen has hatched seeks the water as soon as it has
escaped from the egg, and swims without ever having been
taught. Every being and thing, says St. Augustine, seeks
the place which it ought to occupy in nature. One accom-
plishes its work blindly, another mingles a little intelligence
with its instinct, but all fulfil their destiny necessarily ; to
man alone has been accorded the right of ambition and revolt,
in order that the virtue of ambition should also exist.

MM. Leuret and Gratiolet [1] thus distinctly recognize the
difference between reflex and instinctive actions, and give a
very clear idea of the relations which exist between instinct
and the will.

Müller [2] advances views similar to those of the physiologists just quoted. He regards instinct as innate, as not excited
by impressions made on the senses, and as being due to a determinate purpose, identical with motive organic power.

Dr. J. W. Draper [3] has enunciated several erroneous ideas
relative to instinct. He deems it incapable of improvement,
and not liable to error. Both of these opinions are, as I shall
endeavor to show hereafter, erroneous.

Dr. Dalton [4] evidently considers it as due to impressions
conveyed inwardly from the senses, and does not, I think,
sufficiently discriminate between its manifestations and those
which are of a reflex character. These errors, as we have
seen, have been committed by several authors, and perhaps
the majority of those who have written upon the subject
entertain similar views. There seems to be an indisposition
to recognize the fact that there are innate organic predispositions born with the being exhibiting them, and predominating over all mental and nervous powers.

Lelut, [5] in the main, adopts the theories of Stahl relative
to the differences between instinct and reason, the λόγος—
that is to say, the general formula for all those acts of the
mind in the direction of the body which are vague, intermit-

---

[1] It should be stated that the second volume—the one embracing the remarks
on instinct—of the joint work of these authors was written entirely by M. Gratiolet, the first by M. Leuret.

[2] " Elements of Physiology." Translated by Dr. Baly, London, 1842, vol. ii,
p. 947.

[3] " Human Physiology, Statical and Dynamical," New York, 1856, p. 603.

[4] " A Treatise on Human Physiology."

[5] " Physiologie de la pensée," etc., Paris, 1862, p. 176, *et seq.*

tent, and sensitive, rather than intellectual—corresponding to the instinct, while the λογισμός is that state, that degree of intelligence, where the reason is in the ascendency. His views are more transcendental than philosophical, and do not evince much physiological research.

Fredault [1] considers instinct under the term "animal impulsion," as that faculty which excites sensibility and motion. Exterior causes, in his opinion, influence this faculty.

Dr. McCosh [2] argues with great vigor in favor of the existence of intuitive laws, principles, or rules, which guide the mind. At the same time he denies, with Locke, the existence of innate ideas. I am unable to distinguish between these intuitions of Dr. McCosh and instincts, although he makes no attempt to explain or account for the latter, and even altogether ignores their existence. The following quotation shows the character which he ascribes to intuitions, and their identity with instincts:

"*They are native.* However they have been called—natural, innate, connate, implanted, constitutional—all these phrases point to the circumstance that they are not acquired by practice, nor the result of experience, but are in the mind naturally, as constituents of its very being, and involved in its higher exercises. In this respect they are analogous to universal gravitation and chemical affinity, which are not produced in bodies as they operate, but are in the very nature of bodies, and the springs of their action."

Flourens [3] recognizes three great facts—the instinct, the intelligence of animals, and the intelligence of man. Each of these has its fixed limit. The instinct acts without knowing; the intelligence knows in order to act. The intelligence of man alone knows and is self-conscious. What an animal does through instinct it does without having learned how to do it; what it does through the intelligence it does through experience or instruction. He denies reason to all animals lower in the scale of creation than man.

Flourens is not, I think, consistent in this latter view.

---

[1] "Traité d'anthropologie physiologique et philosophique," Paris, 1863, p. 425.

[2] "The Intuitions of the Mind Inductively Investigated," London, 1860, p. 42.

[3] "De l'instinct et l'intelligence des animaux," 4ième édition, Paris, 1861, p. 103, *et seq.*

The example which he gives of the difference between an instinctive and an intelligential action shows this. I quote his exact language:

"Every one has seen the garden-spider, whose web is made of strands radiating from a centre. I have often seen it, just hatched, begin to weave its web. Here instinct acts alone.

"But if I tear the web the spider repairs it; it repairs the torn part; it does not touch the rest; and this torn place it repairs as often as I tear it.

"There is in the spider the mechanical instinct which *makes* the web, and the *intelligence* (the kind of intelligence which exists in spiders) which advises it of the torn place—of the place where the instinct must act."

M. Flourens might have added that there also exists the *reason* which enables the spider to deduce from the evidence of its senses the conclusion that its web is torn, and that it may be mended by similar operations to those employed in its original construction.

Lord Brougham[1] regards instinct as unchangeable, and does not discriminate between the instincts and the appetites.

Darwin[2] (Charles) asserts that it is in many cases impossible to decide whether certain social instincts have been acquired by natural selection, or are the results of other instincts, or are simply the result of long-continued habit. The whole tenor of his remarks relative to instinct is to the effect that there was a time in the history of every species in which the instincts were different from what they are now. Some have been formed, others have been lost. Briefly stated, his theory is as follows:

If we study the individuals of a species, we perceive that they present certain anatomical and physiological characteristics, and contain mental aptitudes or faculties, manners, or instincts. If, however, we go back into the remote past, and examine, so far as we are able, the ancestors of these individuals, we perceive that there was a period in which they did not possess the same anatomical and physiological characteristics, or the same mental faculties or instincts. The change has been a gradual one, but it has nevertheless been steadily going on.

[1] " Dialogues on Instinct," etc., London, 1844.
[2] " The Descent of Man and Selection in Relation to Sex," New York, 1871. Also, " Origin of Species," New York, 1871.

The influence of habit, transmitted from generation to generation, becomes an instinct in the descendants, and to these influences Darwin attributes most of the instincts which animals possess.

But this mode of origin, though doubtless explanatory of many instinctive actions performed by the lower animals and by man, will not suffice for others. Thus, as Carpenter[1] has pointed out, the offspring of certain of the solitary bees can know nothing of the construction of its nest, either from its own experience or from instruction communicated by its parent, so that, when it makes a nest of the very same pattern, we cannot regard it as anything else than a machine, acting in accordance with its nervous organization.

My own views relative to the nature of instinct have been indicated, to some extent, in the comments I have made on the opinions of other investigators. I will proceed, however, to state them more systematically than I have yet done.[2]

Instinct is that innate faculty which organic beings possess, by which they are enabled, or impelled, to perform certain volitional acts, without being prompted thereto by the perceptions, the intellect, or the emotions, and even in direct opposition thereto, which acts are preservative of the well-being or life of the individual, or of the species to which it belongs.

There are certain qualities and circumstances connected with instinct which require attentive consideration.

In the first place, instinctive acts, so far as the individual exhibiting them is concerned, are not the results of instruction or experience. This is one of the most prominent points wherein the actions in question differ from those which proceed from intelligence and reason, performed for a definite purpose. These latter are necessarily due to impressions conveyed to the mind through the senses and nerves, and are, therefore, of eccentric origin. The former are prompted by a force acting altogether without the agency of intelligential external sensations of any kind, and are of internal origin.

---

[1] "Principles of Mental Physiology," London, 1874, p. 58.

[2] As certain views relative to instinct, published within the last few years, are, in some respects, similar to my own, it may be proper to state that the ideas here expressed were published in an article entitled "Instinct, its Nature and Seat," contained in the *Quarterly Journal of Psychological Medicine* for July, 1867.

Sir James Hall, who was engaged in hatching eggs by artificial heat, saw, on one occasion, a chicken in the act of escaping from its shell. Just as the animal succeeded, a spider ran
along the box, and the young bird immediately darted forward,
seized, and swallowed it.[1] In this case there necessarily could
not have been any but an innate impulse that prompted the
movements. And thus the new-born child does not take its
mother's breast because it smells, or sees, or recognizes it by
the touch, or tastes the milk, or even because it is hungry.
The first time it takes it its movements are wholly instinctive.
It is impelled, by a power which has no element of knowledge
about it, to stretch out its head in search of something, it does
not know what. When the nipple is put into its mouth it
sucks, it does not know why. It will suck anything else,
showing that it is not guided by the evidence of any of its
senses; for, if this were the case, the impression made upon
its mind would be that of this other thing—a finger, for instance—and it would immediately stop sucking. So little has
sensation to do with the action, that the child will even take
nauseous mixtures without perceiving their disagreeable qualities. That hunger is not the immediately impelling force is
very evident, from the facts that the child will suck before
this sensation is formed, and that it will continue to do so
after satiety is reached.

Besides, even admitting that, in the new-born child, impressions are conveyed to its brain through its senses, and
that thus actions are initiated, what possible connection can
there be in its mind between the shape and softness of the
mother's breast and the odor of milk, and the fact that, by
sucking, its life will be maintained? Is it not self-evident
that the senses can only lead to intellectual processes, and to
these solely as the results of experience. For instance, there
is nothing about a lighted cigar that would lead a young
puppy, *a priori*, to a conclusion in regard to the unpleasant
consequences of smelling it. When, however, he has once
made the attempt, with all the simplicity of his confiding
nature, has burnt his nose and been stifled with the smoke,
he has acquired knowledge, and has formed an idea in regard
to a lighted cigar which never deserts him. It is, of course,
impossible that a new-born child sucks at first because of any

[1] "The Ganglionic Nervous System," etc., by Dr. James George Davey,
London, 1858, p. 145.

instruction it may have received, or experience it may have acquired—though, as we have seen, it has been asserted that it learns to suck by practicing on the *liquor amnii* in its mother's womb—and, its mind being more immature than that of a young puppy, more frequent instinctive efforts are necessary before it becomes capable of forming an idea of a necessary relation between the mother's milk and its own sensation of hunger.

The action is, therefore, initiated through instinct; but, with each repetition, two other forces are developed, the one reflex, by virtue of which, whenever an object is placed in the infant's mouth, the lips are closed upon it, and sucking movements begun ; just as the eyes are closed when motions, as if to strike, are made before them, or as coughing takes place when an irritating substance touches the larynx ; the other, based upon the relation of cause and effect, a purely reasoning process carried on by the child's brain. As this latter becomes more completely developed, the two others are gradually extinguished, until finally the action is performed in direct accordance with the intellect, and in obedience to the will.

From what has been said, the reader will perceive that my faith in the power of infantile sensational impressions is not great. It is well known to physiologists that none of the senses are even tolerably developed in the new-born infant. The sight, the hearing, the taste, and the smell, are almost nothing, and the sense of touch is scarcely apparent. The ability to feel pain, in a certain general way, undoubtedly exists, and this the infant probably has even in the womb. It is unphilosophical, therefore, to assume, as have some authors, that the new-born of man comes into the world with its senses in full operation.

It is assumed by some authors that the instinct is incapable of improvement. There is an ambiguity about this expression which is liable to lead to erroneous ideas. It is true that the instinct of any one individual being cannot be improved. The only means by which such an attempt could possibly be made would be by the senses, and then reason, not instinct, would be developed. The one would take the place of the other. But instances of the education of the instinct through a series of generations are common enough. For instance, navigators relate that the duck and other water-birds, of those regions which are not often visited by man, evince, at first, no instinctive fear at his approach. It was, probably, a natural condition of these and many other animals not to be afraid of man. But, as man knocked them over with his oars, and shot them with his guns, a force began to be created which, acting gradually upon successive generations, has become innate, and thus the young shows from the first a fear of man. With the domestic animals, however, this force has been lost, for, during many centuries, an opposite education has been acting upon them. Again, the young of a pair of wild quails run away into the thicket as soon as they have broken the eggs. In such a case there has not been enough time for the natural instinct to become obliterated, but in three or four generations it becomes entirely extinguished. With many varieties of dogs the instincts have been wonderfully developed by long-continued instruction and experience. It would appear, therefore, that the intelligence of former generations becomes converted into instinct in the descendants.

In man, instincts have been developed in accordance with the circumstances in which he has been placed as he has inhabited different parts of the world. This is especially noticeable as regards certain instinctive emotions which are not felt by him in the savage state, but which have become prominent through the power of civilization and refinement, acting through many successive generations. I have seen an infant a year old shudder with disgust at the sight of a hair in its porridge. The universal use of the right hand in preference to the left is evidently the result of education and habit continued through centuries, and leading to the increased development of the left side of the brain over the right.

Instincts can be lost in man, and even more readily than in the lower animals. In illustration of this assertion, it is only necessary to recollect that in the new-born infant, if the breast be withheld for only a few hours, the instinct which prompts to sucking is lost, and the child refuses the breast.

A curious circumstance related by Cabanis[1] is applicable to the question under consideration. He says : "In my district of country, and in several others which border upon it, when hatching hens are needed, it is customary to practice a singular procedure which is worthy of notice. A capon is taken, the feathers are stripped from the breast, and it is rubbed with nettles and vinegar. In the state of local irritation which this

[1] "Rapports du physique et du morale de l'homme," Paris, 1824, p. 215.

operation induces, the capon is placed on the eggs which are to be hatched. At first he remains there mechanically, and, in order to assuage the pain which he experiences. Very soon, however, there is established within him a series of unaccustomed but agreeable impressions, which have the effect of attracting him to the eggs for the time necessary to bring the young to a state of maturity, and which also produce in him a species of factitious maternal love which lasts, as in the hen, as long as the young have any need of his cares. Cocks cannot be thus used ; they have an instinct which leads them in another direction.''

Here we might almost say that an instinct is created in place of the one abolished. It is one, however, which, from its nature and the attendant circumstances, cannot be propagated. But, if cocks could be employed for the purpose in question, say by the method mentioned, I have no doubt that in time the instinct would become permanently created in them. No sufficient efforts have been made in this direction. It is well known that instincts may be entirely destroyed by the action of other instincts more powerful. In the swallow and other migratory birds the instinct to depart when the season arrives is so strong that the parental instinct, strong as it is, is overcome, and they often go, leaving their young to die from neglect. Here we have an instance of an instinct of supreme importance to the preservation of the species overcoming another of less importance. And in regard to the improvement or alteration of the instinct in the lower animals, it must be borne in mind that attempts in that direction by man have not been many. Who can say what would be the result if systematic efforts had been made during several hundred years to change the instinct of bees which prompts them to construct their cells of a hexagonal form ? Doubtless, if left alone, they will never deviate in the slightest degree from the plan which, so far as we know, they have always followed. There is no reason why they should. But, if the formation of hexagonal cells could be rendered impossible for bees during many successive generations, I believe the instinct to make them of that shape would be lost. No instinct is stronger than that of the salmon to return to the place where it was spawned. It will beat itself to death in its frantic leaps to surmount obstacles placed in its way in the river from which it emigrated. But we know that impediments of various kinds have driven them from streams they once frequented to others where no obstacles exist.

It is incorrect, also, to contend for the unerring character of instinct. Instances of its aberration are very common. The beaver, which proceeds to construct a dam across a room in which it may be confined, commits a very serious instinctive error. So does the house-fly, when, hour after hour, it dashes itself against a pane of glass in a window in its efforts to escape toward the light, never learning by experience and intelligence that its attempts are in vain.

In the placental animals lower than man, instinct prompts to the division of the umbilical cord with the teeth. In several species, as the pig and the dog, this impulse is occasionally perverted, and they eat their own young.

In their original state, the horse and the cow eat the placenta. This has been prevented in some countries by the organ being removed as soon as it is born, and the instinct is lost; but in Sweden the mare is allowed its full liberty in this respect, and in that country the placenta continues to be eaten.

In man, the maternal instinct is liable to perversion, and the instinctive love of the mother for her offspring is sometimes turned to indifference and hatred.

In my definition of instinct I have been careful to use the term "organic beings," instead of animals. I did this because I am very sure that plants have instinct; that is, a force, co-existent with their growth and implanted originally in the seed, which impels them to the performance of actions calculated to preserve their existence or secure their well-being. We see this power manifested in those plants which shoot out tendrils in search of a support, in those which send their radicles deep into the earth in dry weather, and in those which open and close their flowers with the rising and setting of the sun. These last-named acts are not the consequence of any physical influence of the light or heat of the sun's rays, for they are performed when both are excluded. The sunflower turns its face to the sun at all periods of the day. It does the same thing, as I have ascertained, when it is entirely covered by an India-rubber tent. There is here another instance of an error of instinct.

It would therefore be unphysiological to deny them the possession of the faculty under consideration—a faculty

THE NATURE OF INSTINCT.

which stands them in place of reason, which they probably have not. So far as I can perceive, the instinct of plants differs in no essential respect from that of animals. Its manifestations are, of course, very different.

As to the essential nature of instinct, it is a fact as much as the mind is a fact. It differs in organic beings in degree and kind, as does the mind. It is implanted in all beings from their beginning, and is a necessary principle of their organization. But, the greater the degree of mental development, the less prominent is the instinct, till, when we reach man, it is lower than in any other animal in which its manifestations have been studied.

CHAPTER II.

THE SEAT OF INSTINCT.

THE brain of man is more highly developed than that of any other animal ; he has reasoning powers in excess of those possessed by any other living being ; his mind governs the world, and, not content with that, seeks for knowledge of those spheres beyond that in which he dwells. But, with all this, he is surpassed by almost every other animal in the ability to perform acts instinctively—by beings, in fact, whose brains are infinitely less perfect than his, and by others which have no organs corresponding to a brain.

If the instinct of man were seated in his brain, he would doubtless exhibit a development of this faculty so great as to place him on that score as high as he now stands as regards his mind.

Going back, for the present, to some of the lower animals, we find that we are able, by certain experimental procedures, to settle some points relative to the seat of instinct with absolute certainty.

1. *It does not reside exclusively in the brain.* The brain of many animals, especially of those belonging to the class of reptiles, can be removed without the animal suffering any very considerable immediate inconvenience. In such cases the instinct remains unimpaired.[1] Thus Maine de Biran

[1] In the president's address delivered before the New York Neurological Society, May 3, 1875, entitled, " The Brain not the Sole Organ of the Mind," I have

states that, according to Perrault, a viper, the head of which had been cut off, moved without deviation to its hole in the wall. It is impossible that the viper could have seen, heard, smelt, tasted, or felt the wall. It could only have gone toward it instinctively, through the action of a force not residing in its brain, and altogether independent of perception.

It is an instinct in certain animals to swim when placed in water. I removed the entire brain of a frog, and, after waiting a few minutes for the animal to recover from the shock of the operation, I placed it in a tub of water. It immediately began to swim. I held my hand so that the animal's head would come in contact with it, and thus further progress be prevented. Continued efforts to swim were made for a few seconds, and then ceased. Removing my hand, the animal again swam.

Of such movements, Vulpian says that when the frog is placed in water an excitation is produced over the entire surface of the body in contact with the water; this excitation provokes the mechanism of swimming, and this mechanism ceases to act as soon as the cause of the excitation has disappeared by the removal of the frog from the water. If this were a true explanation, the movements of swimming would certainly be continued, notwithstanding the interposition of an obstacle; but, as we have seen, they are arrested. Onimus shows very conclusively, and I have verified his experiments, that Vulpian's explanation is not correct; for, as he declares, with frogs without brains placed in water, and from which the skin has been entirely removed, the movements of swimming are continued when they are again placed in the water, which proves that the excitation of the cutaneous surface is not the cause of the movements.

I have repeatedly performed similar experiments with turtles of various kinds, and lately with water-snakes. In all these cases the whole brain was removed from the cranium, yet the animals did not wobble about aimlessly in the water, but swam straight out into the stream or pond apparently with as complete a purpose to escape as though they still

shown that certain faculties of the mind are seated in the spinal cord. The subject of Instinct was not considered, but some of the movements mentioned then will be seen to have been purely instinctive. I have made use of these illustrations with others not therein contained in the present chapter. See *Journal of Nervous and Mental Disease*, January, 1876, for the paper in full.

possessed the full degree of consciousness of the unmutilated animals.

Such experiments show, beyond a doubt, that perception and volition are not seated exclusively in the brain, and thus that instinct is not indissolubly connected with that organ.

It is impossible to make similar investigations in the higher animals with such definite results as those obtained with reptiles, but we may call to mind the fact familiar to all physiologists, and to which reference has been made in an earlier part of this work, of the behavior of a pigeon the brain of which had been removed. Though in such a case most of the actions are the result of perception, yet some, as for instance the act of flying when it is thrown into the air, are purely instinctive. But nature has performed many experiments for us, and these not only on the lower animals, but also on man, which teach us conclusively that even in him instinct does not reside in the brain. They show, too, that certain faculties of the mind are not confined to that organ ; but with that fact we need not at present concern ourselves.

In certain monsters born without a brain, or with impor tant parts of this organ absent, we have interesting examples of the persistence of instinct. Syme[1] describes one of these beings which lived for six months. Though very feeble, it had the faculty of sucking, and the several functions of the body appeared to be well performed. Its eyes clearly perceived the light, and during the night it cried if the candle was allowed to go out. After death the cranium was opened, and there was found to be an entire absence of the cerebrum, the place of which was occupied by a quantity of serous fluid contained in the arachnoid. The cerebellum and pons Varolii were present.

Panizza,[2] of Pavia, reports the case of a male infant which lived eighteen hours. Respiration was established, but the child did not cry. Nevertheless, it was not insensible. Light impressed the eyes, for the pupils reacted to its influence. A bitter juice put into its mouth was immediately rejected. Loud

---

[1] *Edinburgh Medical and Surgical Journal*, vol. xxiv, p. 295. This monster belonged to the genus Thlipsencephalus of Geoffroy Saint-Hilaire, so far as I can determine.

[2] Cited by Gintrac, "Maladies de l'appareil nerveux," Paris, 1867, t. i, p. 51. This was also probably a case of thlipsencephalus.

noises caused movements of the body. On post-mortem examination there was found no vestige of either the cerebrum or cerebellum, but the medulla oblongata and pons Varolii existed. There were no olfactory nerves, the optic nerves were atrophied, and the third and fourth nerves were wanting. All the other cranial nerves were present.

It is not stated of this instance that sucking was or was not performed, but most of the movements mentioned were evidently reflex. The rejection of a bitter juice from the mouth was, however, probably instinctive, as was also the reaction of the pupils to light. This latter could not have been a reflex movement, as the optic nerves were atrophied, and there was no way, therefore, by which a reflex action could have been carried out.

Ollivier d'Angers [1] describes a monster of the female sex which lived twenty hours. It cried, and could suck and swallow. There was no brain, but the spinal cord and medulla oblongata were well developed.

Saviard [2] relates the particulars of a case in which there were no cerebrum, cerebellum, or any other intra-cranial ganglion. The spinal cord began as a little red tumor on a level with the foramen magnum. Yet this being opened and shut its eyes, cried, sucked, and even ate broth. It lived four days. Some of these movements were reflex, but others were clearly instinctive and adapted to the preservation of life.

Dubois,[3] on the authority of Professor Lallemand, of Montpellier, cites the case of a fœtus, born at full term, in which the cerebrum and cerebellum were entirely absent. There were no ganglionic bodies within the cranium but the medulla oblongata and the pons Varolii. This fœtus lived three days; during all this time it uttered cries, exercised suction movements when anything was put into its mouth, and moved the limbs. It was nourished with milk and sweetened water, for no nurse would give it her breast. Dubois cites another case, on the authority of Spessa [4] of Treviso, of a child

[1] "Maladies de la moelle épinière," Paris, 1837, t. i, p. 179.

[2] Cited by Gintrac, op. cit., p. 46. Isidore Geoffroy Saint-Hilaire classes this monster as a nosencephalus. "Histoire générale et particulière des anomalies chez l'homme et les animaux," Bruxelles, 1837, t. ii, p. 235.

[3] "De l'instinct; ou des determinations instinctives. Memoires de l'academie royale de médicine," t. ii, 1833, p. 304. Probably a thlypsencephalus.

[4] Isidore Geoffroy Saint-Hilaire, while classing this case among thlipsencephali, questions some of the anatomical details. Op. cit., p. 252.

born without cerebrum, cerebellum, or medulla oblongata, and which lived eleven hours. It cried, breathed, and moved its limbs, but it did not suck. It is difficult to say of this case to what extent its movements were instinctive, and to what extent reflex.

But all these instances, as well as the experiments referred to as having been performed on lower animals, show that instinct does not reside in the brain.

2. *It is seated exclusively in the medulla oblongata, or in the spinal cord, or in both these organs.* The observations made and experiments cited under the immediately preceding head, apparently lead to the conclusion that the medulla oblongata, or spinal cord, or both these organs, may be the seat of instinct, and further inquiry shows that this view is as correct as that which associates the brain with the mind. It is well known to naturalists that the male frog, in his sexual relations with the female, remains in contact with her for sometimes as long as a month. So powerful is this instinct, and at the same time occasionally so blind, that he will attach himself during the spawning season to anything that is placed between his forelegs—the thumb of the observer, for instance—and is sometimes found adhering strongly to his natural enemy, the pike. Mr. H. Bell[1] states that this instinct of adhesion is in fact sometimes fatal to its legitimate object, as he has taken from the water a large conglomeration of male frogs, amounting to twelve or more, with one solitary female in the middle of the group dead and putrid, and even some of the males toward the centre of the collection pressed into an almost lifeless and shapeless mass.

I have repeatedly cut off the tuberculous thumbs of the male frog, which in the spring take on an increased development; and, though the ability to grasp the female is very considerably lessened thereby, attempts in that direction are made, and with more or less success. Indeed, the ablation of both forelegs does not prevent attempts at the sexual embrace.

These facts demonstrate the intensely powerful character of the instinct of generation in these animals.

Now let us see if we can ascertain, by experiments upon them, where this instinct resides.

[1] "The Cyclopædia of Anatomy and Physiology," vol. i, p. 105, art. "Amphibia."

I have many times cut off the head of the male frog while he was in sexual contact with the female, but never with the effect of causing him to relax his hold till several days had elapsed. If care be taken, by placing them in wet moss, to keep the skin from becoming dry, and to maintain a comparatively low temperature, frogs can be kept alive for over a week after their heads are cut off, and during all this time the male remains in contact with the female. Indeed, if he be forcibly separated from her, and then again brought into contact with her, he at once resumes his former position. In like manner he will attach himself to any other body that may be placed in contact with his abdomen.

But, if the amputation of the head be made so as to include the medulla oblongata, the force of the instinct is very much lessened, and is much sooner abolished than when only the head is removed. The animal will still grasp the thumb, or any substance placed in contact with the under surface of his body, but his hold is not so vigorous, and in a few minutes it is relaxed.

If the head of a frog in the spawning season be cut off, so as not to include the medulla oblongata, and then, taking care not to injure this latter organ, the spinal cord be broken up with a stylet, the instinct in question is not yet abolished. The female is still grasped, and the hold not immediately relaxed if the operations be performed on a male frog attached to the female.

If the head be cut off, and the medulla oblongata and spinal cord be broken up, the grasp is immediately loosened, and cannot again be taken.

And if the head be suffered to remain undisturbed, and the medulla oblongata and spinal cord be destroyed, the instinct of generation is at once abolished ; the male relaxes his grasp of the female, and cannot be made to resume it.

In amyelencephalic monsters[1] of the human species there is neither brain nor spinal cord. There is no authentic instance on record of any one of these creatures being possessed of the

---

[1] Geoffroy Saint-Hilaire (a) and his son (b) gave the title *anencephalic* to those monsters in whom there is neither brain nor spinal cord, making two genera of them. Béclard proposes the name amyelencephalic (without brain and spinal cord), as more correctly describing these monstors.

(a) "Philosophie anatomique des monstruosités humaines," Paris, 1822.
(b) *Op. cit.*

ability to perform any instinctive movement such as that of sucking. The presence in them of a sympathetic system of nerves is sufficient to carry on during their intra-uterine life the several organic functions of the body, and to enable them to live for a few hours after birth, the heart beating and the respiration being performed, though in a sluggish manner. As Isidore Geoffroy Saint-Hilaire [1] remarks, the majority of them are, however, born dead, or only survive a few minutes, or at most a few hours. And I think it may be positively asserted with Dubois [2] that no human being born without brain and spinal cord—that is, an amyelencephalic monster—ever made the least movement either voluntary or instinctive. Reflex actions, and those of organic life, such as the pulsation of the heart and the peristaltic motions of the intestines, are possible for a short time ; but so they are when these organs have been entirely removed from the body.

Another fact tending to show that instinct does not reside in the brain is the fact that it exists in its highest state, in contradistinction to mind, in those animals that have the spinal cord most largely developed. Thus, in the alligator, in which in an animal ten feet or more in length the brain weighs only a fraction of an ounce, the spinal cord is of comparatively great size. In the young of this reptile, as I have repeatedly seen in Florida, the instinct of self-defence is so early manifested, and is so strong, that they place themselves in an attitude of attack immediately on escaping from the egg, if they be poked at with a stick. Dr. John Davy has observed a like circumstance.

In microcephali and other human idiots the instincts are sometimes exceedingly strong, and remain so through life. I have already referred to the instance of one of these creatures, an adult woman holding a rag-baby in her arms as though it were a child, and in whom the maternal instinct must have been strong, and entirely uncontrolled by the intellect. Some idiots also evince a great instinctive talent for music, and for arithmetical calculations, which, although capable of development, as are other instincts, are nevertheless innate.

From these facts, and many others which might be adduced in a work specially directed to the consideration of the many interesting points involved, I think it may be concluded that instinct has at least its chief if not its only seat in the

[1] *Op. cit.*, p. 267.   [2] *Op. cit., p.* 312.

medulla oblongata and spinal cord. It is possible that the cerebrum, the cerebellum, and the pons Varolii have some influence in strengthening the faculty, but this is not essential, and its exercise is not a mental operation.

In the consideration of the subject of insanity I shall have to make many allusions to instinct and its manifestations in the insane, and till then I reserve the further consideration of the question.

SECTION III.

SLEEP.

THE connections of sleep with insanity are so intimate and numerous that the consideration of this important function in some of its normal and abnormal relations cannot fail to aid us in the study of the aberrations of the human mind. The causes of sleep, when thoroughly studied, will be found to have a distinct bearing on the therapeutics of wakefulness and of insanity. The state of the mind during sleep is analogous in some respects to that which exists in some forms of lunacy. Dreams, both healthy and morbid, are sometimes the starting-point of insanity, and often play an important part in its clinical history. Wakefulness is frequently either the obvious cause of mental alienation, or the first sign that the mind is beginning to waver from its normal standards ; and the pathology of this condition throws more light on the pathology of the subsequent state of mental darkness into which the individual passes. I am very sure, therefore, that, in asking the attention of the reader to the chapters in this section, I am rendering a service both to him and the unfortunate persons who may come under his medical charge.

CHAPTER I.

THE CAUSES OF SLEEP.

THE exciting cause of natural and periodic sleep is undoubtedly to be found in the fact that the brain at stated times requires repose, in order that the cerebral substance which has been decomposed by mental and nervous action may be replaced by new material. There are other exciting causes than this, however, for sleep is not always induced by ordinary or natural influences acting periodically. There are many others, which within the strict limits of health may cause such a condition of the brain as to produce sleep.

Authors, in considering sleep, have not always drawn the proper distinction between the exciting and the immediate cause. Thus Macario,[1] in alluding to the alleged causes of sleep, says:

"Among physiologists some attribute it to a congestion of blood in the brain; others to a directly opposite cause—that is, to a diminished afflux of blood to this organ; some ascribe it to a loss of nervous fluid, others to a flow of this fluid back to its source; others again find the cause in the cessation of the motion of the cerebral fibres, or rather in a partial motion in these fibres. Here I stop, for I could not, even if I wished, mention all the theories which have prevailed relative to this subject. I will only add that, in my opinion, the most probable proximate and immediate cause appears to be feebleness. What seems to prove this view is the fact that exhaustive hot baths, heat, fatigue, too great mental application, are among the means which produce sleep."

Undoubtedly the influences mentioned by Macario, and many others which he might have cited, lead to sleep. They do so through the medium of the nervous system, causing a certain change to take place in the physical condition of the brain. We constantly see instances of this transmission of impressions and the production of palpable effects. Under the influence of fatigue, the countenance becomes pale; through the actions of certain emotions, blushing takes place. When we are anxious, or suffering, or engaged in intense thought, the perspiration comes out in big drops on our brow; danger makes some men tremble, grief causes tears to flow. Many other examples will suggest themselves to the reader. It is surely, therefore, no assumption to say that certain mental or physical influences are capable of inducing such an alteration in the state of the brain as necessarily to cause sleep. These influences or exciting causes I propose to consider in detail, after having given my views relative to the condition of the brain which immediately produces sleep.

It is well established as regards other viscera, that during

[1] " Du sommeil, des rêves et du somnambulisme," etc., Lyon, 1857, p. 14.

a condition of activity there is more blood in their tissues than while they are at rest. It is strange, therefore, that, relative to the brain, the contrary doctrine should have prevailed so long, and that even now, after the subject has been so well elucidated by exact observation, it should be the generally received opinion that during sleep the cerebral tissues are in a state approaching congestion. Thus Dr. Marshall Hall,[1] while contending for this view, also advances the theory that there is a special set of muscles, the duty of which is, by assuming a condition of tonic contraction, so to compress certain veins as to prevent the return of the blood from the heart.

Dr. Carpenter[2] is of the opinion that the first cause of sleep in order of importance is the pressure exerted by distended blood-vessels upon the encephalon.

Sir Henry Holland[3] declares that a "degree of pressure is essential to perfect and uniform sleep."

Dr. Dickson[4] regards an increased determination of blood to the cerebral mass, and its consequent congestion in the larger vessels of the brain, as necessary to the induction of sleep.

In his very excellent work on Epilepsy, Dr. Sieveking[5] says:

"Whether or not there is actually an increase in the amount of blood in the brain during sleep, and whether, as has been suggested, the choroid plexuses become turgid or not, we are unable to affirm otherwise than hypothetically; the evidence is more in favor of cerebral congestion than of the opposite condition inducing sleep—evidence supplied by physiology and pathology." Dr. Sieveking does not, however, state what this evidence is.

Barthez[6] is of the opinion that during sleep there is a general plethora of the smaller blood-vessels of the whole body. He does not appear to have any definite views relative to the condition of the cerebral circulation.

Cabanis[7] declares that as soon as the necessity for sleep

[1] "Observations in Medicine," second series, p. 27.

[2] "Cyclopædia of Anatomy and Physiology," art. "Sleep," vol. iv, part i, p. 681.

[3] "Chapters on Mental Physiology," London, 1852, p. 105.

[4] "Essays on Life, Sleep, Pain," etc., Philadelphia, 1852, pp. 63, 64.

[5] "Epilepsy and Epileptiform Seizures," London, 1858, p. 123.

[6] "Nouveaux éléments de la science de l'homme," 3me édition, Paris, 1858, vol. ii, p. 7, et seq.

[7] "Rapports du physique et du morale de l'homme," Paris, 1824, p. 379.

is experienced there is an increased flow of blood to the brain.

To come to more popular books than those from which we have quoted, we find Mr. Lewes,[1] when speaking of the causes of sleep, asserting that "it is caused by fatigue, because one of the natural consequences of continued action is a slight congestion; and it is the *congestion* which produces sleep. Of this there are many proofs." Mr. Lewes omits to specify these proofs.

Macnish[2] holds the view that sleep is due to a determination of blood to the head.

That a similar opinion has prevailed from very ancient times it would be easy to show. I do not, however, propose to bring forward any further citations on this point, except the following, from a curious old black-letter book now before me, in which the views expressed, though obscure, are, perhaps, as intelligible as many met with in books of our own day:

"And the holy scripture in sundrie places doth call death by the name of sleepe, which is meant in respect of the resurrection; for, as after sleepe we hope to wake, so after death we hope to rise againe. But that definition which Paulus Ægineta maketh of sleepe, in my judgment, is most perfect where he saith: Sleepe is the rest of the pores animall, proceeding of some profitable humour moistening the braine. For here is shewed by what means sleepe is caused; that is, by vapours and fumes rising from the stomache to the head, where through coldness of the braine they being congealed, doe stop the conduites and waies of the senses, and so procure sleepe, which thing may plainly be perceived hereby; for that immediately after meate we are most prone to sleepe, because then the vapours ascende most abundantly to the braine, and such things as be most vaporous do most dispose to sleepe, as wine, milke, and such like."[3]

The theory that sleep is due directly to pressure of blood-vessels, filled to repletion, upon the cerebral tissues, doubtless originated in the fact that a comatose condition may be thus induced. This fact has long been known. Servetus, among

[1] "The Physiology of Common Life," New York, 1860, vol. ii, p. 305.

[2] "Philosophy of Sleep," second edition, 1850, p. 5.

[3] "The Haven of Health, chiefly made for the comfort of Students, and consequently for all those that have a care for their health," etc. By Thomas Cogan, Master of Arts and Bachelor of Physic, London, 1612, p. 332.

other physiological truths, distinctly announces it in his
"Christianismi Restitutio," when he says :

"*Et quando ventriculi ita opplentur pituita, ut arteriæ
ipsæ choroidis ea immergantur, tunc subito generatur appo-
plexia.*"

Perhaps the theory which prevails at present—of sleep
being due to the pressure of distended blood-vessels upon
the choroid plexus—is derived from these words of Servetus.

That stupor may be produced by pressure upon the brain
admits of no doubt. It is familiarly known to physicians,
surgeons, and physiologists ; the two former meet with instances due to pathological causes every day, and the latter
bring it on at will in their laboratories. But this form of
coma and sleep are by no means identical. On the contrary,
the chief point of resemblance between the two consists in the
fact that both are accompanied by a loss of volition. It is
true, we may often arrive at a correct idea of a physiological
process from determining the causes and phenomena of its
pathological variations, but such a course is always liable to
lead to great errors, and should be conducted with every
possible precaution. In the matter under consideration it is
especially of doubtful propriety, for the reason stated, that
coma is not to be regarded as a modification of sleep, but as a
distinct morbid condition. Sir T. C. Morgan,[1] in alluding to
the fact that sleep has been ascribed to a congested state of
the brain, for the reason that in apoplectic stupor the blood-
vessels of that organ are abnormally distended, objects to the
theory, on the ground that it assimilates a dangerous malady
to a natural and beneficial process. He states (what was true
at the time he wrote) that the condition of the circulation
through the brain, during sleep, is wholly unknown.

It is important to understand clearly the difference between stupor and sleep, and it is very certain that the distinction is not always made by physicians ; yet the causes of
the two conditions have almost nothing in common, and the
phenomena of each are even more distinct.

1. In the first place, stupor never occurs in the healthy
individual, while sleep is a necessity of life.

2. It is easy to awaken a person from sleep, while it is
often impossible to arouse him from stupor.

[1] "Sketches of the Philosophy of Life," London, 1819, p. 262.

3. In sleep the mind may be active, in stupor it is as it were dead.

4. Pressure upon the brain, intense congestion of its vessels, the circulation of poisoned blood through its substance, cause stupor, but do not induce sleep. For the production of the latter condition a diminished supply of blood to the brain, as will be fully shown hereafter, is necessary.

Perhaps no one agent so distinctly points out the difference between sleep and stupor as opium and its several preparations. A small dose of this medicine acting as a stimulant increases the activity of the cerebral circulation, and excites a corresponding increase in the rapidity and brilliancy of our thoughts. A larger dose lessens the amount of blood in the brain and induces sleep. A very large dose sometimes diminishes the power of the whole nervous system, lessens the activity of the respiratory function, and hence allows blood which has not been properly subjected to the influence of the oxygen of the atmosphere to circulate through the vessels of the brain. There is nothing in the opium itself which produces excitement, sleep, or stupor, by any direct action upon the brain. All its effects are due to its influence on the heart and blood-vessels, through the medium, however, of the nervous system. This point can be made plainer by adducing the results of some experiments which I have lately performed.

Experiment.—I placed three dogs of about the same size under the influence of chloroform, and removed from each a portion of the upper surface of the skull an inch square. The dura mater was also removed, and the brain exposed. After the effects of the chloroform had passed off—some three hours subsequent to the operation—I administered to number one the fourth of a grain of opium, to number two a grain, and to number three two grains. The brain of each was at the time in a perfectly natural condition.

At first the circulation of the blood in the brain was rendered more active, and the respiration became more hurried. The blood-vessels, as seen through the openings in the skulls, were fuller and redder than before the opium was given, and the brain of each animal rose through the hole in the cranium. Very soon, however, the uniformity which prevailed in these respects was destroyed. In number one the vessels remained moderately distended and florid for almost an hour, and then the brain slowly regained its ordinary appearance. In number two the active congestion passed off in less than half an hour, and was succeeded by a condition of very decided shrinking, the surface of the brain having fallen below the surface of the skull, and become pale. As these changes supervened, the animal gradually sank into a sound sleep, from which it could easily be awakened. In number three the surface of the brain became dark, almost black, from the circulation of blood containing a superabundance of carbon; and, owing to diminished action of the heart and vessels, it sank below the level of the opening, showing, therefore, a diminished amount of blood in its tissue. At the same time the number of respirations per minute fell from 26 to 14, and they were much weaker than before. A condition of complete stupor was also induced from which the animal could not be aroused. It persisted for two hours. During its continuance, sensation of all kind was abolished, and the power of motion was altogether lost.

It might be supposed that the conditions present in numbers two and three differed only in degree. That this was not the case is shown by the following experiment:

Experiment.—To the dogs two and three I administered on the following day, as before, one and two grains of opium, respectively. As soon as the effects began to be manifested upon the condition of the brain, I opened the trachea of each, and, inserting the nozzle of a bellows, began the process of artificial respiration. In both dogs the congestion of the blood-vessels of the brain disappeared. The brain became collapsed, and the animals fell into a sound sleep, from which they were easily awakened. If the action of the bellows was stopped, and the animals were left to their own respiratory efforts, no change ensued in number two, but in number three the surface of the brain became dark, and stupor resulted.

In order to be perfectly assured upon the subject, I proceeded as follows with another dog:

Experiment.— The animal was trephined as was the others, and five grains of opium given. At the same time the trachea was opened and the process of artificial respiration instituted. The brain became slightly congested, then collapsed, and sleep ensued. The sleep was sound, but the animal was easily awakened by tickling its ear. After I had continued the process for an hour and a quarter, I removed the nozzle of the bellows, and allowed the animal to breathe for itself. Immediately the vessels of the brain were filled with black blood, and the surface of the brain assumed a very dark appearance.

The dog could no longer be aroused, and died one hour and a quarter after the process was stopped.

I have only stated those points of the experiments cited which bear upon the subject under consideration, reserving for another occasion others of great interest. It is, however, shown that a small dose of opium excites the mind, because it increases the amount of blood in the brain; that a moderate dose causes sleep, because it lessens the amount of blood; and that a large dose produces stupor by impeding the respiratory process, and hence allowing blood loaded with carbon, and therefore poisonous, to circulate through the brain.

It is also shown that the condition of the brain during stupor is very different from that which exists during sleep. In the one case its vessels are loaded with dark blood; in the other they are comparatively empty, and the blood remains florid.

Lately Ecker[1] has confirmed the results of these experiments by repeating them upon dogs and horses.

I think it will be sufficiently established, in the course of these remarks, that sleep is directly caused by the circulation of a less quantity of blood through the cerebral tissues than traverses them while we are awake. This is the immediate cause of healthy sleep. Its exciting cause is, as we have seen, the necessity for repair. The condition of the brain which is favorable to sleep may also be induced by various other causes, such as heat, cold, narcotics, anæsthetics, intoxicating liquors, loss of blood, etc. If these agents are allowed to act excessively, or others, such as carbonic oxide, and all those which interfere with the oxygenation of the blood, are permitted to exert their influence, stupor results.

The theory above enunciated, although proposed in a modified form by Blumenbach several years since, and subsequently supported by facts brought forward by other observers, has not been received with favor by any considerable number of physiologists. Before, therefore, detailing my own experience, I propose to adduce a few of the most striking proofs of its correctness which I have been able to collect, together with the opinions of some of those inquirers who have recently studied the subject from this point of view.

[1] Cited by Marvaud in "Le sommeil et l'insomnie," Paris, 1881, p. 112.

Blumenbach[1] details the case of a young man, eighteen years of age, who had fallen from an eminence and fractured the frontal bone, on the right side of the coronal suture. After recovery took place a hiatus remained, covered only by the integument. While the young man was awake this chasm was quite superficial, but as soon as sleep ensued it became very deep. The change was due to the fact that during sleep the brain was in a collapsed condition. From a careful observation of this case, as well as from a consideration of the phenomena attendant on the hibernation of animals, Blumenbach[2] arrives at the conclusion that the proximate cause of sleep consists in a diminished flow of oxygenated blood to the brain.

Playfair[3] thinks that sleep is due to "a diminished supply of oxygen to the brain."

Dendy[4] states that there was, in 1821, at Montpellier, a woman who had lost part of her skull, and the brain and its membranes lay bare. When she was in deep sleep the brain remained motionless beneath the crest of the cranial bones; when she was dreaming it became somewhat elevated; and when she was awake it was protruded through the fissure in the skull.

Among the most striking proofs of the correctness of the view that sleep is due to diminished flow of blood to the head are the experiments of Dr. Alexander Fleming,[5] late Professor of Medicine, Queen's College, Cork. This observer states that, while preparing a lecture on the mode of operation of narcotic medicines, he conceived the idea of trying the effect of compressing the carotid arteries on the functions of the brain. The first experiment was performed on himself, by a friend, with the effect of causing immediate and deep sleep. The attempt was frequently made, both on himself and others, and always with success. "A soft humming in the ears is heard; a sense of tingling steals over the body, and in a few seconds complete unconsciousness and insensibility supervene, and continue so long as the pressure is maintained."

[1] "Elements of Physiology." Translated by John Elliotson, M. D., etc., fourth edition, London, 1828, p. 191.

[2] *Op. cit.*, p. 282, *et seq.*

[3] *Northern Journal of Medicine*, No. 1, 1844, p. 34.

[4] "The Philosophy of Mystery," London, 1841, p. 283.

[5] *British and Foreign Medico-Chirurgical Review*, Am. ed., April, 1855, p. 404.

Dr. Fleming adds that whatever practical value may be attached to his observations, they are at least important as physiological facts, and as throwing light on the causes of sleep.

Quite recently the subject has been taken up by Dr. J. Leonard Corning,[1] who, in an interesting little book, considers the subject in all its details. Among other cases showing the influence of carotid compression in inducing sleep, is the case he adduces of a man who was suffering from a protracted and most violent attack of acute mania. The instrument devised by Dr. Corning was applied to the arteries, and, after the lapse of a few moments, his cries and struggles ceased, his eyelids drooped, and he began to oscillate to and fro in his chair. In this condition he suffered himself to be led to his bed ; there he remained quietly upon his back, evincing all the symptoms of drowsiness. In a shorter time than it takes to relate it he was wrapt in slumber. This repose had all the characteristics of physiological sleep.[2]

Dr. Bedford Brown,[3] of Alexandria, Virginia, has recorded an interesting case of extensive compound fracture of the cranium, in which the opportunity was afforded him of examining the condition of the cerebral circulation while the patient was under the influence of an anæsthetic, preparatory to the operation of trephining being performed. A mixture of ether and chloroform was used. Dr. Brown says :

"Whenever the anæsthetic influence began to subside, the surface of the brain presented a florid and injected appearance. The hæmorrhage increased, and the force of the pulsation became much greater. At these times so great was the alternate heaving and bulging of the brain that we were compelled to suspend operations until they were quieted by a repetition of the remedy. Then the pulsations would diminish, the cerebral surface recede within the opening of the skull, as if by collapse ; the appearance of the organ becoming pale and shrunken with a cessation of the bleeding. In fact, we were convinced that diminished vascularity of the brain was an invariable result of the impression of chloroform or ether. The changes above alluded to recurred sufficiently often, during the progress of the operation, in connection

[1] "Carotid Compression and Brain Rest," New York, 1882.

[2] *Op. cit.*, p. 24.

[3] *American Journal of the Medical Sciences*, October, 1860, p. 399.

with the anæsthetic treatment, to satisfy us that there could be no mistake as to the cause and effect."

It will be shown, in the course of the present memoir, that Dr. Brown's conclusions, though in the main correct, are erroneous so far as they relate to the effect of chloroform upon the cerebral circulation ; nor does it appear that he employed this agent unmixed with ether in the case which he has recorded so well. He has, probably, based his remarks on this point upon the phenomena observed when the compound of ether and chloroform was used, the action of pure chloroform, as regards its effect upon the quantity of blood circulating through the brain, being the reverse of that which he claims for it.

But the most philosophical and most carefully digested memoir upon the proximate cause of sleep which has yet been published is that of Mr. Durham.[1] Although my own experiments in the same direction, and which will be hereafter detailed, were of prior date, I cheerfully yield all the honor which may attach to the determination of the question under consideration to this gentleman, who has not only worked it out independently, but has anticipated me several years in the publication, besides carrying his researches to a much further point than my own extended.

With the view of ascertaining by ocular examination the vascular condition of the brain during sleep, Durham placed a dog under the influence of chloroform, and removed with a trephine a portion of bone as large as a shilling from the parietal region ; the dura mater was also cut away. During the continuance of the anæsthetic influence, the large veins of the surface of the pia mater were distended, and the smaller vessels were full of dark-colored blood. The longer the administration of the chloroform was continued, the greater was the congestion. As the effects of this agent passed off, the animal sank into a natural sleep, and then the condition of the brain was very materially changed. Its surface became pale, and sank down below the level of the bone ; the veins ceased to be distended, and many which had been full of dark blood could no longer be distinguished. When the animal was roused, the surface of the brain became suffused with a red blush, and it ascended into the opening through the skull.

[1] "The Physiology of Sleep." By Arthur E. Durham. "Guy's Hospital Reports," third series, vol. vi, 1860, p. 149.

11

As the mental excitement increased, the brain became more and more turgid with blood, and innumerable vessels sprang into sight. The circulation was also increased in rapidity. After being fed, the animal fell asleep, and the brain again became contracted and pale. In all these observations the contrast between the two conditions was exceedingly well marked.

To obviate any possible effects due to atmospheric pressure, watch-glasses were applied to the opening in the skull, and securely cemented to the edges with Canada balsam. The phenomena observed did not differ from those previously noticed; and, in fact, many repetitions of the experiment gave like results.

Durham, in the next place, applied ligatures to the jugular and vertebral veins, with the effect—as was to be expected—of producing intense congestion of the brain, attended with coma. This last condition he very properly separates from sleep, which is never caused by pressure from the veins. He likens sleep to the state induced by preventing the access of blood to the brain through the carotids, but does not allude to Fleming's researches on this point.

From his observations, Durham deduces the following conclusions:

"1. Pressure of distended veins upon the brain is not the cause of sleep, for during sleep the veins are not distended; and, when they are, symptoms and appearances arise which differ from those which characterize sleep.

"2. During sleep the brain is in a comparatively bloodless condition, and the blood in the encephalic vessels is not only diminished in quantity, but moves with diminished rapidity.

"3. The condition of the cerebral circulation during sleep is, from physical causes, that which is most favorable to the nutrition of the brain tissue; and, on the other hand, the condition which prevails during waking is associated with mental activity, because it is that which is most favorable to oxidation of the brain substance, and to various changes in its chemical constitution.

"4. The blood which is derived from the brain during sleep is distributed to the alimentary and excretory organs.

"5. Whatever increases the activity of the cerebral circulation tends to preserve wakefulness; and whatever decreases the activity of the cerebral circulation, and, at the same time, is not inconsistent with the general health of the body, tends to induce and favor sleep. Such circumstances may act primarily through the nervous or through the vascular system. Among those which act through the nervous system may be instanced the presence or absence of impressions upon the senses, and the presence or absence of exciting ideas. Among those which act through the vascular system may be mentioned unnaturally or naturally increased or decreased force or frequency of the heart's action.

"6. A probable explanation of the reason why quiescence of the brain normally follows its activity is suggested by the recognized analogical fact that the products of chemical action interfere with the continuance of the action by which they are produced." [1]

Luys,[2] after stating the two opposite views relative to the state of the cerebral circulation during sleep, gives his adhesion on principles of analogy to that which holds to a diminished afflux of blood. Taking the condition of the salivary glands during their periods of inaction as the basis of his argument, he says:

"We are then naturally led, in making the application of known facts to those which are yet unknown, to say that the nervous tissue and the glandular tissue present, between themselves, the closest analogy, so far as circulatory phenomena and the double alternation of their periods of activity and repose are concerned. And that if the period during which the gland reconstitutes its immediate principles corresponds to a period of reduced activity of circulatory phenomena—to a state of relative anæmia—and that when it functionates it is awakened to a state in which its capillaries are turgid with blood, it is very admissible that the same circulatory conditions should be present in the nervous tissue, and that the period of inactivity, or of sleep, should be characterized by an anemic state. Inversely, the period of activity or wakefulness should be marked by an acceleration of the flow

---

[1] As I have recently been accused of doing injustice to Mr. Durham by refusing him the credit belonging to his investigations, it seems proper to state that the foregoing account of his researches is *verbatim* that given by me in a memoir entitled "Sleep and Insomnia," and published in the *New York Medical Journal* for May, 1865, and subsequently in "Sleep and its Derangements," Philadelphia, 1869.

[2] "Recherches sur la système nerveux cerebro-spinal, sa structure, ses fonctions et ses maladies," Paris, 1865, p. 448.

of blood, and by a kind of erethism of the vascular element."

Having thus, in as succinct a manner as possible, brought forward the principal observations relative to the immediate cause of sleep, which up to the present time have been published, I come, in the next place, to detail the result of my own researches.

In 1854 a man came under my observation who had, through a frightful railroad accident, lost about eighteen square inches of his skull. There was thus a fissure of his cranium three inches wide and six inches long. The lost portion consisted of a great part of the left parietal, and part of the frontal, occipital, and right parietal bones. The man, who was employed as a wood chopper, was subject to severe and frequent epileptic fits, during which I often attended him. In the course of my treatment I soon became acquainted with the fact that, at the beginning of the comatose condition which succeeded the fits, there was invariably an elevation of that portion of the scalp covering the deficiency in the cranium. As the stupor passed away, and sleep from which he could easily be aroused ensued, the scalp gradually became depressed. When the man was awake, the region of scalp in question was always nearly on a level with the upper surface of the cranial bones. I also noticed on several occasions that during natural sleep the fissure was deeper, and that in the instant of awaking the scalp covering it rose to a much higher level.

After my attention was thus drawn to this subject, I observed that in young infants the portion of scalp covering the anterior fontanelle was always depressed during sleep and elevated during wakefulness.

During the summer of 1860 I undertook a series of experiments, with the view of ascertaining the condition of the cerebral circulation during sleep, of which the following is a brief abstract:

A medium-sized dog was trephined over the left parietal bone, close to the sagittal suture, having previously been placed under the full anæsthetic influence of ether. The opening made by the trephine was enlarged with a pair of strong bone-forceps, so as to expose the dura mater to the extent of a full square inch. This membrane was then cut away and the brain brought into view. It was sunk below the inner surface of the skull, and but few vessels were visible. Those which could be perceived, however, evidently conveyed dark blood, and the whole exposed surface of the brain was of a purple color. As the anæsthetic influence passed off, the circulation of the blood in the brain became more active. The purple hue faded away, and numerous small vessels filled with red blood became visible; at the same time the volume of the brain increased, and, when the animal became fully aroused, the organ protruded through the opening in the skull to such an extent that, at the most prominent part, its surface was more than a quarter of an inch above the external surface of the cranium. While the dog continued awake, the condition and position of the brain remained unchanged. After the lapse of half an hour sleep ensued. While this state was coming on I watched the brain very attentively. Its volume slowly decreased; many of its smaller blood-vessels became invisible, and finally it was so much contracted that its surface, pale and apparently deprived of blood, was far below the level of the cranial wall.

Two hours subsequently the animal was again etherized, in order that the influence of the ether upon the cerebral circulation might be observed from the commencement. At the time the dog was awake, and had a few minutes previously eaten a little meat and drank a small quantity of water. The brain protruded through the opening in the skull, and its surface was of a pink hue, with numerous red vessels ramifying over it. The ether was administered by applying to the muzzle of the animal a towel folded into the shape of a funnel, and containing a small sponge saturated with the agent.

As soon as the dog began to inspire the ether, the appearance of the brain underwent a change of color, and its volume became less. As the process of etherization was continued, the color of the surface darkened to a deep purple, and it ceased to protrude through the opening. Finally, when a state of complete anæsthesia was reached, it was perceived that the surface of the brain was far below the level of the cranial fissure, and that its vessels conveyed black blood alone.

Gradually the animal regained its consciousness; the vessels resumed their red color, and the brain was again elevated to its former position. In this last experiment there did not appear to be any congestion of the brain. Had this condition existed, it would have been difficult to account for the diminution in bulk, which certainly took place. There was evidently less blood in the cerebral tissue than there had been previously at the etherization; but this blood, instead of being oxygenated, was loaded with excrementitial matters, and, consequently, was not fitted to maintain the brain in a condition of activity.

The following morning, the dog being quite lively, I removed the sutures which had been placed in the skin, covering the hole in the cranium, with the view of ascertaining the effects of chloroform upon the brain when introduced into the system by inhalation. Suppuration had not yet taken place, and the parts were in good condition. The opening in the skull was completely filled by the brain, and the surface of the latter was traversed by a great many small vessels carrying red blood. The chloroform was administered in the same way in which the ether had been given the previous day.

In a few seconds the change in color of the blood circulating in the vessels began to take place, but there was no sinking of the brain below the level of the chasm in the skull. On the contrary, its protrusion was greater than before the commencement of the experiment. There was thus not only unoxygenated blood circulating to too great an extent through the brain, but there was very decided congestion.

The foregoing experiments were frequently repeated on other dogs, and also on rabbits, with like results. Within a short period I have in part gone over the ground again, without observing any essential point of difference in the effects produced.

But, by means of an instrument designed in somewhat different form by Dr. Weir Mitchell and myself, independently of each other, and which I described in 1869,[1] the state of the brain as regards its blood contents can be accurately determined by ascertaining the degree of pressure exerted upon the fluid contained in the tube of the apparatus. The action is that of any other manometer. Many experiments performed with this instrument shows conclusively that sleep is produced by the blood supply of the brain suffering diminution, and not, as some have supposed, the diminution being

[1] *Quarterly Journal of Psychological Medicine and Medical Jurisprudence,* January, 1869, p. 47.

caused by the sleep. Invariably it happens that the fall of the fluid, indicating a lessened amount of blood, takes place before the superinduction of sleep.

I have also performed Fleming's experiment on the human subject in several instances with Corning's instrument, and then sleep was instantaneously produced. As soon as the pressure was removed from the carotids, the individual gained his consciousness. On dogs and rabbits I have performed it frequently, and, though, if the pressure be continued for longer than one minute, convulsions generally ensue, a state of insensibility resembling natural sleep is always the first result. Several years ago I had, through the kindness of my friend, Dr. Van Buren, the opportunity of examining a case which afforded strong confirmation of the correctness of the preceding views. It was that of a lady in whom both common carotids were tied for a cirsoid aneurism, involving a great portion of the right side of the scalp. One carotid was tied by the late Dr. J. Kearney Rogers, and the other by Dr. Van Buren, seven years before I saw the patient, with the effect of arresting the progress of the disease. No peculiar symptoms were observed in consequence of these operations, except the supervention of persistent drowsiness, which was especially well marked after the last operation, and which even then was at times quite troublesome.

It has been alleged by some writers that although it is true that the amount of blood in the brain is reduced during sleep, yet that it is a consequence, not a cause, of the condition. But the experiments performed upon the carotid arteries by Fleming, Corning, and myself, as well as the phenomena of the case just cited, invalidate this hypothesis. Moreover, the instinct which I have described also shows the contrary, for sleep does not ensue before the fluid begins to fall in the tube, but an appreciable time thereafter.

A similar view of the immediate cause of sleep is that of Mr. Moore.[1] He regards it as being produced by the contraction of the arteries, and the consequent diminution of the quantity of arterial blood circulating through the brain.

Dr. Cappie,[2] however, is of the opinion that sleep is the result of a succession of conditions. First, there is a modified nutrition in the nervous texture ; last, a pressure over the sur-

---

[1] "On Going to Sleep."
[2] "The Causation of Sleep," a Physiological Essay, Edinburgh, 1872, p. 36.

face of the brain, caused by an increase in the amount of blood in that part; and, as a connecting link between the two, a weakened capillary circulation through the brain itself. All this is very ingeniously argued, but it is nevertheless pure hypothesis, and cannot be accepted as contradicting positive experiments.

The theory that sleep is due to a diminished amount of blood in the brain is combated by Langlet,[1] mainly on the ground that in sleep the pupils are contracted as established by Müller, while in cerebral anæmia they are dilated. But the fact is, that the contraction of the pupils observed during sleep and their dilatation during the existence of cerebral anæmia are circumstances not resulting from the condition of the brain as regards its blood supply, but due to influences acting on the sympathetic nerve. As Claude Bernard has shown, the fibres of the cervical sympathetic which go to the cerebral vessels do not come from the same part of the spinal cord as those that supply the iris. Vulpian,[2] while doubting the correctness of the theory in question, admits that the state of the pupil affords no argument against its truth, and cites the experiments of Dr. Hughlings Jackson to the effect that ophthalmoscopic examination showed that during sleep the optic papilla was paler than during wakefulness, and that the arteries were smaller and the veins larger.

We thus see that the *immediate* cause of sleep is a diminution of the quantity of blood circulating in the vessels of the brain, and that the *exciting* cause of periodical and natural sleep is the necessity which exists that the loss of substance which the brain has undergone, during its state of greatest activity, should be restored. To use the simile of the steam-engine again, the fires are lowered and the operatives go to work to repair damages and put the machine in order for next day's work.

Whatever other cause is capable of lessening the quantity of blood in the brain is also capable of inducing sleep. There is no exception to this law, and hence we are frequently able to produce this condition at will. Several of these factors have been already referred to, but it will be interesting to consider them all somewhat more at length.

[1] " Étude critique sur quelques points de la physiologie du sommeil," Thèse de Paris, 1872.
[2] " Leçons sur l'appareil vaso-moteur," Paris, 1875, t. ii, p. 149.

Heat.—Most persons in our climate, and in those of higher temperatures, have felt the influence of heat in causing drowsiness, and eventually sleep, if the action is powerful enough and sufficiently prolonged. It is not difficult to understand the mode by which heat acts in giving rise to sleep. During the prevalence of high temperatures the blood flows in increased proportion to the surface of the body and to the extremities, and, consequently, the quantity in the brain is diminished. Sleep accordingly results unless the irritation induced by the heat is so great as to excite the nervous system. Heat applied directly to the head exerts, of course, a directly contrary effect upon the cerebral circulation, as we see in sunstroke. Here there are internal cerebral congestion, loss of consciousness, stupor, etc.

That the effect of heat is to dilate the vessels of the part subjected to its influence can be ascertained by putting the arm or leg into hot water. The swelling of the blood-vessels is then very distinctly seen. It will be shown hereafter that one of the best means of causing sleep in morbid wakefulness is the warm bath.

Cold.—A slight degree of cold excites wakefulness at first, but if the constitution be strong the effect is to predispose to sleep. This it does by reason of the determination of blood to the surface of the body which moderate cold induces in vigorous persons. The ruddy complexion and warmth of the hands and feet produced in such individuals under the action of this influence are well known.

But if the cold be very intense, or the reduction of temperature sudden, the system, even of the strongest persons, cannot maintain a resistance, and then a very different series of phenomena result. Stupor, not sleep, is the consequence. The blood-vessels of the surface of the body contract, and the blood accumulates in the internal organs, the brain among them. Many instances are on record showing the effect of extreme cold in producing stupor, and even death. One of the most remarkable of these is that related by Captain Cook in regard to an excursion of Sir Joseph Banks, Dr. Solander, and nine others, over the hills of Terra del Fuego. Dr. Solander, knowing from his experience in Northern Europe that the stupor produced by severe cold would terminate in death unless resisted, urged his companions to keep in motion when they began to feel drowsy. "Whoever sits down will sleep," said he,

"and whoever sleeps will rise no more." Yet he was the first
to feel this irresistible desire for repose, and entreated his companions to allow him to lie down. He was roused from his
stupor with great difficulty and carried to a fire, when he revived. Two black men of the party, whose organizations were
not so robust as those of the whites, perished. Dr. Whiting[1]
relates the case of Dr. Edward Daniel Clark, the celebrated
traveller, who on one occasion came very near losing his life by
cold. He had performed divine service at a church near Cam-
bridge, and was returning home on horseback, when he felt
himself becoming very cold and sleepy. Knowing the danger
of yielding to the influence which was creeping over him, he
put his horse into a fast trot, hoping thereby to arouse himself from the alarming torpor. This means proving unavailing, he got down and led his horse, walking as fast as he
could. This, however, did not long succeed. The bridle
dropped from his arm, his legs became weaker and weaker,
and he was just sinking to the ground when a gentleman who
knew him came up in a carriage and rescued him.

I have often myself noticed this effect of cold in producing numbness and drowsiness, and on one occasion was nearly
overcome by it. I was crossing the mountain ridge between
Cebolleta and Covero, in New Mexico, when the thermometer
fell in about two hours from 52° to 22° Fahrenheit. So great
was the effect upon me that if I had had much farther to go
I should probably have succumbed. As it was, I reached a
rancho in time to be relieved, though several minutes elapsed
before I was able to speak. The sensations experienced were
rather agreeable than otherwise. There was a great desire to
rest and to yield to the languor which was present, and there
was a feeling of recklessness which rendered me perfectly indifferent to the consequences. I should have dismounted
from my horse and given way to the longing for repose if I
had been able to do so. I have several times experienced
very similar effects from change of air. A few years since
I was so drowsy at the sea-coast, whither I had gone from a
hot city, that it was with difficulty I could keep awake, even
when engaged in active physical exercise.

Another potent cause of sleep, and one of which we generally avail ourselves, is the *diminution of the power of the
attention.* To bring this influence into action generally re-

---

[1] "Cyclopædia of Practical Medicine," art. "Cold."

quires only the operation of the will under circumstances favorable to the object in view. Shutting the eyes so as to exclude light, getting beyond the sound of noises, refraining from the employment of the other senses, and avoiding thought of all kind, will generally, when there is no preventing cause, induce sleep. To think and to maintain ourselves in connection with the outward world by means of our senses require that the circulation of blood in the brain shall be active. When we isolate ourselves from external things, and restrain our thoughts, we lessen the amount of blood in the brain, and sleep results. It is not, however, always easy for us to do this. The nervous system is excited, ideas follow each other in rapid succession, and we lie awake hour after hour vainly trying to forget that we exist. The more the will is brought to bear upon the subject the more rebellious is the brain, and the more it will not be forced by such means into a state of quietude. We must then either let it run riot till it is worn out by its extravagancies, or we must fatigue it by requiring it to perform labor which is disagreeable. Just as we might do with an individual of highly destructive propensities, who was going about pulling down his neighbors' houses. We might, if we were altogether unable to stop him, let him alone till he had become thoroughly wearied with his exertions, or we might divert him from his plan by guiding him to some tough piece of work which would exhaust his strength sooner than would his original labor.

Many ways of thus tiring the brain have been proposed. The more irksome they are, the more likely they are to prove effectual. Counting a hundred backward many times, listening to monotonous sounds, thinking of some extremely disagreeable and tiresome subject, with many other devices, have been suggested, and have proved more or less effectual. Boerhaave[1] states that he procured sleep by placing a brass pan in such a position that the patient heard the sound of water which was made to fall into it, drop by drop. In general terms, monotony predisposes to sleep. Dr. Dickson[2] quotes Southey's experience as related in "The Doctor,"[3] and I also cannot do better than lay it before the reader, particularly as it indicates several methods which may be more effica-

---

[1] "Cyclopædia of Anatomy and Physiology," vol. iv., pt. i, p. 681, art. "Sleep."
[2] "Essays on Life, Sleep, and Pain," Philadelphia, 1852, p. 87.
[3] "The Doctor," etc., edited by Rev. John Wood Warter, London.

cious with others than the one he found to succeed so admirably.

"I put my arms out of bed; I turned the pillow for the sake of applying a cold surface to my cheek; I stretched my feet into the cold corner; I listened to the river and to the ticking of my watch; I thought of all sleepy sounds and of all soporific things—the flow of water, the humming of bees, the motion of a boat, the waving of a field of corn, the nodding of a mandarin's head on the chimney-piece, a horse in a mill, the opera, Mr. Humdrum's conversations, Mr. Proser's poems, Mr. Laxative's speeches, Mr. Lengthy's sermons. I tried the device of my own childhood, and fancied that the bed rushed with me round and round. At length Morpheus reminded me of Dr. Torpedo's Divinity Lectures, where the voice, the manner, the matter, even the very atmosphere and the streamy candle-light, were all alike somnific; when he who, by strong effort, lifted up his head and forced open the reluctant eyes never failed to see all around him asleep. Lettuces, cowslip wine, poppy syrup, mandragora, hop pillows, spider's web pills, and the whole tribe of narcotics, up to bang and the black-drop, would have failed—but this was irresistible; and thus, twenty years after date, I found benefit from having attended the course."

Frequently the power of the attention is diminished by natural causes. After the mind has been strained a long time in one particular direction, and during which period the brain was doubtless replete with blood, the tension is at last removed, the blood flows out of the brain, the face becomes pale, and sleep ensues. It is thus, as Macnish [1] says, that "the finished gratification of all ardent desires has the effect of inducing slumber; hence, after any keen excitement, the mind becomes exhausted and speedily relapses into this state."

A gentleman, recently under my care for a paralytic affection, informed me that he could at any time render himself sleepy by looking for a few minutes at a bright light, so as to fatigue the eyes, or by paying particular attention to the noises in the street, so as to weary the sense of hearing. It is well known that sleep may be induced by gentle frictions of various parts of the body, and doubtless the other senses are capable of being so exhausted, if I may use the expression, as to diminish the power of the attention, and thus lessen the

[1] *Op. cit.*, p. 5.

demand for blood in the brain. As a consequence, sleep ensues.

The cutting off of sensorial impressions aids in lessening the power of the attention, and thus predisposes to sleep. Stillness, darkness, the absence of any decided impression on the skin, and the non-existence of odors and flavors, accomplish this end. In these respects, however, habit exercises great influence, and thus individuals, for instance, who are accustomed to continual loud noises, cannot sleep when the sound is interrupted. As we have already seen, however, the predisposition to sleep is, in healthy persons, generally so great that, when it has been long resisted, no sensation, however strong it may be, can withstand its power.

Digestion leads to sleep by drawing upon the brain for a portion of its blood. It is for this reason that we feel sleepy after the ingestion of a hearty dinner. A lady of my acquaintance is obliged to sleep a little after each meal. The desire to do so is irresistible; her face becomes pale, her extremities cold, and she sinks into a quiet slumber, which lasts fifteen or twenty minutes. In this lady the amount of blood is not sufficient for the due performance of all the operations of the economy. The digestive organs imperatively require an increased quantity, and the flow takes place from the brain, it being the organ with her which can best spare this fluid. As a rule, persons who eat largely, and have good digestive powers, sleep a great deal, and many persons are unable to sleep at night till they have eaten a substantial supper. The lower animals generally sleep after feeding, especially if the meal has been large.

Excessive loss of blood produces sleep. We can very readily understand why this should be so, if we adopt the theory which has been supported in the foregoing pages. It would be exceedingly difficult to explain the fact upon any other hypothesis. I have seen many instances of somnolency due to this cause. It acts not only by directly lessening the quantity of blood in the brain, but also by so enfeebling the heart's action as to prevent a due supply of blood being sent to the cerebral vessels.

Debility is almost always accompanied by a disposition to inordinate sleep. The brain is one of the first organs to feel the effects of a diminished amount of blood or of a depraved quality of this fluid being supplied; and hence in old age,

or under the influence of a deficient quantity of nutritious
food, or through the action of some exhausting disease, there
is generally more sleep than when the physical health is not
deteriorated.

The action of certain medicines, and of other measures
capable of causing sleep, not coming within the range of
ordinary application, will be more appropriately considered
hereafter.

CHAPTER II.

THE NECESSITY FOR SLEEP.

THE state of general repose which accompanies sleep is of
especial value to the organism in allowing the nutrition of the
nervous tissue to go on at a greater rate than its destructive
metamorphosis. The same effect is, of course, produced upon
the other structures of the body ; but this is not of so much
importance as regards them, for while we are awake they
all obtain a not inconsiderable amount of rest. Even those
actions which are most continuous, such as respiration and the
pulsation of the heart, have distinct periods of suspension.
Thus, after the contraction and dilatation of the auricles and
ventricles of the heart, there is an interval during which the
organ is at rest. This amounts to one fourth of the time
requisite to make one pulsation and begin another. During
six hours of the twenty-four the heart is therefore in a state
of complete repose. If we divide the respiratory act into three
equal parts, one will be occupied in inspiration, one in expiration, and the other by a period of quiescence. During eight
hours of the day, therefore, the muscles of respiration and the
lungs are inactive. And so with the several glands. Each
has its time for rest. And, of the voluntary muscles, none,
even during our most untiring waking moments, are kept in
continued action.

But for the brain there is no rest except during sleep, and
even this condition is, in many instances, as we all know, only
one of comparative quietude. So long as an individual is
awake, there is not a single second of his life during which
the brain is altogether inactive ; and, even while he is deprived

by sleep of the power of volition, nearly every other faculty of the mind is capable of being exercised ; and several of them, as the imagination and memory, for instance, are sometimes carried to a pitch of exaltation not ordinarily reached by direct and voluntary efforts. If it were not for the fact that all parts of the brain are not in action at the same time, and that thus some slight measure of repose is afforded, it would probably be impossible for the organ to maintain itself in a state of integrity.

During wakefulness, therefore, the brain is constantly in action, though this action may be of such a character as not always to make us conscious of its performance. A great deal of the power of the brain is expended in the continuance of functional operations necessary to our well-being. During sleep these are altogether arrested, or else very materially retarded in force and frequency.

Many instances of what Dr. Carpenter very happily calls "unconscious cerebration" will suggest themselves to the reader. We frequently find suggestions occurring to us suddenly—suggestions which could only have arisen as the result of a train of ideas passing through our minds, but of which we have been unconscious. This function of the brain continues in sleep, but not with so much force as during wakefulness. The movements of the heart, of the inspiratory muscles, and of other organs which perform either dynamic or secretory functions, are all rendered less active by sleep ; and during this condition the nervous system generally, obtains the repose which its ceaseless activity during our periods of wakefulness so imperatively demands. Sleep is thus necessary in order that the body, and especially the brain and nervous system, may be renovated by the formation of new tissue to take the place of that which by use has lost its normal characteristics.

From what has been said it will be seen that the brain is no exception to the law which prevails throughout the whole domain of organic nature—that use causes decay. Its substance is consumed by every thought, by every action of the will, by every sound that is heard, by every object that is seen, by every substance that is touched, by every odor that is smelled, by every painful or pleasurable sensation ; and so each instant of our lives witnesses the decay of some portion of its mass and the formation of new material to take its place.

The necessity for sleep is due to the fact that during our waking moments the formation of the new substance does not go on so rapidly as the decay of the old. The state of comparative repose which attends upon this condition allows the balance to be restored, and hence the feeling of freshness and rejuvenation we experience after a sound and healthy sleep. The more active the mind, the greater the necessity for sleep, just as with a steamship, the greater the number of revolutions its engine makes, the more imperative is the demand for fuel.

The power with which this necessity can act is oftentimes very great, and not even the strongest exertion of the will is able to neutralize it. I have frequently seen soldiers sleep on horseback during night marches, and have often slept thus myself. Galen on one occasion walked over two hundred yards while in a sound sleep. He would probably have gone farther but for the fact of his striking his foot against a stone, and thus awaking.

The Abbé Richard states that once, when coming from the country alone and on foot, sleep overtook him when he was more than half a league from town. He continued to walk, however, though soundly asleep, over an uneven and crooked road.[1]

Even when the most stirring events are being enacted, some of the participants may fall asleep. Sentinels on posts of great danger cannot always resist the influence. To punish a man with death, therefore, for yielding to an inexorable law of his being, is not the least of the barbarous customs which are still in force in civilized armies. During the battle of the Nile many of the boys engaged in handing ammunition fell asleep, notwithstanding the noise and confusion of the action and the fear of punishment. And it is said that on the retreat to Corunna whole battalions of infantry slept while in rapid march. Even the most acute bodily sufferings are not always sufficient to prevent sleep. I have seen individuals who had been exposed to great fatigue, and who had while enduring it met with accidents requiring surgical interference, sleep through the pain caused by the knife. Damiens, the lunatic who attempted the assassination of Louis XV of France, and who was sentenced to be torn to pieces by four horses, was for an hour and a half before his execution subjected to the most infamous tortures, with red-hot pincers, melted lead,

---

[1] " La théorie des songes," Paris, 1766, p. 206.

burning sulphur, boiling oil, and other diabolical contrivances, yet he slept on the rack, and it was only by continually changing the mode of torture, so as to give a new sensation, that he was kept awake. He complained, just before his death, that the deprivation of sleep was the greatest of all his torments, and he also declared that, had he been bled as he had requested, he would never have committed the crime for which he suffered.

Dr. Forbes Winslow [1] quotes from the *Louisville Semi-Monthly Medical News* the following case :

" A Chinese merchant had been convicted of murdering his wife, and was sentenced to die by being deprived of sleep. This painful mode of death was carried into effect under the following circumstances : The condemned was placed in prison under the care of three of the police guard, who relieved each other every alternate hour, and who prevented the prisoner falling asleep night or day. He thus lived nineteen days without enjoying any sleep. At the commencement of the eighth day his sufferings were so intense that he implored the authorities to grant him the blessed opportunity of being strangled, guillotined, burned to death, drowned, garroted, shot, quartered, blown up with gunpowder, or put to death in any conceivable way their humanity or ferocity could invent. This will give a slight idea of the horrors of death from want of sleep."

In infants the necessity for sleep is much greater than in adults, and still more so than in old persons. In the former the formative processes are much more active than those concerned in disintegration. Hence the greater necessity for frequent periods of repose. In old persons, on the contrary, decay predominates over construction, there is a decreased activity of the brain, the nervous system, and of all other organs, and thus the demand for rest and recuperation is lessened.

The necessity for sleep is not felt by all organic beings alike. The differences observed are more due to variations in habits, modes of life, and inherent organic dispositions, than to any inequality in the size of the brain, although the latter has been thought by some authors to be the cause. It has been assumed that the larger the brain the more sleep is required. Perhaps this is true as regards the individuals of

---

[1] " On Obscure Diseases of the Brain," etc., London, 1860, p. 604, note.

12

any one species of animals, but it is not the case when species are compared with each other. In man, for instance, persons with large heads, as a rule, have large, well-developed brains, and, consequently, more cerebral action than individuals with small brains. There is accordingly a greater waste of cerebral substance, and an increased necessity for repair.

This is not, however, always the case, as some individuals with small brains have been remarkable for great mental activity.

All animals sleep, and even plants have their periods of comparative repose. As Lelut says:[1]

" No one is ignorant of the nocturnal repose of plants. I say repose and nothing else. I do not say diminution or suspension of their sensibility, for plants have no sensibility. I say diminution of their organic actions—a diminution which is evident and characteristic in all, more evident and more characteristic in some. . . .

" Their interior or vital movements are lessened, the flow of the sap and of other fluids which penetrate and rise in them is retarded. Their more mobile parts—the leaves, the flowers—show by their falling, their occlusion, their inclination, that their organic actions are diminished, and that a kind of repose has been initiated, which takes the place of the lying down which, with animals, is the condition and the result of sleep."

CHAPTER III.

THE PHYSICAL PHENOMENA OF SLEEP.

THE approach of sleep is characterized by a languor which, when it can be yielded to, is agreeable, but which, when circumstances prevent this, is far from being pleasant. Many persons are rendered irritable as soon as they become sleepy, and children are especially liable to manifest ill-temper under the uncomfortable feelings they experience when unable to indulge the inclination to sleep. It is somewhat difficult to analyze the various phenomena which go to make up the condition called sleepiness. The most prominent feelings are an

---

[1] " Physiologie de la pensée. Recherche critique des rapports du corps à l'esprit." Deuxième édition, Paris, 1862, t. ii, p. 440.

impression of weight in the upper eyelids, and of a general relaxation of the muscles of the body, but there is besides an internal sensation of supineness, enervation, and torpor, to describe which is by no means easy. This sluggishness is closely allied in character, if not altogether identical, with that experienced before an attack of fainting, and is doubtless due to a like cause—a deficient quantity of blood in the brain. Along with this languor there is a general obtuseness of all the senses, which increases the separation of the mind from the external world, already initiated by the eyelids interposing a physical obstruction to the entrance of light. Even when the eyelids have been removed, or from disease cannot be closed, the sight, nevertheless, is the first of the special senses to be abolished. Some animals, as the hare, for example, do not shut the eyes when asleep ; but even in them the ability to see disappears before the action of the other senses is suspended.

These latter are not altogether abolished during sleep ; their acuteness is simply lessened. Taste is the first to fade, and then the smell ; hearing follows, and touch yields last of all, and is most readily re-excited. To awake a sleeping person, impressions made upon the sense of touch are more effectual than attempts to arouse through any of the other senses ; the hearing comes next in order, smell next, then taste, and the sight is the last of all in capacity for excitation.

During sleep the respiration is slower, deeper, and usually more regular than during wakefulness. The vigor of the process is lessened, and therefore there is a diminution of the pulmonary exhalations. In all probability, also, the ciliated epithelium which lines the air-passages functionates with reduced activity. Owing to this circumstance, and to the general muscular torpor which prevails, mucus accumulates in the bronchial tubes and requires to be expectorated on awaking.

The circulation of the blood is rendered slower. The heart beats with more regularity, but with diminished force and frequency. As a consequence, the blood is not distributed to distant parts of the body so thoroughly and rapidly as during wakefulness, and accordingly the extremities readily lose their heat. Owing to the reduction in the activity of the respiratory and circulatory functions, the temperature of the whole body falls, and coldness of the atmosphere is less easily resisted.

The functions of the several organs concerned in digestion have their activity increased by sleep. The blood which leaves the brain goes, as Durham has shown, to the stomach and other abdominal viscera, and hence the quantities of the digestive juices are augmented, and the absorption of the nutritious elements of the food is promoted.

The urine is excreted in less quantity during sleep than when the individual is awake and engaged in mental or physical employment, because the wear and tear of the system is at its minimum.

The perspiration is likewise reduced in amount by sleep. In warm weather, however, the effort to go to sleep often causes an increase in the quantity of this excretion, just as would any other mental or bodily exertion. This circumstance has led some writers to a conclusion the reverse of that just expressed. Others, again, have accepted the doctrine of Sanctorius on this point without stopping to inquire into its correctness. This author,[1] among other aphorisms relating to sleep, gives the following :

"Undisturbed sleep is so great a promoter of perspiration that, in the space of seven hours, fifty ounces of the concocted perspirable matter do commonly exhale out of strong bodies.

"A man sleeping the space of seven hours is wont, insensibly, healthfully, and without any violence, to perspire twice as much as one awake."

The observations of Sanctorius with his weighing chair led to a good many important results, but they were inexact so far as the function of the skin was concerned, in that they made no division between the loss by this channel and that which takes place through the lungs, for by perspiration in the above quotations he means not only the exhalation from the skin, but the products of respiration—aqueous vapor, carbonic acid, etc. His apparatus was, besides, very imperfect, and could not possibly have given the delicate indications which the subject requires.

Whether the condition of sleep promotes the absorption of morbid growths and accumulations of fluids is very doubtful. Macnish[2] contends that it does, but a priori reasoning would rather lead us to an opposite conclusion. Deficiencies are probably more rapidly made up during sleep than during

[1] " Medicina Statica ; or, Rules of Health," etc., London, 1676, p. 106, et seq.
[2] Op. cit., p. 6.

wakefulness, and thus ulcers heal with more rapidity, owing to the increased formation of granulations which takes place ; but the removal of tumors, etc., by natural process involves the operation of forces the very opposite of those concerned in reparation, and observation teaches us that sleep is a condition peculiarly favorable to the deposition of the materials constituting morbid growths. Some writers have alleged that sleep accelerates the absorption of dropsical effusions, but the disappearance of such accumulations during the condition in question is clearly due to the mechanical causes depending upon the position of the body.

It has also been asserted that there is an exaltation of the sexual feeling during sleep. It is difficult to arrive at any very definite conclusion on this point, but it is probable that here again the position of the body conjoined with the heat of the bed has much to do in producing the erotic manifestations occasionally witnessed. Every physician who has had much to do with cases of the kind knows that sleeping upon the back, by which means the blood gravitates to the generative organs and to the lower part of the spinal cord, will often give rise to seminal emissions with or without erotic dreams, and that such occurrences may generally be prevented by the individual avoiding the dorsal decubitus and resting upon one side or the other while asleep. The erections which the generality of healthy men experience in the morning before rising from bed are likewise due to the fact that the recumbent posture favors the flow of blood to the penis and testicles. Such erections are usually unaccompanied by venereal desire.

The ganglionic nervous system and the spinal cord continue in action during sleep, though generally with somewhat diminished power and sensibility. The reflex faculty of the latter organ is still maintained, and thus various movements are executed without the consciousness of the brain being awakened. Somnambulism is clearly a condition of exaltation in the functions of the spinal cord without the controlling influence of the cerebrum being brought into action. But, aside from this rather abnormal phenomenon, there are others which are entirely within the range of health, and which show that the spinal cord is awake, even though the sleep be most profound. Thus, for instance, if the position of the sleeper becomes irksome, it is changed ; if the feet become cold, they are drawn up to a warmer part of the bed ; and cases are recorded in which individuals have risen from bed and emptied a distended bladder without awaking.

The instances brought forward in a previous chapter, of persons riding on horseback and walking during sleep, show the activity of the spinal cord, and not that the will is exercised ; and Cabanis [1] is wrong in the view which he gives of such phenomena in the following extract.

Speaking of cases like those just referred to, he says :

" These rare instances are not the only ones in which movements are observed to be produced during sleep by that portion of the will which is awake ; for it is by virtue of certain direct sensations that a sleeping man moves his arm to brush away the flies from his face, that he draws the cover around him so as to envelop himself carefully, or that he turns in bed till he has found a comfortable position. It is the will which during sleep maintains the contraction of the sphincter of the bladder, notwithstanding the effort of the urine to escape."

Such examples as the above we now know to be instances of reflex action, and as not, therefore, being due to the exercise of the will.

Sleep favors the occurrence of certain pathological phenomena. Thus, individuals affected with hæmorrhoids have the liability to hæmorrhage increased when they are asleep. Several instances of the kind have come under my notice. In one the patient lost so large a quantity of blood that syncope ensued, and might have terminated fatally had not his condition been accidentally discovered. Bleeding from the lungs is also more apt to occur during sleep in those who are predisposed to it. Darwin states that a man of about fifty years of age, subject to hæmorrhoids, was also attacked with hæmoptysis three consecutive nights at about the same hour—two o'clock—being awakened thereby from a state of very profound sleep. He was advised to suffer himself to be roused at one o'clock, and to leave his bed at that hour. He did so with the result not only of entirely breaking up the hæmorrhagic disposition, but also of curing himself of very violent attacks of headache, to which he had been subject for many years. The contractile power of the sphincter of the bladder is often so weakened during sleep that enuresis is apt to occur, especially in children.

Epileptic fits are also more liable to take place during sleep

[1] *Op. cit.*, t. ii, p. 385.

than at other times, a fact not always susceptible of easy explanation. In a case of epilepsy formerly under my charge, this proclivity is so well marked that the patient, a lady, scarcely ever goes to sleep without being attacked. Her face becomes exceedingly pale just before the fit, and, if then seen, the paroxysm can be entirely prevented by waking her. She is never attacked at other times, and I tried, with excellent results, the plan of making her sleep altogether during the day and of waking her as soon as her face became pallid. It is probable that the fits in her case were due to a diminished amount of blood in the brain, and this supposition is strengthened by the additional fact that bromide of potassium—a substance which, as I have shown, lessens the amount of intracranial blood—invariably rendered her paroxysms more frequent and severe.

Sleep predisposes to attacks of gout in those who have the gouty diathesis, and likewise favors exacerbations in several other diseases which it is scarcely necessary to allude to specifically. The accession of fever toward night and the increase which takes place in pain due to inflammation are generally associated with the approach of night, and have no direct relation with sleep.

Certain other morbid phenomena, such as somnambulism and nightmare, which have a necessary relation with sleep, will be more appropriately considered in another place.

On the other hand, sleep controls the manifestations of several diseases, especially those which are of a convulsive or spasmodic character. Thus, the paroxysms of chorea cease during sleep, as do likewise the spasms of tetanus and hydrophobia. Headache is also generally relieved by sleep, though occasionally it is aggravated.

CHAPTER IV.

THE STATE OF THE MIND DURING SLEEP.

WE have seen that, though during sleep the operations of the senses are entirely suspended as regards the effects of ordinary impressions, the purely animal functions of the body continue in action. The heart beats, the lungs respire, the stomach, the intestines and their accessory organs digest, the skin exhales vapor, and the kidneys secrete urine. With the central nervous system, however, the case is very different; for, while some parts retain the property of receiving impressions or developing ideas, others have their actions diminished, exalted, perverted, or altogether arrested.

In the first place, there is, undoubtedly, during sleep, a general torpor of the sensorium, which prevents the appreciation of the ordinary excitations made upon the organs of the special senses. So far as the nerves themselves are concerned, there is no loss of their irritability or conducting power, and the impressions made upon them are, accordingly, perfectly well conveyed to the brain. The suspension of the operations of the senses is not, therefore, due to any loss of function in the optic nerve, the auditory nerve, the olfactory nerve, the gustatory nerve, or the cranial or spinal nerves concerned in the sense of touch, but solely to the inability of the brain to take cognizance of the impressions conveyed to it. In regard to the cause of this torpor, I have given my views in a previous chapter.

Now, it must not be supposed that, because mild excitations transmitted by the nerves of the special senses are incapable of making themselves felt, that, therefore, the brain is in a state of complete repose throughout all its parts. So far from such a condition existing, there are very decided proofs that several faculties are exercised to a degree almost equalling that reached during wakefulness, and we know that, if the irritations made upon the senses be sufficiently strong, the brain *does* appreciate them, and the sleep is broken. This ability to be readily roused through the senses constitutes one of the main differences between sleep and stupor, upon which stress has been already laid.

Relative to the different faculties of the mind as affected by sleep great variations are observed. It has been thought by some authors that several of them are really exalted above the standard attained during wakefulness, but this is probably a wrong view. The predominance which one or two mental qualities apparently assume is not due to any absolute exaggeration of power, but to the suspension of the action of other faculties, which, when we are not asleep, exercise a governing or modifying influence. Thus, for instance, as regards the imagination—the faculty of all others which appears to be most increased—we find, when we carefully study its manifestations in our own persons, that although there is often great brilliancy in its vagaries, that uncontrolled as it is by the judgment, the pictures which it paints upon our minds are usually incongruous and silly in the extreme. Even though the train of ideas excited by this faculty when we are asleep be rational and coherent, we are fully conscious on awaking that we are capable of doing much better by intentionally setting the brain in action and governing it by our intellect and will.

Owing to the fact that these two faculties of the mind are incapable of acting normally during sleep, the imagination is left absolutely without controlling influence. Indeed, we are often cognizant, in those dreams which take place when we are half awake, of an inability to direct it. The impressions which it makes upon the mind are therefore intense, but of very little durability. Many stories are told of its power— how problems have been worked out, poetry and music composed, and great undertakings planned ; but, if we could get at the truth, we should probably find that the imagination of sleep had very little to do with the operations mentioned. Indeed, it is doubtful if the mind of a sleeping person can originate ideas. Those which are formed are, as Locke[1] remarks, almost invariably made up of the waking man's ideas, and are for the most part very oddly put together ; and we are all aware how commonly our dreams are composed of ideas, or based upon events which have recently occurred to us.

In the previous section to the one just quoted, Locke refers to the exaggeration of ideas which form so common a feature of our mental actions during sleep. "It is true," he says, "we have sometimes instances of perception while we are asleep, and retain the memory of those thoughts ; but, how extravagant and incoherent for the most part they are, how little conformable to the perfection and order of a rational being, those acquainted with dreams need not be told."

And yet many remarkable stories are related which tend to show the high degree of activity possessed by the mind during sleep. Thus, it is said of Tartini,[2] a celebrated musi-

---

[1] "An Essay concerning Human Understanding," book ii, section 17.

[2] "Encyclopædia Americana," Philadelphia, 1832, vol. xii, p. 143, art. "Tartini"; and "L'imagination considérée dans ses effets directs sur l'homme et les animaux," etc. Par J. B. Demangeon. Seconde édition, Paris, 1829, p. 161.

cian of the eighteenth century, that one night he dreamed he had made a compact with the devil, and bound him to his service. In order to ascertain the musical abilities of his servitor, he gave him his violin, and commanded him to play a solo. The devil did so, and performed so admirably that Tartini awoke with the excitement produced, and, seizing his violin, endeavored to repeat the enchanting air. Although he was unable to do this with entire success, his efforts were so far effectual that he composed one of the most admired of his pieces, which, in recognition of its source, he called the "Devil's Sonata."

Coleridge gives the following account of the composition of the fragment, Kublai Khan:

"In the summer of 1797 the author, then in ill-health, had retired to a lonely farm-house, between Perlock and Linton, on the Exmoor confines of Somerset and Devonshire. In consequence of a slight indisposition, an anodyne had been prescribed, from the effects of which he fell asleep in his chair at the moment that he was reading the following sentence, or words of the same substance, in 'Purchas's Pilgrimage': 'Here the Khan Kublai commanded a palace to be built, and a stately garden thereunto. And thus ten miles of fertile ground were enclosed with a wall.' The author continued for about three hours in a profound sleep, at least of the external senses, during which time he had the most vivid confidence that he could have composed not less than from two to three hundred lines, if that, indeed, can be called composition, in which all the images rose up before him as *things* with a parallel production of the corresponding expression without any sensation or consciousness of effort. On awaking, he appeared to himself to have a distinct recollection of the whole; and, taking his pen, ink, and paper, instantly and eagerly wrote down the lines that are here preserved. At this moment he was unfortunately called out by a person on business from Perlock, and detained by him above an hour; and on his return to his room found, to his no small surprise and mortification, that though he still retained some vague and dim recollection of the general purport of the vision, yet, with the exception of some eight or ten scattered lines and images, all the rest had passed away like the images on the surface of a stream into which a stone had been cast, but, alas! without the after-restoration of the latter."

Dr. Cromwell,[1] citing the above instance of poetic inspiration during sleep, states that, having, like Coleridge, taken an anodyne during a painful illness, he composed the following lines of poetry, which he wrote down within half an hour after awaking. These lines, though displaying considerable imagination, are not remarkable for any other quality.

"Lines composed in sleep on the night of January 9, 1857:

"SCENE.— *Windsor Forest.*

"At a vista's end stood the queen one day
Relieved by a sky of the softest hue;
It happen'd that a wood-mist, risen new,
Had made that white which should have been blue.
A sunbeam sought on her form to play;
It found a nook in the bowery nave,
Through which with its golden stem to lave
And kiss the leaves of the stately trees
That fluttered and rustled beneath the breeze;
But it touched not her, to whom 'twas given
To walk in a white light pure as heaven."

In the last two of these instances it is impossible to say whether the individuals were really asleep or not, as the opium or other narcotic taken is a very disturbing factor in both conditions, and doubtless was the exciting cause of the activity in the imagination. No more graphic account of the effects of opium in arousing the imagination to its highest pitch has been written than that given by De Quincey.[2] He says:

"At night when I lay awake in bed, vast processions passed along in mournful pomp; friezes of never-ending stories, that to my feelings were as sad and solemn as if they were stories drawn from times before Œdipus or Priam, before Tyre, before Memphis. And at the same time a corresponding change took place in my dreams; a theatre seemed suddenly opened and lighted up within my brain, which presented nightly spectacles of more than earthly splendor." And then, after referring to the various scenes of architectural magnificence, and of beautiful women which his imagination conceived, and which forcibly recalls to our minds the poetical

[1] The "Soul and the Future Life." Appendix viii. Quoted by Seafield in "The Literature and Curiosities of Dreams," etc., London, 1865, vol. ii, p. 229.
[2] "Confessions of an English Opium-Eater," Boston, 1866, p. 109.

effusions of Coleridge and Cromwell, he gives the details of
another dream, in which he heard music. "A music of preparation, of awakening suspense ; a music like the opening of
the Coronation Anthem, and which like *that* gave the feeling
of a vast march, of infinite cavalcades filing off, and the tread
of innumerable armies."

In reference to this subject, Dr. Forbes Winslow [1] relates
the following interesting case :

"A feeble, sensitive lady, suffering from a uterine affection, writes to us as follows concerning the influence of three
or four sixteenth-of-a-grain doses of hydrochlorate of morphia:
'After taking a few doses of morphia, I felt a sensation of extreme quiet and wish for repose, and, on closing my eyes, visions, if I may so call them, were constantly before me, and as
constantly changing in their aspect: scenes from foreign lands,
lovely landscapes, with tall, magnificent trees covered with
drooping foliage, which was blown gently against me as I
walked along. Then, in an instant, I was in a besieged city
filled with armed men. I was carrying an infant, which was
snatched from me by a soldier and killed upon the spot. A
Turk was standing by with a cimeter in his hand, which I
seized, and, attacking the man who had killed the child, I
fought most furiously with him and killed him. Then I was
surrounded, made prisoner, carried before a judge, and accused
of the deed ; but I pleaded my own cause with such a burst
of eloquence (which, by the by, I am quite incapable of in my
right mind) that judge, jury, and hearers acquitted me at
once. Again, I was in an Eastern city visiting an Oriental
lady, who entertained me most charmingly. We sat together
on rich ottomans, and were regaled with supper and confec-
tionery. Then came soft sounds of music at a distance, while
fountains were playing and birds singing, and dancing girls
danced before us, every movement being accompanied with
the tinkling of silver bells attached to their feet. But all this
suddenly changed, and I was entertaining the Oriental lady
in my own house, and, in order to please her delicate taste, I
had everything prepared as nearly as possible after the fashion with which she had so enchanted me. She, however, to
my no small surprise, asked for wine, and took not one, two,
or three glasses, but drank freely, until at last I became terrified that she would have to be carried away intoxicated.

[1] *Journal of Psychological Medicine and Mental Pathology*, July, 1859, p. 44.

While considering what course I had better adopt, several English officers came in, and she at once asked them to drink with her, which so shocked my sense of propriety that the scene changed and I was in darkness.

" 'Then I felt that I was formed of granite, and immovable. Suddenly a change came again over me, and I found that I consisted of delicate and fragile basket-work. Then I became a danseuse, delighting an audience and myself by movements which seemed barely to touch the earth. Presently beautiful sights came before me, treasures from the depth of the sea, gems of the brightest hues, gorgeous shells, coral of the richest colors, sparkling with drops of water, and hung with lovely sea-weed. My eager glances could not take in half the beautiful objects that passed before me during the incessant changes the visions underwent. Now I was gazing upon antique brooches and rings from buried cities ; now upon a series of Egyptian vases ; now upon sculptured wood-work blackened by time ; and lastly I was buried amid forests of tall trees, such as I had read of but never seen.

" 'The sights that pleased me most I had power to a certain extent to prolong, and those that displeased me I could occasionally set aside, and I awoke myself to full consciousness once or twice while under the influence of the morphia by an angry exclamation that I would not have it. I did not once lose my personal identity.'

" The lady almost invariably suffers more or less from hallucinations of the foregoing character if it becomes necessary to administer to her an opiate ; and, on analyzing her visions, she can generally refer the principal portions of them, notwithstanding their confusion and distortion, to works that she has recently read."

Opium, in certain doses, increases the amount of blood in the brain, and this induces a condition very different from that of sleep. In this fact we have an explanation of the activity of the imagination as one of its prominent effects. That Coleridge should have composed the Kublai Khan under its influence is in no wise remarkable. It is probable, however, that the full influence of his mind was exerted upon it after he awoke to consciousness, and that the wild fancies excited by the opiate, and based upon what he had been previously reading, formed the substratum of his conceptions. In any event, the ideas contained in this fragment are no more fanciful than those which occurred to De Quincey and the lady whose case has just been recorded.

The imagination may therefore be active during sleep, but we have no authentic instance on record that it has, unaided by causes which exercise a powerful influence over the intracranial circulation, led to the production of any ideas which could not be excelled by the individual when awake. Perhaps the most striking case in opposition to this opinion is one detailed by Abercrombie,[1] who says:

"The following anecdote has been preserved in a family of rank in Scotland, the descendants of a distinguished lawyer of the last age. This eminent person had been consulted respecting a case of great importance and much difficulty, and he had been studying it with intense anxiety and attention. After several days had been occupied in this manner, he was observed by his wife to rise from his bed in the night and go to a writing-desk which stood in the bedroom. He then sat down and wrote a long letter, which he put carefully by in the desk and returned to bed. The following morning he told his wife that he had had a most interesting dream; that he had dreamt of delivering a clear and luminous opinion respecting a case which had exceedingly perplexed him, and that he would give anything to recover the train of thought which had passed before him in his dream. She then directed him to the writing-desk, where he found the opinion clearly and fully written out, and which was afterward found to be perfectly correct."

It is probable that this gentleman was actually awake when he arose from the bed and wrote the paper referred to, and that in the morning he mistook the circumstance for a dream. It is not at all uncommon for such errors to be committed, especially under the condition of mental anxiety and fatigue. A gentleman informed me only a short time since that, going to bed after a very exciting day, he thought the next morning that he had dreamt of a fire occurring in the vicinity of his house. To his surprise his wife informed him that the supposed dream was a reality, and that he had got up to the window, looked at the fire, conversed with her concerning it, and that he was at the time fully awake.

[1] "Inquiries concerning the Intellectual Powers and the Investigation of Truth," tenth edition, London, 1840, p. 304.

Brierre de Boismont [1] relates the following instance, which is to the same effect:

"In a convent in Auvergne an apothecary was sleeping with several persons. Being attacked with nightmare, he charged his companions with throwing themselves on him and attempting to strangle him. They all denied the assertion, telling him that he had passed the night without sleeping, and in a state of high excitement. In order to convince him of this fact, they prevailed on him to sleep alone in a room carefully closed, having previously given him a good supper, and even made him partake of food of a flatulent nature. The paroxysm returned; but on this occasion he swore that it was the work of a demon, whose face and figure he perfectly described."

That the imagination may in its flights during sleep strike upon fancies which are subsequently developed by the reason into lucid and valuable ideas, is very probable. It would be strange if, from among the innumerable absurdities and extravagances to which it attains, something fit to be appropriated by the mind should not occasionally be evolved, and thus there are many instances mentioned of the starting-point of important mental operations having been taken during sleep. Some of these may be based upon fact, but the majority are probably of the class of those just specified, or occurred at an age of the world when a belief in the supernatural exercised a greater power over men's minds than it does at the present day. Among the most striking of them are the following:

Galen declares that he owed a great part of his knowledge to the revelations made to him in dreams. Whether this was really the case or not we can in a measure determine by recalling the fact that he was a believer in the prophetic nature of dreams, and states that a man having dreamt that one of his legs was turned into stone, soon afterward became paralytic in this limb, although there was no evidence of approaching disease. Galen also conducted his practice by dreams, for an athlete, having dreamt that he saw red spots, and that the blood was flowing out of his body, was supposed by Galen to require blood-letting, which operation was accordingly performed.

[1] "A History of Dreams, Visions, Apparitions," etc., Philadelphia, 1855, p. 184.

It has been said [1] that the idea of the "Divina Commedia" occurred to Dante during sleep. There is nothing at all improbable in this supposition, though I have been unable to trace it to any definite source.

Cabanis [2] states that Condillac assured him that often during the course of his studies he had to leave them unfinished in order to sleep, and that on awaking he had more than once found the work upon which he was engaged brought to a conclusion in his brain.

These were clearly instances of "unconscious cerebration," of that power which the brain possesses to work out matters which have engaged its attention, without the consciousness of the individual being aroused to a knowledge of the labor being performed. It is not unlikely that this kind of mental activity goes on to some extent during sleep; but, as it is of such a character that the mind does not take cognizance of its operations, I do see how the exact period of its performance can be ascertained.

Jerome Cardan believed that he composed books while asleep, and his case is often adduced as an example of the height to which the imagination can attain during sleep. But this great man was superstitious to an extreme degree; he believed that he had a familiar spirit from whom he received intelligence, warnings, and ideas, and asserted that when awake he frequently saw long processions of men, women, animals, trees, castles, instruments of various kinds, and many figures different from anything in this world. His evidence relative to his compositions and mathematical labors when asleep is not therefore of a trustworthy character.

As regards the memory in sleep, it is undoubtedly exercised to a considerable extent. In fact, whatever degree of activity the mind may then exhibit is based upon events the recollection of which has been retained. But there is more or less error mingled with a small amount of truth. The unbridled imagination of the sleeper so distorts the simplest circumstances as to render their recognition a matter of no small difficulty, and thus it scarcely if ever happens that events are reproduced during sleep exactly as they occurred, or as they would be recalled by the mind of the individual, when awake. Frequently, also, recent events which have made a strong im-

[1] Macario, "Du sommeil, des rêves et du somnambulisme," Paris, 1857, p. 59.
[2] *Op. cit.*, t. ii, p. 395.

pression on our minds are forgotten, as when we dream of seeing and conversing with persons not long dead.

And yet it has sometimes happened that incidents or knowledge which had long been overlooked or forgotten, or which could not be remembered by any effort during wakefulness, have been strongly depicted during sleep. Thus Lord Monboddo[1] states that the Countess de Laval, a woman of perfect veracity and good sense, when ill, spoke during sleep in a language which none of her attendants understood, and which even she was disposed to regard as gibberish. A nurse detected the dialect of Brittany; her mistress had spent her childhood in that province, but had lost all recollection of the Breton tongue, and could not understand a word of what she said in her dreams. Her utterances applied, however, exclusively to the experience of childhood, and were infantile in structure.

Abercrombie[2] relates the case of a gentleman who was very fond of the Greek language, and who, in his youth, had made considerable progress in it. Subsequently, being engaged in other pursuits, he so entirely forgot it that he could not even read the words; often, however, in his dreams he read Greek works, which he had been accustomed to use at college, and had a most vivid impression of fully understanding them.

Many other instances of the action of memory during sleep might be brought forward, but the subject will be more appropriately considered in the chapter on dreams.

The judgment is frequently exercised when we are asleep, but almost invariably in a perverted manner. In fact, we scarcely ever estimate the events or circumstances which appear to occur in our dreams at their real value, and very rarely from correct conceptions of right and wrong. Highminded and honorable men do not scruple during sleep to sanction the most atrocious acts, or to regard with complacence ideas which, in their waking moments, would fill them with horror. Delicate and refined women will coolly enter upon a career of crime, and the minds of hardened villains are filled with the most elevated and noble sentiments. The deeds which we imagine we perform in our sleep are generally inadequate to or in excess of what the apparent occasion re-

[1] " Ancient Metaphysics." Quoted in Dr. Forbes Winslow's *Medical Critic and Psychological Journal*, No. vi, April, 1862, p. 206.

[2] *Op. cit.*, p. 283.

13

quires, and we lose so entirely the ideas of probability and possibility that no preposterous vision appears otherwise than as perfectly natural and correct. Thus, a physician dreamed that he had been transformed into a monolith, which stood grandly and alone in the vast desert of the Sahara, and had so stood for ages, while generation after generation wasted and melted away around him. Although unconscious of having organs of sense, this column of granite saw the mountains growing bald with age, the forests drooping with decay, and the moss and ivy creeping around its crumbling base.[1]

But, although in this instance there was some conception of time, as shown in the association of the evidences of decay with the lapse of years, there is in general no correct idea on this subject. Without going into details which more appropriately belong to another division of this treatise, I quote the following remarkable example from the essay last cited. It appeared originally in a biographical sketch of Lavalette, published in the *Revue de Paris*, and is related by Lavalette as occurring to him while in prison :

" One night, while I was asleep, the clock of the Palais de Justice struck twelve and awoke me. I heard the gate open to relieve the sentry, but I fell asleep again immediately. In this sleep I dreamt that I was standing in the Rue St. Honoré. A melancholy darkness spread around me ; all was still ; nevertheless, a slow and uncertain sound soon arose. All of a sudden I perceived at the bottom of the street, and advancing toward me, a troop of cavalry—the men and horses, however, all flayed. The men held torches in their hands, the red flames of which illuminated faces without skin, and bloody muscles. Their hollow eyes rolled fearfully in their sockets, their mouths opened from ear to ear, and helmets of hanging flesh covered their hideous heads. The horses dragged along their own skins in the kennels, which overflowed with blood on all sides. Pale and dishevelled women appeared and disappeared at the windows in dismal silence ; low, inarticulate groans filled the air, and I remained in the street alone petrified with horror, and deprived of strength sufficient to seek my safety in flight. This horrible troop continued passing along rapidly in a gallop, and casting frightful looks upon me. Their march continued, I thought, for five hours, and

[1] " Dream Thought and Dream Life." *Medical Critic and Psychological Journal*," No. vi, April, 1862, p. 199.

they were followed by an immense number of artillery wagons full of bleeding corpses, whose limbs still quivered ; a disgusting smell of blood and bitumen almost choked me. At length the iron gates of the prison, shutting with great force, awoke me again. I made my repeater strike ; it was no more than midnight, so that the horrible phantasmagoria had lasted no more than two or three minutes—that is to say, the time necessary for relieving the sentry and shutting the gate. The cold was severe and the watchword short. The next day the turnkey confirmed my calculations. I, nevertheless, do not remember one single event in my life the duration of which I have been able more exactly to calculate, of which the details are deeper engraven on my memory, and of which I preserve a more perfect consciousness."

No instance can more strikingly exemplify aberration of the faculty of judgment than the above. There was no astonishment felt with the horror experienced, but all the impossible events which appeared to be occurring were accepted as facts, which might have taken place in the regular order of nature.

An important question connected with the exercise of judgment is : Does the dreamer know that he is dreaming ? Some authors assert that this knowledge is possible, others that it is not. The following account is interesting, and I therefore transcribe it, especially as it has not to my knowledge been heretofore published in this country.

In a letter to the Rev. William Gregory, Dr. Thomas Reid [1] says :

"About the age of fourteen I was almost every night unhappy in my sleep from frightful dreams. Sometimes hanging over a frightful precipice and just ready to drop down ; sometimes pursued for my life and stopped by a wall or by a sudden loss of all strength ; sometimes ready to be devoured by a wild beast. How long I was plagued by such dreams I do not now recollect. I believe it was for a year or two at least ; and I think they had quite left me before I was fifteen. In those days I was much given to what Mr. Addison in one of his 'Spectators' calls castle-building, and, in my evening solitary walk, which was generally all the exercise I took,

---

[1] " Account of the Life and Writings of Thomas Reid, D. D.," p. cxliv, prefixed to " Essays on the Powers of the Human Mind." By Thomas Reid, D. D., etc., Edinburgh, 1803, vol. i.

my thoughts would hurry me into some active scene, where I generally acquitted myself much to my own satisfaction, and in these scenes of imagination I performed many a gallant exploit. At the same time, in my dreams, I found myself the most arrant coward that ever was. Not only my courage, but my strength failed me in every danger, and I often rose from my bed in the morning in such a panic that it took some time to get the better of it. I wished very much to get free of these uneasy dreams, which not only made me unhappy in sleep, but often left a disagreeable impression in my mind for some part of the following day. I thought it was worth trying whether it was possible to recollect that it was all a dream, and that I was in no real danger. I often went to sleep with my mind as strongly impressed as I could with this thought, that I never in my lifetime was in any real danger, and that every fright I had was a dream. After many fruitless endeavors to recollect this when the danger appeared, I effected it at last, and have often, when I was sliding over a precipice into the abyss, recollected that it was all a dream, and boldly jumped down. The effect of this commonly was, that I immediately awoke. But I awoke calm and intrepid, which I thought a great acquisition. After this my dreams were never very uneasy, and, in a short time, I dreamt not at all."

Beattie[1] states that he once dreamt that he was walking on the parapet of a high bridge. How he came there he did not know, but, recollecting that he was not given to such pranks, he began to think it might all be a dream, and, finding his situation unpleasant, and being desirious to get out of it, threw himself headlong from the height, in the belief that the shock of the fall would restore his senses. The event turned out as he anticipated.

Aristotle also asserts that, when dreaming of danger, he used to recollect that he was dreaming, and that he ought not to be frightened.

A still more remarkable narration is that of Gassendi,[2] which he thus relates as occurring to himself:

"A good friend of mine, Louis Charambon, judge of the criminal court at Digne, had died of the plague. One night,

---

[1] "Dissertations, Moral and Critical," London, 1783, art. "Dreaming," p. 222.
[2] "Syntagma philosophicum," pars 71, lib. viii. "Opera omnia," t. i, Lugduni, 1658.

as I slept, I seemed to see him ; I stretched out my arms toward him, and said : ' Hail thou who returnest from the place of the dead ! ' Then I stopped, reflecting in my dream as follows : ' One cannot return from the other world ; I am doubtless dreaming ; but, if I dream, where am I ? Not at Paris, for I came last to Digne. I am, then, at Digne, in my house, in my bedroom, in my bed.' And then, as I was looking for myself in the bed, some noise, I know not what, awoke me."

In all these and like instances it is very probable the individuals were much more awake than asleep, for certainly the power to judge correctly is not exercised in dreams, involving even the most incongruous impossibilities. As Dendy[1] says, " if we *know* that we are dreaming, the faculty of judgment cannot be inert, and the dream would be known to be a fallacy." There would therefore be no occasion for any such management of it as that made use of by Reid and Beattie, or for the recollection of Aristotle. The dream and the correction of it by the judgment would go together, and there would be no self-deception at all—not even for an instant. Dreams would accordingly be impossible. The essential feature of mental activity during sleep—absolute freedom of the imagination—would not exist.

Relative to Gassendi's case, it is impossible to believe that he was fully asleep, and the fact that he was awakened by some noise, the nature of which was unrecognized, and which was therefore probably slight, tends to support this view. Moreover, although he was, as he thought, enabled to detect the fallacy of his dream in one respect, his judgment was altogether at fault in others. Thus, he had great difficulty in making out where he was, and actually so far lost all idea of his identity with the person dreaming as to look for himself in his own bed ! Certainly an individual whose judgment was thus much deranged would scarcely be able to reason correctly as to the fact of his dreaming or not, or to question the possibility of the dead returning to this world.

My opinion therefore is, that during sleep the power of bringing the judgment into action is suspended. We do not actually lose the power of arriving at a decision, but we cannot exert the faculty of judgment in accordance with the principles of truth and of correct reasoning. An opinion may therefore be formed during sleep, but it is more likely to be

[1] " Philosophy of Mystery," London, 1841, p. 208.

wrong than right, and no effort that we can make will enable us to distinguish the false from the true, or to discriminate between the possible and the impossible.

That faculty of the mind—the judgment—which when we are awake is pre-eminently our guide, can no longer direct us aright. The stores of experience go for naught, and the mind accepts as truth whatever preposterous thought the imagination presents to it. We are not entirely rendered incapable of judging, as some authors assert, but the power to perceive the logical force of circumstances, to take them at their true value and to eliminate error from our mental processes, is altogether arrested, and we arrive at absurd conclusions from impossible premises.

But there is no doubt that at times the faculty of judgment is suspended as regards some parts of our mental operations during sleep and this to such an extent that we are, like Gassendi in the case quoted, not capable of recognizing our own individuality. Thus it is related of Dr. Johnson, that he had once in a dream a contest of wit with some other person, and that he was very much mortified by imagining that his opponent had the better of him. "Now," said he, "one may mark here the effect of sleep in weakening the power of reflection; for, had not my judgment failed me, I should have seen that the wit of this supposed antagonist, by whose superiority I felt myself depressed, was as much furnished by me as that which I thought I had been uttering in my own character."

Van Goens dreamt that he could not answer questions to which his neighbor gave correct responses.

An interesting case, in which the judgment was still more at fault, has recently come to my knowledge.

Mrs. C. dreamt that she was Savonarola, and that she was preaching to a vast assembly in Florence. Among the audience was a lady whom she at once recognized to be her own self. As Savonarola, she was delighted at this discovery, for she reflected that she was well acquainted with all Mrs. C.'s peculiarities and faults of character, and would therefore be enabled to give special emphasis to them in the sermon. She did this so very effectively that Mrs. C. burst into a torrent of tears, and, with the emotion thus excited, the lady awoke. It was some time before she was able to disentangle her mixed-up individualities. When she became fully awake she perceived that the arguments she had employed to bring about the conversion of herself were puerile in the extreme, and were directed against characteristics which formed no part of her mental organization, and against offences which she had not committed.

Macario[1] makes the following apposite remarks on the point under consideration. Referring to the preposterous nature of many dreams, he says:

"It is astonishing that all these fantastical and impossible visions seem to us quite natural, and excite no astonishment. This is because the judgment and reflection, having abdicated, no longer control the imagination nor co-ordinate the thoughts which rush tumultuously through the brain of the sleeper, combined only by the power of association.

"When I say that the judgment and reflection abdicate, it should not be inferred that they are abolished and no longer exist, for the imagination could not, unaided by the reason, construct the whimsical and capricious images of dreams."

Relative to the power to work out, during sleep, problems involving long and intricate mental processes, I have already expressed my opinion adversely. In this view I am not alone. Rosenkranz,[2] whose contributions to psychological science cannot be overestimated, and whose clear and powerful understanding has rarely been excelled, has pointed out how such operations of the understanding are impossible; for, as he remarks, intellectual problems cannot be solved during sleep, for such a thing as intense thought, accompanied by images, is unknown, while dreams consist of a series of images connected by loose and imperfect reasoning. Feuchtersleben,[3] referring with approval to this opinion of Rosenkranz, says that he recollects perfectly having dreamed of such problems, and, being happy in their solution, endeavored to retain them in his memory ; he succeeded, but discovered, on awaking, that they were quite unmeaning, and could only have imposed upon a sleeping imagination.

Müller[4] says :

[1] *Op. cit.*, p. 286.

[2] " Psychologie ; oder der Wissenschaft von subjectiven Geist," 2ten Auflage, Elberfeld, 1843, p. 144.

[3] "The Principles of Medical Psychology," etc., Sydenham Society Translation, p. 167.

[4] " Elements of Physiology." Translated from the German, with Notes, by William Baly, M. D., etc., London, 1842, vol. ii, p. 1417.

"Sometimes we reason more or less correctly in dreams. We reflect on problems, and rejoice in their solution. But, on awaking from such dreams, the seeming reasoning is frequently found to have been no reasoning at all, and the solution of the problem over which we had rejoiced, to be mere nonsense. Sometimes we dream that another person proposes an enigma ; that we cannot solve it, and that others are equally incapable of doing so ; but that the person who proposed it himself gives the explanation. We are astonished at the solution we had so long labored in vain to find. If we do not immediately awaken and afterward reflect on this proposition of an enigma in our dream, and on its apparent solution, we think it wonderful ; but if we awake immediately after the dream, and are able to compare the answer with the question, we find that it was mere nonsense."

And in regard to the knowledge that we are dreaming, the same author [1] observes that :

"The indistinctness of the conception in dreams is generally so great that we are not aware that we dream. The phantasms which are perceived really exist in our organs of sense. They afford, therefore, in themselves as strong proof of the actual existence of the objects they represent as our own perceptions of real external objects in the waking state ; for we know the latter only by the affections of our senses which they produce. When, therefore, the mind has lost the faculty of analyzing the impressions on our senses, there is no reason why the things which they seem to represent should be supposed unreal. Even in the waking state phantasms are regarded as real objects when they occur to persons of feeble intellect. On the other hand, when the dreaming approaches more nearly to the waking state, we sometimes are conscious that we merely dream, and still allow the dream to proceed, while we retain this consciousness of its true nature."

Sir Benjamin Brodie,[2] in discussing the subject of wonderful discoveries made in dreams, and abstruse problems worked out, remarks that it would indeed be strange if, among the vast number of combinations which constitute our dreams, there were not every now and then some having the semblance of reality ; and further, that, in many of the stories of great discoveries made in dreams, there is much of either mistake or

[1] *Op. cit.*, p. 1418.
[2] "Psychological Inquiries," part i, London, 1856, p. 153.

exaggeration, and that, if they could have been written down at the time, they would have been found to be worth little or nothing.

Another faculty exercised during sleep has been ascribed to the judgment. It is well known that many persons having made up their minds to awake at a certain hour invariably do so. I possess this power in a high degree, and scarcely ever vary a minute from the fixed time. Just as I go to bed I look at my watch and impress upon my mind the figures on the dial which represent the hour and minute at which I wish to awake. I give myself no further anxiety on the subject, and never dream of it, but I always wake at the desired moment.

Now, I cannot conceive what connection the judgment has with this power. In the case of alarm-clocks set to go off at a certain time, the judgment, as Jouffroy [1] asserts, may take cognizance of the impression made upon the ear, and establish the relation between it and the wish to awake at a certain time. But in cases where the awaking is the result of an idea conceived before going to sleep, and which is not subsequently recalled, the judgment cannot act, for this faculty is only exercised upon ideas which are submitted to it. The brain is, as it were, wound up like the alarm-clock and set to a certain hour. When that hour arrives, an explosion of nervous force takes place, and the individual awakes.

Fosgate [2] asserts that the power of judging during sleep is probably as good as when we are awake, for decisions are made only on the premises presented in either case, and, if those in the former condition are absurd or unreasonable, the conclusion will likewise be faulty. But this is not very accurate reasoning ; for it is as much the province of the judgment to determine the validity of the premises as it is to draw a conclusion from them, and, if it cannot recognize the falsity or truth of propositions the irrational character of which would be readily perceived during wakefulness, there is not much to be said in favor of its power.

In fact, however, the conclusions formed in dreams are often without any logical relation with the premises. Thus,

[1] "Du sommeil—mélanges philosophiques," seconde édition, Paris, 1858, p. 301.

[2] " Sleep psychologically considered with reference to Sensation and Memory," New York, 1850, p. 74.

when an individual dreams, as in the instance previously quoted, that he is a column of stone, it is contrary to all experience to deduce therefrom the conclusion that he can see rocks crumbling around him, and can reflect upon the mutability of all things. The premise of his being a stone pillar being submitted to the judgment, the proper conclusion would be that he is composed of inorganic material, is devoid of life, and, consequently, not possessed of either sensation or understanding.

Why the judgment is not properly exercised during sleep we do not know. Dr. Philip[1] believes that in this condition ideas flow so rapidly that they are not submitted to the full power of the judgment, and that hence the absurdity which characterizes them is not perceived. But this explanation is by no means satisfactory; for a merely swift succession of ideas is no very serious bar to correct judgment, and when the thoughts are as preposterous as those which so often occur in dreams, they present no obstacle at all to a proper estimation of them by the healthy mind. The cause properly resides in some alteration in the circulation of the blood in that part of the brain which presides over the judgment, whereby its power is suspended and the imagination left free to fill the mind with its incongruous and fantastic images.

As regards the will, we find very opposite opinions entertained relative to its activity; but no one, so far as I am aware, appears to have had correct views upon the subject. Without going into a full discussion of the views enunciated, it will be sufficient to refer to the ideas on the point in question which have been expressed by some of the most eminent philosophers and physiologists.

In the course of his remarks on sleep, Darwin[2] repeatedly alleges that during this condition the action of the will is entirely suspended; but he falls into the singular error of confounding volition with the power of motion. Thus he says:

"When by one continued posture in sleep some uneasy sensations are produced, we either gradually awake by the exertion of volition, or the muscles connected by habit with such sensations alter the position of the body; but where the

---

[1] "An Inquiry into the Nature of Sleep and Death," London, 1834, p. 152. (Reprinted from the "Philosophical Transactions" for 1833.)

[2] "Zoonomia; or, The Laws of Organic Life," Am. ed., vol. i, Philadelphia, 1818, p. 153.

sleep is uncommonly profound, and these uneasy sensations great, the disease called the incubus or nightmare is produced. Here the desire of moving the body is painfully exerted ; but the power of moving it, or volition, is incapable of action till we are awake."

In consequence of this misapprehension of the nature of the will, it is not easy to arrive at Darwin's ideas on the subject; and the attempt is rendered still more difficult from the fact that, though he repeatedly states that volition is entirely suspended during sleep, he yet in the first part of the foregoing quotation makes an individual awake by the gradual exercise of the power of the will ; and then in the last part of the same paragraph asserts that volition is incapable of action till sleep is over.

Mr. Dugald Stewart [1] contends that during sleep the power of volition is not suspended, but that those operations of the mind and body which depend on volition cease to be exercised. In his opinion the will loses its influence over all our powers both of mind and body in consequence of some physical alteration in the system which we shall never probably be able to explain. To show in full the views of so distinguished a philosopher as Mr. Stewart, I quote the following extracts from his remarks on the subject :

"In order to illustrate this conclusion [the one above stated] a little further, it may be proper to remark that, if the suspension of our voluntary operations in sleep be admitted as a fact, there are only two suppositions which can be formed regarding its cause. The one is that the power of volition is suspended ; the other that the will loses its influence over those faculties of the mind and those members of the body which during our waking hours are subjected to its authority. If it can be shown, then, that the former supposition is not agreeable to fact, the truth of the latter seems to follow as a necessary consequence.

"1. That the power of volition is not suspended during sleep appears from the efforts which we are conscious of making while in that situation. We dream, for instance, that we are in danger, and we attempt to call out for assistance. The attempt, indeed, is in general unsuccessful, and the sounds that we emit are feeble and indistinct ; but this

[1] "Elements of the Philosophy of the Human Mind," Am. ed., Boston, 1818, vol. i, p. 184.

only confirms, or rather is a necessary consequence of, the supposition that in sleep the connection between the will and our voluntary operations is disturbed or interrupted. The continuance of the power of volition is demonstrated by the effort, however ineffectual.

"In like manner, in the course of an alarming dream we are sometimes conscious of making an exertion to save ourselves by flight from an apprehended danger; but, in spite of all our efforts, we continue in bed. In such cases we commonly dream that we are attempting to escape and are prevented by some external obstacle; but the fact seems to be that the body is at that time not subject to the will. During the disturbed rest which we sometimes have when the body is indisposed, the mind appears to retain some power over it; but as even in these cases the motions which are made consist rather of a general agitation of the whole system than of the regular exertion of a particular member of it with a view to produce a certain effect, it is reasonable to conclude that in perfectly sound sleep the mind, although it retains the power of volition, retains no influence whatever over the bodily organs.

"In that particular condition of the system which is known by the name of *incubus* we are conscious of a total want of power over the body; and I believe the common opinion is that it is this want of power which distinguishes the *incubus* from all the other modifications of sleep. But the more probable supposition seems to be that every species of sleep is accompanied with a suspension of the faculty of voluntary motion; and that the incubus has nothing peculiar in it but this—that the uneasy sensations which are produced by the accidental posture of the body, and which we find it impossible to remove by our own efforts, render us distinctly conscious of our incapacity to move. One thing is certain, that the instant of our awaking and of our recovering the command of our bodily organs is one and the same.

"2. The same conclusion is confirmed by a different view of the subject. It is probable, as was already observed, that when we are anxious to procure sleep, the state into which we naturally bring the mind approaches to its state after sleep commences. Now, it is manifest that the means which nature directs us to employ on such occasions is not to suspend the powers of volition, but to suspend the exertion of those powers whose exercise depends on volition. If it were necessary that volition should be suspended before we fall asleep, it would be impossible for us by our own efforts to hasten the moment of rest. The very supposition of such efforts is absurd, for it implies a continued will to suspend the acts of the will.

"According to the foregoing doctrine with respect to the state of the mind in sleep, the effort which is produced on our mental operations is strikingly analogous to that which is produced on our bodily powers. From the observations which have been already made, it is manifest that in sleep the body is in a very inconsiderable degree, if at all, subject to our command. The vital and involuntary motions, however, suffer no interruption, but go on as when we are awake, in consequence of the operation of some cause unknown to us. In like manner it would appear that those operations of the mind which depend on our volition are suspended, while certain other operations are at least occasionally carried on. This analogy naturally suggests the idea that all our mental operations which are independent of our will may continue during sleep; and that the phenomena of dreaming may, perhaps, be produced by these, diversified in their apparent effects in consequence of the suspension of our voluntary powers."

A very little reflection will suffice to convince the reader that Mr. Stewart has altogether mistaken the nature of sleep. There is no evidence to support his view that the body is not subject to the action of the will during sleep. No change whatever is induced by this condition in the nerves or muscles of the organism. The first are just as capable as ever of conducting the nervous fluid, and the muscles do not lose any of their contractile power. The reason why voluntary movements are not performed in sleep is simply because the will does not act; and Mr. Stewart is again wrong in asserting that volition is not then suspended. We do not will any actions when we are asleep. We *imagine* we do, and that is all. The difficulties which encompass us in sleep are, it must be recollected, purely imaginary, and the efforts we make to escape from them are likewise the products of our fancy. Herein lies the main error which Mr. Stewart has committed. He appears to accept the dream for a reality, and to regard the seeming volitions which occur in it as actual facts, whereas they are all entirely fictitious.

An example will serve to make this point still clearer.

Not long since I dreamed that I stood upon a very high perpendicular table-land, at the foot of which flowed a river. I thought I experienced an irresistible desire to approach the brink and to look down. Had I been awake, such a wish would have been the very last to enter my mind, for I have an instinctive dread of standing on a height. I dreamed that I threw myself on my face and crawled to the edge of the cliff. I looked down at the stream, which scarcely appeared to be as wide as my hand, so great was the altitude upon which I was placed. As I looked I felt an overpowering impulse to crawl still farther and to throw myself into the water below. I imagined that I endeavored with all my will to resist this force, which appeared to be acting by means altogether external to my organism. My efforts, however, were all in vain. I could not control my movements, and gradually I was urged farther and farther over the brink, till at last I went down into the abyss below. As I struck the water I awoke with a start. During my imaginary struggle I thought I experienced all the emotions which such an event if real would have excited, and I was painfully conscious of my utter inability to escape from the peril of my situation. Here were circumstances such as, according to Mr. Stewart, demonstrate the activity of volition, but at the same time show its inability to act upon the body. But clearly they show no such thing, for the imaginary volition was to refrain from crawling over a precipice which did not exist, and over which, therefore, I was not hanging. Such an act of the will, if real, could not, in the very nature of the real conditions of the situation, have been carried out ; the volition was just as imaginary as all the other circumstances of the dream.

Again, it is not always the case that the imaginary acts of the will are not executed during sleep ; and hence it would follow from Mr. Stewart's argument that the power of the will over the body is not then suspended. Assuming for the moment that the volitions of sleep are real, as Mr. Stewart supposes; if it can be shown that they are satisfactorily performed, it results from his line of reasoning that the will has power over the body during sleep. Every one who has ever dreamed has at times had his will carried out to his entire satisfaction. He has ridden horses when pursued, and has urged them forward with whip and spur so as to escape from his enemies. Or he has executed the most surprising feats both with his mind and body, and has performed voluntary deeds which have excited the admiration of all beholders. Such acts are, of course, entirely the product of the imagination, and all the volitions which accompany them have no firmer basis than the unbridled fancy ; but, according to Mr. Stewart, they would be evidence of the power of the will over the body—a power which in reality does not exist; not, however, as Mr. Stewart supposes, from any impediments in the nerves or muscles, but because it is never exerted.

So far as relates to movements performed during sleep, such as turning in bed and assuming more comfortable positions, they have nothing whatever to do with the will. They are dependent upon the action of the spinal cord, an organ that is never at rest, and the functions of which were not known as well when Dr. Darwin and Mr. Stewart wrote as they are now. The same is true of more complex and longer-continued actions, such as those already mentioned of individuals riding on horseback, or even walking, during sleep.

Cabanis[1] contends that the will is not entirely suspended during sleep; but, as will be perceived from the following quotation, he bases his argument upon the fact that movements are produced which he attributes erroneously to the action of the will, but which, like those previously referred to, are accomplished by the agency of the spinal cord. He says, speaking of the instances of persons walking while asleep:

"These rare cases are not the only ones in which during sleep movements are produced by what remains of the will; for it is by virtue of certain direct sensations that a sleeping man moves his arm to brush away the flies that may be on his face, that he draws up the bedclothes so as to cover himself carefully ; or, as we have already remarked, that he turns over and endeavors to find a more comfortable position. It is the will which during sleep maintains the contraction of the sphincter of the bladder, notwithstanding the effort of the urine to escape; it is the same power which directs the action of the arm in seeking for the *vase de nuit*, which knows where to find it, and enables the individual to use it for several minutes and to return it to its place without being awakened. Finally, it is not without reason that some physiolo-

---

[1] *Op. cit.*, t. ii, p. 376, *et seq.*, art. "Du sommeil en particulier."

gists have made the will concur in the contraction of several muscles, the movements of which are necessary to the maintenance of respiration during sleep.''

All these movements, and many others of a similar character, are entirely spinal, and are altogether independent of cerebral influence. Even when we are awake, we constantly execute muscular actions through the power of the spinal cord, when the mind is intently occupied with other things. Take, for instance, the example of a person playing on the piano, and at the same time carrying on a conversation. Here the brain is engaged in the one act and the spinal cord in the other. So long as the player is not expert in the fingering of the instrument, he cannot divert his attention from his performance; for the whole power of the mind is required for the proper appreciation and execution of the music. But after the spinal cord has become educated to the habit, and he has attained proficiency in the necessary manipulations, the mind is no longer required to control the actions, and may be directed to other subjects. The arguments of Cabanis, therefore, in favor of the partial exercise of the will during sleep, are of no force.

But the power of the will over the muscles of the body is only one of the ways in which this faculty is shown. It regulates the thoughts and the manifestations of emotion when we are awake. How utterly incapable it is of any such action during sleep we all know. A gentleman, remarkable for the ability he possesses for controlling his feelings, tells me that when he is asleep he frequently weeps or laughs at imaginary events, which, if they really had occurred to him during wakefulness, would give rise to no such disturbance. He often desires to stop these emotional manifestations, but is entirely powerless to do so. Most individuals have had similar experiences.

The theory that the will is in action during sleep is, therefore, to my mind untenable. It has probably had its origin in the idea that confounds it with desire, from which it differs so markedly that it seems strange the distinction should ever fail of being made. Locke [1] points out very clearly the differences between the two faculties. In fact, they may be exerted in directly opposite ways. Desire often precedes volition; but we all, at times, will acts which are contrary to

[1] " An Essay concerning Human Understanding," chap. xxi, section 30.

our desire, and desire to perform others which we are unable to will.

Reid [1] writes with great perspicuity on this distinction between desire and will. He says:

"Desire and will agree in this, that both must have an object of which we must have some conception; and, therefore, both must be accompanied with some degree of understanding. But they differ in several things.

"The object of desire may be anything which appetite, passion, or affection leads us to pursue; it may be any event which we think good for us, or for those to whom we are well affected. I may desire meat or drink, or ease from pain. But to say that I will meat, or will drink, or will ease from pain, is not English. There is, therefore, a distinction in common language between desire and will. And the distinction is, that what we will must be an action, and our own action; what we desire may not be our own action, it may be no action at all.

"A man desires that his children may be happy, and that they may behave well. Their being happy is no action at all; their behaving well is not his action, but theirs.

"With regard to our own actions, we may desire what we do not will, and will what we do not desire; nay, what we have a great aversion to.

"A man athirst has a strong desire to drink; but for some particular reason he determines not to gratify his desire. A judge, from a regard to justice, and to the duty of his office, dooms a criminal to die, while, from humanity or particular affection, he desires that he should live. A man for health may take a nauseous draught, for which he has no desire, but a great aversion. Desire, therefore, even when its object is some action of our own, is only an incitement to will; but it is not volition. The determination of the mind may be not to do what we desire to do. But, as desire is often accompanied by will, we are apt to overlook the distinction between them."

That desire is manifested during sleep there can be no doubt; and Mr. Stewart, although insisting as he does on the distinction between this faculty and volition, confounds them in his remarks already quoted. A person suffering from nightmare has a most intense desire to escape from his im-

[1] "Essays on the Powers of the Human Mind," vol. iii, Edinburgh, 1803, p. 77.

14

aginary troubles. In my own dream, to which reference has been made, my desire to restrain myself from crawling over the precipice was exerted to the utmost; but the will could not be brought into action. Darwin,[1] when he says that in nightmare "the *desire* of moving the body is painfully exerted, but the *power of moving it, or volition,* is incapable of action till we awake," makes the proper distinction between desire and will; but, as I have already shown, confounds the latter with another very different faculty.

From the foregoing observations it will be seen that during sleep the three great divisions of the mind are differently affected.

1. Feeling, embracing sensation and emotion, is suspended, so far as the first is concerned; but is in full action as regards the second. We do not see, hear, smell, taste, or enjoy the sense of touch in sleep, although the brain may be aroused into activity and we may awake through the excitations conveyed to it by the special senses. The emotions have full play, unrestrained by the will, and governed only by the imagination.

2. The Will or Volition is entirely suspended.

3. The Thought or Intellect is variously affected in its different powers. The imagination is active, and the memory may be exercised to a great extent; but the judgment, perception, conception, abstraction, and reason are weakened, and sometimes altogether lost.

CHAPTER V.

THE PHYSIOLOGY OF DREAMS.

THE subject of the foregoing chapter is so intimately connected with the phenomena of dreaming, and I have expressed my views in regard to it at such length, that but few psychological points remain to be considered in the present discussion. What I have to say, therefore, in regard to the physiology of dreaming must be read in connection with the chapter on "The State of the Mind during Sleep," in order that the whole matter may be fully understood.

[1] *Op. cit.*, p. 155.

It is contended by some writers that the mind is never at rest, and that even during the most profound sleep dreams take place, which are either forgotten immediately, or which make no impression on the memory. That this view is erroneous is, I think, very evident. If it were correct, the first object of sleep—rest for the brain—would not be attained. We all know how fatigued we are, and how indisposed to exertion the brain is, after a night of continued dreaming, and we can easily imagine what would be the consequences if such a condition were kept up night after night. To say that we really do dream not only every night, but every instant of the night—in fact, always and continually when we sleep—but that we forget our dreams as soon as they are formed, remembering solely those which are most vivid, is making assertions which not only are without proof, but which are impossible of proof. For, if, as Locke [1] remarks, the sleeping man on awaking has no recollection of his thoughts, it is very certain that no one else can recollect them for him.

The observations of Locke on this point are extremely appropriate, and, to my mind, very philosophical and logical. After insisting that, sleeping or waking, a man cannot think without being sensible of it, he says : [2]

"I grant that the soul of a waking man is never without thought, because it is the condition of being awake ; but whether sleeping without dreaming be not an affection of the whole man, mind as well as body, may be worth a waking man's consideration, it being hard to conceive that anything should think and not be conscious of it. If the soul doth think in a sleeping man without being conscious of it, I ask, whether during such thinking it has any pleasure or pain, or be capable of happiness or misery ? I am sure the man is not, any more than the bed or earth he lies on, for to be happy or miserable without being conscious of it seems to me utterly inconsistent and impossible. Or if it be possible that the soul can, while the body is sleeping, have its thinkings, enjoyments, and concerns, its pleasure or pain, about which the man is not conscious of nor partakes in, it is certain that Socrates asleep and Socrates awake is not the same person ; but his soul when he sleeps and Socrates the man, consisting of body and soul when he is waking, are two persons, since wak-

[1] " An Essay concerning the Human Understanding," book ii, section 17.
[2] *Op. et loc. cit.*, section 11.

ing Socrates has no knowledge of or concernment for that happiness or misery of his soul which it enjoys alone by itself while he sleeps without perceiving anything of it, any more than he has for the happiness or misery of a man in the Indies whom he knows not; for if we take wholly away all consciousness of our actions and sensations, especially of pleasure and pain, and the concernment that accompanies it, it will be hard to know wherein to place personal identity."

In a subsequent section of the same chapter Locke asserts that most men pass a great part of their lives without dreaming, and that he once knew a scholar who had no bad memory, who told him he had never dreamed in his life till after the occurrence of a fever in the twenty-fifth or twenty-sixth year of his age.

Examples of persons who have not ordinarily dreamed are adduced by the ancient writers. Pliny [1] refers to men who never dreamed. Plutarch [2] alludes to the case of Cleon, who, in living to an advanced age, had yet never dreamed; and Suetonius [3] declares that before the murder of his mother Nero had never dreamed.

A lady who was under my care for a serious nervous affection declared to me that she never had had but one dream in her life, and that was after receiving a severe fall in which she struck her head.

And yet, notwithstanding the experience of every one that sleep often happens without the accompaniment of dreams, the great majority of writers hold the view that the brain is never at rest. Doubtless this opinion has its origin partly in the doctrine that the mind is a something altogether independent of and superior to the brain. They appear to be incapable of appreciating the fact that when the brain is in a state of complete repose there can be no mental manifestation, and that all intellectual phenomena are the results of cerebral activity. Another cause for their belief is the fact that they make no distinction between dreaming and thinking, whereas it is very evident that the two are not to be placed in the same category. Thinking is an *action* which requires cerebral effort, and which is undertaken with a determinate purpose. We will to think, and we think what we please; but it is very

---

[1] " Historia naturalis," lib. x, cap. lxxv, " De somno animalium."
[2] " De defectu oraculorum."
[3] " De vita xii. Cæsarum," " Nero," cap. xlvi.

different with our dreams, which come and go without any power on our part to regulate or direct them. To think requires all the faculties of the mind; to dream necessitates only the memory and the imagination. In thinking, the brain is active in all its parts; in dreaming, it is nearly entirely quiescent.

Writers who contend for the doctrine of constant mental activity regard the brain as the organ or tool of the mind, a structure which the mind makes use of in order to manifest itself. Such a theory is certain to lead them into difficulties, and is contrary to all the teaching of physiology. The full discussion of this question would be out of place here; I will, therefore, only repeat what has been said in the first chapter, that this work is written from the stand-point of regarding the mind as nothing more than the result of cerebral action. Just as a good liver secretes good bile, a good candle gives good light, and good coal a good fire, so does a good brain give a good mind. When the brain is quiescent there is no mind.

Lemoine[1] begins his chapter "On the State of the Mind during Sleep" with the assertion that "there is no sleep for the mind." He is obliged, however, to admit that, "when the organs of the body are benumbed by sleep, the mind appears to be in a particular state; it seems to be submitted to other laws than those which govern it during wakefulness; it seems to have lost for a time its most precious faculties."

During sleep the mind is, as he supposes, in a particular state, for, as has been shown in the previous chapter, it has lost many of its chief parts. The laws which govern it are, however, the same which always regulate it. The body from which its power is primarily derived—the brain—is not in the same condition during sleep as during wakefulness, and hence the differences in the evidences of cerebral activity.

Sir William Hamilton[2] is generally considered to have determined affirmatively the question of the continuance of the action of the brain during sleep. He caused himself to be aroused from sleep at intervals through the night, and invariably found that he was disturbed from a dream, the particulars of which he could always distinctly recollect. But a full knowledge of the subject he was investigating would have sufficed to convince Sir William that the conclusion he drew from his experiments was altogether fallacious. It is well

[1] *Op. cit.*, p. 63.   [2] "Lectures on Metaphysics," vol. i, p. 323.

known that dreams are excited by strong impressions made upon the senses, or by irritations arising in the internal organs. Thus Baron Trenck relates that when confined in his dungeon he suffered the pangs of hunger almost continually, and that his dreams at night were always of delicate meats and sumptuous repasts, spread before him on luxuriously furnished tables. The mere excitation of waking a sleeping person is generally sufficient to give rise to a dream. Maury, in his very interesting work, to which reference has already been made, and which will hereafter be more specifically considered, adduces many examples of dreams produced by sensorial impressions. I have myself performed many experiments with reference to this point, and have generally found ample confirmation of Maury's investigations. It may therefore, I think, be assumed, without any violence to the actual facts of the cases, that the brain is not always in action, and that there are times when we sleep without dreaming.

In the previous chapter the idea is sought to be conveyed that we originate nothing in our dreams. We may conceive of things which never existed, or of which we have heard or read, but the images we make of them are either composed of elements familiar to us, or else are based upon ideal representations which we have formed in our waking moments. Thus, before the discovery of America no Europeans ever dreamed of American Indians, for the reason that nothing existed within their knowledge which could give any idea of the appearance of such human beings. It is possible that Columbus and his companions may have dreamed of the continent of which they were in search, and of its natives, but the images formed of the latter must necessarily have resembled other beings they had seen, or which they had heard described. After the discovery, however, it was no unusual thing for the Spaniards and others to have correct images of Indians appear to them in their dreams.

Dreams, therefore, must have a foundation, and this is either impressions made upon the mind at some previous period, or produced during sleep by bodily sensations. These impressions, however they may be formed, are subjected to the unrestrained influence of the imagination.

At first sight it may seem that we often have dreams not excited by actual sensations, and which have no relation to any events of our lives, or any ideas which have passed through our minds, but thorough investigation will invariably reveal the existence of an association between the dream and some such ideas or events. For instance, some time ago I dreamed that a gentleman, a friend of mine, had invented what he called a "dog-cart ambulance," a vehicle which he declared was the best ever made for the transportation of sick or wounded men. On awaking, all the particulars were fresh in my mind, but I could not for some time perceive why I had had such a dream. At last I recollected that the morning before a gentleman had given me a very full description of Prospect Park, in Brooklyn. The friend of whom I dreamed has charge of the construction of this park. His presence was, therefore, fully explained, and, as dog-carts are driven in parks, this link was also accounted for. The ambulance part was due to the fact that I had that same morning found the card of a gentleman upon my table who really had invented an ambulance. The imagination had, therefore, taken these data supplied by the memory, and had combined them into the incongruous web constituting my dream.

Dreams are also frequently built upon circumstances which have occurred many years previously, and which have long since apparently passed from our recollection. A very striking instance of this kind is related by Abercrombie,[1] on the authority of Sir Walter Scott.

"Mr. R. J. Rowland, a gentleman of landed property in the vale of Gala, was prosecuted for a very considerable sum, the accumulated arrears of teind (tithe), for which he was said to be indebted to a noble family the titulars (lay impropriators of the tithe). Mr. R. was strongly impressed with the belief that his father had, by a form of process peculiar to the law of Scotland, purchased these teinds from the titular, and, therefore, that the present prosecution was groundless. But, after an industrious search among his father's papers, an investigation of the public records, and a careful inquiry among all persons who had transacted law business for his father, no evidence could be discovered to support his defence. The period was now near at hand when he conceived the loss of his lawsuit to be inevitable, and he had formed his determination to ride to Edinburgh next day and make the best bargain he could in the way of compromise. He went to bed

[1] "Inquiries concerning the Intellectual Powers and the Investigation of Truth," tenth edition, London, 1840, p. 283.

with this resolution, and, with all the circumstances of the case floating upon his mind, had a dream to the following purpose. His father, who had been many years dead, appeared to him, he thought, and asked him why he was disturbed in his mind. In dreams men are not surprised at such apparitions. Mr. R. thought that he informed his father of the cause of his distress, adding that the payment of a considerable sum of money was the more unpleasant to him because he had a stray consciousness that it was not due, though he was unable to recover any evidence in support of his belief. 'You are right, my son,' replied the paternal shade; 'I did acquire right to these teinds, for payment of which you are now prosecuted. The papers relating to the transaction are in the hands of Mr. ——, a writer (or attorney), who is now retired from professional business, and resides at Inveresk, near Edinburgh. He was a person whom I employed on that occasion for a particular reason, but who never, on any other occasion, transacted business on my account. It is very possible,' pursued the vision, 'that Mr. —— may have forgotten a matter which is now of a very old date; but you may call it to his recollection by this token—that when I came to pay his account there was difficulty in getting change for a Portugal piece of gold, and that we were forced to drink out the balance at a tavern.'

"Mr. R. awoke in the morning with all the events of the vision impressed on his mind, and thought it worth while to ride across the country to Inveresk, instead of going straight to Edinburgh. When he came there he waited on the gentleman mentioned in the dream, a very old man; without saying anything of the vision, he inquired whether he remembered having conducted such a matter for his deceased father. The old gentleman could not at first bring the circumstance to his recollection, but, on mention of the Portugal piece of gold, the whole returned upon his memory; he made an immediate search for the papers and recovered them, so that Mr. R. carried to Edinburgh the documents necessary to gain the cause which he was on the verge of losing."

A friend has related to me some circumstances in his own case similar to the above, and illustrating the same points. In the course of his practice as a lawyer it became necessary for him to ascertain the exact age of a client, who was also his cousin. Their grandfather had been a rather eccentric personage, who had taken a great deal of notice of both his grandsons—his only direct descendants. He died when they were boys. My friend often told his cousin that if his grandfather were alive there would be no difficulty at getting at the desired information, and that he had a dim recollection of having seen a record kept by the old gentleman, and of there being some peculiarity about it which he could not recall. Several months elapsed, and he had given up the idea of attempting to discover the facts of which he had been in search, when, one night, he dreamed that his grandfather came to him and said: "You have been trying to find out when J—— was born; don't you recollect that one afternoon when we were fishing I read you some lines from an Elzevir Horace, and showed you how I had made a family record out of the work by inserting a number of blank leaves at the end? Now, as you know, I devised my library to the Rev. —— ——. I was a d——d fool for giving him books which he will never read! Get the Horace, and you will discover the exact hour at which J—— was born." In the morning all the particulars of this dream were fresh in my friend's memory. The reverend gentleman lived in a neighboring city; my friend took the first train, found the copy of Horace, and at the end the pages constituting the family record, exactly as had been described to him in the dream. By no effort of his memory, however, could he recollect the incidents of the fishing excursion.

Dr. Macnish,[1] in stating his opinion that dreams are uniformly the resuscitation or re-embodiment of thoughts which have formerly, in some shape or other, occupied the mind, relates the following example from his own experience:

"I lately dreamed that I walked upon the banks of the great canal in the neighborhood of Glasgow. On the side opposite to that on which I was, and within a few feet of the water, stood the splendid portico of the Royal Exchange. A gentleman whom I knew was standing upon one of the steps, and we spoke to each other. I then lifted a large stone and poised it in my hand, when he said that he was certain I could not throw it to a certain spot, which he pointed out. I made the attempt, and fell short of the mark. At this moment a well-known friend came up whom I knew to excel at *putting* the stone; but, strange to say, he had lost both his

[1] *Op. cit.*, p. 10.

legs, and walked upon wooden substitutes. This struck me as exceedingly curious, for my impression was that he had only lost one leg, and had but a single wooden one. At my desire he took up the stone, and, without difficulty, threw it beyond the point indicated by the gentleman upon the opposite side of the canal. The absurdity of this dream is extremely glaring, and yet, on strictly analyzing it, I find it to be wholly composed of ideas which passed through my mind on the previous day, assuming a new and ridiculous arrangement. I can compare it to nothing but to cross-reading in the newspapers, or to that well-known amusement which consists in putting a number of sentences, each written on a separate piece of paper, into a hat, shaking the whole, then taking them out, one by one, as they come, and seeing what kind of medley the heterogeneous compound will make when thus fortuitously put together. For instance, I had, on the above day, taken a walk to the canal along with a friend. On returning from it, I pointed out to him a spot where a new road was forming, and where, a few days before, one of the workmen had been overwhelmed by a quantity of rubbish falling upon him, which fairly chopped off one of his legs, and so much damaged the other that it was feared amputation would be necessary. Near this very spot there is a park, in which, about a month previously, I practiced throwing the stone. On passing the Exchange, on my way home, I expressed regret at the lowness of its situation, and remarked what a fine effect the portico would have were it placed upon more elevated ground. Such were the previous circumstances, and let us see how they bear upon the dream. In the first place, the canal appeared before me. 2. Its situation is an elevated one. 3. The portico of the Exchange occurring to my mind as being placed too low became associated with the elevation of the canal, and I placed it close by on a similar altitude. 4. The gentleman I had been walking with was the same whom in the dream I saw standing upon the steps of the portico. 5. Having related to him the story of the man who lost one limb and had a chance of losing another, this idea brings before me a friend with a pair of wooden legs who, moreover, appears in connection with putting the stone, as I knew him to excel at that exercise. There is only one other element in the dream which the preceding events will not account for, and that is the surprise at the individual referred to having more than one wooden leg. But why should he have even one, seeing that in reality he is limbed like other people? This also I can account for. Two years ago he slightly injured his knee while leaping a ditch, and I remember jocularly advising him to get it cut off. I am particular in illustrating this point with regard to dreams, for I hold that, if it were possible to analyze them all, they would invariably be found to stand in the same relation to the waking state as the above specimen. The more diversified and incongruous the character of a dream, and the more remote from the period of its occurrence the circumstances which suggested it, the more difficult does its analysis become; and, in point of fact, this process may be impossible, so totally are the elements of the dream often dissevered from their original sense, and so ludicrously huddled together."

A dream which Professor Maas,[1] of Halle, relates as having occurred to himself affords an excellent example of the dependence of dreams upon actual events, and shows how these latter are distorted and perverted by the imagination of the sleeper.

"I dreamed once," he says, "that the Pope visited me. He commanded me to open my desk, and he carefully examined all the papers it contained. While he was thus employed, a very sparkling diamond fell out of his triple crown into my desk, of which, however, neither of us took any notice. As soon as the Pope had withdrawn I retired to bed, but was soon obliged to rise on account of a thick smoke, the cause of which I had yet to learn. Upon examination, I discovered that the diamond had set fire to the papers in my desk and burned them to ashes."

In analyzing the circumstances which gave rise to this dream, Professor Maas relates the following events, which constituted its basis:

"On the preceding evening I was visited by a friend with whom I had a lively conversation upon Joseph II's suppression of monasteries and convents. With this idea, though I did not become conscious of it in the dream, was associated the visit which the Pope publicly paid the Emperor Joseph, at Vienna, in consequence of the measures taken against the clergy; and with this again was combined, however faintly, the representation of the visit which had been paid me by my

[1] Quoted in Dendy's "Philosophy of Mystery," London, 1841, p. 225.

friend. These two events were, by the subreasoning faculty, compounded into one, according to the established rule—that things which agree in their parts also correspond as to the whole; hence the Pope's visit was changed into a visit paid to me. The subreasoning faculty, then, in order to account for this extraordinary visit, fixed upon that which was the most important object in my room—namely, the desk, or rather the papers which it contained. That a diamond fell out of the triple crown was a collateral association, which was owing merely to the representation of the desk. Some days before, when opening the desk, I had broken the crystal of my watch, which I held in my hand, and the fragments fell among the papers; hence no further attention was paid to the diamond being a representation of a collateral series of things. But afterward the representation of the sparkling stone was again excited, and became the prevailing idea; hence it determined the succeeding association. On account of its similarity it excited the representation of fire, with which it was confounded; hence arose fire and smoke. But in the event the writings only were burned, not the desk itself, to which, being of comparatively little value, the attention was not directed."

Feuchtersleben[1] takes the same view of dreaming as that enunciated in this chapter. Thus he says:

"Dreaming is nothing more than the occupation of the mind in sleep with the pictorial world of fancy. As the closed or quiescent senses afford it no materials, the mind, ever active, must make use of the store which memory retains; but as its motor influence is likewise organically impeded, it cannot independently dispose of this store. Thus arises a condition in which the mind looks, as it were, on the play of the images within itself, and manifests only a faint or partial reaction."

Locke[2] contends that "the dreams of a sleeping man are all made up of the waking man's ideas oddly put together."

Observation and reflection show us that the mind originates nothing during sleep; it merely remembers—and often in the most chaotic manner—the thoughts, the fancies, the impressions which have been imagined or received by the

---

[1] "The Principles of Medical Psychology," etc., Sydenham Society Translation, London, 1847, p. 163.

[2] *Op. cit.*, book ii, section 17.

individual when awake.   Sometimes ideas are reproduced in dreams exactly as they have occurred to us in our waking moments, and this may take place night after night with scarcely the alteration of a single circumstance.   A friend informs me that he is very subject to dreams of this character, and that on some occasions the repetition has taken place as many as a dozen times.

A very striking instance of this kind occurred to me a few years since, and made a deep impression on my mind.   I had just read Schiller's ode to Laura, as translated by Sir E. Bulwer Lytton, beginning,

"Who and what gave to me the wish to woo thee?"
and admired it as a striking piece of versification, conveying some noted philosophical ideas in a forcible and beautiful manner.   The following night I had a very vivid dream of a condition of pre-existence, in which I imagined myself to be. The connection between the dream and the poem I had been reading was sufficiently well marked, and did not astonish me.   I was, however, surprised to find that the next night I had exactly the same dream, and that it was repeated three times subsequently on consecutive nights.

The dependence of dreams upon ideas which we have had when awake was well known to the ancients. ⸪ Thus Lucius Accius,[1] a poet who lived more than a hundred and fifty years before the Christian era, says :

"Quae in vita usurpant homines, cogitant, curant, vident
Quaeque agunt vigilantes, agitantque casi cui in somno accidant,

.   .   .   .   .   Minus mirum est."
Lucretius[2] declares that during sleep we are amused with things which have made us weep when awake ; that circumstances which have pleased us are recalled to our minds ; that objects are presented to us which occupied our thoughts long before ; and that recent events appear still more vividly before us.

Petronius Arbiter[3] cites Epicurus to the same effect.   Tryphæna having declared that she had had a dream in which there appeared to her the image of Neptune she had seen at Baiæ, "Hence you may perceive," observed Eumolpus, "what

---

[1] Cited by M. l'Abbé Richard in "La Théorie des Songes," Paris, 1766, p. 32.
[2] "De Rerum Natura," l. iv, v. 959.
[3] "Satyricon," Bohn's edition, London, 1854, p. 307.

a divine man is Epicurus, who so ingeniously ridiculed these
sports of fancy.

   " ' When in a dream presented to our view
      Those airy forms appear so like the true,
      No prescient shrine, no god the vision sends,
      But every breast its own delusion lends.
      For when soft sleep the body wraps in ease,
      And from the inactive mass the fancy frees,
      What most by day affects, at night returns ;
      Thus he who shakes proud states, and cities burns,
      Sees showers of darts, forced lines, disordered wings,
      Blood-reeking fields, and deaths of vanquished kings ;
      He that by day litigious knots untied,
      And charmed the drowsy bench to either side,
      By night a crowd of cringing clients sees,
      Smiles on the fools and kindly takes their fees ;
      The miser hides his wealth, new treasure finds ;
      Through echoing woods his horn the huntsman winds ;
      The sailor's dream wild scenes of wreck describes ;
      The wanton lays her snares ; the adulteress bribes ;
      Hounds in full cry, in sleep, the hare pursue ;
      And hapless wretches their old griefs renew.' " [1]

It is related of an ancient tyrant that one of his courtiers
described to him a dream in which the courtier had assassinated his master. "You could not," exclaimed the tyrant,
"have dreamed this without having previously thought of
it," and then ordered his immediate execution.

Now, besides this foundation of dreams upon circumstances
which have happened during our waking moments, they may
arise, as has already been intimated, from impressions made
upon the mind during sleep. Sensations may be so intense as
to be partially appreciated by the brain, and yet not strong
enough to cause sleep to be interrupted. In such cases the
imagination seizes the imperfect perception and weaves it into
a tissue of incongruous fancies, which, however, generally
bear a more or less definite relation to the character of the
sensorial impression. Many examples of dreams thus produced are on record, and many others have come under my
own observation. The interest which attaches to phenomena

---

[1] In the above quotation I have slightly altered Kelly's version in Bohn's
edition of Petronius. The original Latin is fully as forcible and true to nature as
the translation.

of this character must be my excuse for quoting some of the more remarkable instances of this kind which have been brought to my attention.

The following are related by Abercrombie : [1]

During the alarm excited in Edinburgh by the apprehension of a French invasion, almost every man was a soldier, and all things had been arranged in expectation of the landing of the enemy. The first notice was to be given by the firing of a gun from the castle, and this was to be followed by a chain of signals calculated to arouse the country. The gentleman to whom the dream occurred was a zealous volunteer, and, being in bed between two and three o'clock in the morning, dreamt of hearing the signal gun. He imagined that he went at once to the castle, witnessed the proceeding for displaying the signals, and saw and heard all the preparations for the assemblage of the troops. At this time he was roused by his wife, who awoke in a fright, in consequence of a similar dream. The origin of both dreams was ascertained in the morning to be the noise produced by the falling of a pair of tongs in the room above.

A gentleman dreamt that he had enlisted as a soldier, joined his regiment, deserted, was apprehended, carried back, condemned to be shot, and at last led out to execution. At this instant a gun was fired, and he awoke, to find that a noise in the adjoining room had both produced the dream and awakened him.

The next is a very extraordinary case.

The subject was an officer in the expedition to Louisburg, in 1758. During his passage in the transport his companions were in the habit of amusing themselves at his expense. They could produce in him any kind of dream by whispering in his ear, especially if this was done by a friend with whose voice he was familiar. Once they conducted him through the whole process of a quarrel which ended in a duel, and when the parties were supposed to have met, a pistol was put into his hand, which he fired, and was awakened by the report. On another occasion they found him asleep on the top of a locker in the cabin, when they made him believe he had fallen overboard, and exhorted him to save himself by swimming. Then they told him that a shark was pursuing him, and entreated him to dive for his life. He instantly did so,

[1] *Op. cit.*, p. 275, *et seq.*

and with so much force as to throw himself from the locker upon the cabin floor, by which he was much bruised, and awakened, of course. After the landing of the army at Louisburg, his friends found him one day asleep in his tent, and evidently much annoyed by the cannonading. They then made him believe that he was engaged, when he exhibited great fear, and showed a decided disposition to run away. Against this they remonstrated, but at the same time increased his fears by imitating the groans of the wounded and the dying ; and when he asked, as he often did, who was hit, they named his particular friends. At last they told him that the man next himself in his company had fallen, when he instantly sprang from his bed, rushed out of his tent, and was roused from his danger and his dream by falling over the tent-cords.

A friend informs me that he has a brother who will carry on a conversation with any person who whispers to him in his sleep, and that his emotions are then very readily excited by any pitiful story that may be told him. Upon awaking, he has a distinct recollection of his dreams, which are always connected with the ideas communicated.

I recollect very distinctly the particulars of a dream which I had several years since, and which was due to an impression conveyed to the brain through the ear. The dream also illustrates the point previously brought forward, that a definite conception of time does not enter into the phenomena of dreams.

I dreamed that I had taken passage in a steamboat from St. Louis to New Orleans. Among the passengers was a man who had all the appearance of being very ill with consumption. He looked more like a ghost than a human being, and moved noiselessly among the passengers, noticing no one, though attracting the attention of all. For several days nothing was said between him and any one, till one morning, as we approached Baton Rouge, he came to where I was sitting on the guards and began a conversation by asking me what time it was. I took out my watch, when he instantly took it from my hand and opened it. "I too once had a watch," he said ; "but see what I am now." With these words he threw aside the large cloak he habitually wore, and I saw that his ribs were entirely bare of skin and flesh. He then took my watch, and, inserting it between his ribs, said it would make a very good heart. Continuing his conversation, he told me that he had resolved to blow up the vessel the next day, but that, as I had been the means of supplying him with a heart, he would save my life. "When you hear the whistle blow," he said, "jump overboard, for in an instant afterward the boat will be in atoms." I thanked him, and he left me. All that day and the next I endeavored to acquaint my fellow-passengers with the fate in store for them, but discovered that I had lost the faculty of speech. I tried to write, but found that my hands were paralyzed. In fact, I could adopt no means to warn them. While I was making these ineffectual efforts, I heard the whistle of the engine; I rushed to the side of the boat to plunge overboard, and awoke. The whistle of a steam saw-mill near my house had just begun to sound, and had awakened me. My whole dream had been excited by it, and could not have occupied more than a few seconds.

The following account [1] shows how a dream may be set in action by the sense of smell.

"On one occasion during my residence at Birmingham I had to attend many patients at Coventry, and for their accommodation I visited that place one day in every week. My temporary residence was a druggist's shop in the market-place. Having on one occasion, now to be mentioned, a more than usual number of engagements, I was obliged to remain one night, and a bed was provided for me at the residence of a cheese-monger in the same locality. The house was very old, the rooms very low, and the street very narrow. It was summer-time, and during the day the cheese-maker had unpacked a box or barrel of strong old American cheese; the very street was impregnated with the odor. At night, jaded with my professional labors, I went to my dormitory, which seemed filled with a strong, cheesy atmosphere, which affected my stomach greatly, and quite disturbed the biliary secretions. I tried to produce a more agreeable atmosphere to my olfactory sense by smoking cigars, but did not succeed. At length, worn out with fatigue, I tried to sleep, and should have succeeded, but for a time another source of annoyance prevented me doing so; for in an old wall behind by head, against which my ancient bed stood, there were numerous rats gnawing away in real earnest. The crunching they made was in-

[1] *Journal of Psychological Medicine*, July, 1856.

deed terrific, and I resisted the drowsy god from a dread that these voracious animals would make a forcible entrance, and might take personal liberties with my flesh.

"But at length 'tired nature' ultimately so overpowered me that I slept in a sort of fever. I was still breathing the cheesy atmosphere, and this, associated with the marauding rats, so powerfully affected my imagination that a most horrid dream was the consequence. I fancied myself in some barbarous country, where, being charged with a political offence, I was doomed to be incarcerated in a large cheese. And although this curious prison-house seemed most oppressive, it formed but part of my sufferings; for scarcely had I become reconciled to my probable fate than, to my horror, an army of rats attacked the monster cheese, and soon they seemed to have effected an entrance, and began to fix themselves in numbers upon my naked body. The agony I endured was increased by the seeming impossibility to drive them away, and, fortunately for my sanity, I awoke, but with a hot head and throbbing temples, and a sense of nausea from the extremely strong odor of the cheese."

I have on two occasions that I recollect had dreams which were due to odors. On one of them, the smell of gas escaping in the room excited the dream of a chemical laboratory; on the other, the smell of burning cloth caused me to dream of a laundry, and of one of the women ironing a blanket, which she scorched with a hot iron. A lady informs me that a similar odor produced in her a dream of the house being on fire, and the impossibility of her escaping by reason of all her clothes being burned up.

Dreams are very readily excited through impressions made on the special nerves of sensation. Instances are given of persons sleeping with bottles of hot water applied to their feet dreaming of walking on burning lava, or some other hot substance. A patient related to me the particulars of a dream which occurred to him while he was asleep with a vessel of hot water applied to the soles of his feet. He had, just before going to sleep, read in the evening paper an account of the capture of an English gentleman by Italian brigands. He dreamt that while crossing the Rocky Mountains he had been attacked by two Mexicans, who, after a long fight, had succeeded in taking him alive. They conveyed him very hurriedly to their camp, which was situated in a deep gorge.

Here they told him that, unless he revealed to them the means of making gold from copper, they would submit him to torture. In vain he pleaded ignorance of any such process. Pulling off his boots and stockings, they held his naked feet to the fire till he shrieked with agony, and awoke to find that the blanket which was wrapped around the tin vessel containing the hot water had become disarranged, and that his feet were in direct contact with the hot metal.

In another case, that of a lady whose lower limbs were paralyzed, artificial heat was applied during the night to her feet. Frequently her dreams had reference to this circumstance. On one occasion she dreamed that she was transformed into a bear, and was being taught to dance by being made to stand on hot plates of iron. On another, that the house was on fire, and that the floors were so hot as to burn her feet in her efforts to escape. Again, that she was wading through a stream of water which came from a hot spring in the Central Park.

Another patient, a lady, subject to neuralgic attacks of great severity, frequently had the lancinating pains give rise to dreams in which she was stabbed with daggers, cut with knives, torn with pincers, etc.

Not long since I had an attack of erysipelas in which the disease included the head and face. The pain was not severe, and yet it was sufficient to give rise to the following dream:

I dreamed that I was taking a cold bath, and that while thus engaged a Turk, armed with a pair of long pincers, came into the room and began to pull the hair out of my head. I remonstrated, but was unable to offer any material resistance, for the reason that the water in which I was lying suddenly froze, leaving me embedded in a solid cake of ice. In order to facilitate his operations, the Turk sponged my head with boiling water, and then, finding the use of the pincers rather slow work, shaved the hair off with a red-hot razor. He then rubbed an ointment on the naked scalp, composed of sulphur, phosphorus, and turpentine, to which he immediately applied fire. Taking me in his arms, he rushed down stairs into the street, lighting his way with the flame from my burning head. He had not gone far before he fell down in a fit, and in his struggles gave me a severe blow between the eyes which instantly deprived me of sight.

When I awoke in the morning I had a very distinct recol-

lection of this dream. The incidents were in part due to the
fact that I had, two or three days previously, been reading an
account of the insanity of Mohammed, and of his being subject to attacks of epilepsy.

The sense of taste is not, for obvious reasons, so productive of dreams as the other senses, but the experiments of M.
Maury and myself, to which fuller reference will presently
be made, show that strong excitations made upon it are transmitted to the brain ; and the following instance, which has
recently come under my immediate observation, is an interesting case in point.

A young lady had, in her early childhood, contracted the
habit of going to sleep with her thumb in her mouth. She
had tried for several years to break herself of the practice,
but all her attempts were in vain, for even when by strong
mental effort she succeeded in getting to sleep without the
usual accompaniment, it was not long before the unruly member was in its accustomed place. Finally she hit upon the
plan of covering the offending thumb with extract of aloes
just before she went to bed, hoping that if she put it into
her mouth she would instantly awake. But she slept on
through the night, and in the morning found her thumb in
her mouth and all the extract of aloes sucked off. During the
night, however, she dreamed that she was crossing the ocean
in a steamer made of wormwood, and that the vessel was
furnished throughout with the same material. The plates,
the dishes, tumblers, chairs, tables, etc., were all of wormwood, and the emanations so pervaded all parts of the ship
that it was impossible to breathe without tasting the bitterness. Everything that she ate or drank was likewise, from
being in contact with wormwood, so impregnated with the
flavor that the taste was overpowering. When she arrived
at Havre, she asked for a glass of water for the purpose of
washing the taste from her mouth, but they brought her an
infusion of wormwood, which she gulped down because she
was thirsty, though the sight of it excited nausea. She went
to Paris and consulted a famous physician, M. Sauve Moi,
begging him to do something which would extract the wormwood from her body. He told her there was but one remedy, and that was ox-gall. This he gave her by the pound,
and in a few weeks the wormwood was all gone, but the ox-
gall had taken its place, and was fully as bitter and disagree-

able. To get rid of the ox-gall she was advised to take counsel of the Pope. She accordingly went to Rome, and obtained an audience of the Holy Father. He told her that she must make a pilgrimage to the plain where the pillar of salt stood, into which Lot's wife was transformed, and must eat a piece of the salt as big as her thumb. During her journey in search of the pillar of salt she endured a great many sufferings, but finally triumphed over all obstacles, and reached the object of her journey. What part to take was now the question. After a good deal of deliberation she reasoned that, as she had a bad habit of sucking her thumb, it would be very philosophical to break off this part from the statue, and thus not only get cured of the bitterness in her mouth, but also of her failing. She did so, put the piece of salt into her mouth, and awoke to find that she was sucking her own thumb.

It might be supposed that the brain during sleep is not excitable through the sense of sight. Many examples, however, are on record of dreams being thus produced, and several very interesting cases have come under my own observation. Among them are the following :

A gentleman of a nervous and irritable disposition informed me that he had dreamed of being in heaven and being dazzled by the brilliancy of everything around him. So great was the light that he hastened to escape from the pain which it caused in his eyes. In the efforts which he made he struck his head against the bedpost, and awoke to find that the fire which he had left smouldering on the hearth had kindled into a bright flame, the light from which fell full in his face.

Another, who had been under my care for epilepsy, dreamed that his room was entered by burglars, and that, with lighted candles in their hands, they were searching his drawers and trunks. He related his dream the following morning, and was told by his mother that she had gone into his room the previous night, and had held a lighted candle close to his face in order to see whether or not he was sound asleep.

No one has more philosophically studied the mode of production of dreams than M. Maury [1] in his remarkable work to which reference has already been made. I propose, therefore, to place a brief outline of his experiments and views before the reader.

[1] "Le sommeil et les rêves; études psychologiques," etc., troisième édition, Paris, 1865.

Just before falling asleep, and immediately before becoming fully awake, many persons are subject to hallucinations partaking of many of the characteristics belonging to dreams. To them the name of hypnagogic (ὕπνος, sleep, and ἀγωγεύς, leader) hallucinations has been given—i. e., hallucitions which lead to sleep. Previous to M. Maury's investigations, the phenomena in question had attracted some attention from German and French physiologists, but M. Maury's investigations, many of which were performed upon himself, throw more light upon the subject than it has hitherto received.

According to M. Maury, the persons who most frequently experience these hypnagogic hallucinations are those who are of an excitable constitution, and are generally predisposed to hypertrophy of the heart, pericarditis, and cerebral affections. This may be true, but in two most remarkable instances which have come under my observation the type of organization was the very reverse of this.

In M. Maury's own case, he finds that the hallucinations are more numerous and more vivid when he experiences, as is frequent with him, a disposition to cerebral congestion. Thus, when he has headache, nervous pains in the eyes, the ears, and the nose, and vertigo, the hallucinations make their appearance as soon as he closes his eyelids. Loss of sleep and severe intellectual exertions invariably produce them, as do also café noir and champagne, which, by causing headache and insomnia, strongly predispose him to the hypnagogic hallucinations. On the contrary, calmness of mind, rest, and country air lessen his liability to them. From the inquiries made of others by M. Maury, the results of his own experience, as well as from my own observations, I am well convinced that the hypnagogic hallucinations are directly the result of an increase in the amount of blood circulating through the brain rather than to actual congestion, as he supposes. They therefore indicate the existence of a condition unfavorable to sound sleep.

The theory which M. Maury proposes in order to account for the existence of hypnagogic hallucinations further presupposes that, as the power of the attention immediately before sleep begins to be diminished, and the mind cannot therefore voluntarily and logically arrange its thoughts, it abandons itself to the imagination, and that thus fancies arise and disappear unchecked by the other mental faculties. This absence of the attention need not be of long duration, a second, or even a shorter period, being sufficient. Thus he lay down, and the attention which had been fully aroused soon became weakened ; images appeared, and these partially reawakened the attention, and the current of his thoughts was resumed, to be replaced again by hallucinations, and this continued till he was fully asleep. As an example, he states that on the 30th of November, 1847, he was reading aloud the "Voyage dans la Russie Méridionale," by M. Hommaire de Hell. He had just finished a line when he closed his eyes instinctively. In this short instant of sleep he saw hypnagogically, but with the rapidity of light, the figure of a man clothed in a brown robe, and with a hood on his head like a monk. The appearance of this image reminded him that he had shut his eyes and ceased reading. He immediately opened his eyelids and resumed his book. The interruption was practically nothing, for the person to whom he was reading did not perceive it.

M. Maury gives numerous examples of these hypnagogic hallucinations, all tending to show that they are induced by a congested condition of the cerebral vessels, and that thus, according to the views I have set forth relative to the condition of the brain in sleep, they are not to be regarded as precursors of that state, but of stupor.

In two very interesting cases of these hallucinations, which have come under my notice, they were brought about by any cause which increased the quantity of blood in the brain, or retarded the flow of blood from this organ. Thus, a glass of champagne or a few drops of laudanum would induce them, as also would the recumbent posture, with the head rather low.

As showing how readily dreams can be excited by impressions made upon the senses, M. Maury caused a series of experiments to be performed upon himself when asleep, which afforded very satisfactory results, and which are interesting in connection with the points already discussed in the present chapter.

First Experiment.—He caused himself to be tickled with a feather on the lips and inside of the nostrils. He dreamed that he was subjected to a horrible punishment. A mask of pitch was applied to his face, and then torn roughly off, taking with it the skin of his lips, nose, and face.

Second Experiment.—A pair of tweezers was held at a little distance from his ear, and struck with a pair of scissors. He dreamed that he heard the ringing of bells ; this was soon converted into the tocsin, and this suggested the days of June, 1848.

Third Experiment.—A bottle of eau de Cologne was held to his nose. He dreamed that he was in a perfumer's shop. This excited visions of the East, and he dreamed that he was in Cairo in the shop of Jean Marie Farina. Many surprising adventures occurred to him there, the details of which were forgotten.

Fourth Experiment.—A burning lucifer match was held close to his nostrils. He dreamed that he was at sea (the wind was blowing in through the windows), and that the magazine of the vessel blew up.

Fifth Experiment.—He was slightly pinched on the nape of the neck. He dreamed that a blister was applied, and this recalled the recollection of a physican who had treated him in his infancy.

Sixth Experiment.—A piece of red-hot iron was held close enough to him to communicate a slight sensation of heat. He dreamed that robbers had got into the house, and were forcing the inmates, by putting their feet to the fire, to reveal where their money was. The idea of the robber suggested that of the Duchess d'Abrantes, who he supposed had taken him for her secretary, and in whose memoirs he had read some account of bandits.

Seventh Experiment.—The word *parafagaramus* was pronounced in his ear. He understood nothing, and awoke with the recollection of a very vague dream. The word *maman* was next used many times. He dreamed of different subjects, but heard a sound like the humming of bees. Several days after, the experiment was repeated with the words *Azor, Castor, Léonore.* On awaking, he recollected that he had heard the last two words, and had attributed them to one of the persons who had conversed with him in his dream.

Another experiment of the same kind showed, like the others, that it was the sound of the word, and not the idea it conveyed, which was perceived by the brain. Then the words *chandelle, haridelle,* were pronounced many times in rapid succession in his ear. He awoke suddenly, saying to himself, *c'est elle.* It was impossible for him to recall what idea he had attached to this dream.

Eighth Experiment.—A drop of water was allowed to fall on his forehead. He dreamed that he was in Italy, that he was very warm, and that he was drinking the wine of Orvieto.

Ninth Experiment.—A light, surrounded with a piece of red paper, was repeatedly placed before his eyes. He dreamed of a tempest and lightning, which suggested the remembrance of a storm he had encountered in the English Channel in going from Merlaix to Havre.

These observations are very instructive. They show conclusively that one very important class of our dreams is due to our bodily sensations. I have frequently performed analogous experiments on others, and had them practiced on myself, and have rarely failed in obtaining decided results. They strongly inculcate the truth of the conclusions arrived at in the foregoing chapter, and they serve as important data in enabling us to understand the division of the subject next to be considered.

In regard to the immediate cause of dreams the opinions of authors are very diverse. The older writers ascribe them to the rise of vapors from the stomach, to the visitation of demons, and other fanciful causes. Bishop Bull[1] declares that he knows from his own experience that dreams are to be ascribed " to the ministry of those invisible instruments of God's providence that guide and govern our affairs and concerns, viz., the angels of God " ; and Bishop Ken held a similar view.

It would neither be possible nor profitable to refer at greater length to views which positive physiology has overturned. Observation and experiment have aided us greatly in arriving at definite conclusions on this subject, and the instances quoted on page 159 of this treatise, even if standing alone uncontradicted, would go far toward guiding us in the right path. On page 164 I have referred to the case of a man who, some time after receiving a severe injury of the head by which a considerable portion of the skull was lost, came under my professional care. Standing by his bedside one evening, just after he had gone to sleep, I observed the scalp slightly rise from the chasm in which it was deeply depressed. I was sure he was going to awake, but he did not, and very

[1] Sermon on the Office of the Holy Angels toward the Faithful, quoted by Seafield, *op. cit.*, vol. i, p. 157.

soon he became restless and agitated, while continuing to sleep. Presently he began to talk, and it was evident that he was dreaming. In a few minutes the scalp sank down to its ordinary level when he was asleep, and he became quiet. I called his wife's attention to the circumstance, and desired her to observe this condition thereafter when he slept. She subsequently informed me that she could always tell when he was dreaming from the appearance of the scalp.

My opinion, therefore, is that dreams are directly caused by an increased activity of the cerebral circulation over that which exists in profound sleep. This activity is probably sometimes local and at others general, and never equals that which prevails in the condition of wakefulness, when the functions of the brain are at their maximum of energy. This view is further supported by a consideration of the state of the brain in sleep and wakefulness, the condition of dreaming being, in a measure, an intermediate one. Illustrations of the effects produced by a notable increase in the quantity of blood circulating through the brain will be given in the chapter on illusions and hallucinations. All of these, it will be perceived, have a direct bearing on the question now under consideration.

CHAPTER VI.

MORBID DREAMS.

MORBID or pathological dreams are divided by Macario [1] into three classes: the prodromic, or those which precede diseases; the symptomatic, or those which occur in the course of diseases; and the essential, or those which constitute the main features of diseases. As this classification is natural and simple, I propose to follow it in the remarks I shall have to make on the subject.

Prodromic Dreams.—There appears to be no doubt that diseases are sometimes preceded by dreams which indicate, with more or less exactitude, the character of the approaching morbid condition. Many instances of the kind which have been reported—especially by the earlier authors—are, however, in all probability, merely coincidences; and in others

[1] *Op. cit.*, p. 86.

the relation between the character of the dream and that of the disease is by no means clear.

Many cases of dreams indicating the nature of a malady which had not yet developed itself are referred to by Macario.[1] The instance of Galen's patient, who dreamed that his leg had become converted into stone, and who was soon afterward paralyzed in that member, has already been cited.

The learned Conrad Gesner dreamed that he was bitten in the left side by a venomous serpent. In a short time a severe carbuncle appeared on the identical spot, and death ensued in five days.

M. Teste, formerly minister of justice and then of public works under Louis Philippe, and who finally died in the Conciergerie, dreamed three days before his death that he had had an attack of apoplexy. Three days afterward he died suddenly of that disease.

A young woman saw in a dream objects apparently confused and dim, as through a thin cloud, and was immediately thereafter attacked with amblyopia, and threatened with loss of sight.

A woman, who had been under the care of M. Macario, dreamed, at about the period of her menstrual flow, that she spoke to a man who could not answer her, for the reason that he was dumb. On awaking, she discovered that she had lost her voice.

Macario himself dreamed one night that he had a severe pain in his throat. On awaking, he felt very well; but a few hours subsequently was attacked with severe tonsillitis.

Arnold, of Villanova, dreamed that a black cat bit him in the side. The next day a carbuncle appeared on the part bitten.

Dr. Forbes Winslow[2] gives several similar instances. A patient had, for several weeks before an attack of apoplexy, a series of frightful dreams, in one of which he imagined he was being scalped by Indians. Others dreamt of falling down precipices, and of being torn to pieces by wild beasts. One gentleman dreamed that his house was in flames, and that he was gradually being consumed to a cinder. This occurred a few days before an attack of inflammation of the brain. A

[1] *Op. cit.*, p. 88, *et seq.*
[2] "On Obscure Diseases of the Brain and Disorders of the Mind," etc., London, 1860, p. 611, *et seq.*

person, prior to an attack of epilepsy, dreamt that he was severely lacerated by a tiger ; and another, just before a seizure, dreamt that he was attacked by murderers, and that they were knocking out his brains with a hammer.

A barrister, for several years before an attack of cerebral paralysis, was in the habit of awaking from sleep in a condition of great alarm and terror without being able to explain the reason for his apprehension. Dr. Beddoes attended a patient whose first fit succeeded a dream of being crushed by an avalanche.

Gratiolet[1] cites additional examples. Thus, Roger d'Oxteryn, Knight of the Company of Douglas, went to bed in good health. Toward the middle of the night he saw in a dream a man affected with the plague and entirely naked, who attacked him with fury, threw him to the ground after a severe contest, and, holding him between his thighs, vomited into his mouth. Three days afterward he was seized with the plague and died. He also alludes to a case detailed by Gunther, in which a woman dreamt that she was being flogged with a whip, and, on awaking, found that she had marks on her body resembling the scars made by the lash.

The existence of diseases of the heart and larger vessels is often revealed by frightful dreams when there is no other evidence of their presence. Macario states that a young lady was under his care in whom violent palpitations of the heart were preceded by painful dreams. She subsequently died of disease of the heart.

Moreau (de la Sarthe),[2] in a very elaborate treatise on dreams, relates the case of a French nobleman, whom he had attended during several months for threatened chronic pericarditis, and who was at first tormented every night by painful and frightful dreams. These dreams, attracting attention, gave the earliest indication of the real condition, and excited fears as to the result, which were soon verified.

He cites another case in illustration of the fact that periodical hæmorrhages are sometimes preceded by morbid dreams. A physician had, in his youth, been subject to periodical hæmorrhages, but without dreams or other trouble during sleep. As he advanced in years the hæmorrhages

---

[1] " Anatomie comparée du système nerveux," etc. Par MM. Leuret et Gratiolet, Paris, 1839–'57, t. ii, 517, *et seq.*

[2] Art. "Rêves," in " Grand dictionnaire de médecine."

were not so frequent, but were always preceded by a condition of general irritation, characterized during wakefulness by heat of skin and frequency of the pulse, and during sleep by painful dreams. These dreams almost always related to violent actions, such as giving and receiving heavy blows, walking on a volcano, or being precipitated into lakes of fire.

Many cases of insanity being preceded by frightful dreams are on record. Falret,[1] in calling attention to the remarkable analogy which exists between mental alienation and dreams, says that it is an incontestable fact that insanity is often preceded by significant dreams, and that these constitute the whole essence of the disorder by becoming firmly fixed in the patient's mind. Thus, he relates that Odier, of Geneva, was consulted, in 1778, by a lady, who, during the night preceding the outbreak of her insanity, dreamed that her step-mother approached her with a dagger in order to kill her. This dream made so strong an impression upon her that she ultimately accredited it as true, and thus became the victim of a delusion which rendered her a lunatic. He declares that numerous similar instances have come under his observation, and refers to the case of a young lady, subject to periodical attacks of mental derangement, whose paroxysms are always preceded by notable dreams.

Morel[2] affirms that many patients, before becoming completely insane, have frightful dreams, which they regard as evidences that they are about to lose their reason. Sometimes they are afraid to go to sleep on account of the terrifying apparitions which then visit them.

The following cases, related by Dr. Forbes Winslow,[3] are interesting in this connection:

"A gentleman, who had previously manifested no appreciable symptoms of mental disorder, or even of disturbed and anxious thought, retired to bed apparently in a sane state of mind. Upon arising in the morning, to the intense terror of his wife, he was found to have lost his senses! He exhibited his insanity by asserting that he was going to be tried for an offence which he could not clearly define, and of the nature of which he had no right conception. He declared that the

---

[1] "Des maladies mentales et des asiles d'aliénés," etc., Paris, 1864, p. 221.

[2] "Traité des maladies mentales," Paris, 1860, p. 457.

[3] "On Obscure Diseases of the Brain and Disorders of the Mind," etc., London, 1860, p. 614.

officers of justice were in hot pursuit of him—in fact, he maintained that they were actually in the house. He begged and
implored his wife to protect him. He walked about the bedroom in a state of great agitation, apprehension, and alarm,
stamping his feet, and wringing his hands in the wildest agony
of despair. Upon inquiring into the history of the case, his
wife said that she had not observed any symptoms that excited her suspicions as to the state of her husband's mind, but,
upon being questioned very closely, she admitted that during
the previous night he appeared to have been under the influence of what she considered to be the nightmare, or a frigthful
dream. While apparently asleep he cried out several times,
evidently in great distress of mind, 'Don't come near me!'
'Take them away!' 'Oh, save me; they are pursuing me!'
It is singular that in this case the insanity which was clearly
manifested in the morning appeared like *a continuation of
the same character and train of perturbed thought that existed during his troubled sleep*, when, according to the wife's
account, he was evidently dreaming."

Dr. Winslow's second case is equally to the point: "I am
indebted to a medical friend for the particulars of the following case. During the winter of 1849 he was called to see
H. B., about five or six o'clock in the morning. The patient
was the wife of a tailor, and mother of three children. At
this time she was rather emaciated and debilitated in bodily
health, and anæmic in appearance. She was of a religious
turn of mind, and belonged to the Wesleyan persuasion. On
the morning of the narrator's visit, he found the woman in a
state of great mental excitement, and under the influence of
hallucinations. She had gone to bed apparently well, but
during the night was the subject of a vivid dream, imagining
that she saw her sister, long since dead and to whom she was
much attached, suffering the pains of hell. When quite
awake, no one could persuade her that she had been under
the influence of an agitated dream. She stoutly persisted in
maintaining the reality of her vision. During the whole of
that day she was clearly insane, but on the following morning her mind appeared to have recovered its balance. She
continued tolerably well, mentally, for four years, with the
exception of her occasionally having moments of despondency, arising from real or fancied troubles." . . .

The further particulars of this case, relating as they do to another division of the subject—"sleep-drunkenness," as the Germans designate it—will be considered under that head.

Without pretending to endorse all the conclusions of Albers—as set forth in the following summary, and which I quote from a very learned and philosophical writer [1]—there is no doubt that some of his dicta are well founded.

"Lively dreams are in general a sign of the excitement of nervous action.

"Soft dreams are a sign of slight irritation of the head; often in nervous fevers announcing the approach of a favorable crisis.

"Frightful dreams are a sign of determination of blood to the head.

"Dreams about fire are, in women, signs of an impending hæmorrhage.

"Dreams about blood and red objects are signs of inflammatory conditions.

"Dreams about rain and water are often signs of diseased mucous membranes and dropsy.

"Dreams of distorted forms are frequently a sign of abdominal obstructions and diseases of the liver.

"Dreams in which the patient sees any part of the body especially suffering, indicate disease in that part.

"Dreams about death often precede apoplexy, which is connected with determination of blood to the head.

"The nightmare (*incubus ephialtes*), with great sensitiveness, is a sign of determination of blood to the chest."

A very interesting paper on dreaming, by Dr. Thomas More Madden,[2] has been recently published, and from it I make the following extract:

"Intermittent fever is often announced, several days before any of the recognized symptoms set in, by persistent dreams of terrifying character. I have experienced this in my own person, and heard it confirmed by other sufferers on the African coast. The following case of morbid dreaming, ushering in yellow fever, I subjoin in the words of the gentleman to whom it occurred, himself a medical man hold-

---

[1] "The Principles of Medical Psychology." Being the Outlines of a Course of Lectures by Baron Ernst von Feuchtersleben, M. D. Sydenham Society Translation, p. 198.

[2] *Medical Press and Circular*; also, *Quarterly Journal of Psychological Medicine and Medical Jurisprudence*, vol. i, p. 276.

ing a high official position on the Gold Coast, where it occurred.

" 'In the early part of 1840 I was an inmate of Cape Coast Castle, and, as some repairs were then being made in the castle, the room assigned to me was that in which the ill-fated L. E. L. (Mrs. Maclean), the wife of the governor of Cape Coast, had been found dead, poisoned by prussic acid, not very long previously. I had known her in London, and had been intimately acquainted with her history and much interested in it. Her body had been found on the floor near the door and in front of a window. After a fatiguing excursion to some of the adjoining British settlements on the coast, having retired to rest, I awoke, disturbed by a dream of a very vivid character, in which I imagined that I saw the dead body of the lady, who had died in that chamber, lying on the floor before me. On awaking, the image of the corpse kept possession of my imagination. The moon was shining brightly into the part of the room where the body had been found, and there, as it seemed to me on awaking, it lay, pale and lifeless, as it appeared to me in my dream.

" 'After some minutes I started up, determined to approach the spot where the body seemed to be. I did so, not without terror, and, walking over the very spot on which the moon was shining, the fact all at once became evident and obvious that no body was there — that I must have been dreaming of one. I returned to bed, and had not long fallen asleep when the same vivid dream recurred ; the same waking disturbance occurring while awake. As long as I lay gazing on the floor I could not dispossess my mind of that appalling vision ; but, when I started up and stood erect, it vanished at the first glance.

" 'Again I returned to bed, dozed, dreamt again of poor L. E. L.'s lamentable end, and of her remains in the same spot ; again awoke, and arose with the same strange results.

" 'There was no more disturbance that night of which, at least, I was conscious, but when morning came fever was on me in unmistakable force in its worst form, and partial delirium set in the same night. I was reduced to the last extremity about the third or fourth night of my illness, when a conviction seized on my mind that it was absolutely essential to my life that I should not pass another night in Cape Coast Castle. I caused the negro servant I had fortunately brought out with me from England to have a litter prepared for me at dawn, and, stretched on this litter, hardly able to lift hand or foot, I was carried out of my bed by four native soldiers, and was conveyed to the house of a merchant, and countryman of mine, to whose care and kindness I owe my life. So much for a visionary precursor of fever on the west coast of Africa.'

" In neuralgia, disturbed dreaming is occasionally a prominent symptom. In an obscure case I was led to make what I believe to be a true diagnosis from the indications furnished by the patient's dreams. The individual in question is a man, aged about forty-five, of an anæmic habit, confined by a sedentary occupation, who, for many years, had suffered from hemicrania, which lately had become more intense, and the intervals shorter. A couple of days before the attack his sleep becomes broken by unpleasant dreams, and, when the paroxysm has attained its height, he invariably dreams that he is the helpless victim of a persecutor, who finishes a series of torments by driving a stake through his skull. During his recovery from each attack he states that his dreams are of a most agreeable character, though so vague that he cannot give any account of them. The frequent repetition of his dreams leads me to conclude that there is some osseous growth within the cranium, and that the vascular distention accompanying the neuralgic attack occasions pressure upon this, giving rise to the sensation I have referred to, while the subsequent feeling of comfort results from that pressure being removed."

A case has been recently published [1] in which the dream immediately preceded, or perhaps even accompanied, the morbid action. A German, aged forty-five, of a nervo-sanguineous temperament, went to bed at 11 P. M., feeling as well as usual. Between 12 and 1 o'clock he dreamed that he saw his child lying at his side, dead. He was very much frightened, and at once awoke, to find that his tongue was paralyzed, and that he could not talk. The faculty of speech and the ability to move the tongue remained impaired for four months.

For several years past I have made inquiries of patients and others relative to their dreams, and have thus collected a large amount of material bearing upon the subject. With

---

[1] *Medical Investigator;* also, *Quarterly Journal of Psychological Medicine,* etc., April, 1868, p. 405.

reference to the point under consideration, the data in my
possession are exceedingly important and interesting. Among
the cases which have come under my observation of diseases
being preceded by morbid dreams are the following :

A gentleman, two days before an attack of hemiplegia,
dreamed that he was cut in two exactly down the mesial line,
from the chin to the perinæum. By some means, union of the
divided surfaces was obtained, but he could only move one
side. On awaking, a little numbness existed in the side
which he had dreamed was paralyzed. This soon passed off,
and ceased to engage his attention. The following night he
had a somewhat similar dream, and the next day, toward
evening, was seized with the attack which rendered him hemi-
plegic.

Another dreamed one night that a man dressed in black and
wearing a black mask came to him and struck him violently
on the leg. He experienced no pain, however, and the man
continued to beat him. In the morning he felt nothing, with
the exception of a slight headache. Nothing unusual was
observed about the leg, and all went on well, until on the
fifth day he had an apoplectic attack, accompanied with
hemiplegia, including the leg which he had in his dream imagined to have been struck.

A lady, aged forty, who had been a great sufferer from
rheumatism for many years, dreamt one afternoon, while sitting in her chair in front of the fire, that a boy threw a stone
at her, which, striking her on the face, inflicted a very severe
injury. The next day violent inflammation of the tissues
around the facial nerve as it emerges from the stylo-mastoid
foramen set in, and paralysis of the nerve followed, due to
effusion of serum, thickening, and consequent pressure.

A young lady dreamt that she was seized by robbers and
compelled to swallow melted lead. In the morning she felt
as well as usual, but toward the middle of the day was attacked with severe tonsillitis.

A young man informed me that, a day or two before being attacked with acute meningitis, he had dreamed that he
was seized by banditti while travelling in Spain, and that they
had taken his hair out by the roots, causing him great pain.

A lady of decided good sense had an epileptic seizure,
which was preceded by a singular dream. She had gone to
bed feeling somewhat fatigued with the labors of the day,

which had consisted in attending three or four morning receptions, winding up with a dinner party. She had scarcely fallen asleep when she dreamed that an old man, clothed in black, approached her, holding an iron crown of great weight in his hands. As he came nearer, she perceived that it was her father, who had been dead several years, but whose features she distinctly recollected. Holding the crown at arm's length, he said : "My daughter, during my lifetime I was forced to wear this crown ; death relieved me of the burden, but it now descends to you." Saying which, he placed the crown on her head and disappeared gradually from her sight. Immediately she felt a great weight and an intense feeling of constriction in her head. To add to her distress, she imagined that the rim of the crown was studded on the inside with sharp points which wounded her forehead, so that the blood streamed down her face. She awoke with agitation, excited, but felt nothing uncomfortable. Looking at the clock on the mantel-piece, she found that she had been in bed exactly thirty-five minutes. She returned to bed, and soon fell asleep, but was again awakened by a similar dream. This time the apparition reproached her for not being willing to wear the crown. She had been in bed this last time over three hours before awaking. Again she fell asleep, and again, at broad daylight, she was awakened by a like dream.

She now got up, took a bath, and proceeded to dress herself with her maid's assistance. Recalling the particulars of her dream, she recollected that she had heard her father say one day that in his youth, while being in England, his native country, he had been subject to epileptic convulsions consequent on a fall from a tree, and that he had been cured by having the operation of trephining performed by a distinguished London surgeon.

Though by no means superstitious, the dreams made a deep impression upon her, and, her sister entering the room at the time, she proceeded to detail them to her. While thus engaged, she suddenly gave a loud scream, became unconscious, and fell upon the floor in a true epileptic convulsion. This paroxysm was not a very severe one. It was followed in about a week by another ; and, strange to say, this was preceded, as the other, by a dream of her father placing an iron crown on her head, and of pain being thereby produced. Since then several months have elapsed, and she has had no other attack, owing to the influence of the bromide of potassium, which she continues to take.

In the case of a gentleman now under my treatment for epilepsy, the fits are invariably preceded by dreams of difficulties of the head, such as decapitation, hanging, perforation with an auger, etc.

A lady, previous to an attack of sciatica, dreamed that she had caught her foot in a spring-trap, and that before she could be freed it was necessary to amputate the member. The operation was performed; but, as she was released, a large dog sprang at her and fastened his teeth in her thigh. She screamed aloud, and awoke in her terror. Nothing unusual was perceived about the leg; but, on getting up in the morning, there was slight pain along the course of the sciatic nerve, and this before evening was developed into well-marked sciatica.

Insanity is frequently preceded by frightful dreams, and I have advanced several examples to this effect from the experience of others. We should naturally expect that very often the first manifestations of a diseased brain should appear during sleep. But dreams are of such a varied character, and so thoroughly irreconcilable with the normal mental phenomena of the wakeful state, that it is difficult to say that such or such a dream is evidence of a diseased mind. As, in some of the cases I have brought forward, a dream may take so firm a hold of the reason as to be the exciting cause of insanity, and not simply a sign of its approach, I am disposed, from my own experience, to regard the frequent repetition of the same dream as often indicative of a disordered mind, when very close observation would fail to reveal other evidences. There are, however, exceptions to this statement, as has been shown in the previous chapter.

Several cases, in which insanity was preceded by terrifying dreams, have come under my observation. In one of them a lady dreamed that she had committed murder, under circumstances of great atrocity. She cut up the dead body, but could not, with all her efforts, divide the head, which resisted the blows, with an axe and other instruments. Finally she filled the nose, eyes, and mouth with gunpowder, and applied a match. Instead of exploding, smoke issued slowly from the orfices of the skull, and was resolved into a human form, which turned out to be that of a police officer sent to arrest her. She was imprisoned, tried, and sentenced to execution, by being drowned in a lake of melted sulphur. While the preparations were being made for the punishment she awoke. She related the particulars of her dream to several friends, but it apparently made no great impression on her mind. The next night she dreamed of somewhat similar circumstances, and for several nights subsequently. On the sixth day, without any premonition, she attempted to kill herself by plunging a pair of scissors into her throat, and since that time to her death, which took place a few months subsequently, was constantly insane.

In this case there was no direct analogy between the character of her dream and the type of insanity which ensued. It cannot, therefore, be said that the dream produced the mental aberration. On the contrary, the dream was, in all probability, the first evidence of deranged cerebral action, a condition which subsequently became developed into positive insanity.

The following case is similar to the foregoing in its general features :

A gentleman, who had been unfortunate in some business speculations, shortly afterward became insane. Previous to this event he was troubled with frightful dreams, which gave him a great deal of annoyance, and frequently caused him to awake in terror. One of them occurred several times, and was of the following character ; He dreamed that he was engaged to be married to a lady of beauty and wealth, and who was, moreover, possessed of great musical talent. One evening, as he in his dream was paying her a visit, she placed herself at the piano and began to sing. He remarked that he did not admire the piece of music she was singing, and asked her to sing something else. She indignantly refused. Angry words followed, and in the midst of the dispute she drew a dagger from her bosom and stabbed herself to the heart. As he rushed forward, horror-struck, to her assistance, her friends entered the room, and found him with the dagger in his hand. He was accused of murdering the lady, and, notwithstanding his protestations of innocence, was tried, found guilty, and sentenced to be hanged. He always awoke at the point when preparations were being made for his execution.

A dream may make such a strong impression on the mind as to subsequently constitute the essential feature of the in-

sane condition. This point has already been elucidated to
some extent in the preceding pages. The following cases,
however, are from my own records of practice:

A gentleman awoke in the middle of the night, and, calling his wife, told her he had dreamed that a large fortune
had been left him by a miner in California. He then went to
sleep again, but in the morning again repeated the dream to
his wife, and said that "there might be something in it." She
laughed, and remarked that she "hoped it might prove true."
About the time the California steamer was expected, the gentleman was observed to become very anxious and excited, and
was continually talking of his expected fortune. At last the
steamer arrived. He then began asking the postman for letters from California, went several times a day to the post-
office to make like inquiries, and finally went aboard the
steamer and questioned the officers on the same subject.
Then he was sure the letter had miscarried, and would sit
for hours in the most profound melancholy. He was now
recognized by his family as a monomaniac, and strenuous
efforts were made to cure him of his delusion, but they were
unsuccessful; and, although now apparently sane on other
subjects, he still holds the erroneous idea which was first
given him in his dream of several years ago.

A young lady was brought to me in July, 1868, who had
been rendered insane by a dream which took place a few
months before I saw her. She went to bed one night in good
health and spirits, though somewhat fatigued in consequence
of having skated a good deal the previous afternoon. In the
morning she told her mother she had committed the "unpardonable sin," and that there was consequently no hope of her
salvation. She based her idea on a dream she had had, in
which an angel appeared to her, and sorrowfully informed
her of her sin and her destiny. When asked to tell what her
sin was, she refused to do so, saying it was too shocking and
atrocious to talk about. She kept to her delusion, and soon
settled into a sort of melancholic stupor, from which it was
impossible entirely to rouse her. Under the use of arsenic
and the acid phosphate of lime she gradually recovered her
reason.

The manner in which prodromic dreams are excited is very
simple. The ancients and some modern writers have regarded
them as prophetic; but the true explanation does not require

so severe a tax on our powers of belief. In the previous chapter, it was shown that very slight impressions made upon the senses during sleep are exaggerated by the partially awakened brain. The first evidence of approaching paralysis may be a very minute degree of numbness—so minute that the brain, when awake and engaged with the busy thoughts of active life, fails to appreciate it. During sleep, however, the brain is quiescent, till some exciting cause sets it in uncontrollable action, and dreaming results. Such a cause may be the incipient numbness of a limb. A dream of its being turned into stone, or cut off, or violently struck, is the consequence. The disease goes on developing, and soon makes its presence unmistakable.

This explanation applies *mutatis mutandis* to all prodromic dreams. They are invariably based upon actual sensations, unless we except the rare cases which are simply coincidences.

Symptomatic Dreams. — Morbid dreams are so generally met with in the course of disease, especially in that of the brain and nervous system, that I never examine a patient without questioning him closely on this point. The information thus obtained is always valuable, and sometimes constitutes the most important feature of the investigation.

Fevers are very often accompanied by frightful dreams. According to Moreau (de la Sarthe),[1] their occurrence indicates that the attack will be long, and that there is probably some organic affection present. My own experience agrees with that of Macario,[2] to the effect of not confirming these opinions. I have, however, generally observed that the frequency and intensity of the morbid dreams were in proportion to the severity of the fever.

Diseases of the heart are very generally attended with disagreeable dreams. They are usually short, and, as Macario remarks, relate to approaching death. The patient starts from sleep in terror, and sometimes it is difficult to convince him of the unreality of his visions.

Dyspepsia and other diseases of the intestinal canal often give rise to morbid dreams. They are usually accompanied by a sense of impending suffocation, and ordinarily consist of frightful images, such as devils, demons, strange

---

[1] *Op. cit.*, art. "Rêves." [2] *Op. cit.*, p. 95.

animals, and the like. The presence of worms in the intestines is likewise a frequent cause of such dreams.

In *chlorosis*, dreams are very common. Occasionally they are of a pleasant character, but in the majority of cases they are the reverse of this.

It would be difficult to mention a disease which is not, at some time or other of its career, an exciting cause of morbid dreams. The most interesting examples, however, are met with in cases of *insanity and other cerebral affections*, and frequently the delusions of the dreams are so mixed up with those which arise during the waking condition that the patient is unable to separate them and to determine which are the consequence of erroneous sensations received when awake, and which are the results of dreams. The careful examination of almost any insane persons will also show that they incorporate the fancies of their dreams with the realities of every-day life. Indeed, the relations of dreaming to insanity are so interesting and important as to have attracted the marked attention of alienists and psychologists.

Cabanis [1] gives Cullen the credit of being the first to point out the similarity between the phenomena of dreaming and those of delirium, and himself enters at length into the full discussion of the several questions involved. A very little reflection will suffice to convince the reader that the two conditions are strikingly alike. In dreams we never distinguish the false from the real; the judgment, if exercised at all, acts in the most erratic manner; we are rarely surprised at the occurrence of the most improbable circumstances; our characters for the time being often undergo a radical change, and we perform imaginary acts in our sleep which are altogether at variance with our actual dispositions. The hallucinations of sleep we accept as realities just as the insane individual believes in all the erroneous impressions made upon his senses. The dreaming person is, in fact, the victim of delusions which, during the existence of his condition, have a firm hold on his mind, and render him in no essential particular different from the one who suffers from mental unsoundness. The incoherence present in dreams and the evident dependence of the various images upon the suggestion of previous images are likewise phenomena of the insane state.

Even in persons perfectly sane, dreams often produce a

---

[1] " Rapports du physique et du morale de l'homme," Paris, 1824, t. ii, p. 359.

very powerful influence on the mind. Most of us have, on awaking, felt pleased or disturbed from reflecting upon the circumstances of a dream we have had during the night, and occasionally the impression has remained through the entire day. With children this influence is still more strongly shown. As Sir Henry Holland[1] remarks, the corrections from reason and experience are less complete in them than in adults. As a consequence, they not infrequently confuse their dream-visions with the facts of their lives, and regard the former as real events. The hallucinations of dreams are also occasionally continued during wakefulness, and hence some persons have, on awaking, seen the images which had been present to them in their sleep.

The celebrated Benedict de Spinoza[2] was once the subject of an illusion which had its starting-point in a dream. He dreamed that he was visited by a tall, thin, and black Brazilian, diseased with the itch. He awoke, and thought he saw such an image standing beside him.

Muller,[3] in referring to such instances, says:

"I have myself also very frequently seen these phantasms, but am now less liable to them than formerly. It has become my custom, when I perceive such images, immediately to open my eyes, and direct them upon the wall or surrounding objects. The images are then still visible, but quickly fade. They are seen whichever way the head is turned, but I have not observed that they moved with the eyes. The answers to the inquiries which I make every year of the students attending my lectures, as to whether they have experienced anything of the kind, have convinced me that it is a phenomenon known to comparatively few persons. For, among a hundred students, two or three only, and sometimes only one, have ob-

[1] "Chapters on Mental Physiology," London, 1852, p. 126.

[2] B. D. S. "Opera Posthuma," 1677, Epistola xxx, p. 471. In the course of this letter to his friend, Peter Balling, Spinoza says :

"Quum quodam mane, lucesente jam cælo, ex somnio gravissima evigilarem imagines, quæ mihi in somnio occurrerant, tam vividè ob oculos versabantur, ac si res finissent veræ, et præsertim cujusdam nigri et scabiosi Brasiliani, quem nunquam antea videram. Hæc imago partem maximam disparebat, quando, ut me alia re oblectarem, oculus in librum, vel aliud quid defigibam ; quamprimium verò oculos à tali objecto rursus avertebam, sine attentione in aliquid oculos defigendo, mihi eadem ejusdem Æthiopis imago eâdem vividètate, et per vices apparebat, donec paulatim circa caput disparetet."

[3] "Elements of Physiology," translated by Baly, vol. ii, p, 1394.

served it. This rarity of the phenomena is, however, more apparent than real. I am satisfied that many persons would perceive these spectres if they learned to observe their sensations at the proper times. There are, however, undoubtedly, many individuals to whom they never appear, and in my own case they now sometimes fail to show themselves for several months at a time, although in my youth they occurred frequently. Jean Paul recommended the watching of the phantasms which appear to the closed eyes as a means of inducing sleep."

If such phenomena take place in persons of healthy brains, the greater liability of the insane to experience them will readily be admitted.

The character of dreams, as Macario[1] remarks, varies according to the type of insanity to which the patient is subject. In melancholia they are ordinarily sad and depressing, and leave a deep and lasting impression; in expansive monomania they are gay and exciting; in mania they give evidence of the extraordinary mental excitement and activity of the subject, and in duration they are vague, fleeting, and occur but seldom.

Essential Morbid Dreams.—Under this head are comprehended the various forms of frightful dreams which are ordinarily designated under the name of nightmare. It has been my good fortune to have had the opportunity of carefully studying the phenomena of this singular affection in several persons of intelligence, and I propose, therefore, detailing the results of my own experience, after a short historical retrospect, which I hope will not prove uninteresting.

Nightmare is characterized by the existence during sleep of a condition of great uneasiness, the principal features of which are a sense of suffocation, a feeling of pain or of constriction in some part of the body, and a dream of a painful character. There are thus two essential elements of the affection—the bodily and the mental.

At a very early period the phenomena of nightmare attracted the attention of physicians. Hippocrates[2] describes it in the following words : "I have often seen persons in their sleep utter groans and cries, appear as if suffocated, and throw themselves wildly about until they finally waked.

[1] *Op. cit.*, p. 93.   [2] Περὶ ἱερῆς νόσο.

Then they were in their right minds, but were, nevertheless, pale and weak."

The general opinion held at that time was that the phenomena of nightmare were due to excess of bile and dryness of the blood. This view originated with Hippocrates, but was more or less modified by subsequent writers.

After the establishment of Christianity, the conviction began to prevail that during an attack of nightmare the subject was visited by a demon, who, for the time being, took possession of his body. Oribasius, in the fourth century, combated this idea, and endeavored to show that it was a severe disease, which, if not cured, might lead to apoplexy, mania, or epilepsy. He located it in the head.

Aetius also denied the existence of demoniacal agency in nightmare. He considered it as a prelude to epilepsy, mania, or paralysis.

During the middle ages nightmare was attributed to the power of the devil. Imps, male and female, called incubi and succubi, respectively, were supposed to be the active agents in producing the affection. The treatment was in accordance with the theory, and consisted of prayers and exorcisms. Not unfrequently the subject of the disease perished at the stake for the alleged crime of having sexual intercourse with incubi or succubi, according to sex.

Even in later times many persons have been found who believed implicitiy in the reality of the visions which they experienced during an attack of nightmare. Thus, Jansen[1] relates that a clergyman came to consult him. "Monsieur," said he, "if you do not help me I shall certainly go into a decline, as you see I am thin and pale—in fact, I am only skin and bone ; naturally I am robust, and of good appearance ; now I am scarcely more than the shadow of a man."

" What is the matter with you?" said Jansen. "And to what do you attribute your disease?"

"I will tell you," answered the clergyman, "and you will assuredly be astonished at my story. Almost every night a woman, whose figure is not unknown to me, comes and throws herself on my breast, and embraces me with such power that I can scarcely breathe. I endeavor to cry out, but she stifles my voice, and the more I try, the less successful I am. I can

[1] Quoted from I. Franck by Macario, *op. cit.*, p. 100.

neither use my arms to defend myself, nor my legs to escape. She holds me bound and immovable."

"But," said the doctor, " what you relate is not in the least surprising. Your visitor is an imaginary being, a shade, a phantom, an effect of your imagination."

" Not so ! " exclaimed the patient. " I call God to witness that I have seen with my own eyes the being of whom I speak, and I have touched her with my hands. I am awake, and in the full possession of my faculties, when I see this woman before me. I feel her as she attacks me, and I try to contend with her, but fear, anxiety, and languor prevent me. I have been to every one, asking for aid to bear up against my horrible fate, and, among others, I have consulted an old woman who has the reputation of being very skilful, and something of a sorceress. She directed me to urinate toward daylight, and to immediately cover the *pot de chambre* with the boot of my right foot. She assured me that on the very day I would do this the woman would pay me a visit.

"Although this seemed to me very ridiculous, and although my religion was altogether against my making any such experiment, I was finally induced, by reflecting on my sufferings, to follow the advice I had received. I did so, and, sure enough, and on the same day, the wicked woman who had so tormented me came to my apartment, complaining of a horrible pain in the bladder. All my entreaties and threats, however, were unavailing to induce her to cease her nocturnal visits."

Jansen at first could not turn this gentleman from his insane idea, but, finally, after two hours' conversation, he made him have some just conception of the nature of his disease, and inspired him with the hope of a cure.

Epidemics of nightmare have been noticed, and it likewise sometimes prevails endemically under certain peculiar forms. Thus, vampirism, a belief in which exists in different parts of the world, is nothing but a kind of nightmare. Charles Nodier[1] gives some interesting details on this point, which I do not hesitate to transcribe.

In Morlachia there is scarcely a hamlet which has not several *vukodlacks* or vampires, and there are some, every family of which has its *vukodlack*, just as every Alpine family has its cretin. The cretin, however, has a physical infirmity,

[1] " De quelques phénomènes du sommeil." Œuvres complets, t. v, p. 170–175.

and with it a morbid state of the brain and nervous system, which destroys his reason, and prevents him appreciating his degraded condition. The *vukodlack*, on the contrary, appreciates all the horror of his morbid perception; he fears and detests it; he combats it with all his power; he has recourse to medicine, to prayers, to division of a muscle, to the amputation of a limb, and sometimes even to suicide. He demands that after his death his children shall pierce his heart with a spike, and fasten his corpse to the coffin, so that his dead body, in the sleep of death, may not be able to follow the instinct of the living body. The *vukodlack* is, moreover, often a man of note, often the chief of the tribe, the judge, or the poet.

Through the sadness which is due to the recollection of his nocturnal life, the *vukodlack* exhibits the most generous and lovable traits of character. It is only during his sleep, when visited with his terrible dreams, that he is a monster, digging up the dead with his hands, feeding on their flesh, and waking those around him with his frightful cries.

The superstition is that during this state of morbid dreaming the soul of the sleeper quits the body to visit the cemeteries, and feast upon the remains of the recently dead.

In Dalmatia the belief is current that there are sorcerers whose delight is to tear out the hearts of lovers, and to cook and eat them. Nodier relates the story of a young man about to be married, who was the constant victim of nightmare, during which he dreamed that he was surrounded by these sorcerers, ready to pluck his heart from his breast, but who often awakened just as they were about to proceed to extremities. In order to be effectually relieved from their visitations, he was advised to avail himself of the company of an old priest, who had never previously heard of these horrible dreams, and who did not believe that God would give such power to the enemies of mankind. After using various forms of exorcism, the priest went peacefully to sleep in the same room with the patient whom he was commissioned to defend against the sorcerers. Hardly, however, had sleep descended upon his eyelids than he thought he saw the demons hovering over the bed of his friend, alight, and, laughing horribly, throw themselves on his prostrate body, and with their claws tear open his breast, and, seizing his heart, devour it with frightful avidity. Unable to move from his bed, or to utter a sound, he was forced to witness this terrible scene. At last he awoke, to see no one but his companion, pale and haggard, staggering toward him, and finally falling dead at his feet.

These two men, adds Nodier, had had similar attacks. What the one dreamed he saw, the other dreamed he had experienced.

As an instance of like dreams occurring to many persons at the same time, the circumstances related by Laurent [1] are worthy of notice.

"The first battalion of the regiment of Latour d'Auvergne, of which I was surgeon-major, while in garrison at Palmi, in Calabria, received orders to march at once to Tropea in order to oppose the landing from a fleet which threatened that part of the country. It was in the month of June, and the troops had to march about forty miles. They started at midnight, and did not arrive at their destination till seven o'clock in the evening, resting but little on the way, and suffering much from the heat of the sun. When they reached Tropea, they found their camp ready and their quarters prepared, but as the battalion had come from the farthest point, and was the last to arrive, they were assigned the worst barracks, and thus eight hundred men were lodged in a place which, in ordinary times, would not have sufficed for half their number. They were crowded together on straw placed on the bare ground, and, being without covering, were not able to undress. The building in which they were placed was an old, abandoned abbey, and the inhabitants had predicted that the battalion would not be able to stay there all night in peace, as it was frequented by ghosts, which had disturbed other regiments quartered there. We laughed at their credulity ; but what was our surprise to hear, about midnight, the most frightful cries issuing from every corner of the abbey, and to see the soldiers rushing terrified from the building. I questioned them in regard to the cause of their alarm, and all replied that the devil lived in the building ; that they had seen him enter by an opening into their room, under the figure of a very large dog, with long black hair, and, throwing himself upon their chests for an instant, had disappeared through another opening in the opposite side of the apartment. We laughed at their consternation, and endeavored to prove to them that the phenomenon was due to a very simple and natu-

[1] "Grand dictionnaire de médecine," t. xxxiv., art. "Incubi," par M. Parent.

ral cause, and was only the effect of their imagination; but we failed to convince them, nor could we persuade them to return to their barracks. They passed the night scattered along the sea-shore, and in various parts of the town. In the morning I questioned anew the non-commissioned officers and some of the oldest soldiers. They assured me that they were not accessible to fear; that they did not believe in dreams or ghosts, but that they were fully persuaded they had not been deceived as to the reality of the events of the preceding night. They said they had not fallen asleep when the dog appeared, that they had obtained a good view of him, and that they were almost suffocated when he leaped on their breasts. We remained all day at Tropea, and, the town being full of troops, we were forced to retain the same barracks, but we could not make the soldiers sleep in them again without our promise that we would pass the night with them. I went there at half past eleven with the commanding officer; the other officers were, more for curiosity's sake than anything else, distributed in the several rooms. We scarcely expected to witness a repetition of the events of the preceding night, for the soldiers had gone to sleep, reassured by the presence of their officers, who remained awake. But about one o'clock, in all the rooms at the same time, the cries of the previous night were repeated, and again the soldiers rushed out to escape the suffocating embrace of the big black dog. We had all remained awake, watching eagerly for what might happen, but, as may be supposed, we had seen nothing.

"The enemy's fleet having disappeared, we returned next day to Palmi. Since that event we have marched through the kingdom of Naples in all directions and in all seasons, but the phenomena have never been reproduced. We are of opinion that the forced march which the troops had been obliged to make during a very hot day, by fatiguing the organs of respiration, had weakened the men, and, consequently, disposed them to experience these attacks of nightmare. The constrained position in which they were obliged to lie, the fact of their not being undressed, and the bad air they were obliged to breathe, doubtless aided in the production."

A gentleman was, not long since, under my professional charge who was very subject to attacks of nightmare. Though remarkable for his personal courage, he confessed that during his paroxysms he was the most arrant coward in the world. Indeed, so powerful an impression had his frequent frightful dreams made upon him that he was afraid to go to sleep, and would often pass the night engaged in some occupation calculated to keep him awake.

The dreams which he had were always of such a character as to inspire terror, and generally related to demons and strange animals, which seated themselves on his chest, and tried to tear open his throat. They came on a few minutes after he fell asleep, and lasted sometimes for more than an hour. During their continuance he remained perfectly still and quiet, giving no evidence of the tumult within beyond the appearance of a cold sweat over the whole surface of the body. When he awoke, as he always did when the climax was reached, he started from the bed with a bound, and with all the evidences of intense fright. After that he was safe for the remainder of the night.

I am acquainted with another case in which there are no very obvious physical symptoms.

Ordinarily, however, the sufferer groans, and tosses about the bed ; he appears to be endeavoring to speak, and to escape from his imaginary danger ; his face, neck, and chest are flushed ; a cold perspiration appears, especially on his forehead, and he is sometimes seized with a general trembling of the whole body. The respiration appears to be particularly disturbed ; he gasps for air, and occasionally the breathing is stertorous. As to the pulse, strange as it may appear, there is rarely any marked change from the healthy standard beyond the slight irregularity induced by the disorder of the respiration.

Among the mental symptoms, in addition to the fear with which he is filled, the sufferer is strongly impressed with a sense of his utter helplessness. His will is actively engaged in endeavoring to bring his muscles into action, but they cannot be made to obey its behests, and he consequently feels himself powerless to escape from the enemies which attack him.

In regard to the kind of images which make their appearance, there is more or less uniformity. Generally they consist of animals, such as hogs, dogs, monkeys, or nondescripts created by the imagination of the dreamer. At other times they are demons of various forms. A gentleman, whose

case came under my notice, was visited almost nightly by a
huge black walrus, which appeared to roll off of a large cake
of ice, and, crawling up the bed, to throw itself on his chest.
Another was tormented by an animal, half lion and half mon-
key, which seemed to fasten its claws in his throat while
seated on his breast.

At other times there are no images, but only painful delusions, in which the dreamer is placed in dangerous positions,
or suffers some kind of torturing operation. Thus, a lady informs me that she is subject to frequent attacks of nightmare,
during which she imagines she is standing on the top of a
high mast, and in extreme fear of falling off. Again, she is
dragged through a key-hole by some invisible power; and
again has her nose and mouth so tightly closed that she can
get no breath of air.

The *causes* of nightmare may be divided into the *exciting*
and the *immediate*. The *exciting causes* are very numerous.
Unusual fatigue, either of mind or of body, recent emotional
disturbance, such as that produced by fright, anxiety, or anger, and intense mental excitement of any kind, may produce
it. I have known a young lady to have a severe attack the
night after a school examination, in which she had been unduly tasked. Another young lady is sure to be attacked
after witnessing a tragedy performed. A young man, who was
under my care for a painful nervous affection, always had a
paroxysm of nightmare during the first sleep after delivering
an address, which he was obliged to do every month for a
year or more.

Fulness of the stomach, or the eating of indigestible or
highly stimulating food late in the evening, will often cause
nightmare. As Motet[1] remarks : " One of the best-established
causes is repletion of the stomach, and slowness and difficulty of digestion. Let an individual habitually systematic
depart for one day from the accustomed regularity of his
meals, let him change the hour of his dinner, and go to bed
before the work of digestion is completed, and it is probable
that his sleep will be troubled, and that nightmare will be
the consequence of his indiscretion. The painful feeling will
be induced by distention of the stomach, by anxiety, and by
the restraint given to the movements of the diaphragm."

[1] "Nouveau dictionnaire de médecine et de chirurgie pratiques," t. 6ième,
Paris, 1867, art. "Cauchemar."

17

Feculent food would appear to be especially powerful in causing nightmare, and, according to Motet, strong liquors and sparkling wines and coffee are equally so. I have several times known it produced by the New England dish of baked pork and beans, and by green Indian corn eaten just before going to bed.

Various morbid affections, such as diseases of the heart, aneurism of the large arteries, affections of the brain or spinal cord, and diseases of the digestive or urinary apparatus, are often exciting causes of nightmare. It may originate from painful sensations in any part of the body. Some women, about the time of the menstrual flow, are particularly liable to paroxysms of this morbid dreaming.

Whatever interferes with the respiration or the easy flow of blood to and from the head may bring on an attack of nightmare. I have known it caused by the collar of the night-gown being too tight, and by the pillow being under the head and not under the shoulders, thus putting the head at such an angle with the body as to constrict the blood-vessels of the neck, and by the head falling over the side of the bed. I have not been able to ascertain that sleeping upon the back or on the left side predisposes to the affection, unless in those cases in which the former position causes snoring from relaxation of the soft palate.

The *immediate cause* of nightmare is undoubtedly the circulation of blood through the brain which has not been sufficiently aërated. The appearance of the sufferer is sufficient to indicate this, as the condition of the cerebral vessels and all the exciting causes act either by retarding the flow of the venous blood from the brain or by impeding the respiratory movements. The effects of emotion, of mental fatigue, and of severe and long-continued muscular exertion, are such that the nervous influence to the muscles of respiration is increased or the muscles themselves are debilitated through this general fatigue of the organism. Fulness of the stomach acts mechanically, by interfering with the action of the diaphragm, and constriction about the neck directly increases the flow of blood through the brain. Certain diseases of the heart and lungs act upon the function of respiration, and thus interfere with the due oxygenation of the blood.

The *treatment* of morbid dreams presents no points of any difficulty. When they are the result of impressions made upon the nerves during sleep, and are the forerunners of disease, it is not very likely that physicians will be consulted as to their cure. Undoubtedly, however, much can be done to abate them when they belong to the category of prodromic dreams, as well as when they are symptomatic of existing disease. Hygienic measures, such as open-air exercise, attention to diet, and warm baths, and the use of the oxide of zinc and some one of the bromides, will do much to lessen the irritability of the nervous system, and to diminish any hyperæmic condition of the brain.

Nightmare often requires more active management, though even here we will ordinarily find the measures above mentioned the most effectual that can be taken for its treatment. Of course, the exciting cause must be ascertained if possible, and means taken to remove it. This is not always an easy matter, and frequently cannot be accomplished without a considerable alteration in the course of life followed by the patient, and more or less sacrifice on his part. Among hygienic measures, I have several times found relief follow a sojourn at the sea-shore and ocean bathing. Change of air is almost invariably beneficial, and moderate physical exercise, just to the point of fatigue, can scarcely be dispensed with. A gentleman, at this moment under my care, has been cured by a course of gymnastic training, which he took at my instance. The food of those subject to nightmare should always be plain, easily digestible, and moderate in quantity. Alcoholic beverages should always be sparingly taken, especially just before going to bed. Any article of food or drink known to produce the paroxysm should, of course, be omitted altogether.

As to medicines, the whole round of so-called anti-spasmodics is usually tried by routine physicians. I have never seen them do any good. Iron and bitter tonics are indicated in cases of anæmia or exhaustion. As the disease is sometimes induced in children by the presence of worms in the alimentary canal, diligent inquiry should be made relative to symptoms indicating irritation from these parasites, and, if they are found to exist, anthelmintics should be administered.

A case of intermittent nightmare, occurring every alternate night, in a young lady, was recently under my care. No exciting causes could be discovered, except the probable one of malaria. The affection yielded at once to the sulphate of quinia.

Ferrez[1] has published the details of a case of intermittent nightmare occurring in the person of a Spanish officer, who was attacked after passing forty-two nights at the bedside of a sick daughter. Every night, at the same hour, he was awakened by frightful dreams, which, irritating his brain, produced cramps, convulsive movements, an afflux of blood to the cerebral tissues, a sadness which he could not conquer, and a continual and powerful feeling of approaching death.

The patient, though of strong constitution, became enfeebled and emaciated. His countenance was pale, the pupils contracted, and his whole appearance showing the exhaustion consequent upon the battle which he was obliged continually to fight with his disease. He composed at this time some verses, describing in graphic terms the deplorable condition of his mind and body.

Gymnastics, temperance in eating and drinking, and the study of poetry, failed to give him relief. Finally he consulted Dr. Ferrez, who advised him to reveal his state to his family, who hitherto had been kept in ignorance of his malady, to continue his gymnastics moderately, not to eat in the evening, to drink only cold water, to use friction over the whole surface of the body, to apply mustard plasters to the extremities, to sleep with his head elevated and uncovered, to bathe his head frequently during the night with cold water, to give up the study of poetry, and to devote himself to mathematics and political economy. These measures were rigorously carried out; but his daughter, who had been the involuntary cause of his disease, prescribed a better remedy than all the others. She had him waked at midnight, before the occurrence of his paroxysm, and thus broke up the habit.

Perhaps no one medicine is so uniformly successful in the ordinary forms of nightmare as the bromide of potassium or of sodium, administered in doses of from twenty to forty grains, three times a day. I have seen a number of cases which have resisted all hygienic measures, and the simple removal of the apparent cause, yield to a few doses of this remedy.

When the affection has lasted a long time, it is more difficult to break up the acquired habit. In these cases, the plan

[1] "Gazette médicale de Lyon," 15 Mai, 1856; also, Macario, *op. cit.*, p. 104.

so successfully employed by the daughter of the Spanish officer will almost invariably succeed.

Finally, persons subject to nightmare should so train the mind as to employ the intellectual faculties systematically by engaging in some study requiring their full exercise. The action of the emotions should be as much as possible controlled, and the reading of sensational stories, or hearing sensational plays, should be discouraged. By severe mental training, individuals can do much to regulate the character of their dreams. It is a well-recognized fact that intense thought upon subjects which require the highest degree of intellectual action is not favorable to the production of dreams of any kind.

SECTION IV.
DESCRIPTION AND TREATMENT OF INSANITY.

CHAPTER I.

DEFINITIONS AND DESCRIPTIONS.

NOTHING is more essential to a proper understanding of a subject, especially of so abstruse a one as insanity, as to have clear ideas of the meanings of the terms employed in its consideration ; and this is particularly necessary when there are wide-spread errors existing in regard to the signification of several of the words used to designate some of the most important symptoms of the disease. It will be well, therefore, to start with exact notions of what we mean when these words are employed.

Definition of Insanity.—Every medical witness who appears in a case involving the mental capacity or responsibility of an individual is expected to give a definition of insanity. It is extremely difficult to do this satisfactorily, as it is also with a good many other terms which are applied to complex forces, for the definition should cover all possible cases of deficiency or aberration of the mental faculties, and yet not include those instances of cerebral disease which cannot properly be classed under this head. For the purpose of showing how authors have varied in their ideas of the signification of the word, as well as for the instruction of the reader seeking for information on the point, I quote a number of definitions from some of the most eminent authorities.

Dr. John Haslam,[1] who has written one of the most lucid treatises on insanity in the English language, and who was

[1] "Observations on Madness and Melancholy," etc., London, 1809, p. 37.

for many years one of the physicians to Bethlehem Hospital, confesses his inability to give a thoroughly comprehensive, and yet a sufficiently exhaustive, definition of madness; and Dr. Prichard [1] frankly admits that it is better to give up the attempt to define insanity in general terms. Notwithstanding the reluctance of these and other medical authorities to formularize the phenomena of insanity, the attempt has frequently been made with more or less approach to completeness. If the word can be even imperfectly defined in simple language without conveying erroneous ideas, it is certainly advisable to make an effort in this direction.

According to Hoffbauer, [2] an individual is insane when the understanding is diverted or changed in its operations; when he is powerless to avail himself of his intellectual faculties, or to make known his wishes in a suitable manner.

This definition neither embraces all kinds of insanity, nor excludes certain cerebral disorders which are not properly classed under this head. For instance, it does not comprehend morbid impulse, the subjects of which often evince no derangement of the understanding or intellect, and it includes apoplexy, and concussion and compression of the brain.

Dr. Bucknill [3] defines insanity as "a condition of the mind in which a false action of conception or judgment, a defective power of the will, or an uncontrollable violence of the emotions and instincts, has separately or jointly been produced by disease."

According to this definition, the individual who is comatose from the effects of a cerebral hæmorrhage or a blow on the head, and who certainly has a "defective power of the will" produced by disease, is insane.

Dr. Guislain, [4] an eminent Belgian authority, says that insanity is

"A chronic disease, free from fever, in which the ideas and the acts are under the control of an irresistible power, a change taking place in the manner of feeling, conceiving, thinking, and acting peculiar to the individual, in his character and in his habits; a state which contrasts with the sentiments, the

---

[1] Art. "Insanity" in "Cyclopædia of Practical Medicine."

[2] "Untersuchungen über die Krankheiten der Seele," Halle, 1803, p. 11.

[3] "Unsoundness of Mind in relation to Criminal Acts," second edition, 1857.

[4] Leçons orales sur les phrenopathies," etc., Gand—Paris, 1880, second edition, t. i, p. 52.

thoughts, and the acts of those about him ; an affection which renders it impossible for him to act so as to provide for his preservation, and with a sense of his responsibility to God or to society."

The objections to this definition are, that insanity is not necessarily unaccompanied by fever, that it is not always a chronic affection, and that it, like the others mentioned, includes too much.

Drs. Bucknill and Tuke,[1] in the first edition of their work on insanity, quoting from Maimon, say that "mental health consists in that state in which the will is free, and in which it can exercise its empire without obstacle. Any condition different to this is *a disease of the mind*. And if it be asked, What is the Will? it may be replied, according to the definition of Marc, that it is in health a moral faculty, which originates, directs, prevents, or modifies the physical or moral acts which are submitted to it."

More recently, however, they[2] state that they believe it impracticable to propose any definition entirely free from objection, and which shall comprise every form of mental disorder. They, therefore, omit the partial definition above given, and announce[3] a qualified adherence to the one previously given by Dr. Bucknill.

The late Professor Gilman,[4] of this city, who had given a great deal of study to the subject, declared that the best definition he had been able to make was, that "insanity is a disease of the brain by which the freedom of the will is impaired."

This definition neither covers the subject nor excludes other diseases.

Dr. Thomas K. Cruse[5] has given a definition of insanity far in advance of any of those cited. For him "insanity is a psychic manifestation of brain disease." The only objection to be urged against this definition, which, in a few words, embraces every form of insanity, is, that it includes too much. A man insensible from the effects of cerebral hæmorrhage

---

[1] "A Manual of Psychological Medicine," etc., London, 1858, p. 79.

[2] "A Manual of Psychological Medicine," etc., fourth edition, London, 1879, p. 19.   [3] *Op. cit.*, p. 23.

[4] "The Relations of the Medical to the Legal Profession," p. 20.

[5] "A New Definition of Insanity," *Journal of Psychological Medicine*, April, 1872, p. 267.

exhibits a "psychic' manifestation of brain disease," but he certainly is not insane.

Dr. E. C. Spitzka[1] has proposed a very comprehensive definition, which, with some modifications, may be made sufficiently complete and satisfactory. It is:

"Insanity is either the inability of the individual to correctly register impressions and experiences in sufficient number to serve as rational guides to rational behavior in consonance with the individual's age, time, and circumstances, or, such impressions and experiences being correctly accumulated in sufficient number, a failure to co-ordinate them, and thereon form logical conclusions, or any other gross mental incongruity with the individual's surroundings in the shape of subjective manifestations of cerebral disease or defect, excluding the phenomena of sleep, trance, somnambulism, the ordinary manifestations of the neuroses, such as epilepsy and hysteria, of febrile delirium, coma, acute intoxication, and the ordinary immediate results of nervous shock and injury." This definition, however, excludes all morbid impulses, and all emotional and volitional manifestations of mental derangement.

It would be easy to go on and quote numerous other authorities on this point, but enough have been cited to show the general import which physicians give to the word "insanity." I will, therefore, dismiss the further consideration of this division of the subject by stating that my own idea of insanity is based entirely on the fact that as a healthy mind results from a healthy brain, so a disordered mind comes from a diseased brain. Insanity, therefore, strictly speaking, is only a symptom of cerebral disease, and I would define it as—

A manifestation of disease of the brain, characterized by a general or partial derangement of one or more faculties of the mind, and in which, while consciousness is not abolished, mental freedom is weakened, perverted, or destroyed.[2]

An essential feature of the definition here given is, that it is directly the result of a diseased condition of the brain. This is the immediate cause, and may consist of structural changes due to injury, disease, or malformation; or malnutrition, the result of excessive intellectual exertion, the ac-

---

[1] "A Practical Definition of Insanity," *Chicago Medical Review*, July 15, 1882.

[2] See "A Treatise on Diseases of the Nervous System," first edition, 1871, p. 334; also, subsequent editions up to and including the sixth.

tion of powerful emotions, irritations in distant parts of the body, the sudden stoppage of the digestive process, the introduction into the system of certain drugs—such as opium, alcohol, belladonna, etc.—the retention in the organism of substances poisonous in character, but which, in health, are excreted as some of the constituents of the bile or the urine, and of other factors capable of altering the quantity or quality of the blood circulating through the cerebral vessels, or of accelerating or retarding the metamorphosis of tissue which the brain undergoes in common with all the other organs of the body.

This definition, so far as I can perceive, excludes no form of insanity, nor does it include diseases which are not insanity. It rests upon the basis of brain disease, without which there can, in my opinion, be no insanity.

But, with a little modification, Dr. Cruse's definition, previously cited, can be made to exclude the manifestations of brain disease which are not usually comprehended under the term insanity. I would propose to add to it the words *unattended by loss of consciousness*. It will then read: "A psychic manifestation of brain disease unattended by loss of consciousness." In this form, it is shorter than and as comprehensive as my own, and perhaps is, on these accounts, to be preferred.

Illusion.—An illusion is a false perception of a real sensorial impression. Thus, a person seeing a ball roll over the floor, and obtaining from it the perception that it is a mouse, has an illusion of the sense of sight; another, hearing the pattering of the rain on the roof, and perceiving in this sound the voice of some one calling him, has an illusion of the sense of hearing; another, having some bitter substance placed on his tongue, and forming the perception of a sweet flavor, has an illusion of the sense of taste; another, smelling a bottle of Cologne-water, and receiving the impression of turpentine in the nostrils, has an illusion of the sense of smell; and another, rubbing the tips of his fingers over a smooth plate of glass and obtaining a sensation like that derived from contact with sand-paper, has an illusion of the sense of touch. In all such cases there is a material basis for the perception, but, owing to disorder or disease of the sensorial organ, the nerves by which the impression received is conveyed to the brain, or of the perceptional ganglion, an erroneous perception is produced—and, consequently, the normal relation between the cause and the effect is disturbed.

Illusions are not always indicative of the existence of insanity, or even of cerebral disorder. It is, perhaps, never the case that the perception is precisely in accordance with the real properties of the substance making the sensorial impression. We never see, hear, taste, smell, or feel things exactly as they are. This imperfection may be due to the fact that the surrounding circumstances are not favorable. Insufficient light may thus make our vision imperfect ; a thing, for instance, may seem to be of a green color when it is in reality blue ; loud noises may make us incapable of perfectly appreciating the character of gentle sounds ; a strongly sapid substance rubbed over the tongue and fauces prevents us distinguishing delicate flavors ; a powerful odor may make such an impression on the Schneiderian membrane that other odors for a long time smell like it ; and exposure to very cold weather interferes markedly with the discriminating power of the sense of touch.

Imperfect perceptions are often formed in consequence of the perceptive ganglia being otherwise occupied. Thus, if we are looking intently at some object of interest, we are not apt to attend to the sounds that reach our ears, and, consequently, no clear perception of them is formed.

Illusions of all the senses, but especially of sight and hearing, are met with in insanity, and particularly in those acute forms characterized by the presence of delirium. They may also exist as diseases without the higher faculties of the mind being involved, but this is not a common circumstance. Usually the persistent presence of illusions is evidence of brain disease, which, if not already involving the intellect, the emotions, or the will, is particularly liable so to do at no very distant date.

Hallucination.—A hallucination is a false perception, without any material basis, and is, therefore, centric in its origin. It is more, therefore, than an erroneous interpretation of a real object, for it is entirely formed by the mind. An individual, who on looking at a blank wall perceives it to be covered with pictures, has a hallucination of the sense of sight ; another, who, when no sounds reach his ears, hears voices whispering to him, has also a hallucination, but it is of the sense of hearing—and such false perceptions may be created as regards all kinds of sensorial excitations. The organs of the senses are, in fact, not necessary to the existence of hallucinations. Thus, if the eyes be closed, images may still be seen ; if the hearing be lost, voices may still be heard, and the reason for this is found in the fact that the erroneous perception constituting the hallucination is found in that part of the brain which ordinarily requires the excitation of a sensorial impression for its functionation. A remarkable instance of this fact has come under my observation, in which an old lady, absolutely deaf, not being able, in fact, to hear thunder or the noise caused by the discharge of a cannon, was constantly troubled by imaginary voices whispering in her ears. The blind are very often subject to hallucinations of sight.

But hallucinations of any sense cannot exist unless the individual has, at some time or other, possessed the use of that sense. A person, for instance, born blind or deaf, cannot have hallucinations of sight or hearing until the one or other of these senses has been given to him ; and, if they are never given, he will remain all his life incapable of having hallucinations of the kind referred to. I have had the opportunity of studying the case of a man born with double cataracts, who remained blind till his fourteenth year, when he was operated upon by a surgeon in Berlin. Previous to that time he had never had hallucinations of sight, but, after the operation, he became subject to these false perceptions. Coming to this country, he was again rendered blind by ophthalmic inflammation, caused by the premature explosion of a blast, but the hallucinations persisted, though he was unable to tell light from darkness.

Hallucinations are always evidence of cerebral derangement, and are common phenomena of insanity. They may be excited by emotions of various kinds, by which the character and quantity of blood circulating within the cranium are changed, by excessive intellectual exertion, by mechanical impediments to the return of blood from the brain, by various diseases which, directly or indirectly, affect the encephalon, by certain drugs, and by other factors presently to be more fully considered.

Delusion.—Illusions and hallucinations may exist, and the individual be perfectly sensible that they are not realities. In such cases the intelligence is not involved. But, if he accepts his false perceptions as facts, his intellect participates, and he has delusions. A delusion, therefore, may be based upon an illusion or a hallucination. It may also result from false reasoning in regard to real occurrences, or be evolved out of the intellect spontaneously, as the result of imperfect information, or of an inability to weigh evidence, or to discriminate between the true and the false. Delusions are not a test of insanity, as most lawyers and many physicians believe. If they were, one half the world would be trying to put the other half into lunatic asylums. They may be present without coexistent insanity, and many cases of mental aberration run their course without them.

To be indicative of the existence of insanity, a delusion must relate to a matter of fact, be contrary to the customary mode of thought of the individual, and held in opposition to such evidence as is logically opposed thereto. Beliefs in regard to matters of faith, however ridiculous they may be, are not necessarily proofs that the individual holding them is insane. Thus, a believer in spiritualism may be perfectly sane, for his belief is one not capable of proof or disproof. It is a part of his mentality to believe in the existence of spirits, and in the possibility of calling them so as to see and talk with them; moreover, he has probably at some time or other been deceived by impostors, who have passed off material objects upon him as immaterial and spiritual, and he has not had the opportunity or the desire to investigate the matter and to expose the fraud. But, if a non-believer in the system of spiritualism, should imagine that he was in the habit of seeing spirits and of conversing with them, the fact would be good evidence of his insanity. There would hence be hallucinations, and a delusion resulting from them and relating to a matter of fact; and, further, though the spiritualist might believe in the existence of spirits capable of making themselves visible, wearing textile fabrics, and talking, and still be sane, yet, if he believed, without foundation and contrary to positive evidence, that his brother had tried to poison him, he would have a delusion sufficient to indicate his insanity.

At a former period of the world's history a belief in the possibility of seeing devils and demons of various kinds, and of suffering from their torments, was commonly entertained. Indeed, it is religiously held now by a good many otherwise sensible people. Such a belief is, according to my mode of thought, a delusion ; and probably nine tenths of those who read this treatise will agree with me in so regarding it. But it certainly would not be safe to consider every one holding such a creed as insane. The number who accept such a belief is daily becoming smaller, and eventually the time will come when, from a change of the modes of thought due to progressive enlightenment, an educated person, believing that there are evil spirits commissioned by a sovereign, the devil, to afflict mankind with various ills, will be regarded as a lunatic. The acceptance of such a belief will be considered as showing the existence of a state of mind incompatible with a healthy condition of the brain. At the present day the brain of man has not acquired such an average advanced state of development as to enable us to declare that a belief of the kind mentioned is any indication of the presence of disease, however much it may be evidence of deficient education and training.

A like reasoning applies to the holders of every other form of belief accepted as an article of faith not susceptible of proof.

A delusion, therefore, to be an indication of the existence of insanity, must relate to a matter of fact, must be such a belief as would not be entertained in the ordinary normal condition of the individual, must have been formed without such evidence as would have been necessary to convince in health, and must be held against such positive testimony as would in health have sufficed for its eradication.

As above stated, a delusion, to be evidence of the existence of insanity, must relate to a matter of fact in regard to which testimony may be taken and its truth or falsehood demonstrated. A normally constituted mind cannot refuse to accept a demonstration if its elements are of such a character as to be within the degree of development of the brain of the individual. Thus, a person of ordinary intelligence and education will comprehend a demonstration of one of the problems of Euclid, which a man with a brain free from disease, but which has not been educated, will not be able to understand. Nevertheless, he has the capacity for comprehension, and this capacity only requires education. If another, who at one time fully understood all the problems of geometry, should lose this power, it would be very strong evidence of his insanity ; and if another, not accustomed to believe impossible or improbable things, imbibes a belief without there being any evidence to support it, and clings tenaciously to it, notwithstanding its improbability and the facts which are brought to show its untruth, he would certainly be insane.

But, no matter how improbable or absurd the religious belief of an individual may appear to us to be, it would not show him to be insane, for it would relate altogether to a matter of faith in regard to which certain knowledge could not be brought to bear. Thus, in the case of Louis Bonard, a Frenchman, who died a few years ago in this city, it was in evidence that the deceased had entertained the belief of metempsychosis, and the attempt was made before the surrogate of the city and county of New York to set aside the will by which he bequeathed his tolerably large estate to the Society for the Prevention of Cruelty to Animals, on the ground that metempsychosis was a delusion, and that an individual brought up in a Christian community who believed in it was insane. My opinion on the subject was requested by the proponents of the will, and I stated in the Surrogate's Court that "no religious belief, no matter how absurd it may be, is of itself sufficient evidence of a man's insanity. I base that answer upon the investigation of a large number of cases, and likewise upon a very thorough reading of the subject. As regards the doctrine of the transmigration of souls and the doctrine of metempsychosis—because, I think, there is a distinction between them—both have been held, at various times of the world's history, by the most enlightened nations then on the earth. They were, and are at the present day, held by the Hindoos, by the people of Siam, by the people of Thibet, by the Chinese. They were held by the ancient Egyptians, Greeks, Persians, Scythians, by the Druids, and by the Celts generally, to some extent. They are held now by the North American and South American Indians, as I know of my own knowledge in regard to the North American Indians. They were held by various heretical sects among the early Christians, and especially by the Gnostics and Manicheans, who were early heretical sects. They have likewise been held by several distinguished European men—Pythagoras, Plato, Pericles, Plotinus; by Origen, by Fourier, by Lessing; and among writers of the present day by Pierre Leroux; and Fourier has written extensively on the subject. I know of my own knowledge that they are held at the present day by people in the city of New York. I may say that Mr. Alger, in his very learned work, 'The Doctrine of a Future Life,' declares from his own knowledge that these beliefs, in some form or other, are largely held in this country and in Europe at the present day."

In deciding to admit the will to probate, the surrogate, in adopting these views, said :

" It appears to me that, if a judicial officer should assume that merely because a man believed in that doctrine [metempsychosis] he was insane, or acted under an insane delusion or monomania incapacitating him from making a will, if prompted by that faith, but though consistent with it, wholly rational in its provisions, it would not fall far short in principle of assuming that all mankind who do not believe in the particular faith which the judge accepts respecting a future state are more or less insane, or the victims of an insane delusion.

" This question is entirely within the domain of opinion or faith, and not of knowledge. A man may properly be assumed insane upon evidence that he is governed by hallucinations which are physically impossible to the knowledge of all sane men, and which are contrary to the evidence of the senses, or who is influenced by delusions which are the creation of diseased reflective faculties.

" Hence, the opinion as to a future state, of which no man has positive knowledge, and in regard to which mankind have always differed, and so widely differ to-day, even in the most civilized communities and among the most intellectual of men, cannot in any respect be deemed evidence of insanity, the only rule by which the insanity of one of certain opinions can be determined being by some test founded on positive knowledge." [1]

I have considered this point at some length, for the reason that I am aware that a good deal of misapprehension exists in the minds of physicians and lawyers relative to the essential nature of a delusion which is to be evidence of an individual's insanity. The distinction between a belief founded on faith and one founded on fact is not always recognized, and we are all more or less apt, unless we guard ourselves closely, to look upon those who hold what we consider erroneous convictions as being the victims of insane delusions, when, in reality,

---

[1] " Abbot's Reports of Practice, Cases determined in the Courts of the State of New York," vol. xvi, Nos. 2 and 3, p. 128, *et seq.*

the matter in question is entirely beyond the pale of investigation by the rules of evidence.

But there are certain delusions, mostly of a religious character, which, though partly based on faith, may urge the subject to the perpetration of some act of criminal violence. An individual may, for instance, imbibe the belief that God has ordered him to kill his son on a certain day, and when the time comes round he murders his child. Such a belief cannot be controverted by evidence, because there is no attainable testimony which can be brought to bear upon the matter. The man persists that he knows it to be true, that he was told what to do in a dream, and he adduces text after text from the Bible to prove that there is nothing in his conduct unbecoming a believer in God, and of one acknowledging his power. Such a man, if really holding to the belief in question, must, nevertheless, be pronounced insane, for it is one not only of faith, but of fact also. He might believe in God's power to order him to kill his son, and in his right to do so : that would be entirely a matter of faith ; but when he adds to this the belief that God actually did order him to do so, the element of fact is brought in, and an insane delusion exists.

As I have said, insanity may exist without delusions being at any time present. Some physicians doubt this fact, but this is due to the circumstance that they have no clear conception of what a delusion is. I have heard the superintendent of a lunatic asylum state that all attempts of the insane to commit suicide or homicide were the results of delusions, and, when I requested to be informed as to the understanding in his mind of the nature of a delusion, he replied that "any notable deviation of the mind from its usual and accustomed standard was a delusion." We see, therefore, how necessary it is that we should have in the study of insanity exact ideas of the meaning of the words we employ.

Incoherence.—There are two kinds of incoherence :

1. That in which the words used in speaking or writing are without proper relation to each other.

2. That in which the ideas are without logical arrangement, or are incompletely expressed.

Not infrequently both kinds exist in the same individual.

As an example of the first-named variety of incoherence, I cite the following letter :

18

"IN THE NECK, *January* 7, 1871.

"DEAR SIR : I said he was in my own conscience that the book was confined. I quote the long time with eccentricity in the common way. This is in memory to my upshot, which was incorrect in the final oblivion. Dogs and money, consistency with foundlings without antebellum, which was in *statu quo.*

"This is passive in contiguity with the works met in the creation of existence.   "Very commingle,

"In good faith,

"J. S. W——."

The patient who wrote this was at the time suffering from an attack of acute mania. Although no one not familiar with his case can obtain an idea of what he was thinking of when he wrote this letter, or rather of what he was endeavoring to think, I—knowing the cause of his insanity, and the predominating thoughts present with him at the time he became insane, and during the prodromatic stage, when his mind was not yet overthrown—can discover here and there the vestige of an idea. He was a young man who had, without much preliminary training, entered upon the task of refuting Darwin's views relative to the "Descent of Man," and who had written quite a large volume on the subject. He had labored very assiduously at his undertaking, and had consulted a large number of authorities, frequenting the public libraries, and sitting up late at night at his work. Finally he broke down. His letter refers indistinctly to his book, and the words "dogs" and "works met in the creation of existence" indicate subjects that he had been engaged in studying.

The following "poem" was written by a lady who was also suffering from acute mania, with slightly erotic tendencies. As is seen, the words used to express each idea are logically arranged, but there is no proper relation between the ideas. Each is, in fact, entirely independent of the others:

"I stood upon the awful height
To be my funeral shroud ;
Oh, how can Heaven reveal its light,
And then to him she bowed.

"Come, come with me, my gentle youth,
Sleep wafted o'er my soul,
I am a maid, called Ruby Ruth,
So sadly I condole."

The following is from the "Evening Post" of about three years ago. It is an excellent example in the first part of incoherence of ideas, and in the latter of incoherence of words. I cite it, with the editor's remarks, as printed at the time:

"[For the 'Evening Post.']

"LES OISCANY SOLITAIRES.

"[Usually we have an opinion about the verse sent to us. The following piece, which appears to be of noble origin, goes beyond our comprehension. We leave it to the judgment of the reader.]

"Closely watch'd—Juvenile Bridal Dress :
Arch summer smiles. Dreaming ever of thee.
My desolate heart no longer throbs
Lifted hand—sad—why wearily ?
I listen in spirit the Sea Gull's call.
The story runs, that, dishearten'd the child ran away—Gone !
Worn-cast-down-look. September evening breeze,
Gray Mist dissolves. Peeps ! Love's honey'd kiss, chaste as the
   dawn.

"Lord of the Dead Sea : more by right ! Crisp hair
Beams ! Filigree, Shabby Dress ! Soothing idle hours—
Hopes cunning chaplet. Little Baggage, wreaths,
Enchanted, Immaculate Flowers.
Temp'rate Isles yield Candy tuft. Daysparkles
Turning Fickle Youth : Ma Foi ! Time Glides ! Unmerited disdain !
Toy Baskets surfeit unruly sycophants : Ruffle Green, violet chène,
Polands advance, white Parasols, dépôts John Leach haunts. No
   longer seen.
                        "COUNTESS OF BRIGHTWELL.
"BROOKLYN, *October* 3, 1879."

It often happens that insane persons, who exhibit incoherence in their writings, nevertheless converse without any marked manifestation of this symptom. They seem to require the stimulus of intercourse with others in order to arrange their words or ideas correctly, and when left to themselves are unable to do so. Again, some will express themselves with entire coherence until they begin to get tired, when they break down, and their words and ideas become disarranged, or the like result may ensue from gradually advancing excitement as the conversation goes on. Morel[1] refers to the case

[1] Cited by Dagouet. "Nouveau traité elementaire et pratique des maladies mentales," Paris, 1876, p. 49.

of a lunatic who, at the beginning of a conversation, was calm and reasonable, but who, if it was continued, became excited little by little; his eyes shone brightly, his countenance assumed an expression impossible to describe, and very soon his words, his ideas, his gestures—in short, his whole appearance and all his actions—became those of a maniac in a violent paroxysm. Excitement produces a similar effect, though, of course, not to so great an extent, in many persons of perfectly sane minds.

Incoherence is a prominent feature in delirium. It is generally present at some time or other in cases of acute mania, and is common in imbecility, and in chronic insanity of any kind. It appears to be directly due either to the impossibility of keeping the attention sufficiently long on one idea for its full consideration, or to a difficulty of co-ordinating those parts of the brain which are concerned in the formation and expression of thoughts so as to obtain continuity of mental action.

Delirium.—Delirium is that condition in which there are illusions, hallucinations, delusions, and incoherence, together with a general excess of motility, an inability to sleep, and acceleration of pulse. The derivation of the word, *de*, out of, and *liro*, a rut or furrow, sufficiently indicates the idea entertained by the ancients of the essential nature of the condition in question.

Foville[1] has described two species of delirium: that which occurs in acute diseases generally, and in other conditions not insanity, and that which is met with in cases of mental aberration. The first class, however, embraces many different kinds, such as the delirium of starvation, the delirium due to toxic agents taken into the system, that which follows on wounds and injuries, and that which is sometimes met with in extreme old age. However, we need not at present concern ourselves with these varieties. A few words, nevertheless, relative to the characteristics of the delirium of insanity will not be out of place.

The condition may make its appearance suddenly, but usually it is of gradual development, being preceded by many signs of mental and physical disturbance. The perceptions, the intellect, the emotions, and the will may, singly or in

[1] Art. " Delire," *Nouveau dictionnaire de médicine et de chirurgie pratiques*, t. xi, p. 1.

combination, be involved. Generally speaking, illusions and hallucinations are the most prominent features, the patient being entirely aware of their true character, conversing of them rationally, and willing to take proper measures to get rid of them. Erroneous ideas are at first distinctly recognized as abnormal, he laments the emotional disturbance of which he may be the subject, and regrets that he cannot better restrain himself from perpetrating disorderly or eccentric acts. With this implication of the mental faculties there is a disposition to talk incessantly, and, of course, somewhat wildly ; there is an exaggeration of motility, extravagant and excessive gestures are employed, and the patient is up and down through the day and night, now in this place and now in that, button-holing those he knows, and often those with whom he has no acquaintance, and telling them of the schemes he has in hand, or the persecution of which he is the victim. The delusion of persecution is a common phase of the disorder, and, to escape from the enemies which he imagines are conspiring against him, he may wander off unintelligently, or depart secretly for some distant place.

Esquirol[1] has given a short description of delirium which, so far as its mental manifestations are concerned, is very accurate.

"A man," he says, "is in a state of delirium when his sensations are not in relation with exterior objects, when his ideas are not in relation with his sensations, when his judgments and his determinations are not in relation with his ideas, and when his ideas, his judgments, and his determinations are independent of his will."

Delirium may be the first stage of any variety of insanity, though it is most common in the beginning of acute mania. I have seen several cases in which it was the first obvious sign of the existence of general paralysis of the insane. In one of them, the patient, a gentleman engaged in a large mercantile business, left his office at about three o'clock in order to take a drive in the Central Park. Up to that time, no one who had had any relations with him had noticed the slightest evidence of mental derangement. He drove up town in a cab, and never left it till he arrived at his own door. His wife was in the library waiting for him, but, as soon as he reached the room, she perceived that he was not right. His clothes were

[1] "Des maladies mentales," Paris, 1838, t. i, p. 5.

in disorder, his eyes were extraordinarily bright, he was gesticulating violently, he was alternately laughing and crying, and she could not understand a word of his incoherent and voluble speech. From that time on the signs of serious mental disorder became more apparent, and eventually there was no doubt of the existence of general paralysis.

In such cases as the foregoing, there were probably earlier symptoms, which from their lightness escaped observation, but of which the patient was himself fully aware.

Although the erroneous perceptions and ideas may succeed each other with great rapidity, there is not always such a degree of incoherence as to prevent the patient being understood. Still, I think there is always some disturbance in the faculty of speech. Words are misplaced or mispronounced, or entirely forgotten, or the individual, attempting to make his articulation keep pace with his ideas, only succeeds in making himself difficult to be understood.

If the patient has in his or her normal condition been musically inclined, the proclivity is very apt to be increased in delirium, and hours are spent at the piano or some other musical instrument, or in singing at the top of the voice. Bergman [1] has called attention to a singular tendency, occasionally manifested by individuals in delirium, to the formation of rhymes. One case of the kind has come under my observation in which the patient, a clergyman of about forty years of age, began to show evidences of mental aberration by excitement of mind and body, and in a short time by speaking and writing altogether in rhymes, or, as he called it, "rhythmical inspiration." The following is a portion of a letter I received from him at the time he was advised to consult me:

"Dear Sir : If thus you'll allow me to call you,
I write to inform you that my friend Mr. Ballou
Has advised me to see you in regard to my health,
If my means will admit ; for I have but small wealth ;
I'm a preacher, and have but little of this world's goods
Beyond a small salary and a little house in the backwoods.
I shall leave here on the 4th—that is, Wednesday next—
And will be in your city, if by railroads not vexed,
On the following Saturday, and hope there you to meet
At your city residence in Fifty-fourth Street,

[1] "Nasse's Zeitschrift für psychologischen Aerzte," 1823, B. II, s. 419.

Say at ten o'clock, if that hour suits,
And if it does not, it makes little difference to me, for I
  shall be entirely at your disposal.''
He even went so far as to prepare a sermon in rhyme, and
was with difficulty prevented preaching it. I quote a few
lines from this production :
  '' I see before me many a face
    That but for God Almighty's grace
    Would sink into the depths of hell,
    And there in endless torments dwell.
    You sit regardless of your fate,
    Perhaps you'll stay till it is too late
    To save your weak and sinful souls
    From the lake that in fire and sulphur rolls.
    The devil and all his fiends are there,
    Waiting to seize you by the hair,
    To drag you down to the deepest pit
    And keep you there by God's permit.''
And so on for thirty-one pages.
  Whatever we may think of the poetry of this sermon, it
must be admitted that its orthodoxy is unquestionable.
  When he entered my consulting-room, he advanced, hold-
ing out his hand, and, with a smile on his face, said :
  ''Good-morning, Dr. Hammond, I hope you are well,
    I've come a long distance my story to tell :
    They say I'm insane, but that's an inanity,
    I've a rhyming inspiration, but that's not insanity.''
  His whole conversation was in rhyme, or the attempt
at it, for occasionally he failed to get the word he wanted,
and then he would ''drop into prose'' for a few sentences.
He lost his rhyming inspiration in a few days after I saw
him, and passed through an attack of acute mania and dementia, eventually recovering and returning to his duties with
his congregation.
  Lucid Interval.—By the term lucid interval is to be understood a condition in which there is a total cessation of the
symptoms of mental aberration and a complete restoration
to reason occurring between any two paroxysms of insanity.
With this understanding of a lucid interval it must be regarded as a rare occurrence. In fact, it probably does not exist except in the recurrent and epileptic forms of insanity, and
in certain varieties of monomania and of morbid impulses. As

thus defined, it differs essentially from those remissions which occur in the violence of all kinds of mental aberration, and in which, while to a superficial observer the patient is sane, careful investigation by a skilful physician will not fail to reveal the evidences of unsoundness of mind. It is necessary to draw the line closely between these two conditions, and this is especially necessary in many medico-legal cases, in which it is important to show the state of an individual's mind at the time certain acts are alleged to have been done.

Shelford[1] defines a lucid interval as "not a remission of the complaint, but a temporary and total cessation of it, and complete restoration to the perfect enjoyment of reason upon every subject upon which the mind was previously cognizant"; and he adds: "The determination as to the existence of a lucid interval requires attentive observation and long and repeated examination by a person acquainted with the subject of the patient's insanity."

Taylor[2] says, with apparently less decision: "By a lucid interval we are to understand, in a legal sense, a temporary cessation of the insanity, or a perfect restoration to reason. This state differs entirely from a remission in which there is a mere abatement of the symptoms. It has been said that a lucid interval is only a more perfect remission, and that although a lunatic may act rationally and talk coherently, yet his brain is in an excitable state, and he labors under a greater disposition to a fresh attack of insanity than one whose mind has never been affected. Of this there can be no doubt, but the same reasoning would tend to show that insanity is never cured, for the predisposition to an attack is undoubtedly greater in a recovered lunatic than in one who is and has always been perfectly sane. Even admitting the correctness of this reasoning, it cannot be denied that lunatics do occasionally recover, for a longer or shorter period, to such a degree as to render them perfectly conscious of and legally responsible for their actions with other people."

All this is very true, but a cure is a very different thing from a lucid interval, for the latter, properly speaking, if it

---

[1] "A Practical Treatise on the Law concerning Lunatics, Idiots, and Persons of Unsound Mind," London, 1833, p. lxx.

[2] "The Principles and Practice of Medical Jurisprudence," vol. ii, second edition, London, 1873, p. 484.

exists at all, must be a part of the disease, during which the tendency to a return is present to such a degree that the paroxysms will almost certainly recur. A complete restoration to mental health may be followed by a recurrence of the insanity, but then the period of cessation is scarcely a lucid interval in the true sense of the term, and the return should be regarded as a fresh attack. If the period during which an individual is entirely well, and extending, as it may, over several years, is to be regarded as a lucid interval, nearly every kind of insanity exhibits it.

A patient, for instance, suffers with an attack of acute mania for several months, is restored to health, goes about his business, and attends to it as well as he ever did, perhaps marries, and has children. Undoubtedly a predisposition to another attack exists, but this may never be excited into action, and the person is regarded by every one as permanently cured. But, on the other hand, the tendency may, through some sufficiently exciting cause, be roused into activity, and another paroxysm, after many years of perfect health, mental and physical, be developed. Is it not stretching the point a good deal to call this period a lucid interval? Dr. Taylor, while avoiding the Scylla of remission, runs foul of the Charybdis of cure.

The case of Cartwright *vs.* Cartwright was adjudicated upon the presumption that the patient, a lunatic, had a lucid interval when she wrote her will. The testatrix had for some time been, as all acknowledged, insane. There were no collateral circumstances to indicate the existence of a lucid interval. She was in restraint at the time she made her will, and her hands were unbound so that she could hold a pen. She was alone when she performed the act, though observed through an aperture by persons in an adjoining room, who deposed that, while engaged in doing it, she frequently left off writing, threw the pieces of paper into the fire, and walked about the room in a disordered manner. But the paper itself had no mark of irritation. Whatever outward appearance of disorder there may have been, it had no effect upon the writing itself, which was a perfectly steady and correct performance, entirely consistent with her attachments, impressions, and habits when in a sane condition, and written without a single mistake or blot. The will was planned and completed by the testatrix without any assistance, and afterward recognized by her.[1] Sir William Wynne, in deciding in favor of the will, said : "The strongest and best proof that can arise as to a lucid interval is that which arises from the act itself, which is the thing to be first examined, and, if it can be proved and established that it is a rational act rationally done, that is sufficient." But, if the performance of "a rational act in a rational manner" is sufficient to establish the existence of complete sanity—for that is what a lucid interval is—nearly every lunatic is sane. To go to the fire for warmth, to put butter on bread, to wash clothes, to dig in the garden, to make baskets, are "rational acts rationally done," but they do not establish the existence of complete sanity. For this purpose, not only a single act or a dozen acts must be "rational and done rationally," but *all* the acts must come under this category. The idea that during a paroxysm of acute mania a person can be sane enough to make a valid will, the period of so-called lucidity lasting at most an hour, is simply absurd. Even a much longer duration of apparent sanity is frequently only a superficial glaze of rationality, which may be broken through by the slightest impression. A case which is of striking application to the point under notice is within my knowledge. A gentleman of this city became, during a period of great excitement, temporarily insane. After a not very long attack of acute mania, he was apparently restored to reason, and was about resuming his business, when he conceived the idea of making his will. He sent for his lawyer, and dictated clearly and fully all the provisions which he wished inserted in this document. His property was large, but he made such a disposition of it as his legal friend thought rational if not just. The will was signed, witnessed, and committed to the lawyer's hands for safe keeping. Soon afterward the gentleman had a relapse ; he recovered, however, and was finally pronounced cured. Two years afterward, meeting the lawyer in the street, he requested him to come to his house that evening, as he wished him to draw up his will. His friend asked him if he desired to cancel the will already made, and which he had in his safe. "I have never made a will," replied the gentleman. "Yes," answered the lawyer, "I drew one up for you more than two years ago ; you signed it ; it was witnessed, and is now in my safe." The gentleman was astonished. He had no recol-

[1] Shelford, *op. cit.*, p. 290.

lection of the matter, and, when the will was shown to him, he expressed the utmost surprise and regret at some of the provisions, which, as he said, were altogether different from those he would have made had he been of sane mind at the time. The will was destroyed, and a new one executed, differing essentially from that which he had dictated during his so-called lucid interval.

In a review of Redfield's "Law of Wills," [1] Dr. Isaac Ray makes some excellent remarks relative to the theory of lucid intervals, which, I think, fairly express the prevailing doctrine on the subject among the most intelligent physicians of the present day. He says:

"No phenomenon of insanity has played a wider part in medical jurisprudence than lucid intervals, so called, and no one, we may also say, has been more differently understood. And the fact is not surprising, for they indicate a phase of the disease which none but those who have been long and intimately connected with the insane can correctly appreciate. The descriptions of it in books serve to make the matter very clear, and leave the impression that lucid intervals are frequent occurrences, and easily distinguished from other remissions of the disease ; and here lies the mischief, that of using a phenomenon which is complicated with many conditions not easily discernible for any important practical purpose. It is to be regretted that the phrase, implying as it does a foregone conclusion, ever found its way into the law. It certainly has led to mistakes, and will lead to many more before it ceases to influence the decisions of the courts. One author (Judge Redfield) inclines to believe that there is no essential difference between a lucid interval and a remission of the disease, and such we suppose to be the view generally entertained by those who are specially acquainted with the subject. The idea of a lucid interval being a temporary cure is now confined, we apprehend, to the writings of those whose notions of the disease have been derived from books rather than from the wards of a hospital. Like most other diseases, insanity is subject to remissions more or less complete, and there is no more propriety in regarding them as recoveries than there would be in considering the intervals between the paroxysms of a quotidian fever as a temporary recovery. And, if the disease remained in any condition whatever, it is

[1] *American Journal of Insanity*, April, 1865, p. 515.

mere presumption to say that the operations of the mind are entirely beyond its influence. This effect may not be very obvious, but the fact of its possible existence should render us cautious how we regard the acts of the insane during a lucid interval. In criminal cases the occasion will seldom arise, but in the matter of wills and contracts the decision will often depend on the speculative views that prevail on the subject."

It is thus seen that Dr. Ray doubts the existence of lucid intervals in the sense in which they are commonly understood by lawyers, and as defined in the beginning of this description.

Relative to the subject, Dr. George Combe[1] says : "But, however calm and rational the patient may be during the lucid intervals, as they are called, and while enjoying the quietude of domestic society or the limited range of a well-regulated asylum, it must never be supposed that he is in as perfect possession of his senses as if he had never been ill. In ordinary circumstances and under ordinary excitement, his perceptions may be accurate and his judgment perfectly sound, but a degree of irritability remains behind which renders him unable to withstand any unusual emotion, any sudden provocation, or any unexpected or pressing emergency. Were not this the case, it is manifest that he would not be more liable to a fresh paroxysm than if he had never been attacked, and the opposite is notoriously the fact ; for relapses are always to be dreaded, not only after a lucid interval, but even after perfect recovery ; and it is but just, as well as proper, to keep this in mind, as it has too often happened that the lunatic has been visited with the heaviest responsibility for acts committed during such an interval which previous to the first attack of the disease he would have shrunk from with horror."

Dagonet[2] declares that "the lucid interval is no more health than the intermission between the attacks of ague is a cure. However much restored the reason may apparently be, the individual is placed in a special situation which the least circumstance may easily and instantaneously transform into one of disease. Doubtless the distinction is often difficult to establish ; it belongs to the physician, and, above all, to the

[1] "Observations on Mental Derangement," Edinburgh, 1831, p. 221.

[2] "Nouveau traité elementaire et pratique des maladies mentales," Paris, 1876, p. 111.

physician who has devoted himself to the study of insanity, to fix the character after an attentive examination in certain special cases. Thus, it is not rare to observe, in the asylums for the insane, some patients, in the moments of remission in their affections, show themselves to be calm and rational to such a degree that it would be difficult to prove that they were at all in an insane condition. If, however, they were in any way to be subjected to the excitements of life, they would immediately return to their state of intellectual derangement."

There is a great deal more that might doubtless be adduced relative to lucid intervals, were it not for the fact that the subject in most of its relations appertains to the domain of medical jurisprudence. Enough has, however, been said to show that full, complete intervals in the course of an attack of insanity, during which the individual is well, and would so be pronounced by competent observers, are exceedingly rare. They are only to be found, in my opinion, in recurrent mania and the other forms previously mentioned. Remissions are common enough, but a remission is not a restoration to health, and the patient in whom it is exhibited ought not to be regarded as being possessed of legal responsibility.

CHAPTER II.

CLASSIFICATION.

THE systems of classification of the several forms of insanity are almost as numerous as the writers on mental alienation. To detail at length the various arrangements which have been proposed would be of little service to the student, and, indeed, would mostly only confuse his mind. It will be sufficient to indicate the principles upon which some of the more important have been constructed, and to specify more minutely a few of those which appear to be of most importance.

There are six different methods which may be employed in the classification of mental diseases :

1. *The Anatomical,* in which the forms are classified according to the part of the brain affected.

This is the method which is to be preferred to all others, but, unfortunately, our knowledge is not yet sufficient to enable us to adopt it to any considerable extent.

2. *The Physiological*, in which an attempt is made to classify mental diseases according to the part of the encephalon involved, as determined by our knowledge of its functions.

The objection to this method, which has been proposed by Professor Laycock,[1] of Edinburgh, is similar to that urged against the anatomical method—lack of sufficient knowledge to enable us to make one that would be much more than guess-work.

3. *The Etiological.*—In this system the different forms of insanity are arranged according to the supposed causes. Morel[2] and Skae[3] have proposed elaborate schemes of classification in accordance with this method. Thus, we have the toxic insanity, such as is caused by alcohol, malaria, ergot, mercury, etc.; hysterical insanity, epileptic insanity, etc., of Morel; and the amenorrhœal mania, post-connubial mania, ovario mania, traumatic mania, and even the mania of oxaluria and phosphaturia of Skae.

4. *The Psychological.*—A classification from a psychological stand-point is one in which the pathology of the mind is arranged in accordance with the several categories of mental faculties. Hence, there is a perceptional, an intellectual, an emotional, and a volitional insanity, corresponding to the four divisions of the mind. There are some advantages belonging to this system, but there are disadvantages which more than overbalance them. It has been followed, in whole or in part, by many authors, among them being Crichton,[4] Arnold,[5] Hoffbauer,[6] Heiiroth,[7] Griesinger,[8] and Despine.[9] It was the one

[1] " Mind and Brain," etc., Edinburgh, 1869.

[2] " Traité des maladies mentales," Paris, 1860.

[3] *Journal of Mental Science*, 1863 and 1873.

[4] " An Inquiry into the Nature and Origin of Mental Derangement," etc., London, 1798.

[5] " Observations on the Nature, Kinds, Causes, and Prevention of Insanity," second edition, London, 1806.

[6] " Untersuchungen über die Krankheiten der Seele," Halle, 1802, 5–7.

[7] " Lehrbuch der Störungen des Seelensbebens," Leipzig, 1818.

[8] " Die Pathologie und Therapie der psychischen Krankheiten," Stuttgart, 1863, 2te Auflage.

[9] " De la folie du point de vue philosophique ou plus spécialment psychologique," Paris, 1875.

which was adopted in the earlier editions of my "Treatise on the Diseases of the Nervous System," in which insanity was considered. Mature reflection has, however, convinced me that it cannot be exclusively followed, although it may very properly be the basis for a satisfactory classification—satisfactory, that is, in the present state of our knowledge of brain anatomy, physiology, and pathology.

5. *The Pathological.*—In this method of arrangement the various forms of insanity are classified according to the morbid conditions of the brain, which are supposed to be in immediate relation with them as causes and effects. This basis is that adopted by Luys[1] in his recent work on insanity, who divides all forms of mental derangement into three classes— those which result from cerebral hyperæmia, those due to cerebral anæmia, and those in which both conditions exist simultaneously in different parts of the brain.

It was still more elaborately laid out by M. Aug. Voisin,[2] who, in addition to the recognition of congestion and anæmia as pathological states acting as the immediate causes of insanity, designated also atheroma of the cerebral arteries and tumors of various parts of the encephalon as giving rise to mental derangement.

According to M. Aug. Voison, all insanity may be divided into six classes : [3]

"1. *Acquired Insanity.*—That which supervenes in the course of the life of the individual, and which has been preceded by a state of ordinary intelligence.

"2. *Native Insanity.*—That in which the intellectual troubles are shown at an early age, especially under the influence of heredity.

"3. *Insanity by intoxication, or virus,* the nature of which is indicated by its name.

"4. *Cretinism, idiocy, and imbecility,* under which head are embraced a great number of forms of mental derangement, characterized either by a weakness of the will and the understanding, giving rise to feebleness of mind to the extent, perhaps, of an almost complete abolition of the mental faculties, with or without lesions of the skeleton.

"5. *General Paralysis.*—The best studied form of insan-

---

[1] "Traité clinique et pratique des maladies mentales," Paris, 1881.
[2] "Leçons cliniques sur les maladies mentales," Paris, 1876.
[3] *Op. cit.*, p. 15.

ity—one in which the lesions and the symptoms have been placed intimately in relation with each other, and with our actual knowledge of the physiology of the nervous system.

"6. *Senile Dementia.*"

The class of acquired insanity embraces *primitive or idiopathic insanity, secondary insanity, sensorial insanity,* and *sympathetic insanity.*

The essential part, however, of M. Aug. Voisin's classification is that any variety of insanity may be due to congestion, anæmia, atheroma, or tumors, and the condition, whichever it may be, determines the character of the symptoms of any one variety. Thus, a case of primitive insanity belonging to his first class may be due either to congestion or to anæmia of the brain. If the former, the type will be one of mental exaltation ; if the latter, of mental depression. He is, however, obliged to admit that it may be the result of inappreciable lesions ; that is, without congestion, anæmia, atheroma, or tumors being present. The same may be said of his other forms ; so that while the classification is ingenious, and is a good basis for further investigation, it cannot be accepted as a finality, or as tending to simplify the study of the subject of mental derangement.

6. *The Clinical or Symptomatological Classifications,* based on the clinical features or symptoms exhibited by the varieties of insanity, are those which are most in vogue at the present time. As insanity as a whole is only a symptom of brain disease, it follows that such classifications are merely arrangements of the phenomena or symptoms into groups for study, investigation, and treatment. Perhaps, notwithstanding this fact, such systems, in some form or other, are about the best which are attainable in the present state of our knowledge. A very simple grouping is that of Leidesdorf [1] and other writers—namely, *states of mental depression, states of mental excitement, states of mental weakness.* Under the first head are embraced all the forms of melancholy ; under the second, mania in general and monomania in particular ; under the third, imbecility, dementia, and idiocy.

One of the most recent classifications is that of Kraft Ebing. [2] On account of the recognized position of its author, as

[1] " Lehrbuch der psychischen Krankheiten," Erlangen, 1865.
[2] " Lehrbuch der Psychiatrie," u. s. w., Stuttgart, 1880.

also of the fact that it is put forth as representing the present state of psychological medicine, I give it entire :

A. Psychical Diseases of the Fully Developed Brain.

I. THE PSYCHO-NEUROSES.

1. Primary Curable Conditions.
   a. Melancholia.
      aa. Melancholia passiva.
      bb. Melancholia attonita.
   b. Mania.
      aa. Maniacal exaltation.
      bb. Acute mania (Tobsucht).
   c. Primary dementia (Stupidität).
2. Secondary Incurable Conditions.
   a. Chronic mania (secondär Verrücktheit).
   b. Terminal dementia.
      aa. Dementia with excitement.
      bb. Dementia with depression.

II. PSYCHICAL DEGENERATIONS.

a. Constitutional affective insanity (folie raisonnante).
b. Moral insanity.
c. Primary mania.
   aa. With delusions of persecution.
   bb. With exaltation (erotic and religious mania).
   cc. Imperative conceptions (morbid impulses ?).
d. Insanity from constitutional neuroses.
   aa. Epileptic insanity.
   bb. Hysterical insanity.
   cc. Hypochondriacal insanity.
   dd. Periodical insanity.

III. BRAIN DISEASES WITH PREDOMINATING PSYCHICAL DISTURBANCES.

a. Dementia paralytica.
b. Cerebral syphilis.
c. Chronic alcoholism.
d. Senile dementia.
e. Acute delirium.

B. PSYCHICAL STATES OF ARRESTED DEVELOPMENT, IDIOCY,
AND CRETINISM.

The objections to this arrangement are mainly that it is too full in some respects and too meagre in others. In fact, it is not consistent with the principles upon which it is founded. Thus, while moral insanity is recognized, there is no mention of that form of mental derangement in which there is an inability to exert the will. If alcoholic insanity is introduced into psychological nosology, why should absinthine insanity be left out? There is no mention of puerperal insanity, circular insanity, hebephrenia, and other well-known forms. Moreover, the system is radically imperfect which makes classes of conditions depend for their arrangement on their presumed curability or incurability.

Far better is the simpler arrangement proposed by Dr. Spitzka,[1] in which, while there is no attempt at a systematic classification into groups or genera, the several forms which he recognizes are enumerated in an order which is itself not a necessary feature. It is as follows:

1. Progressive paresis.
2. Senile dementia.
3. Chronic confusion of ideas. Chronic mania proper.
4. Chronic mania with imbecility.
5. Monomania.
6. Hebephrenia.
7. Katatonia.
8. Circular insanity.
9. Epileptic insanity.
10. Periodical insanity.
11. Acute mania.
12. Lypemania.

So far as it goes, no classification could be better than this, but the objections to it are that it does not embrace all known forms of insanity, and that the psychological element is not recognized. Perhaps its extension in its present line would be amply sufficient for purposes of study and practical application, but as a treatise on insanity should be something more than a mere manual of practice, so a system of classification upon which the treatise is based should also be more. It

[1] " On the Scientific Necessity for a Clinical Demarkation of the Various Forms of Insanity," *Medical Gazette*, May 15 and 29, 1880.

should not only, as far as practicable, embrace all well-established varieties of mental alienation, but it should, at least, make the attempt to arrange them in groups, according to whatever philosophical idea may exist in the mind of its author. The system adopted may be wrong, it may be artificial and strained, it may lack exactness and sharpness in its boundaries; but, nevertheless, it is better than none, and will at least, by exciting thought in the mind of the reader, lead to discussion, and, perhaps, a better system.

Influenced by these ideas, I venture to propose the following arrangement. It is not claimed that it is perfect; it is not asserted that the several groups are in all cases clearly separated from each other; on the contrary, I know very well that they are not. There are, perhaps, for instance, few if any of the forms which I have classed under the head of "Intellectual Insanities" which do not show emotional disturbance also. I have placed them where they are for the reason that the chief manifestations of mental disorder which they exhibit relate to the intellect. It may be true that not a single one of the forms which are designated as "Emotional Insanities" are not constantly marked by intellectual derangement, but I do contend that their most prominent characteristics are connected with the emotions, and I have classified them in accordance with that view. Similar remarks are applicable to the varieties which I have placed under the head of "Volitional Insanities," though not to the same extent.

The division of "Compound Insanities" embraces those forms which are either so constituted that no predominance of intellectual, emotional, or volitional derangement can be determined, or which manifest themselves in these respects differently with different individuals.

The group of "Constitutional Insanities" comprises those varieties which are either the result of some pre-existing physiological or pathological condition, or which owe their origin to a general toxic state of the system.

Under the head of "Arrest of Mental Development" are placed those states which are due to deficient brain and nervous development.

Relative to the first-named group, "Perceptional Insanities," I have to say that as the perceptions in health form the basis of all higher mental processes, so in mental derangement they are the groundwork on which most of the various forms of insanity are constructed. That they may be the seat of disorder without the other categories of mental faculties being affected admits of no doubt, and there is hence no good reason why their aberrations should not be included in a classification intended to embrace all well-established forms of mental derangement.

I have not placed such forms as alcoholic mania, malarial mania, absinthine mania, podagral mania, and many others of the kind in this classification, for I do not believe that the cause in such cases exercises any influence as a modificator of the type. Malarial mania, for instance, is not distinguishable, so far as the symptoms are concerned, from the mania produced by alcohol. Moreover, of several cases, for instance, of malarial mania, and many of alcoholic mania, which have come under my observation, some were characterized by mental exaltation, others by mental depression, and others again were well-marked instances of primary dementia. Alcohol, malaria, gout, rheumatism, etc., act as causes, but do not give rise to specific types of insanity.

I. **Perceptional Insanities.**—Insanities in which there are derangements of one or more of the perceptions.

a. Illusions.

b. Hallucinations.

II. **Intellectual Insanities.**—Forms in which the chief manifestations of mental disorder relate to the intellect, being of the nature of false conceptions (delusions), or clearly abnormal conceptions.

a. Intellectual monomania with exaltation.

b. Intellectual monomania with depression.

c. Chronic intellectual mania.

d. Reasoning mania.

e. Intellectual subjective morbid impulses.

f. Intellectual objective morbid impulses.

III. **Emotional Insanities.**—Forms in which the mental derangement is chiefly exhibited with regard to the emotions.

a. Emotional monomania.

b. Emotional morbid impulses.

c. Simple melancholia.

d. Melancholia with delirium.

e. Melancholia with stupor.

f. Hypochondriacal mania, or melancholia.

g. Hysterical mania.

h. Epidemic insanity.

IV. **Volitional Insanities.**—Forms characterized by derangement of the will, either by its abnormal predominance or inertia.

a. Volitional morbid impulses.

b. Aboulomania (paralysis of the will).

V. **Compound Insanities.**—Forms in which two or more categories of mental faculties are markedly involved.

a. Acute mania.

b. Periodical insanity.

c. Hebephrenia.

d. Circular insanity.

e. Katatonia.

f. Primary dementia.

g. Secondary dementia.

h. Senile dementia.

i. General paralysis.

VI. **Constitutional Insanities.**—Forms which are the result of a pre-existing physiological or pathological condition, or of some specific morbid influence affecting the system.

a. Epileptic insanity.

b. Puerperal insanity.

c. Pellagrous insanity.

d. Choreic insanity, etc.

VII. **Arrest of Mental Development.**

a. Idiocy.

b. Cretinism.

As each particular form is brought under consideration, the subdivisions of which it is capable will be indicated. This course is not followed now, in order to avoid any possible confusion which might arise from the necessarily intricate construction of the table.

Although *arrests of mental development* are necessary to be considered in the classification of the several forms of derangement of the mind, it is not the intention to discuss them in the present treatise. The treatment which they require is quite special, and it is such as is not within the province of the medical practitioner, unless he gives himself up to the work and to that alone.

CHAPTER III.

I.

PERCEPTIONAL INSANITIES.

In uncomplicated perceptional insanities those parts only of the brain are disordered which are concerned in the formation of perceptions. They constitute the primary form of mental aberration, and of themselves are not of such a character as to lessen the responsibility of the individual or to warrant any interference with his rights. They consist entirely of false perceptions; and if the intellect should be for a moment deceived, the error is immediately corrected. As already stated, there are two forms of false perceptions—illusions and hallucinations. In some cases they coexist in the same individual. They may be related to any one or more of the special senses, but are especially common as regards sight and hearing.

a—ILLUSIONS.

Illusions, as already mentioned, are not necessarily due to any central disturbance, though such an origin is common. It is, of course, only when they have such an origin that they are an indication of mental derangement. Thus, it is an illusion if a person, on looking at one object, sees two images, or if, when a single sound strikes the ears, he hears two sounds, and often pitched on different keys. In the first case, the result is due to some cause destroying the parallelism of the visual axes, and may be produced by a tumor of the orbit or by paralysis of one or the other of the ocular muscles. In the latter, it is caused by disease of the middle ear, producing a different degree of pressure upon the fluid in the labyrinth of each ear. A gentleman who has this symptom informs me that at first it was difficult for him to avoid the belief that two persons were talking to him at the same time and saying the same thing, one being a little slower than the other in his speech, and having a voice pitched in a slightly lower key.

Illusions may also result from a combination of circumstances unfavorable to perfect sensation. Thus, when the light is insufficient there may be illusions of the sense of sight. This is especially apt to be the case in the mystifying light of the moon, in which objects are more or less disturbed from their natural appearance. Under such a condition a roadside bush may appear to be an animal of some kind or other, and a guide-post look like a man on horseback. The state of mind of the individual has great influence in modifying the images which form on the retina, the words which reach the tympanum, the odors which impinge on the Schneiderian membrane, the flavors which touch the tongue, or the objects which come in contact with the tips of the fingers, and this strictly within the limits of health. It is well known that many people, for instance, can see what they wish to see. Falret cites a story, from Fontenelle's "Pluralité des Mondes," of a priest and a young lady talking together in the light of the moon, and examining the lights and shadows on the face of that luminary. "Do they not look to you like cloisters?" said the clergyman. "Oh, no," she answered, "not in the least; I should rather say like two lovers."

But illusions such as these, and many others that might be mentioned, do not now require consideration. We have rather to give attention to those which, resulting from central derangement, belong to the domain of mental pathology.

Illusions of this character, without the implication of the higher categories of mental faculties, are rare. Still, there is no doubt that they do exist. That is, that there are illusions not the results of derangement of the organs of sense, or of circumstances unfavorable to exact perception, but which are due to a morbid condition of the perceptional ganglia, and the unreal nature of which is clearly recognized by the individual.

Illusions of *sight* often relate merely to the size of objects. Thus, a young lady who had overtasked herself at school saw everything of enormous size at which she looked. The head of a person seemed to be several feet in diameter, and little children looked like giants. When I took out my watch, while examining her pulse, she remarked that it was as large as the wheel of a carriage. The room in which she sat appeared to her to be several acres in extent. So far as her own person was concerned there were no illusions. Her own hands appeared of the natural size, but, as soon as she turned her eyes to the hands of other people, she at once saw those of enormous proportions. Saurages refers to a somewhat similar case, in which a young woman suffering from epilepsy had the illusion of seeing objects greatly magnified in size. A fly seemed to her to be as large as a chicken, and a chicken appeared to be as big as an ox. In the case which came under my observation, the unreal character of the perception was fully recognized, and hence the intellect was not involved.

A gentleman who had met with severe pecuniary losses, and who had consequently endured great anxiety and distress, consulted me for an illusion of the sense of sight with which he was troubled every night as he was about going to bed. The banister-post—technically called a newel-post—at the head of the stairs was large, and, notwithstanding the fact that the hall was well lighted, this post always appeared to him like a very tall and thin woman, who stood leering at him with a diabolical expression of countenance. The moment he touched the post the illusion ceased, but until then, from the time he came within sight of the object, it persisted. His only way to escape from it was to shut his eyes and to keep them closed till he had passed it. If he kept them open, he felt impelled by a force he could not resist to turn them toward the post, and then instantly it assumed the form of the tall and thin woman. At any time after dining, if he went upstairs, he had the illusion as soon as he came within sight of the post, but a night's rest, or even a little sleep, seemed to have the power of dispelling it, or at least generally so, for he rarely saw it on his way down stairs in the morning. Upon one occasion he sat down, and, fixing his eyes on the post, resolved that he would, if possible, tire out his adversary, but the longer he looked the more distinct she became, until after three or four minutes his head began to ache violently, and he gave up the attempt. The next morning his head was still painful, and then, as he passed by on his way down stairs, he had the illusion. With this evidence of intracranial derangement there were others which clearly pointed to cerebral hyperæmia, to which condition the illusion was doubtless due. His intellect did not for a moment accept the false perception as real.

In another case the patient, a lawyer of a neighboring city, was so subject to illusions of the sense of sight that he found it very difficult to determine the true from the false images which he perceived, and, as a consequence, he made many mistakes. He would often take a stranger for an intimate friend, and address him as such, and again would pass his acquaintances, and even his relatives, without recognizing them. If one of the latter would say, "Why, J., don't you know me?" he would stop, look his questioner in the face, and answer, "So far as I know, I never saw you before, but I'll take your word for it; who are you?" And, when told, would say, "All right! I suppose you are; but you don't look like any one I ever knew." This gentleman had also great difficulty occasionally in estimating distances by the eye; but this he was able to correct by his judgment.

St. Theresa states that she often saw the wooden cross of her rosary changed into another cross composed of four precious stones of supernatural beauty.

Illusions of *hearing*, due to derangement of the perceptional ganglia, but unaccompanied by derangement of the intellect, are not very common. One case only has come under my observation, but this was a very interesting one. It was that of a gentleman to whom the ticking of a clock on the mantle-piece was resolved into articulate words. At first he only had this illusion at night after he went to bed, but after a few weeks the ticking of any clock sounded to him like human speech. There was no uniformity either of the tone or of the language employed, but sometimes a particular phrase would be repeated hundreds of times. As soon as he got beyond the range of the sound from the clock, the words were no longer heard.

Generally the expressions were in the form of commands. For instance, if at dinner, they would be, "Eat no soup!" "Drink no wine!" or, "Eat your soup!" "Drink some wine!" and so on. One day he made the discovery that, if he closed the right ear firmly, the illusion disappeared; but, if the left ear were closed, the words were still distinctly heard. It was hence clear that the centre for hearing on the right side was the one affected, and that that on the left side was normal. On neither side was there the slightest impairment of the capacity for hearing other sounds. A watch could be readily heard to tick at the distance of three feet from either ear.

For a long time this gentleman resisted accepting any of these illusions as facts, but after a time he began to be influenced by them to the extent of regarding them as guides, though he tried to conceal the circumstance. When asked, for instance, whether or not he was going to the theatre that evening, he would reply, in a *nonchalant* way, to the effect that he had not thought about it, and then, after a little while, when he thought the matter forgotten, he would saunter toward where the clock stood, and shortly afterward give his answer, either affirmatively or negatively, according to the words conveyed to him by the clock. Eventually he put clocks in every room in his house, and professed to be governed altogether by the directions they gave him. Not, as he said, from any belief that the ticks were real words, but because there was probably some influence, spiritual or other, that caused them to seem like words to him.

Illusions of *touch*, as Michea[1] says, may relate to temperature, movement, weight, and the character of surfaces. Thus, to some patients, substances that are hot feel cold, and *vice versa;* others feel the things on which they sit or lie glide from under them.

Cabanis[2] states that a man who had an abscess of the corpus callosum several times told him that during the course of his disease he felt his bed sink away from his body. Illusions in regard to temperature and weight are common with the subjects of locomotor ataxia, but in these cases the lesion is in the spinal cord. There is, however, reason for thinking that the cord is to some extent a centre for perceptions of touch.

Various abnormal sensations existing on the surface of the body become illusions with some persons. Thus, one feels a tight band encircling the head, another has a sensation such as would be produced by the claw of a bird scratching the vertex, and another as if a fly were crawling over the face.

Illusions connected with the internal viscera, and analogous to those of external touch, are quite common, especially with hypochondriacs; and again they may be of a general character as regards the whole body—giving the sensation of extreme weight or lightness—or as if the body were immensely lengthened or shortened.

The sensation of lightness has induced some hyperæsthetic or hysterical persons to believe that they have actually been raised from the ground. St. Theresa[3] frequently

[1] "Des hallucinations," etc., "Mémoires de l'académie royale de médecine," t. xii, p. 252.

[2] "Rapports du physique et du moral de l'homme," Paris, 1824, t. i, p. 148.

[3] "The Lives of the Fathers, Martyrs, and other Principal Saints," London, S. A., vol. x, p. 385, *et seq.*

experienced this sensation. This remarkable woman was born in 1515. From a very early age she was afflicted with frequent fits of fainting and violent pain at her heart, which sometimes deprived her of her senses. Sharp pains were frequent through her whole frame, her sinews began to shrink up, and finally, in August, 1537, she fell into a lethargic coma or trance which lasted four days. At one time she was thought to be dead, and her grave was actually dug. During this attack she bit her tongue in several places, and was for a long time unable to swallow. Sometimes her whole body seemed as if her bones were disjointed in every part, and her head was in extreme disorder and pain. It is quite evident from all this that St. Theresa was a hystero-epileptic.

Speaking of the elevation of her soul, she says that sometimes her whole body was lifted up with it from the ground, though this was seldom, and that when she tried to resist the elevation there seemed to be a mighty force under her which raised her up in spite of all her efforts. Hundreds of such cases are given in the lives of the saints, and many of less holy personages.

Madame d'Arnim, Goethe's friend, in speaking of the sensation in question as experienced by herself, says: "I was certain that I flew and floated in the air. By a simple elastic pressure of the toe, I was in the air. I floated silently and deliciously at two or three feet above the earth. I alighted, mounted again, flew from side to side, and then returned. A few days after, I was taken with fever, I went to bed and slept. It happened two weeks after I was confined." [1]

The following instances are within my own experience :

A lady of strongly marked hysterical temperament and of most fanatical religious tendencies often had the sensation that she was raised from the ground while she was in the act of saying her prayers. She usually spent several hours each day in these exercises, and during the whole time was in a state of fervid exaltation, which rendered her insensible to all that was passing around her. While in this condition she would exclaim, "I rise! I rise! I see angels!" and, with her hands raised on high, her head elevated, her face turned upward, and her countenance illuminated with ecstatic radiance, she really did seem to some superficial and sympathetic ob-

---

[1] "Correspondence de Goethe et de Bettina," translated by M. Sebast. Albin, t. i, p. 63.

servers to be lifted up. A young married lady, formerly under my professional care, was very confident that, during the cataleptic seizures to which she was subject, she was raised from her bed. In neither of these cases was there any permanent deception of the intellect, and both eventually lost their illusions.

As Brièrre de Boismont[1] remarks: "The sensation of flying is rather common. Frequently in dreams we feel ourselves carried along with the rapidity of an arrow; we accomplish great distances, just lightly touching the ground. We have noticed this fact in a literary man of our acquaintance whom we have several times found with fixed eyes, and who said to us, 'I am flying, do not stop me.' On returning to himself, he described his sensations, and it seemed to him that he really had flown."

The sensation of amplification of the body is also an occasional illusion. Thus, Görres[2] states that the blessed Ida of Lorraine, who lived in the convent of Rosenthal, was so filled with the desire to render herself acceptable to the Lord that one night, as she occupied a bed with a very devout nun, her intense longing so filled her soul that very soon all the members of her body began to swell, and quickly assumed monstrous proportions. The skin of one of her legs burst, so great was the strain, and she ever afterward had the cicatrix. The poor nun, her bedfellow, did not know what to think of this enormous amplification of the saintly Ida, and her situation in addition was rendered very uncomfortable, for the swelling saint went on enlarging till she occupied all but a very narrow strip of the bed. Suddenly, however, things changed. Ida's body diminished little by little, till at last it was reduced to an extremely minute size. This phenomenon was reproduced as she was returning from the church with her friend.

In such a case, and in many others which have helped to enlarge the ranks of the credulous, the statements of the illusionated individuals are so strongly expressed that they serve to deceive many of those who hear them. Nothing is easier than to make others perceive things which they are emphatically told they must perceive.

---

[1] "A History of Dreams, Visions, Apparitions, Ecstasy, Magnetism, and Somnambulism," American edition, Philadelphia, 1855, p. 94.

[2] "La mystique, divine, naturelle et diabolique," Paris, 1861, t. i, p. 349.

Illusions of *taste* and of *smell*, except with persons who are otherwise insane, are not common. No instance of an illusion of smell of the kind under notice has occurred within my personal experience ; several cases of illusions of taste are, however, within my knowledge. To one of these, a lady, everything she put into her mouth tasted like cauliflower ; in another instance, the flavor was that of strong Roquefort cheese, and in another of pears.

As regards frequency, illusions of the sense of touch occupy the front rank ; next are those of sight, and next those of hearing. Illusions of smell and taste are less frequent than the others.

Illusions as symptoms of higher forms of mental alienation will engage our attention further on.

b—HALLUCINATIONS.

Bearing in mind what has been previously said, the student will have no difficulty in recognizing the difference which exists between illusions and hallucinations, and will, therefore, recall the fact to his recollection that the latter are entirely cerebral in origin, and do not require, as do the former, a material basis. That they may and often do exist without the implication of the intellect is not a question in dispute at the present day. They cannot be produced by any defects or derangements of the sensory organs, or by any external circumstances tending to interfere with the regular and normal actions of these organs. When present, therefore, they are always an evidence of cerebral disorder. We have to consider them now as resulting from disorder of the perceptional ganglia without the implication of those parts of the brain which are concerned in the production of intellect, emotion, or will.

Beginning with the consideration of hallucinations of *sight*, the case of M. Andral,[1] the distinguished French physician, is interesting. "At the beginning of my medical studies," he says, "I was intensely interested in seeing, in a corner of the dissecting-room at La Pitié, the dead body of a child half devoured by worms. The following morning, on going to the fireplace to kindle my fire, I saw this corpse. It was distinctly before my vision, and I even smelled its putrid odor, although all the time I kept telling myself that the thing was impossible. This hallucination lasted about a quarter of an hour."

[1] "Cours de pathologie interne," t. iii, p. 184.

Here there was nothing to show the implication of the intellect. The false appearance was not even for an instant accepted as a reality. Its origin was clearly in the brain, and was a projection of an impression made upon it the previous day in the dissecting-room.

The case of Nicolai, the German bookseller, is another striking instance of the existence of hallucinations of sight without intellectual disturbance.

During the ten latter months of the year 1790 he had been the subject of a good deal of emotional disturbance in consequence of the supervention of several melancholy incidents. A customary bloodletting was omitted, and added to all was an unusual press of business matters, and a sharp altercation which took place on the morning of the day on which the hallucinations supervened. Suddenly he perceived, at apparently the distance of ten steps, a form like that of a deceased person. He pointed at it, asking his wife if she did not see it. She saw nothing, but his question alarmed her so much that she sent for a physician. The phantom continued for about ten minutes. In a short time he grew more calm, and fell asleep. But at four in the afternoon the form he had seen in the morning reappeared. He arose and went to another room, the apparition accompanying him, disappearing, however, at intervals, and always maintaining the erect posture. At about six o'clock there appeared other figures unlike the first.

After the first day the figure of the deceased person no longer appeared, but its place was supplied by many other phantoms, sometimes representing acquaintances, but mostly strangers. They seemed to be equally clear and distinct at all times and under all circumstances, both when he was alone and in company, and as well in the day as at night, and in his own house as well as abroad. They were, however, less frequent when he was in the house of a friend, and rarely appeared to him in the street. When he shut his eyes these phantasms would sometimes vanish entirely, though there were instances when he beheld them with his eyes closed. When they disappeared from this cause, they generally returned when he opened his eyes. Generally he saw human forms of both sexes, but they usually did not appear to take the least notice of each other, moving as in a market-place, where all are eager to pass through the avenue ; at times, however, they seemed to be transacting business with each other. He saw also, on several occasions, people on horseback, dogs, and birds. All these phantoms appeared to him of their natural size, and as distinct as though alive, exhibiting different shades of carnation in the uncovered parts, as well as different colors and fashions in their dresses. Though the colors seemed somewhat paler than in real nature, none of the figures appeared particularly terrible, comical, or disgusting, most of them being of an indifferent shape, and some presenting a pleasing aspect. The longer these phantoms continued to visit him, the more frequently did they return, while at the same time they increased in number. After about four weeks had elapsed he began to hear them talk.

The application of leeches to the arms relieved him promptly of his hallucinations.

Michea[1] cites from St. Gregory of Tours the case of a man of his time who was overwhelmed by an impulse to commit suicide. He made ready with a rope, but, not having quite determined on the act, he implored the assistance of the apostle St. Paul. He had no sooner uttered his invocation than he perceived before him a figure of sinister and diabolical aspect, who thus addressed him: "Courage; do not longer defer the execution of the resolution you have taken." The unfortunate man at once placed the rope around his neck, but, before he could execute his project, he saw another figure, which said to the other form: "Get out, wretch! This man has called upon St. Paul for aid, and the great apostle has heard him; he is here." At these words the two figures disappeared, and the man was relieved of his temptation.

This story is given, not as being entitled to much credit—for it is supposed to refer to an event which took place over thirteen hundred years ago—but as an example which, having all the elements of probability about it, seems well adapted to illustrate the character of the hallucinations of a remote period.

Pascal saw a cavern constantly yawning at his side, and, though it did not impose on his intellect, he felt more comfortable with a screen so arranged that he could not see it. Other instances of hallucinations of sight existing with intellectual integrity are cited in the chapters on sleep and dreams.

[1] "Des hallucinations," *op. cit.*, p. 253.

I have had experience in my practice of many cases of like character. In one of these, a young lady of good mental development, but of delicate physical organization, was for several months almost constantly troubled with apparitions of various kinds of faces, which she saw no matter where she turned her eyes. She had, while looking through her father's library a few weeks before they first appeared, come across a book containing many engravings of Roman and Grecian masks, and these had made a great impression on her. The false faces beset her on all sides. Sometimes they would peep at her from around the corners of the streets as she was driving or walking. Again she would see them coming out of the shelves in the shops she visited, and again they would start up from the street just before her. They never passed out of her range of vision suddenly, but gradually faded away without changing their positions. If she closed one eye she saw fewer, and if she shut both eyes at the same time, they disappeared altogether for a time. If, however, she kept the eyes closed for a few minutes, they reappeared, but less distinctly, and, when she opened her eyes, this set vanished at once, and a new series came on the field. They were of all colors and nationalities, and a good many were of the same appearance as the grotesque masks of the ancients. She never saw them after dark except in well-lighted rooms or other places. The gas-light of the streets was not sufficient to develop them, but the electric light brought them out very distinctly. By repeating the experiment of Sir David Brewster—pressing on the outside of the globe of either eye so as to produce temporary strabismus— she could make any face appear double, but this was only when it had been visible for several minutes. A newly appearing face she could not duplicate in this way.

In another case, occurring in a young man who had received a severe blow on the head just above the left ear a few weeks previously, the hallucination consisted of a large black cat that followed him wherever he went, and sometimes jumped on his lap or his shoulder. He was clearly aware of the fact that the appearance was unreal, but it nevertheless gave him a good deal of annoyance. Being possessed of a considerable degree of intelligence, he had, by observation and experiment, settled several interesting points to his satisfaction. Thus, he found that the image was always larger and more distinct in the evening than soon after getting out of bed. Occasionally at this latter time it was altogether absent, but not often. Again, it was always clearer, larger, and apparently nearer to him when he suffered from pain at the seat of the injury—as he did in paroxysms several times a day. At the times that he was free from pain, it disappeared when he shut his eyes, but, when the paroxysms were present, he saw it just as well with his eyes closed as when they were open. Pressing on either eyeball so as to destroy the parallelism of the visual axes did not cause the production of two images, and then he made the discovery, by alternately shutting the eyes, that the hallucination only existed on the side corresponding to that on which he had been injured. He had, therefore, a unilateral hallucination such as those to which M. Regis[1] has recently called attention. I proposed trephining, but he declined to submit to the operation, and I finally lost sight of him.

Hallucinations of *hearing* coexistent with integrity of the intellect are more common than those of any other of the special senses, and, according to my experience, are more apt to lead to further mental disorder. As Michea[2] says, quoting Theophrastus and Plutarch, the hearing is that one of the senses through which the passions are most readily excited. It, is through the hearing that speech is perceived, without which the intelligence would be greatly restricted, through which the memory and the imagination are so extensively supplied with food, and through which, from childhood to old age, the mind is stimulated by recitals calculated to stir the emotions to their utmost pitch. Undoubtedly the mind is more capable of being influenced through the hearing than through any other sense by the continual repetition of the sensorial excitation. Far more people kill themselves under the influence of hallucinations of hearing than from those of all the other senses combined. The reiteration in the ears, during every minute of the day, of the command to commit suicide, to jump into the river, to blow the brains out, to take poison, to plunge a convenient knife into the heart, and so on, day in and day out, without intermission, is calculated to shake the power of control of the strongest minded, and it often does shake it. Few suicides or other acts of violence,

[1] " Des hallucinations unilatérales," *L'Encephale*, Mars, 1881.
[2] *Op. cit.*, p. 268.

20

comparatively, are perpetrated through hallucinations of the other senses. Those from hallucinations of sight are almost invariably connected with the idea of self-defence.

Instances of hallucinations of hearing in those not otherwise insane abound in psychological literature, and are constantly coming under the observation of medical men. In their simplest form they consist of voices of various kinds ; in their more complex character they are words, sentences, and even long discourses.

A patient of my own is subject to the hallucination—frequently repeated through the day and sometimes awaking him at night—of a sound close to his ears like that produced by striking two heavy books violently together. Another hears a tea-kettle hissing at a distance of a few feet from him, and another, a lady, is much annoyed by long-drawn sighs and moans like those which might come from a person in mental or physical suffering. Such hallucinating sounds must not be confounded with those intra-cranial or intra-aural noises produced by disturbances of the auditory apparatus. The latter always appear to be where they really are—in the head or ears, while the former are invariably referred to a position at some distance from the body.

Baillarger[1] states that, during one of the street-fights in Paris, in April, 1831, the wife of a workman, returning to her home, saw her husband mortally wounded by a bullet. A month later she was confined, but on the tenth day after her accouchement delirium set in. In the very beginning of her mental disturbance she heard the sound of cannon, the firing of the platoons, the whistling of the balls. To avoid these sounds, she fled to the country, but was arrested and placed in the Salpêtrière, where in a month she was cured. During the ensuing ten years she had six relapses, which always began by her hearing the discharges of cannon and muskets, and the hissing of bullets around her.

Sometimes a single word or a few words constitute the hallucination. These are very apt to be of an obscene or profane character, or to consist of epithets of abuse. Thus, a gentleman of education and refinement is constantly tormented by hearing a coarse word for sexual intercourse spoken into his ears in all tones, from a whisper to the voice of a stentor.

[1] " Des hallucinations," etc., " Mémoires de l'académie royale de médecine," t. xii, p. 279.

Another hears himself called "brigand," and another is constantly being told that he is a "damned fool."

Again, they are commanded to do some particular act which it is repugnant to the individual to perform. Thus, one is told to hang himself, to throw himself from a precipice, to go up in a balloon, to kill a certain person, perhaps a near friend or relation, to commit arson or burglary, to blow up a house with dynamite, and a hundred other things mostly of the nature of crimes. Such hallucinations as these very often succeed eventually in overcoming the reason and with leading to the perpetration of the act ordered, or to some other incongruity indicative of advanced insanity.

But no instance that has come under my observation equals that of a lady who hears recited to her long pieces of original poetry or prose, which, if not brilliant compositions, are still coherent, and sometimes above mediocrity. Usually they seem to come from a man speaking, as if addressing an audience, and again they are whispered in a low tone like the voice of a child. She has repeatedly written down these recitations and brought them to me. I select the following as one of the best and shortest, premising that she wrote it in my presence after it had been, as she said, whispered into her ears all the morning :

"Ah me, how sad and drear I feel,
What withering fancies o'er me steal,
And load my weary brain !

"I sit and dream from day to day
Of that fair death for which I pray—
For which I pray in vain.

"Oh, God of fate, make sharp thy dart
And pierce my aching, breaking heart,
And set my spirit free.

"My race on earth is nearly run,
My thread of life is nearly spun,
Oh, God, I long for thee."

This lady had a strong hereditary tendency to insanity, and, shortly after the development of the hallucinations referred to, she imbibed the delusion that she had committed the "unpardonable sin." She made two attempts at suicide, one by throwing herself into the water from a boat in which she was sailing with some friends, and another by taking laudanum. The last came very near being successful, but her life was saved, though with difficulty. She is still insane, but has—an unusual circumstance—lost the delusion of the "unpardonable sin," and contracted the idea that she has no bowels. She has no hallucinations of any kind, unless the sensations which she says she feels in her abdomen, and which, she describes, are those indicating the existence of a vacuum.

As hallucinations of sight often exist while the eyes are closed, or in persons who are totally blind, so hallucinations of hearing continue though the ears be stopped, or originate in persons who are entirely deaf. I have already, in a previous chapter, cited the case of a deaf old lady who heard voices whispering to her. Another instance is that of a deaf-mute who came to my clinique at the University Medical College during the last session, and who was constantly subject to hallucinations of hearing of various kinds. Baillarger[1] mentions the cases of five women, patients in the Salpêtrière, who, being deaf, are yet subject to hallucinations of hearing. One of these, the deafest, hears the voices most distinctly. It is said that in the last years of his life Beethoven became completely deaf, but that he heard his compositions as distinctly as when he actually listened to them when performed by an orchestra.

Hallucinations of hearing, like those of sight, are sometimes unilateral—that is, heard by only one ear. Baillarger[2] cites several examples of the kind.

Calmet,[3] in relating the events which ensued at St. Maur, near Paris, in consequence of the supposed appearance of a ghost, gives some interesting details relative to hallucinations. A M. de S. was the observer, and he is described as a young man, short in stature, and well made for his height. After mentioning several circumstances connected with the apparition, Calmet goes on to state that, one afternoon, M. de S. entered his study, and, returning toward the door to go to his bedroom again, was much surprised to see it shut of itself and barricade itself with the two bolts that belonged to it. At the same time the two doors of a large press opened behind

---

[1] *Op. cit.*, p. 310.   [2] *Op. cit.*, p. 260.
[3] "The Phantom World; or, The Philosophy of Spirits, Apparitions," etc., by Augustus Calmet. Edited by Rev. Henry Christmas, London, 1850, p. 291.

him and rather darkened his study, because the window which was open was behind these doors.

"At this sight the fright of M. de S. is more easy to imagine than to describe ; however, he had sufficient calmness left to hear, in his left ear, a distinct voice which came from a corner of the closet, and seemed to him to be about a foot above his head. This voice spoke to him in very good terms during the space of half a miserere, and ordered him, *thee-ing* and *thouing* him, to do some one particular thing which he was commanded to keep secret."

Calmeil[1] states that persons have told him that the sounds which they seemed to hear came to them sometimes by the right and sometimes by the left ear.

Again, the voices appear to come from various parts of the body, such as the abdomen, the chest, the uterus, etc. These facts, however, in my experience, only occur with the subjects of well-marked insanity affecting other faculties of the mind besides the perceptions. They do not, therefore, come within the range of our consideration at present.

Hallucinations of *smell*, though not so common as those of sight and hearing, are yet often met with independently of any aberration of the intellect. A gentleman of my acquaintance was almost constantly subject to the hallucination of smelling paint or turpentine, another had the odor of coffee ever present in his nostrils, and another, a physician, was always annoyed with the smell of the dissecting-room. It is well known that some epileptic seizures are preceded by the sensation of a horrible stench, which, as a gentleman subject to epileptic paroxysms told me, was in his case like that of rotten fish. Hallucinations of smell are not so readily corrected by the intellect as those of sight and hearing, and it may sometimes be impossible for the subject of them to assure himself, in the beginning, of their unreality. The persistency which they evince while serving to convince some persons that they cannot be actualities, will, on the other hand, have a contrary effect with individuals who may have a hereditary predisposition to insanity, or who are under the influence of some other cause. Thus, a patient whom I occasionally saw several years ago, and who suffered from hypochondriacal mania, had a hallucination of the odor of fresh blood. For a long time he resisted the sensation, and endeavored in

[1] Art. " Hallucinations," " Dictionnaire de médecine," en 25 volumes.

various ways to account for it, but at last it gained such an ascendency over him that he became convinced that his nose was continually bleeding, and that the blood was flowing down his throat. This made him very unhappy, and was the cause of his using all kinds of astringent douches and gargles for the purpose of stopping the flow. He wanted me to tie the carotid arteries in order to prevent him bleeding to death, a process which he was confident was going on rapidly. He almost starved himself in the endeavor to lower the action of the heart, and to this end also took various debilitating medicines. The hallucination had thus become a veritable delusion, although through its whole course not a single drop of blood had escaped from his nose or mouth. He neglected his business—that of a merchant tailor—and spent his whole time swabbing out his nostrils and gargling his throat. Somebody finally persuaded him that a journey across the plains would be of service to him. Fortunately he took the advice, and, after an absence of several months in Colorado and California, returned, entirely cured of his hallucination and delusion.

Ecstatics, especially those of a religious character, are sometimes under the hallucination that delicious odors are being wafted to their nostrils, and they sniff the air with every manifestation of delight.

Hallucinations of *taste* are not common. Indeed, it is sometimes difficult to say whether they exist or not, as various visceral irregularities may cause the production of tastes by modifications impressed upon the saliva. Mental excitement will cause a like effect in some persons. I am acquainted with a gentleman who cannot participate in any engrossing conversation without having a bitter taste developed in his mouth. An exciting dream will, as he tells me, produce it.

Hallucinations of the sense of *touch* are, on the other hand, very frequently met with, not only in the insane, but in individuals of otherwise complete mental integrity. Sensations apparently not based on any real impression are experienced in various parts of the body. It is difficult, however, to discriminate between illusions and hallucinations of touch. Probably the majority of the false perceptions connected with touch belong to the first-named category. This seems to be especially the case with visceral sensations, and the feeling of lightness or weight of body, to which reference has already been made. The former, whether of the nature of illusions or hallucinations, are common symptoms of hypochondriacal mania, and are often the starting-point of this disorder.

Baillarger[1] was the first to describe a peculiar kind of hallucination, generally of hearing, in which the individual has the impression derived from words being spoken to him, but in which he does not hear sounds. It is a kind of intellectual hallucination, not being directly connected with the organ of sense to which it is referred. The voices, which appear to come from various parts of the body, such as the chest or stomach, are, according to Baillarger, not recognized by the individual as real sounds, but are only ideas of sounds, which, however, impress him with as much force as though they were spoken directly into his ear. I am quite sure that this is not always the case. I have under my care at this time a patient who hears voices speaking to him from his epigastrium, and to whom they appear as real sounds ; moreover, these psychical hallucinations are never found except in those lunatics in whom the intellect is involved.

Occasionally persons have the power of voluntarily producing hallucinations of various kinds. A practice, fraught with danger for the time, is apt to come, sooner or later, at which they cannot get rid of their false perceptions. As an instance of the facility with which hallucinations, especially of vision, may be formed, and of the ill consequences which may result from the practice, I cite the following case from Wigan.[2] The painter referred to is Blake.

"A painter, who inherited much of the patronage of Sir Joshua Reynolds, and believed himself to possess a talent superior to his, was so fully engaged that he told me he had painted three hundred large and small portraits in one year. The fact appeared physically impossible, but the secret of his astonishing success was this: he required but one sitting of his model. I watched him paint a portrait in miniature in eight hours of a gentleman whom I well knew ; it was carefully done, and the resemblance was perfect. I begged him to detail to me his method of procedure, and he related what follows.

"When a sitter came, I looked attentively on him for half an hour, sketching from time to time on the canvas. I did

[1] *Op. cit.*, p. 383.

[2] "A New View of Insanity. The Duality of the Mind." London, 1844, p. 123.

not require a longer sitting. I removed the canvas and passed to another person. When I wished to continue the first portrait, I recalled the man to my mind; I placed him on the chair, where I perceived him as distinctly as if he were really there, and, I may add, in form and color more decided and brilliant. I looked from time to time at the imaginary figure, and went on painting, occasionally stopping to examine the posture as though the original were before me. Whenever I looked toward the chair I saw the man.

"This method made me very popular, and, as I always caught the resemblance, the sitters were delighted that I spared them the annoying sittings of other painters. In this way I laid by much money for myself and my children.

"By degrees I began to lose all distinction between the imaginary and the real figure, and I sometimes insisted to my sitters that they had set the day before. Finally I was persuaded that it was so, and then all became confusion; I recollect nothing more. I lost my reason, and remained for thirty years in an asylum. With the exception of the last six months of my confinement, I recollect nothing; it, however, appears to me that, when I hear persons speak of their visits to the establishment, I have a faint recollection of them."

It is related of Talma, the great actor, that he could, by the power of his imagination, cause the audience to appear like skeletons, and that, when the hallucination was complete, his histrionic genius was at its height, through the effort produced upon his emotions, and he produced the most vivid effects upon all who heard him.

Goethe states that he had the power of giving form to the images passing before his mind, and upon one occasion saw his own figure approaching him. Wigan states that he knew a very intelligent man who also had this power.

Abercrombie [1] refers to the case of a gentleman who had all his life been affected by the appearance of spectral figures. To such an extent did this peculiarity exist that, if he met a friend in the street, he could not at first satisfy himself whether he saw a real or an imaginary person. By close attention he was able to determine that the outline of the false was not so distinct as that of the real figure, but generally he used other means—such as touch, or speech, or listening for the footsteps—to verify his visual impressions. He had also

[1] "Inquiries Concerning the Intellectual Powers," etc., London, 1840, p. 380.

the power of calling up spectral figures at will, by directing his attention steadily for some time to the conceptions of his own mind, and these either consisted of a figure or a scene he had witnessed or a composition created by his imagination. But, though he had the faculty of producing hallucinations, he had no power of banishing them, and, when he had once called up any particular person or scene, he could never say how long it would continue to haunt him. This gentleman was in the prime of life, of sound mind, in good health, and engaged in business. His brother was similarly affected.

Several like cases have come under my own observation. In one, the power was directly the result of attendance at spiritual meetings, and of the efforts made to become a good "medium." The patient, a lady, was of a very impressionable temperament, and was consequently well disposed to acquire the dangerous faculty in question. At first she thought very deeply of some particular person, whose image she endeavored to form in her mind. Then she assumed that the person was really present, and she addressed conversation to him, at the same time keeping the idealistic image in her thoughts. At this period she was not deceived, for she clearly recognized the fact that the image was not present.

One day, however, she was thinking very intently of her mother, and picturing to herself her appearance as she looked when dressed for church on a particular occasion. She was reading a book at the time; happening to raise her eyes, she saw her mother standing before her exactly as she had imagined her. At first she was somewhat startled, and, in her agitation, closed her eyes with her hands. To her surprise she still saw the phantom, but yet, not being aware of the centric origin of the image, she conceived the idea that she had really seen her mother's spirit. In a few moments it disappeared, but she soon found that she had the ability to recall it at will, and that the power existed in regard to many other forms—even those of animals and of inanimate objects.

During the spiritualistic meetings she attended, she could thus reproduce the image of any person upon whom she strongly concentrated her thoughts, and was for a long time sincere in her belief that they were real appearances. At last she lost control of the operations, and became constantly subject to hallucinations of sight and hearing. She was unable to sleep, and complained of vertigo, pain in the head, and of

other symptoms indicating the existence of cerebral hyperæmia. The application of ice to the vertex and nape of the
neck, and other suitable medication, saved her from an attack of insanity of a higher grade than that from which she
was suffering, but her nervous system was for several months
in a state of exhaustion, from which she rallied with difficulty.

A young lady once informed me that she was able to bring
visually before her the images of any novel she may have
been reading, or of any striking play she may have witnessed.

It is probable that many of the visions of Jerome Cardan
and of Swedenborg were induced in much the same way. No
one presumes to question the honesty of either of these distinguished men, but both were impressionable to an extreme
degree, and, doubtless, mental concentration of an intense
character, and long continued, was the agent in the production of the visions of which they were the subjects. In some
persons very slight thought is sufficient to cause hallucinations of great distinctness.

Thus, a married lady consulted me for hallucinations of
sight and hearing, from which she had suffered for several
months. It was only necessary for her to think of some particular person, living or dead, when she immediately saw the
image of the person thought of, who spoke to her, laughed,
wept, walked about the room, or did whatever other thing
she imagined. In fact, to such an extent had her proclivity
reached that it was often impossible for her to avoid thinking of persons, and immediately having their figures brought
to her perception.

At first she religiously believed in the reality of her visions, and that she really saw the spirits of the various individuals of whom she happened to think. But, as the hallucinations became more common, she lost her faith, and ascribed
them to their true cause—disease. Upon examination, I found
that she was pre-eminently of a hysterical type of organization, and was then laboring under other symptoms of its presence besides the hallucinations. Thus, she had hysterical
paralysis of motion and sensibility in the right leg to such
an extent that she could neither move it nor feel a pin
thrust through the skin. Her pulse was small and weak, her
appetite capricious, and her complexion pale. Not the least
of her afflictions was an almost perpetual headache. Under

the administration of treatment directed to the relief of what I considered to be an anæmic brain, she entirely recovered.

Quite recently, Mr. Francis Galton,[1] in a paper which, though interesting to the lay reader, cannot but excite, on some accounts, a feeling of disapproval in the minds of neurologists, advises the cultivation of the faculty of forming mental images. The ability to recall desirable impressions is one which is developed in different degrees in different people, and it is one which may be exercised not only without detriment but with advantage to the individual. It is simply an instance of the power of memory, and its exercise leads to close and exact observation. But this is a very different thing from forming images which are not transmitted to the brain through the retina and optic nerve, and the perception of which is therefore purely imaginary. It is, in fact, the voluntary production of a hallucination. As Mr. Galton says, the power is very high in some young children, who seem to spend years of difficulty in distinguishing between the subjective and the objective world. Undoubtedly the high cultivation of this faculty by adults would lead to like inconvenience, and probably disease. My own experience, as well as that of others to whom I have referred, is sufficient to assure me of the great danger of developing a power which we all possess to some extent, and it would be very easy to adduce other instances, besides those given, of the disastrous results likely to ensue from the indiscriminate adoption of Mr. Galton's views.

Perceptional insanity, either in the form of illusions or hallucinations, or both these varieties of sensorial derangement, may make its appearance suddenly, the first evidence of its presence being the illusion or hallucination. Usually, however, there are prodromata indicating the existence of cerebral derangement. These are, pain in the head, irritability of temper, suffusion of the eyes, noises in the ears, a general restlessness, inability to sleep, unpleasant and vivid dreams, and some febrile excitement. The skin is generally dry, the mouth parched, the bowels costive, and the urine high colored. If not arrested, it may pass into a higher form of mental derangement.

Causes.—The causes of central illusions and hallucinations are generally to be found in derangements of some kind in the

[1] "Mental Imagery," *Fortnightly Review*, September, 1880.

blood circulating in the brain.   These may either relate to its quantity or its quality.

Physical influences calculated to produce cerebral hyperæmia or congestion may give rise to illusions or hallucinations. Brierre de Boismont[1] refers to a case, on the authority of Moreau, in which an individual was able to obtain hallucinations of sight by inclining his head a little forward.   By this movement the return of blood from the brain was impeded, and the functions of the ganglia for vision were unduly exalted. A similar case was not long since under my own care.   A gentleman, while sitting at his table writing, happened to raise his eyes from the paper without moving his head, and was astonished to see before him the figure of an old woman with black cloak and hood.   Throwing himself back in his chair in his amazement, he was again surprised to find that the image slowly disappeared ; and, as often as he repeated these movements, a like series of phenomena occurred.   A few days afterward he repeated the circumstances to me, and, on examining him, I found that he wore a very high old-fashioned stock, which, as he sat at the table with his head bent forward, compressed the large veins of the neck, and prevented for a time the return of blood from the brain.   On changing his neck-wear for other of more modern fashion, he was enabled to bend his head and raise his eyes without encountering the apparition.

An instance showing the influence of position in giving rise to false perceptions is given in *Nicholson's Journal :*[2] "I know a gentleman," says the narrator, "in the vigor of life, who, in my opinion, is not exceeded by any one in acquired knowledge and originality of deep research, and who, for nine months in succession, was always visited by a figure of the same man threatening to destroy him, at the time of his going to rest.   It appeared on his lying down, and instantly disappeared when he resumed the erect position."

A gentleman who stands high as an author consulted me for a similar trouble.   For several weeks he had been visited, just as he lay down, by the figure of a very old man, who stood by the side of his bed grinning and beckoning to him with one finger.   At first he was deceived, and, starting suddenly from his bed, endeavored to seize his visitor, but he

---

[1] " A History of Dreams, Visions, Apparitions," etc., American edition, Philadelphia, 1855, p. 370.   [2] Vol. vi, p. 166.

was gone before he could fairly stretch out his hands. He again laid down, and again the figure appeared. He reached out with one arm and convinced himself that he could touch the very place where the image apparently stood, but he grasped nothing. He shut both eyes, and then each eye alternately, but it still remained. He was then entirely satisfied as to its real character, and so, like a sensible man, tried to get to sleep, but in this attempt he succeeded badly. He allowed this to go on for several weeks before he concluded to seek medical advice.

Dendy[1] mentions the case of a gentleman of high attainments who was constantly haunted by a spectre, when he retired to rest, which seemed to attempt his life. When he raised himself in bed, the phantom vanished, but reappeared as he resumed the recumbent posture.

The explanation of such cases is very simple. The recumbent posture facilitates the flow of blood to the brain, and at the same time tends, in a measure, to retard its exit. Hence, the appearances were due to the resulting congestion. As soon as the individuals rose in bed, or stood erect, the reverse conditions existed, the congestion disappeared, and the apparitions went with it.

Hallucinations of hearing are also sometimes produced by like causes. I had occasion recently to treat a lady suffering from epilepsy, and one of the means I advised for her relief was the wearing of an elastic band around the neck so as to compress the veins. After wearing it a few days, she complained of great fulness of the head and continual noises in the ears. Sometimes these were of a soft, moaning character, and at others like the hissing of a tea-kettle. I advised her, however, to persevere, which she did for another week, when she returned to say that she constantly heard voices singing all kinds of ribald words to familiar tunes. At first she had rather liked this, but it soon began to grow tiresome, and had kept her from sleeping. She had, accordingly, taken off the band, and at once the sounds had ceased.

In another case, the patient, a young man, heard a voice whispering to him in the ear which rested on the pillow. When he turned over in bed, the voice at once disappeared, but in about a minute was heard in the ear which was then in contact with the pillow.

[1] "The Philosophy of Mystery," London, 1841, p. 290.

The influence of cerebral *hyperæmia* in causing hallucinations would, therefore, seem to be clearly established by actual experiment. Ferriar[1] wrote a treatise with the special object of proving that this is the only cause; but this is an extreme view which cannot be sustained, for, as we shall presently see, the very opposite condition, cerebral anæmia, may give rise to them in a very marked degree.

That cerebral *anæmia* is an immediate cause of hallucinations is seen in the facts that during starvation, and other conditions producing great bodily exhaustion, hallucinations are common occurrences. As I have said in another work:[2] "Hallucinations and illusions are common in the slowly developed forms of cerebral anæmia, and may affect any one or all of the senses. Those of sight and hearing are, however, more prominent. In the case of a young lady under my care, and whose only marked disease was that [cerebral anæmia] under consideration, the hallucination that she saw a black man was almost constantly present. At times she conversed with this imaginary being, told him not to trouble her, that she no longer feared him," etc.

A more striking instance has, however, recently come under my observation, which shows, undoubtedly, that a reduction in the amount of blood circulating within the cranium may give rise to hallucinations. A young woman affected with epilepsy was of a very gross habit of body, and suffered from many attacks of the *petit mal* every day. While in my consulting-room, she had repeated seizures, and, with the view of arresting them, I exerted strong pressure on both carotid arteries, according to the method recommended by Dr. Corning, of this city. Her face instantly became pale, and, without losing consciousness, she uttered a loud shriek, and pointed with her finger at an object which she apparently saw near her. I at once discontinued the pressure, when she informed me that she had seen an immense negro man rushing toward her with a club, and that as soon as I had stopped pressing on her neck the figure had disappeared. I assured her it was a hallucination, and, after much persuasion, induced her to let me repeat the experiment. As soon as the pressure on the arteries was made, she saw the figure ap-

[1] " An Essay toward a Theory of Apparitions," London, 1813.

[2] " A Treatise on the Diseases of the Nervous System," first edition, New York, 1871, and subsequent editions.

proaching her with a club. "There he is! there he is!" she exclaimed. I continued to press, and she soon became insensible. On removing the pressure, she at once regained consciousness, and explained that the figure was exactly the same as she had at first seen. I now exerted moderate pressure, with the view of keeping it up for some little time. In about half a minute she said that she saw the figure, but not very distinctly. I made more pressure, and then she stated that she saw him very clearly. I found that I could make the figure distinct or indistinct by varying the degree of pressure.

Michea[1] divides the causes of hallucinations—embracing under this term illusions also—into two classes, *material* and *psychological.* In the first category are included electricity, great variations of temperature, the abuse of alcoholic liquors, or the sudden deprivation of these agents with persons accustomed to them, large doses of sulphate of quinine, digitalis, belladonna, stramonium, hyoscyamus, opium and its compounds, Indian hemp, nux vomica, camphor, lead, nitrous oxide (when inhaled), suspension by the neck, simple pressure upon or mechanical irritation of any of the organs of the special senses, cerebral shock, starvation, heredity, intestinal worms, diminution or total absence of light, the middle period of life, and notably that between thirty-five and forty-five years, in the female sex.

These data rest almost entirely on the dicta of other persons, and many of the alleged causes are probably more fanciful than real.

The psychological causes are, according to the same author, the prolonged continuance of the same sensation, a too vivid impression made upon any organ of sense, revery, or the prolonged concentration of the faculty of attention, solitude, remorse, fright, sorrow, extreme ambition, humiliation.

In looking over these lists of causes, it is perceived that many of them refer to illusions which are not of centric origin, and which, therefore, have nothing to do with mental aberration. Hallucinations can never be produced by irritations applied to an organ of sense, except by such irritation producing centric disturbance, as it sometimes does. I have seen several cases of illusions and hallucinations of hearing produced by impacted cerumen, but in all these cases there were

[1] *Op. cit.,* p. 264.

unmistakable evidences of the existence of cerebral hyperæmia, to which the sensorial disturbances were directly due.

Baillarger,[1] speaking of the influence of certain drugs in causing hallucinations, mentions the fact that hashish (Indian hemp) produces the sensation of an elongation of the limbs and a swelling of the body such as we may suppose was experienced by the blessed Ida, whose case I have cited. I have repeatedly noticed this fact, and likewise the additional circumstance also mentioned by Baillarger, that opium and stramonium give rise to similar sensations. Peculiar illusions and hallucinations are said to be caused by other drugs, but I have never found any marked degree of uniformity in this respect, except as regards the bromide of potassium and other bromides, which certainly, when carried to extreme points in administration, often cause hallucinations of seeing dead or dying persons.[2] Moreover, all the sensorial aberrations produced by these drugs are of distressing or sorrowful character.

As Baillarger[3] has pointed out, the state between sleeping and waking is that during which hallucinations are particularly apt to occur, and he cites many cases in illustration of the fact. I have already in a previous chapter, "The Physiology of Dreams," called attention to this interesting circumstance, which, under the name of "hypnagogic hallucinations," has been so thoroughly studied by M. Maury.

Children are very liable to be subject to hallucinations, and frequently give circumstantial accounts of apparitions and incidents which they believe have occurred to them, of voices they have heard, etc.—and this with an earnestness of expression and attention to detail which show that they are sincere in the stories they tell. It is often impossible for them to discriminate between the true and the false, and I am afraid they are often punished for lying by ignorant parents when they have told nothing but what they have had the evidence of their senses for believing. The explanation of this proclivity is to be found in the fact that they are possessed of a

[1] Op. cit., p. 353.

[2] See paper, by the author, "On some of the Effects of the Bromide of Potassium when administered in Large Doses," Quarterly Journal of Psychological Medicine, vol. iii, 1869, p. 46.

[3] "De l'influence de l'état intermédiaire à la veille et au sommeil sur la production et la marche des hallucinations," "Mémoires de l'académie royale de médecine," t. xii, p. 476.

degree of nervous development out of proportion to that of the rest of their body, and are hence impressionable to a high degree. Moreover, they have not the necessary experience in the use of their sensorial organs or the intellectual development essential to the discrimination between the unreal and the real.

Pathology and Morbid Anatomy.—A great deal has been written relative to the physiology of hallucinations, but without much result so far as any explanation of the process is concerned. As we cannot elucidate the question of the perception of real images and of other sensorial impressions by any experiments or investigations we can make, so we equally fail in our attempts to unravel the mystery of false images, false voices, tastes, smells, and tactile impressions. In the normal state of the brain we obtain perceptions which we believe to be true; in the abnormal state we form perceptions which sometimes we ourselves, and again those about us, are convinced are erroneous. The difference is to be ascribed to the change which has taken place in the perceptional centres. This change may consist of a state of temporary or permanent congestion, temporary or permanent anæmia, the circulation of blood through them which has acquired toxic properties, or the existence of structural disease.

There is some evidence to show that the thalami optici are the centres for all real perceptions, and that hence they are the organs which, through their disease, give rise to all centric illusions and hallucinations. If these bodies be divided centrally antero-posteriorly, they will be seen to have embedded in their substance four ganglionic masses. Of these, three are ranged along the superior surface of each thalamus, and from their positions may be designated the *anterior*, *middle*, and *posterior*, while the other, more deeply placed, may be called the *central*.

Luys,[1] who has studied the formation of the thalami optici with great thoroughness, designates these nuclei, from alleged anatomical and physiological relations, respectively, the *olfactive*, the *optic*, the *acoustic*, and the *sensitive*, or ganglion of general sensibility.

It is true that Meynert[2] only half acknowledges their ex-

---

[1] " Recherches sur le système nerveux," etc., Paris, 1865, p. 108, *et seq.*

[2] Article on "The Brain of Mammals," in " Stricker's Manual of Histology," American edition, p. 690.

istence, contending that the appearance of distinct nuclei is due to the mode of distribution of the fasciculi of fibres which enter and leave the thalamus, and that Huguenin[1] adopts this view of the subject. Really, however, this point is of no special importance so far as its bearing on the pathology of illusions and hallucinations is concerned. That the optic thalami, either by distinct nuclei or by themselves as bodies composed of ganglionic cells, are distinctly connected with the organs of the special senses referred to, in the relation of being their nervous centres, is, I think, a matter capable of complete demonstration.

The connections of the optic thalami with sensibility were first pointed out by Magendie,[2] who ascertained that their irritation in animals produced excessive pain, while the other parts of the brain might be invaded without causing evidences of suffering.

Although Todd, Carpenter, and others have regarded the optic thalami as centres for sensorial impressions, Luys[3] more than any other physiologist has elaborated this idea, and has adduced arguments in its support which it is difficult to overlook. His doctrine is that the optic thalami are reservoirs for all sensorial impressions coming from the periphery of the nervous system, and that, like other ganglionic masses, they elaborate these impressions, and that, by means of the fibres of the corona radiata, they transmit them to the cortex, to be still further perfectionated by being converted into ideas. In his own language : [3]

"All sensorial impressions, after having been received and concentrated in the gray substance of the optic thalami, are irradiated toward the different regions of the cortical periphery. The white central substance transmits them, and the gray substance of the convolutions receives and elaborates them."

Many facts in morbid anatomy go to support this view of the relation between the sensorial organs and the optic thalami. Twenty-six cases have been collected by Ritti[4] from Hunter, Treviranus, Serres, Lancereaux, Cruveilhier, Andral, Marcé, Lallemand, Laborde, Luys, Voisin, and others, to the effect of sensorial disturbances existing during life in connec-

---

[1] "Anatomie des centres nerveux," French translation by Heller, Paris, 1879, p. 104.   [2] Op. cit., p. 344, et seq.   [3] Op. cit., p. 346.
[4] "Théorie physiologique de l'hallucination," Paris, 1874, p. 37.

tion with disease involving the optic thalami discovered after death.

But it is not alone to morbid anatomy that we are to look for evidence of this relation. Experimental physiology equally tends to its establishment, and, though the position of the optic thalami is such as to make it a matter of difficulty to act upon them as in the case of the cortex, the obstacle has been in a great measure overcome by Fournié, and we are thus placed in possession of data which have a distinct connection with the point at issue.

Fournié's [1] method consisted in injecting, by means of a hypodermic syringe, caustic solutions—such as a strong solution of the chloride of zinc—into the brain of a dog, observing the resulting phenomena, and then, after death, carefully noting the part of the organ in which the injection had been deposited. Seven of his experiments related to the optic thalami, and, without referring to the other results, it may be stated that in every one there was a more or less complete loss of sensation.

Thus, in Case XV, the left side was operated upon. The needle traversed the cornu ammonis, and the injection was thrown out in the centre of the optic thalamus. As a consequence, there was complete abolition of all sensibility.

Such being apparently the physiological relations of the optic thalamus, we come in the next place to discuss, with something more of fulness, the consequences, so far as sensation is concerned, of certain abnormal states of these organs. As I have said, Ritti has collected from various sources many cases proving that injury or disease of the optic thalami leads to sensorial derangement, or the entire loss of one or more of the special senses. He has also gathered together, from the works of Calmeil, Lagardelle, and others, instances tending to establish the fact that hallucinations are the result of disease of one or both optic thalami. Several of the cases were supplied to him by M. Aug. Voisin, and had not previously been published. Of these latter I quote the following:

" A woman, aged forty-one, entered the Salpêtrière, January 30, 1867. Since 1865, she has been subject to hallucinations of sight, accompanied at times by some excitement and partial alienation. At her admission she had partial

[1] " Sur le fonctionnement du cerveau," Paris, 1873.

hallucinations of sight and hearing, and others connected with the genital organs. There were also delusions of perception. Latterly the sense of hearing has been impaired. She died, April 17, 1869, of typhoid fever.

"*Autopsy.*—Neither thickening nor adhesions of the membranes; no sub-arachnoid effusion; cranial nerves normal, with the exception of the eighth pair, which were rotten. At the most posterior and internal part of the two lobes of the cerebellum, and in the region nearest to the olivary bodies, there were collections of little granulations such as are seen in the choroid plexus. These were continued as far as the floor of the fourth ventricle, where they covered its cerebellar wall. Nothing was found wrong with the left optic thalamus, but the gray anterior centre of the right thalamus was more than normally vascular, and in the part immediately subjacent to the olfactive centre of gray matter there was a spot the color of the dregs of wine, due to a globiform extravasation of blood. In the middle region there was a lacuna."

This case is instructive, not only on account of the situation of the lesion, but for the reason, also, that there was no other intracranial disease to which the symptoms could have been ascribed.

In a case that came under my own observation, a patient had hallucinations of sight and hearing, while at the same time he was both blind and deaf. The blindness and deafness had existed for several years, but there were no hallucinations or other abnormal mental disturbances till, in the month of October, 1877, on successive days, the 12th and 13th, there were paralytic seizures without coma, on each occasion soon after waking in the morning. The motor paralysis was slight, and almost entirely disappeared in a few days, but the cutaneous anæsthesia was persistent to the day of his death, on December 10th following. The examination of the brain was made by me on December 11th. There was a clot the size of a small bean in each optic thalamus. These were apparently several weeks old, and were, doubtless, the cause of the paralytic attacks and hallucinations in October. The immediate cause of death was a fresh hæmorrhage into the pons Varolii, which had broken through the substance of the organ into the sub-arachnoid space. There was no other evidence of brain disease.

That the optic thalamus is the centre for perception, as

the cortex is for intellection, is, to say the least, exceedingly probable. Every sense has these two stages in its full action. Something is *perceived;* that is one stage. It is more or less thoroughly *understood;* and that is the second stage. A pigeon, for instance, from which the cerebrum has been removed, leaving only the basal ganglia, perceives, but does not understand. A light may be held before the eyes, and the head is turned if the light be moved, so that it can still be seen. If a loud noise be made near by, the animal starts or turns its head in the direction of the sound. These phenomena show *perception*, but they just as clearly show the absence of *intellection*, for the animal does not do the thing which, if it understood, it would do ; it obtains no idea from the sensorial impression, and it is equally incapable of originating an idea, for it is deprived of consciousness. Consequently, it gives no evidences of alarm, no matter how intense the visual or auditory excitation may be. It *perceives*, as is very evident from its actions, but these actions are such as to show that there is no further elaboration of the impression.

The intrinsic starting-point of every real sensorial impression is an organ of sense, such as the eye, the ear, or the terminal ramifications of the olfactory nerves. The starting-point of an erroneous sensorial impression—illusion or hallucination—may be either the organ of sense concerned therein or the sensory ganglion—the optic thalamus. The cortex, or intellectual centre for any sense, cannot form a real or false sensorial impression. It can only elaborate the impressions which reach it from the sensory ganglion, and these are either true or false, real or unreal, according as they come originally from the ganglion or are transmitted through it from an organ of sense receiving real impressions from without ; and according as the cortex is in a normal or an abnormal condition will the ideas or beliefs which it forms from these transmitted impressions be normal or abnormal. It is true the cortex can recall former impressions and construct ideas from them, but here the idea is based on a recollection and not on a sensorial impression. Till, for instance, the eye and the optic thalamus had received the image of an American Indian and perceived it, the cortex could not have formed an idea of such a being. All, therefore, that the cortex does is to take cognizance of present or former sensorial impressions which it receives or has received from the optic thalamus, and to form

ideas from them. It does this normally when we bring the
memory into action in a reasonable and logical manner; it
does it abnormally, for instance, in delirium without hallucinations, but in which there is a constant recurrence, in a disorderly manner, of ideas previously formed from former sensorial impressions. The accompanying diagram (Fig. 5) will
tend to the elucidation of the views here expressed.

A is an organ of sense, the eye. Through the optic nerve

Fig. 5.

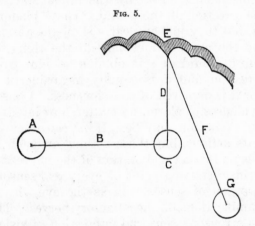

B an impression received on the retina is transmitted to the
sensory ganglion, the optic thalamus *C*, when it becomes a
perception. From the optic thalamus it is transmitted by
fibres of the corona radiata *D* to the cortex *E*, where it is
elaborated into an idea; and from the cortex another form of
force may be evolved, and an intelligent action may take
place in consequence of the transmission through another set
of fibres, *F*, of a motor impulse to a muscle, *G*. If there is no
organ of sense, there can be no normal sensorial impression;
if the optic nerve be divided, the sensation cannot be transmitted to the optic thalamus; if there be a diseased optic
thalamus, the sensorial impression will be perverted, and there
will be an illusion of centric origin; if the cortex be in a normal condition, this illusion will be corrected and understood
as such erroneous perception; if, however, the cortex be diseased, the illusion will be accepted as true, and a false idea, or
delusion, will be formed. If the organ of sense receives no impression from without, but if such impression be formed in
the optic thalamus, then there is a hallucination; if, again,

the cortex be healthy, this hallucination is appreciated at its full value, and there is a true idea in regard to it ; if, on the other hand, the cortex be in an abnormal state, the hallucination is accepted for reality, and a delusion is the result.

Such is, I think, the pathology of perceptional insanity. The lesions of the optic thalamus necessary to the production of a false sensorial impression may be of varied character. Congestion is probably that which most commonly exists, especially in the early stages, and in those cases which are not accompanied by derangements of the other categories of mental faculties. Anæmia is likewise a condition of frequent occurrence. At later periods, as Luys[1] says, the optic thalami are the seats of degenerations which show that there have been frequent perturbations of the circulation. Sometimes there is a little hæmorrhagic focus in different stages of regression, and, again, various stages of sclerosis. This sclerosis is accompanied by partial hyperæmia and the production of a large number of amyloid corpuscles. The nerve cells are correspondingly diminished in number, and those which remain have undergone degeneration and atrophy.

Luys[2] appears to have established the point that in old cases of hallucinations there is a special form of cortical disease affecting the paracental lobe, and which consists of a hypertrophy of this part of the cerebrum on one or both sides. The region in question, therefore, is raised up above the surrounding parts, and presents a gibbous appearance. Incision into the affected portion shows that the convolutions are increased in size, and that a state of hyperæmia exists. Again, there may be atrophy, especially of the frontal convolutions, or a general diminution of the weight of the brain may exist.

But he is very strong in his conviction that there are secondary changes, which are the cause of the transformation of psycho-sensorial hallucinations into those which Baillarger designated psychic, and to which attention has already been called. In my opinion, they are the cause of the hallucination becoming a delusion, and, indeed, between a psychic hallucination and a delusion there is very little difference. The former cannot exist without the involvement of the intellect.

[1] " Traité clinique et pratique des maladies mentales," Paris, 1881, p. 305.
[2] *Op. cit.*, p. 392.

CHAPTER IV.

II.

INTELLECTUAL INSANITIES.

THE intellectual insanities are characterized by the pre-dominance of intellectual derangement. It is not to be con-sidered for a moment that the perceptions, the emotions, and the will are not also often involved to a marked degree ; but, in the forms which I have placed under this head, the intellect is that part of the mind which is pre-eminently·dis-turbed. They are mainly characterized by the existence of delusions, and, if the reader will bear in mind what has been said in regard to delusions, he will at once perceive that they involve the intellect directly and necessarily, without the es-sential implication of the other categories of mental facul-ties. Again, there may be conceptions which, though not false, are yet abnormal.

INTELLECTUAL MONOMANIA.

A perversion of the intellect characterized by the exist-ence of delusions limited to a single subject or to a small class of subjects.

Two forms of this affection are met with. In the one there is mental exaltation, in the other there is mental depression.

a—INTELLECTUAL MONOMANIA WITH EXALTATION.

Although the most prominent symptoms of intellectual monomania with exaltation may appear with suddenness, there is almost always a characteristic prodromatic stage, marked by very decided evidences of mental aberration. These usually consist of erroneous conceptions relative to the importance of the affected individual, the attention which others show him, the observation he attracts as he walks the street or enters a room, the unfitness of a man of his parts for the perhaps humble occupation he follows, and the dispo-sition he evinces to talk about his many superior accomplish-ments or bodily perfections. Gradually these become so pro-nounced that they attract the attention of those with whom he comes in contact ; but, as he continues to transact his business properly, and behaves himself well in other respects, his condition is rarely, by the superficial observer, regarded as being one of incipient insanity. It is usually supposed at first that what he says of himself is simply an exaggerated style of speaking, and it is remarked of him that he is becoming vain, and otherwise disagreeable. The physician, however, meeting with such a case, will scarcely fail to see that the change of character, or the abnormal development of traits, which previously existed only in light degree, is one of the strongest and most common manifestations of mental derangement.

With these symptoms connected with the mind, there are others of a physical character. There is almost always insomnia, there is sometimes pain or discomfort in the head, there is excessive motility and restlessness, the bowels are constipated, the skin is dry, the eyes are brighter than usual, the speech is hurried, but there is no incoherence of either words or ideas.

Gradually the mental symptoms develop in intensity and definiteness, and one or more delusions become firmly established. They may be based on illusions or hallucinations, or they may arise from purely imaginary premises not connected with the senses. Sometimes they are spontaneous, and at others they appear to come from dreams. In a former chapter I have adduced several examples of delusions obviously the result of strong mental impressions made by dreams.

As instances of the existence of perceptional derangement before the occurrence of delusions of fixed character, and apparently leading logically to the intellectual derangement, I cite the following from my note-books :

The patient, a master plumber, had for several weeks been a little excited in his manner, and disposed to exaggerate his importance as a plumber, contending, with great earnestness, that no one understood the business as well as he did. He had cards printed, announcing himself as having more practical experience than any other plumber in the United States, and that his work could not be excelled, as he had devised new methods of soldering which absolutely did away with all possibility of leaks. He had a large business, and it was known that he had been experimenting with solders, so that, though his statements were regarded as extravagant, they were not looked upon as much more than smart advertising devices.

But one morning he announced to his wife that he had received a communication from a deceased plumber, by which he was informed of a still greater improvement to be made in soldering and in the manufacture of lead pipes. His story was that, while sitting in his shop reflecting on the best method of making lead pipes and solder, he heard a whisper telling him to soak the lead in shark's blood and the solder in shark's urine, and that then neither could ever give way. Steamships, it was told him, could be made of large pipes soldered together. He expressed some surprise that he could not see the individual who spoke to him, and who, he said, called himself the "boss plumber of eternity"; but he did not attempt to account for the invisibility. He was promised by the voice a pre-eminence over all other plumbers, and a degree of wealth such as the most sanguine member of the craft never dreamed it possible to obtain.

All this put him into a state of the greatest good humor. His face wore a continual smile ; he talked to every one he met of his great luck, and he joked about the envy of the other plumbers, and of the attempts they would doubtless make to rob him of the honor and profit to accrue to him. As he did no harm to anybody, and as he was perfectly willing to let his son attend to his real business while he worked at his experiments, he was not confined in an asylum. Finally he became less exact in his delusion ; he began to be rambling and incoherent, and is now, after over ten years' duration of his insanity, in a condition of chronic mania approaching dementia.

In another case, that of a young lady eighteen years of age, there had been for several weeks a slight degree of mental excitement, which was attributed to suppressed menstruation. But there were no marked signs of insanity till she announced to her mother that angels had been whispering to her all night that the Virgin Mary would soon pay her a visit, and that she must be prepared to receive her august guest with due honor. From that time she became greatly impressed with a sense of her own dignity, and insisted on writing letters to the cardinal and to several bishops, inviting them to be present on the occasion of the visit. The time for this was not fixed ; she was informed by the angels that she must be "always ready," for, as "Christ would come as a thief in the night, so would his mother." She therefore always kept herself, as much as her friends would allow, in full dress, and even went to bed with all the jewellery on her person that she could collect, and with a gorgeously decorated silk dress by the side of her bed, ready to be slipped on at the least warning that the virgin was coming. She recovered in a few months, and has remained well.

Even when illusions or hallucinations are not among the first symptoms, very few cases of the affection in question run their course without sensorial aberrations. Occasionally, however, this is the case. In a patient under my own charge, who imagined himself to be Charles XII of Sweden, and who strutted about with all the finery he could gather together, fastened in the most incongruous manner to various parts of his person, there were no illusions or hallucinations of any of the senses, so far as could be discovered. In the following case, which I take from Dr. Parsons's records, the like condition apparently existed :

E. H., female, thirty-six years old, a native of France, and by occupation a "clairvoyant," says that Louis Napoleon was her father, and Antoinetta, a daughter of Queen Victoria, her mother. Has known that she was Napoleon's daughter since she was four years old, but said nothing about it till about a year ago. Got into some trouble in Pittsburg, and threatened to have the mayor deposed if he did not attend to his business. Came to New York to get her rights. A hundred thousand dollars are due her. Says all the shopkeepers in New York ought to make her presents ; says the sun and the moon come down and walk with her, but seems to mean by this that they shine on her in a peculiar way in honor of her nobility.

As the delusions in monomania with exaltation usually relate to the greatness, the honor, the wealth, the beauty, or some other ennobling quality or desirable condition of the individual, the bearing and attitude of the patient are in logical accordance therewith, though at the same time are carried to such an extreme point as to show the most decided aberration of judgment. The individual, for instance, who imagines himself to be an emperor, and who stalks about in the most pompous manner, his head thrown far back, his lips compressed, and his eyes expressing the sense of his grandeur, not only overacts his part in these directions, but renders himself still more ridiculous with a piece of tin on his head for a crown, a cane for a sceptre, a rush-bottomed chair for a throne, and bits of tawdry finery pinned to his coat to represent the orders he is entitled to wear.

"In ambitious monomania," says Marcé,[1] "the patient declares that he comes of an illustrious ancestry ; he invents a history of himself and family which excites wonder by the minutiæ and precision of its details. He speaks of his education and of his surroundings, and brings together, in harmony with his ideas, all the persons and incidents which he can imagine. He wearies the authorities with his demands, and finally, when placed in an asylum, he never ceases to protest against what he considers to be his arbitrary detention, and the outrage of which he is the victim."

A colored man, as black as a bit of charcoal, had the delusion that he was white, and that he was "King of the North Pole." He fastened a lot of metallic labels from sardine-boxes together, and wore them for a coronet, while a pair of old epaulets dangled from his coat-tails. The gait, the pose, the expression of these people, are often sufficient of themselves to indicate the general character of the delusions they entertain.

Some forms of *religious monomania*, as it is called, and others of *erotomania*, in which there are delusions of an exalted character, are to be embraced under the present head. In the one, the patient, if a man, imagines that he is God or Christ, or some noted prophet or saint, or that he has a special mission from the Almighty to declare his purposes to mankind. If a woman, she may consider herself to be the Virgin Mary, or the "bride of Christ," or about to give birth to a second son of God. Such cases in either sex are embraced under the term "theomania," and they include some of the most remarkable to be met with in the annals of insanity.

Thus, there is the instance of Joanna Southcote, an ignorant woman, who, some eighty years ago, persuaded a large number of persons that Christ was to be born again of her, and that he was his own father. She called herself the Bride, the Lamb's wife, clothed with the sun. Day and night she had hallucinations or visions, as she called them, which she accepted as realities, and which formed the basis of her prophecies and system of religion. Meetings were held

[1] "Traité pratique des maladies mentales," Paris, 1862, p. 365.

to inquire into the truth of her pretensions, and, a court of investigation being organized, she was accepted for all she assumed to be. Among others of her hallucinations was one that Christ had occupied the same bed with her, and that she had seen and conversed with him. Such sexual orgasms were frequently misinterpreted by the mystical women of the middle ages into acts of intercourse with angels and members of the Godhead, so that Joanna's experience was not isolated.

In her sixty-fifth year she gave out that she was pregnant, and that Christ would soon be born again. She was examined by several medical men, who certified that she was actually pregnant. A crib was procured, which, with the elaborate bedding, cost over two hundred pounds, but which was nevertheless called a manger. The faithful waited in vain for the heavenly infant; but excuses were made, and she continued to have followers till her death, several years afterward.

A somewhat similar case has occurred in my own experience, in which the patient, the wife of a stone mason, fancied that she was pregnant by the Holy Ghost, and that she was about to give birth to a second Christ, who was to revolutionize the world. As a matter of fact, she was pregnant. She insisted that the child left her womb every night, and conversed with her relative to the wonderful things he was going to do when he had accomplished the full term of his intrauterine life. Under the head of "Epidemic Mania" the subject in some of its relations will receive further consideration.

In erotomania of the intellectual variety there are delusions in which the subjects imagine either that their personality is changed, and that they are enacting the part of some noted historical individual, whose life was full of romantic episodes, or that they were and are violently beloved by a real personage, whom they consequently annoy with their importunities. The case of a young lady occurs to me in this connection who had the delusion that her hand had been requested in marriage by a distinguished statesman, and whom she continually annoyed with letters asking for interviews, and begging that a day might be fixed for their marriage. Subsequently, she had the hallucination that he had passed the night with her in a hotel in Jersey City, and, as she talked freely of the supposed circumstance, trouble would have been caused but for the fact that the gentleman was able to show that he was in California for several weeks before and after the alleged seduction. She was taken to Europe by her father and placed in a lunatic asylum in Germany, where she still remains.

Though not generally disposed to do serious mischief, the subjects of monomania with exaltation are always ready to defend their imaginary rights, and to quarrel with those who dispute their claims to distinction. Hence, they are more or less troublesome and offensive to those with whom they come in contact. A word, however, in recognition of the truth of their delusions, generally suffices to restore them to equanimity. A not uncommon form of the affection is that in which the delusions relate to some wonderful or useful discovery or invention which the patient·imagines he has made. One thinks he has devised a machine for converting water into wine. According to him, it is only necessary to pour the water into a receptacle attached to the apparatus, and to turn a crank, when wine of the best quality flows out of a spout at the other end. Another conceives that he has discovered a powder which, when administered to women, will cause them to fall in love with the giver. The following remarkable instance I take from the *New York Tribune* of July 2, 1880 :

A man had the delusion that lead would float on the surface of water, and his faith in his false belief led to his death. For several days he had been acting very strangely, when suddenly he disappeared. Before doing so, however, he sent a letter to his wife to this effect :

" MY DEAR WIFE : I have finally struck something which will bring in money, and I hope happiness, to all of us. I have invented a life-preserver, on an entirely new principle, and am so sanguine as to its results that I am going to try it to-night. I find that it is a fallacy that cork or any wood that absorbs water is lighter than lead. Lead does not displace as much water, but, when submerged, I find that it has three times the lifting power of cork. I have got some lead cut in strips three quarters of an inch wide, and can make a jacket of it, for two dollars and a half, that any one can float in for days and days. Everybody has always said that, because lead was in air heavier than cork, it would be in water ; but I have three times tried it, and find lead in water will, in proportion to its weight, float ten times its weight in cork.   Cork costs fifty cents a pound, lead six cents, and I can put life-preservers on all boats, ships, and steamboats in the world at half price.   I am sure of a hundred thousand dollars to-morrow.   I have everything ready for the trial.   I will go out to-night on a Goodrich steamer, and I will be back at 9 A. M., and show everybody that they can make lead float as well or better than cork.   The result will be that when I come home to-morrow I can sell the right for one hundred thousand dollars, and get rid of all the trouble I am in.   I will leave my clothes in the boat—watch, money, etc.—for fear I may have the lake to cross ; but the way the wind looks now, I can get home by 12 M.   As I shall not go more than forty miles out, and if the wind is right, with my armor I can get in in two hours.   I will get rid of my debts, and fit you and the children out nicely on what I can get when I get in town to-morrow.   Don't worry.''

The poor man had made either a life-preserver or a jacket of lead, and had jumped overboard from the steamer into the water, expecting to float on the surface for hours or days till he could be rescued.

The delusions of intellectual monomania with exaltation sometimes relate to a change of sex which the individual supposes to have taken place in his or her organization, and which is regarded with great pride and satisfaction.   In these cases, the manners, customs, and dress of the sex into which they imagine themselves to be changed are assumed, and their actions are regulated as nearly as possible in accordance with the erroneous belief.   These cases are not to be confounded with those which, occurring in males, are due to injury purposely inflicted on the generative organs, and to which I have called attention in a recently published memoir.[1]   They are instances of true monomania, characterized by the existence of delusions, which the others are not, and may exist either in males or females.   In those which have come under my observation there was no degeneration or exaltation of the sexual feeling, the subjects behaving not only with perfect decorum, but with excessive modesty.

In one of these, the patient, a young man of good family and finished education, but with a strong hereditary tendency

[1] '' The Disease of the Scythians and Certain Analogous Conditions,'' *American Journal of Neurology and Psychiatry*, August, 1882.

to insanity on his mother's side, obtained the idea that he had become a woman, from seeing, as he imagined, his own image looking like a woman, and in the dress of the female sex. At the same moment a voice said to him, "Go thou and do likewise"; and this was repeated to him many times during the day. Without at the time believing that his sex was changed, he put on woman's apparel, and remained in his room all day, surveying himself in the glass with great satisfaction, and walking up and down the floor, aping the gait and attitudes of the other sex. Little by little, however, the idea that his sex was changed took possession of him, and he came to me for an examination, which he was confident would confirm him in his belief. He was somewhat surprised to find that my opinion was different from his own, but no demonstration sufficed to shake him in the strength of his conviction. He congratulated himself that, being a woman, his emotional nature, which, as he said, had up to that time been very coarse and undeveloped, would now be delicate and refined.

A man, named Binns, died recently in the Philadelphia Almshouse, at the age of sixty-nine years, who had for a long time been a notorious character in that institution, in consequence of entertaining the delusion that he was a woman. He affected woman's ways, and was known by the name of "Sally Binns." When a young man, he had joined a theatrical club as an amateur, and the height of his ambition was to play female characters. He became a monomaniac on this subject, his infatuation at last took upon itself a mild form of insanity, and for the greater part of his life he entertained the belief in question. At all times, and on all occasions, he believed himself to be a dashing beauty, at whose feet scores of ardent admirers knelt, and upon whom society smiled with favor. Clad in feminine attire, whenever a ball or concert was given for the patients he was the centre of attraction. He affected an effeminate voice in conversation, and acted in every respect like one of the female sex. The air of a woman never deserted him, and everybody who visited the Almshouse called on "Sally."

The late Dr. James R. Wood informed me that he had several years ago observed the case of a young woman who, without any exaggeration of the sexual feeling, imagined herself to be a man, and who dressed herself, whenever she could do so without being prevented, in men's clothing. It was a veritable delusion, and not one of those cases in which the individual, while having no delusion of a change of gender, evinces erotic propensities toward members of his or her sex. Delusions of this character are sometimes, as in the instance first mentioned, preceded and accompanied by hallucinations, but usually there is no sensorial aberration. In Dr. Wood's case the woman admitted that she had the breasts and the genital organs of a member of the female sex, but she contended that these were not true marks of sexual difference, which were really to be found in a certain organ or part of the brain. She insisted that she knew of several persons who, though having the sexual organs common to women, were in reality men. She had an idea that all unfruitful women were really men, and that all men with blue eyes and light hair were women.

Again, the delusions of the intellectual monomaniac may relate to changes which he supposes have taken place in various parts of his body. One believes that his hand is made of glass, and he carries it enclosed in a stout leathern case to prevent its being broken by contact with other substances. Another imagines that his teeth are of pearls, and he struts about, in the most bombastic manner, with open mouth, descanting on the beauty and value of its contents, or with his lips tightly closed, for fear some one may rob him of his treasures. And another believes herself to be endowed with such a supernatural degree of procreative power that she becomes spontaneously impregnated, and is delivered of a child every night, which is at once taken to an emperor's palace and brought up as a prince of the imperial blood. On all other subjects than those directly connected with these delusions, intellectual monomaniacs reason with such a degree of lucidity as readily to pass for sane persons with most observers, and often even with skilled physicians. As Guislain [1] says, they preserve more or less fully the appearance and manners of normally constituted individuals ; the memory remains intact, they retain their knowledge of arithmetic, they know how to distinguish that which is right from that which is wrong, they judge correctly of passing events, and they can, up to a certain point, conduct themselves well in the world, and even sometimes manage their own business

[1] "Leçons orales sur les phrénopathies," etc., Paris, 1880, t. i, p. 229.

22

matters with promptness and discretion. Moreover, it may be added that they very often have the power, especially in the earlier stages of the malady, before the mind becomes markedly enfeebled, of concealing their delusions under the most rigid examination. But, while able to perceive the ludicrous character of the delusions of their fellow-lunatics, they cling tenaciously to their own, which are, perhaps, still more ridiculous. " Look at that poor woman," said a gentleman to me as we walked together through the grounds of an asylum; "she has lost her baby, and she thinks she has it in that bundle of rags she is nursing." Yet he was himself under the delusion that he was General Grant.

As we have seen, the form of mental derangement under notice may be unaccompanied by illusions or hallucinations. Even when the existing delusion is of such a character as apparently to be connected with some one of the senses, and thus to be based upon a false perception, full inquiry will often show that there is no error of the sensorial processes, centric or eccentric. Thus, a lady under my care had the delusion that she had lost her palate. I held a mirror to her face, and, while she opened her mouth, I pointed out to her that all the parts were present. "Yes," she replied, "I see all that; the form is there, I know very well, but the substance is gone," and no arguments could convince her to the contrary. A gentleman conceived that his right hand was made of glass, and, therefore, to prevent its being broken, he kept it carefully enclosed in a stout case, made to fit it accurately. On my calling his attention to the physical qualities of his hand, and pointing out how they differed from those of glass, he said: "I once thought just as you do. My brain was then incapable of appreciating minute differences as well as it can now; and though I confess that my senses still convey to me the idea that my hand is like other people's, yet I know that the conception is erroneous, and I correct it at once by my reason. My hand looks like flesh and blood, but it is glass for all that. Nothing is more calculated to deceive than the senses." On my asking another monomaniac, who believed that she was the Princess of Wales, whether she thought her prototype would be seen walking about in a pink muslin frock, trimmed with copper wire, from which dangled buttons of various shapes and sizes, she replied: "Certainly not; when I lived in England I was at court, and I was obliged to wear my grandest jewels; but in this republican country I am not allowed to dress as I would like, and hence I put on these symbols. The copper wire stands for gold cord, and the buttons for diamonds and pearls."

Remissions are not very common in intellectual monomania with exaltation, and intermissions are still rarer. Occasionally the patient may hold to his delusions with less tenacity than at other times; he may even express some doubt as to their reality, but such manifestations are of short duration, and it is quite certain that often he is not sincere in his declarations, having some object in view which he thinks he may gain by dissimulation. As Haslam[1] says:

"They have sometimes such a high degree of control over their minds that, when they have any particular purpose to carry, they will affect to renounce their opinions, which shall have been judged inconsistent, and it is well known that they have often dissembled their resentment until a favorable opportunity has occurred of gratifying their revenge. Of this restraint, which madmen have sometimes the power of imposing on their opinions, the remark has been so frequent that those who are more immediately about their persons have termed it, in their rude phrase, 'stifling their disorder.'"

During the course of intellectual monomania with exaltation there may be intercurrent attacks of extreme excitement, during which there is active delirium, characterized by great volubility, incoherence, and excessive motility. At such times the patient may become combative, not only in defence of his delusions, but offensively. There is usually at these periods slight febrile exacerbation, and the sleep is disturbed more than ordinarily. These paroxysms become less frequent as the disease advances, until finally they no longer occur. Under the head of "Scheming Insanity," Arnold,[2] a hundred years ago, described a form of mental derangement which is embraced within the limits of intellectual monomania with exaltation.

"The patient," he says, "thinks himself either endowed with better natural talents, and with more penetration and sagacity, or improved with greater acquisitions of knowledge and experience, or more enlightened by the special favor of

---

[1] "Observations on Madness," etc., London, 1809, p. 53.

[2] "Observations on the Nature, Kinds, Causes, and Prevention of Insanity," second edition, London, 1806, p. 170. First edition published in 1782.

Heaven, or more secure of success by the happy concurrence of power, interest, opportunity, or some other advantageous circumstance, than most other men, and, either by his superior knowledge or cunning, capable of doing great things, which few or none but himself are able to accomplish ; or at least feels an irresistible inclination to be engaged in some schemes or traffic ; and, as he thinks himself, if not actually the most knowing, at least among the most knowing of mankind, so he is secure of that success which the simple and ignorant may wish for, but the wise and provident alone can command."

Many cases of the monomania of Esquirol, and the megalomania of Dagonet and others, are also comprehended under the head of intellectual monomania with exaltation.

b—INTELLECTUAL MONOMANIA WITH DEPRESSION.

This mental disorder is not to be confounded with the emotional form of insanity known as lypemania, or melancholia, with which, though entirely distinct, it has naturally many relations. It is the *monomanie triste* of Marcé, and, as this author has pointed out, is characterized by the fact that, although the patient has fixed delusions of a melancholic character which influence him in his actions, he can, nevertheless, reason well in regard to other subjects, and is often able to conduct himself with entire propriety in all the relations of life, outside of his own particular erroneous beliefs. In melancholia, on the other hand, the emotions are involved to an extreme degree ; the false conceptions assume entire control of the mind and render the individual altogether incapable of the systematic performance of rational acts, whether they are or are not connected with his delusions.

Like the preceding affection, intellectual monomania with depression may arise suddenly, or may be preceded by prodromatic symptoms. These latter, instead of being of the expansive character peculiar to intellectual monomania with exaltation, are depressing in their nature, and hence present an entirely different *ensemble* from that met with in the other form of the disorder. Usually they consist of ill-defined ideas that people are conspiring against the person in whom they exist. He accordingly becomes suspicious of those about him, looks around uneasily, watches every movement in others, takes unusual means to protect himself from imaginary attacks upon his person or property, imagines that conversations which occur in his presence, and which he does not hear, relate to him and to plans for injuring him in various ways. He conceives the idea that his friends and relatives are wanting in proper respect for him, that he is neglected by them and by his servants, and, if he is sufficiently ignorant, that certain persons have laid a spell on him or bewitched him. A patient from the interior of this State, who consulted me a short time since, had the notion that his wife one morning had looked at him in a peculiar way, and that instantly he felt a thrilling sensation pass through his brain. He was also under the impression that, being jealous, she had endeavored to render him impotent, in order that a condition of forced faithfulness might be induced. As he walked the streets, he conceived that the people he met, not one of whom did he know, looked at him as if they were aware of the fact that he was deprived of virile power. He had not been in the city longer than a few days when he contracted the delusion that his testicles had disappeared, and this was followed by the idea that he had been castrated by order of the Pope, in order that he might be put in the choir at St. Peter's in Rome.

The most singular fact connected with the case was that his sexual powers were unusually strong for a man of his age, and that he had intercourse, on an average, once in twenty-four hours during the whole time that he was under my observation—a period of ten days.

Illusions and hallucinations may be present at a very early period, and these very generally relate to the sense of hearing, though by no means exclusively. In a case that came to my clinique at the University Medical College several years ago, the patient, a man of adult age, had imbibed the delusion that people were endeavoring to poison him with noxious vapors, and this idea had clearly arisen in consequence of the long-continued presence of a hallucination of the sense of smell. I have also seen several cases in which illusions of taste have given rise to similar delusions.

Sometimes the apprehensions of impending evil which the individual experiences are vague and indefinable. He feels that something is going to happen, but what, he does not know, and often an accidental circumstance gives form to the fears which he entertains.

Thus, a young man employed in a counting-house had

been for several weeks tormented with morbid fancies of some great catastrophe being about to occur by which he and all his friends would be destroyed. He was unable to sleep with comfort, or to procure a sufficient amount, for, as soon as he got to sleep, he was awakened by some terrible vision, and would often spring from the bed in his terror and rush into his father's room imploring protection.

During all this period he continued to attend at his place of business, and to perform the duties required of him. One morning, however, soon after taking his seat at his desk, a stranger entered the room, and, inquiring his name, occupation, and residence, proceeded to record the items in a book, and soon afterward took his departure. At once the idea took possession of the young man's mind that the stranger was a detective, sent to obtain information preparatory to making his arrest on the charge of murder, and to this conception the fact that the stranger had said something about a dead man contributed in no small degree. The man was in reality an agent for the publishers of a directory; but this fact could not be made clear to the patient, and the delusion that he was "wanted" on the charge of murder took full possession of him. He consequently locked himself up in his room, and refused to come out for any purpose whatever. At last, however, he sent a notice to a newspaper announcing his death, and this appeared to relieve his apprehensions to such an extent that he left his room and walked about the house, and, even after nightfall, took a little exercise in the open air. But ere long his fears were renewed, delusions of persecution became firmly established, and it was necessary to send him to an asylum in order to prevent suicide or homicide, both of which he gave signs of contemplating.

In another case the patient, a married lady, thirty years of age, had for several weeks experienced an indefinable dread for which she could assign no adequate cause. Her sleep became disturbed, her appetite capricious, her bowels constipated, and there were frequent sharp pains in various parts of the head. Her temper, which previously was remarkably mild and equable, was now irritable and fretful. The least thing was sufficient to derange her equanimity and to cause her to indulge in invectives and complaints to a degree that rendered her a very troublesome inmate of the house in which she resided.

But the most prominent symptoms were those connected with the fear that something terrible was about to happen. This delusion took such a firm hold of her mind that she passed the greater part of her time when alone in weeping and wringing her hands, though, when some noted occasion, such as receiving visits or taking her meals in presence of others, required her to restrain herself, no one could be more composed. Things went on in this way for several weeks, till one day, as she was drinking her coffee at breakfast, she suddenly exclaimed that it was poisoned, and, throwing the cup on the floor in her fright and agitation, she refused to eat anything more. From this time on, the idea that poison would be administered to her became a fixed delusion, which was often accompanied by illusions and hallucinations of taste, hearing, and sight.

In both these cases there was present a condition which has attracted a good deal of attention from alienists, and which is one of the most important in all its relations of the several phases of the form of insanity under consideration, and that is the *delirium of persecution*.

Generally this state begins with illusions and hallucinations which for a time may be strenuously resisted by the individual, but which usually end by obtaining a complete mastery over his reason. The sense of hearing is that which is generally the root of these false perceptions, which appear either as vague, uncertain sounds, or isolated words, or as well-defined sentences. These are in the form of threats or warnings, or advice as to the best way of escaping from imaginary enemies or dangers. The sense of sight is not so frequently affected, though occasionally the patient sees a policeman or other person in seach of him in every one who looks at him a little closely. In order to escape from these imaginary enemies he makes complaint to the officials, or seeks safety in flight, or may even proceed to the extent of perpetrating suicide or homicide. Sometimes the individual labors under the delusion that organized bodies of men have banded together for the purpose of destroying him, or of inflicting severe bodily injury upon him. These may, in his imagination, be the whole police force, or the clergy, or the medical profession, or the masonic fraternity, or the members of some nationality. A patient of mine was sure that all the clergymen had entered into a conspiracy to "pray him into hell."

He went to the churches to hear what they had to say, and discovered adroit allusions to himself, and hidden invocations to God for his eternal damnation in the most harmless and platitudinous expressions. He wrote letters to various pastors of churches denouncing them for their uncharitable conduct toward him, and threatening them with bodily damage if they persisted in their efforts to secure the destruction of his soul.

Another was constantly dodging around the corners of the streets and hiding himself in doorways to avoid detectives, for whom he mistook all who happened to look at him with more than a passing glance, and who, he conceived, were seeking to arrest him on the charge of attempting to take the life of the mayor. "I never even saw the mayor," he would exclaim, with tears in his eyes, "and God knows I never wished him any harm, and yet these scoundrels are endeavoring to imprison me for shooting a pistol at him. There is another one of them!" and instantly he darted down an area to hide till a bland-looking old gentleman, whom he took for a disguised detective, had passed. "That man," he continued, when he emerged from his place of seclusion, "is the sharpest one of the whole lot. He looks seventy years old, but he's only twenty-five. His hair is a wig, and his beard is false. I can go nowhere without just managing to escape. Of course, he'll catch me at last, and then I shall go to prison for life."

C. B.,[1] after separating from her husband, and remaining absent six years, came to the United States from Ireland, and then married again. Shortly afterward a daughter by her first husband came over, and then the mother seemed to realize for the first time that she had two living husbands. This idea seemed to be the exciting cause of her insanity, which first showed itself in unfounded suspicions that her daughter was leading an improper life. Hallucinations of hearing next supervened, and these were that people were talking about her night and day. Heard a young man say that she was a bad woman, had stolen laces, committed forgeries, and was the mistress of a Mr. Welsh. Also heard him say that a play founded on her life was being performed at a theatre. Says that people look crossly at her, and point their fingers toward her. Is very positive about all she heard and saw, and says her opinion could not be changed if all the circum-

[1] From Dr. Parsons's MS. "Notes of Cases in Blackwell's Island Asylum."

stances should be denied by the persons who spoke about her and pointed at her. This patient remained in the asylum for several years in about the same condition as when she entered it.

It is not at all uncommon for the victims of delusions of persecution to imagine that they are being acted upon by some occult influence, or by some one of the forces of nature, as heat, magnetism, or electricity. "Spells" are laid on them by certain individuals whom they know, or by invisible persons who only make themselves known by their speech. In one case that was under my charge, the patient, a stationer, doing business in this city, had the delusion that unknown enemies — freemasons — were acting on him by electricity, which they sent into his brain, through the top of his head, by powerful batteries which they had in their lodge-rooms. In another, a woman, who kept a small shop in the Bowery, and who came to my clinique at the Bellevue Hospital Medical College for the purpose of getting relief, conceived that all the iron railings and railway tracks had been charged with electricity in order to injure her, and that, whenever she touched one of them or even came near it, she received a severe shock. A case of like character is cited by Seme-laigne.[1]

Very slight causes are sometimes sufficient, in a patient suffering from intellectual monomania with depression, to excite hallucinations which have been for some time absent. Poterin du Motel[2] cites the case of a woman who had become melancholic, lost sleep, had pains in her head, and bleeding from the nose, in consequence of some insignificant family disagreement. She contracted the delusion that her sisters, who were in reality devoted to her, had conspired to injure her. Had also illusions and hallucinations. Saw a black head, and heard voices speaking against her. The mere opening or shutting of a door, a step on the floor, or the slightest sound, was sufficient to excite these hallucinations.

A somewhat similar case was at one time under my observation, in which the subject, a lady thirty years old, whose mother had died insane, and who was herself of a strongly

---

[1] "Du diagnostic et du traitement de la mélancolie," *Mémoires de l'académie impériale de médecine*, t. xxv, p. 235.

[2] "Études sur la mélancolie," etc., *Mémoires de l'académie impériale de médecine*, t. xxi, p. 462.

marked nervous temperament, suddenly became affected with hallucinations of hearing, by which she was told that her servants had entered into a conspiracy to burn the house and her with it. Although she never had any hallucination of seeing the persons from whom the noises were supposed to come, she was quite sure that they proceeded from real individuals, concealed in various parts of the house, or under the steps of the houses she passed in the street. Night and day, while awake, she heard the voices. Finally the continuity of the hallucinations ceased, but the delusion remained, and she was constantly watching her servants, frequently changing them, and invoking the aid of the police in order to ensure her safety. But if at any time she heard a very loud noise, such as the rumbling of a heavy wagon in the street, or the explosion of a blast, the hallucinations at once returned.

Lasègue[1] states that he has never witnessed a case of delirium of persecution in a person under twenty-eight years of age, or over seventy. In an instance recently under my observation, the patient, a male, had not reached the age of eighteen when well-marked symptoms of the condition in question made their appearance. He had the idea that the workmen employed with him in a paper factory were hatching a conspiracy to poison him, and several times ran away from his home in order to escape from his imaginary danger. Finally it became necessary to confine him in a lunatic asylum.

The hallucinations and delusions to which persons affected with intellectual monomania with depression are subject sometimes lead them to falsely accuse themselves of having perpetrated various crimes. Instances of the kind are constantly occurring, and are of much interest, not only from their medical but from their legal relations. Gradually the false beliefs which have become a part of their mentality produce such a degree of remorse for the offences that are supposed to have been committed, or excite such a high sense of duty, or awaken a desire to be executed, so as to escape from a life of weariness, that the individual delivers himself up to justice, and makes a full and perfectly coherent confession of his guilt.

In former times, many persons, who had not even been ob-

[1] "Du délire de persécution," *Archives générales de médecine*, février, 1852, p. 129.

jects of suspicion, were executed for sorcery, witchcraft, and analogous crimes, on no other evidence than that which they themselves supplied by confession. A man was brought to me, only a few weeks ago, to be treated for insanity, and who had prepared a carefully written statement to the effect that he had been the instigator of Guiteau in his assassination of the President. He had left his home for the purpose of giving himself up to the authorities at Washington, but had been stopped by his friends. He talked very calmly and intelligently of his imaginary crime, and went into all the details of his interviews with Guiteau with a surprising degree of minuteness and consistency. And yet it was a matter of absolute certainty that he had never seen Guiteau, or been outside the limits of the small village in which he lived for over two years before the President was shot. He felt no great sorrow for what he supposed he had done, but was, he said, actuated by an exalted sense of the duty of a citizen to suffer the proper penalty for any crime he may have committed. He was sorry to be imprisoned, but it was his duty to suffer, and suffer he would. He was in great terror lest the people should find out what he had done and lynch him, and, accordingly, his great anxiety was to get to the protection of a jail as soon as possible. As the case was one in which there was no premonitory tendency to insanity, and had clearly arisen from excessive mental work, I gave a favorable prognosis, and advised his being treated at home.

I saw another case in which the patient, a man, confessed to having wrecked several railway trains and caused the sacrifice of many lives. He said that he had, among other like crimes, cut the beams of the railway bridge at Harlem, and that he kept them together by the mere force of his will till such time as he was ready to destroy a train.

In the majority of such cases the insanity has existed for a long time, and the occurrence of a disaster or the perpetration of a crime is the exciting cause of the peculiar delusion which seizes on the patient. Continued thought in any one direction is liable to produce more or less mental disturbance in the minds of the sanest persons. Repeatedly telling the same lie eventually induces the liar himself to believe in its truth.

It is quite commonly the case in intellectual monomania with depression that the chief delusions which the patient experiences are connected with the idea of approaching pauperism. Although he may be in comfortable, or even affluent circumstances, he is quite sure he is on the high-road to beggary, and that his wife and children are about to become inmates of the almshouse. He is influenced by these erroneous conceptions to such an extent that he denies himself and family the commonest necessaries of life, and sits by the hour moaning over the sad fate in store for him and those dependent upon him. While entertaining the delusions in question he continues to transact his business well, though perhaps with increased caution, and in all other respects appears to be perfectly sane. Inquiry, however, will almost invariably reveal the fact that he suffers more or less from the somatic symptoms already mentioned.

As in intellectual monomania with exaltation, so in the depressant form of the disorder, religion is capable of giving a peculiar impress to the phenomena manifested. There are no delusions of being great prophets, or saints, or members of the Godhead, but there are convictions which are accepted as absolute truths, that some great sin has been committed for which continual prayer must be offered, or that the offence has been so great that not even this remedy is effectual. I have already alluded to the delusion of the "unpardonable sin," and have cited one of the cases that have come under my notice in which it was the predominating feature. The following is interesting in this connection: Several years ago a young man was brought to me by his father for examination. The moment he entered the room he fell on his knees before me, and, with clasped hands, implored my intercession with God for his forgiveness. It seems that he took me for a bishop. He entertained the delusion that he had committed thousands of heinous sins, and that his eternal punishment was not only assured, but was deserved. Nevertheless, it was his duty to pray. He had several times attempted suicide. I advised his committal to an asylum, and he was taken to Sanford Hall, at Flushing. As soon as he entered the parlor of the establishment, and before any of the attendants were aware of his purpose, he plunged his naked hand into the midst of a glowing anthracite fire in the grate, and would have held it there till it was entirely consumed but that he was instantly seized and dragged away. He did this as an act of atonement. But, while entertaining the belief mentioned, and making frequent attempts at bodily injury and destruction, there was not the lamentation and supreme unhappiness which would naturally have resulted in a sane person had his imaginary condition been a reality, or such as would have been experienced in some forms of emotional monomania or of acute melancholia.

In regard to such cases Wachsmuth [1] says : " It is not uncommon to see these unfortunate people commit the most hurtful acts, not only against others, but often mutilations of their own bodies. They are well skilled in deception, and know how to elude the vigilance of their attendants. Not only do they torture themselves, cut their throats, swallow knives, nails, or whatever else will injure them, but they commit all kinds of violent and offensive actions against persons and things. To do wrong and to perpetrate crimes is in some manner a justification of the horrible accusations they bring against themselves. To humiliate themselves they must be abased in their own eyes and in the eyes of others. They must not only be full of wickedness, but they must show the world that they are wicked, and for this purpose they select as victims for their misdeeds those to whom they owe the most affection. The more infamous an action is, the more pleasure they take in its perpetration."

Delusions connected with the relations of the sexes, and constituting a species of *erotomania*, are sometimes met with in intellectual monomania with depression. But, unlike those met with in the previously described form with exaltation, they are of a sad or melancholic character. The subjects believe that they are persecuted by various persons who are endeavoring to prevent them making eligible marriages, or they imagine that they are being pursued by persons for whom they have no affection, and who are constantly watching them and seeking to entrap them so as to carry them off to some place where a violation will be committed or a false marriage performed. In a case which I saw in August, 1882, with Dr. Leale, of this city, the patient, a single woman of about thirty-five years of age, had delusions of persecution of which those of an erotic character were prominent. In order to prevent the violation of her person, of which she imagined she was in continual danger, she not only went to bed in her day-clothes, but fastened

[1] " Pathologie der Seele," p. 98.

her legs together with straps and napkins so as to give as much trouble as possible to the anticipated violator. A physician, whose name has escaped me, informed me some time ago of a like instance occurring in his practice, and in which the patient had a tin case so constructed as to fit the perinæum and close the vulva, and which she fastened with lock and key whenever she went to bed.

There is a species of intellectual monomania with depression in which, while the delusions are of a sad character, there is little or no melancholy. This was, so far as I am aware, first described by Billod[1] under the name of "lypemania with predominance of depressing ideas, but without reaction of sadness." It is, in fact, the purest of all the varieties of the form under notice, for it consists mainly of intellectual aberration with the minimum of emotional disturbance.

As Billod[1] says, the patient is neither sad nor gay. He seems indifferent to the ideas which have their seat in his mind, and he speaks of them without the least disturbance of his emotions.

He gives the case of a lady who was not in the least melancholic, although she was constantly giving utterance to the most disquieting ideas. Sometimes she imagined that her nose was growing, or wås about to become detached from her face ; sometimes that her countenance was otherwise deformed, and sometimes believing that she was possessed of the elasticity of caoutchouc, she was afraid to take a step lest she should be bounced off into space. Then she imagined that she was affected with the most mortal and incurable of diseases. When expressing these ideas there was not the least emotion, and her countenance did not exhibit the slightest trace of sadness. Her indifference, in fact, was such that no one would have thought that she was speaking of herself.

In another case the patient, a man, believed himself the victim of a society of demoniacs, and yet his equanimity of manner was not in the least disturbed. And another was constantly on the defensive against an imaginary enemy, whom he accused of inflicting a thousand tortures upon him —for example, abstracting from his body millions of kilogrammes of blood, but who spoke of his misfortunes without exhibiting the slightest emotion.

[1] " Des diverses formes de lypemanie," " Annales médico-psychologiques," juillet, 1856 ; also, " Des maladies mentales," etc., Paris, 1882, t. i, p. 350.

I have had occasion to observe many such cases. In one very interesting instance the patient, a lady, who had some hereditary tendency to insanity, her grandmother on her mother's side having died in an asylum, had the delusion that her husband was continually endeavoring to poison her. She watched everything on the table, and would eat or drink nothing till he had first partaken of it, and yet, while living in this constant apprehension of losing her life, she spoke of the matter with the most perfect unconcern. In all other respects she was, so far as I could ascertain, entirely free from mental aberration. She was fond of music, and went regularly to the opera; she was a leader in several charitable and literary societies, and always conducted herself in public with the utmost decorum. Indeed, even at home there was neither disorderly conduct nor violent language, and no one but her husband was aware of the false belief which she entertained. "H——," she would say to him, while her face expressed no more interest than if she was talking of the most indifferent subject, "you will never succeed in your horrible attempts so long as I possess my reason. I may lose my mind and be unable to watch you, and that is my greatest fear, but, so long as I preserve that, I will circumvent all your nefarious schemes. I saw you drop that powder into the soup-tureen before dinner, but I took it out as soon as you had sneaked out of the room. I heard you creep down stairs this morning to put your vile doses in the coffee-urn; but if you are able to afford two or three makings of coffee every morning, I have no objection. Perhaps you will wear me out at last, and then you will put me in an asylum; any keeper would poison me for five dollars." Finally she became convinced that her husband thought her insane, and that he was making arrangements to place her in an asylum; so one day she quietly secured passage, under an assumed name, in a steamer for Europe, and on the appointed day left her house as though she were going out for a morning's shopping, and, going aboard the vessel, took her departure for Liverpool. It was not known where she had gone till a letter was received from her, in which she stated her intention of returning as soon as she had paid a visit to Trouville and taken twenty-one sea baths. It was thought best by her friends not to interfere with her; she took her twenty-one baths, and came back entirely cured. This was five or six years ago, and she is still in good mental health. The absence from all causes of excitement, especially from her husband, the change of air and scene, and the hygienic influence of the sea bathing, had effected a cure. In such cases it is difficult to say whether the delusion or the incongruity between the false belief and the emotions constitutes the chief feature. It would almost seem as if there was, so to speak, a paralysis of the emotions, but examination shows that, as regards other ideas outside of the delusion which the patient may entertain, there is a normal degree of emotional activity.

It is not at all uncommon for the subjects of intellectual monomania with depression to refuse all nourishment. This is generally the logical consequence of the delusions they entertain. For, believing as they often do that the food offered them is poisoned or is otherwise unfit for use, it is, of course, from their stand-point, a legitimate action for them to refuse to eat. Occasionally, however, they persist in not eating from a desire to die of starvation ; again, simply because they have no appetite, and, therefore, do not care to eat, and at times from a whim or a pure spirit of obstinacy. Again, the patient persists in remaining mute. A man who came to my clinique at the University several years ago refused to speak, but would write what he wanted to say. His reason was that he was surrounded by invisible enemies who could not see, but who were gifted with very acute powers of hearing, and that if he spoke, even in a whisper, they would know where he was and inflict bodily injury upon him. Sometimes it was said he would not even write, being convinced that several of his enemies, who were endowed with very acute powers of hearing, were listening with their ears on the paper so as to detect by the sound of the pen the thoughts he was expressing.

Again, the delusion which actuates the patient may be of such a character as to urge him to refrain from doing other acts, the regular performance of which is essential to the well-being of the organism. Thus, a professor in a college, after passing through a period of great excitement, began to exhibit symptoms of insanity, and these soon took the form of intellectual monomania with depression. Among other delusions which he entertained was one that the kidneys were acting altogether too freely, and that the phosphorus of his brain was being removed so rapidly as to bring him to the verge of idiocy. He talked of the matter with entire calmness, but nevertheless took such measures as he thought would be effectual to arrest the elimination of the urine. He drank scarcely any fluid, and deferred the act of urination as long as was possible. Finally, nature, as he said, being too strong for him, he fastened a leather strap around the penis in such a way as to effectually prevent a drop of urine passing. For a whole day he endured, without complaint, the agony induced by this procedure. At last he began to groan, and to show other signs of extreme suffering, but, as none of those about him were aware of his act, and as he still refused to explain the cause, no intelligent efforts were made for his relief. The time came, however, when he could hold out no longer. He went into the closet for the purpose of removing the strap, and, being followed and watched, the nature of his torment was at once discovered. The penis had, however, become so swollen that the strap could scarcely be seen, and it was found to be impossible to unbuckle it. I saw him a few minutes afterward, and with great difficulty succeeded in cutting the ligature. The urine dribbled out drop by drop, owing to the paralysis of the bladder from over-distention, but a catheter brought it away to the extent of nearly two quarts. He made a good recovery, but suffered for several months from paresis of the bladder.

An interesting case is that of Jean Matthias Klug,[1] who had been Governor of the Department of Truchssée, and then secretary of a commission of the ministry of war in Prussia, and who was well skilled in the sciences of medicine, law, divinity, and physics. He was also acquainted with several ancient and modern languages, but, having written a book which contained religious sentiments contrary to those held by the King, or which he thought were of this character, lost his reason. He imagined that he had irritated his sovereign, and that orders had been given for his arrest and trial. He therefore shut himself up with his nephew in an isolated house, strongly barricaded it, and never left it. His nephew dying, Klug put the corpse outside the door, with an inscription on it asking that it might be buried. He received his food through a grating. He wrote out his dreams, believing them to be inspirations. He died of apoplexy, at the age of sixty.

[1] " La folie considerée sur tout dans ses rapports avec la psychologie normale," etc., par J. Tissot, Paris, 1877, p. 268.

Marcé[1] states that in *monomanie triste*—which, so far as I can determine from his not very full description of the condition, does not differ essentially from that under consideration—the patients are prone to exhibit suicidal or homicidal tendencies. I do not think this view is correct, so far as suicide is concerned, though occasionally a proclivity to this act is shown. But, as regards other acts of violence, I think there can be no difference of opinion among alienists. Within a recent period several such cases have occurred in this city, one of which I had the opportunity of investigating. It was that of a Frenchman, named Dubourque, who, having for several years been affected with delusions of wrongs and injuries being done to him, and having made several assaults on persons whom he imagined had conspired against him, finally rushed through a crowded street, striking right and left with a pair of carpenter's compasses at every woman he met. Some seven persons were stabbed by him, one of whom died. The only reason he could give me for his conduct was that "the women were talking about him."[2] As Marcé further states, the affection is often transformed into melancholia, and it is then, doubtless, that the tendency to suicide is exhibited.

The most common termination of both the forms of intellectual monomania which have been considered in the foregoing pages is chronic intellectual mania, and to that affection the attention of the reader is now invited.

c—CHRONIC INTELLECTUAL MANIA.

By chronic intellectual mania is to be understood a condition in which there is a general disturbance of the intellect characterized by the existence of varying or non-systematized delusions, and accompanied by periods of either mental excitement or depression, with more or less incoherence and mental weakness. It may arise protopathically, or may be the sequence of either of the affections just described, of an attack of acute mania, or of some other form of insanity.

Under the head of chronic mania, asylum medical officers usually include every form of mental derangement the course of which is slow, or which they regard as permanent. The

---

[1] "Traité pratique des maladies mentales," Paris, 1862, p. 369.
[2] "A Case of Intellectual Monomania with Mental Depression," *Illustrated Journal of Medicine and Surgery*, April, 1883.

present section is, however, to be regarded as restricted to the consideration of a mental disorder, the chief features of which are the presence of delusions, a defective power in the association of ideas, incoherence, and mental weakness.

Chronic intellectual mania, as I have said, may show itself as a primary disorder. In such a case there is often a prodromatic series of symptoms not essentially different from those met with in intellectual monomania. Thus, there are wakefulness, morbid dreams, illusions and hallucinations, and an unnatural state of mental and physical excitement, which, perhaps, of all the phenomena, most attracts the attention of the observer, and which may be present several weeks before the development of any marked degree of mental derangement.

Thus, a young man, a salesman in a large mercantile house in this city, from having been rather slow in his movements both of mind and of body, and late in arriving at his office, suddenly exhibited a complete change in all these respects. He became remarkably assiduous in the performance of his duties, was the first to arrive in the morning, and seemed not only anxious to do his own work, but that of almost every other person in the establishment. During the day he was bustling about the rooms, packing and unpacking cases, apparently aimlessly running down into the cellar to see that the steam was all right, and giving orders to one and another as if the whole establishment belonged to him. For a while it was thought that all this activity proceeded from the fact that he had at last become aware of his deficiencies, and was striving, by an excess of zeal, to make amends for previous shortcomings; but it was soon perceived that his show of work really amounted to nothing, and that his meddlesomeness caused only confusion and delay. At the same time it was noticed that his appearance was wild and haggard, and, upon inquiry, it was ascertained that he was irregular in his hours for coming home, that frequently he was out all night, and could give no clear or satisfactory account of his whereabouts. Before there were any other manifestations, his brother brought him to me and gave me the foregoing particulars. I also ascertained that he had suffered for several months with wakefulness, and that hallucinations of sight and hearing had existed for a like period. These, however, he had kept to himself, and it was only with considerable difficulty that I succeeded in establishing the fact of their presence; of their unreality he was at this time fully aware, and he attributed them to the circumstance of his not sleeping well. I could detect no evidence of the existence of delusions strictly so called, though there was certainly an idea in his mind that he was of great use to his employers, and that he did more work in the establishment than all the other salesmen combined. But on my asking him what he did that rendered him of so much importance he laughed, and replied that there was scarcely a thing about the house that he did not attend to. In reality this was not very far from the truth, so far as his intentions and efforts went. If he had been allowed to do as he pleased, nothing would have escaped him. I advised a residence for a month or two at some quiet place in the country under the immediate care of a physician, the use of the bromide of sodium, and, as his bowels were obstinately constipated and the liver inactive—as they usually are in those cases—a course of Carlsbad water. He promised to follow my instructions; he did not, however, and, as was to have been expected, his symptoms grew rapidly worse. He sold the goods under his charge for less than they had cost, made presents of whole cases to the wives of purchasers, reported sales which had never been made, and behaved otherwise in such an unbusiness-like way that his employers were obliged to dispense with his services. I then saw him for the second time. He was then agitated in manner, incoherent in his speech and in his ideas, talked ramblingly about his business, and seemed to feel keenly the fact of his dismissal. At the same time, if his attention was engaged, he was able to converse with clearness and precision, and to assume a degree of physical and mental composure which left nothing to be desired. In a few minutes, however, he was off again with his long and pointedless discourses about his business, the state of the markets, etc. His brother informed me that he had many delusions, no one of which was held for more than a day or two, and often only for a few minutes. Thus he told me in one breath, that he had been summoned to Zurich to take charge of a large silk factory in that city, and that he had taken passage in a steamer to sail the following day, and in the next that he had been requested by the government of Japan to start a cotton mill at Yokohama, and that he was going to leave that very afternoon for that country *via* San Francisco. Then he informed me that he was going to open a store in New York which was to be different from any other in the whole world. Every customer was to receive a present of a book by some distinguished author. In this way, he said, trade and literature would be encouraged, and the purchaser would not only be benefited materially, but would at the same time have his mind improved. And so he went on, forgetting one delusion almost as soon as it was formed, and concocting others, to be in their turn forgotten in a few moments.

But with all this there was a sense of the proprieties of life, and a general condition of good behavior altogether different from what we meet with in cases of acute mania. There was no such excitement of mind and body, no tendency to violence, no tearing of the hair or stripping off of the clothing, no shouting or leaping, or indulgence in obscenity or profanity, so characteristic of that type of insanity. On the contrary, many persons would have failed to see anything in his conduct indicative of mental derangement; and one physician whom he consulted told him he was as sane a man as there was in the city of New York, and that all he wanted was Turkish baths and salt-water injections. I could not persuade his brother that it was necessary to place him in such a place as that of Dr. Parsons, at Sing Sing. He proposed to keep him in the city, but finally he decided to take him home to England. He was in an asylum there for a couple of years, and then, as he was much improved, he was brought back to this country. On his return, I found that, though mentally and physically better, there was still a tendency to wildness in conversation, an inaptitude for intellectual exertion, and an inability to sleep. By my advice he crossed the plains to California, stopping at various places on the way, and on his return, several months afterward, he was in almost a normal condition. To a skilful observer, however, it is quite evident that there is still a proclivity to the formation of delusions, though he is able to correct the tendency. As he says, it would not take much to throw him on the other side of the line.

L. B., a woman, aged forty-three, entered the Blackwell's Island Lunatic Asylum with the diagnosis of chronic mania. On her admission she talked a great deal, but connectedly, and had no very evident delusions, but a good many erroneous beliefs scarcely distinguishable from them. Thus, she thought her landlord had had her committed to the asylum because she could not pay her rent. In her manner she was excited, but not violent, and gave no trouble. For several days she continued in a pleasant frame of mind, talking almost continuously but coherently, and behaving herself well; but about ten days subsequently she became depressed in spirits, and wanted a priest sent for. Then she became noisy and abusive, talked in a loud voice, and had various delusions, among them one that the attendants had stolen her children. A year subsequently she was still in the asylum, at times having well-marked delusions, and at others apparently free from them. During the subsequent four years she had alternations of excitement and depression, without there being any marked change in her condition. The last entry in the case-book is dated February 13, 1875: " Fell on the ice yesterday and bruised her hand and knee ; mental condition unimproved, physical health good." [1]

J. M., a woman, thirty-five years old, was brought to me by her husband, December 18, 1882, to be treated for insanity. She had first become affected three years previously, and had passed two years in a lunatic asylum without any improvement having been effected. Her husband, a remarkably intelligent man, had, from the very beginning, kept full notes of her case, and, as he put them at my disposal, I have used them in the preparation of this synopsis :

During the autumn of 1879 a series of excitements and misfortunes of a family nature occurred, which resulted in disturbing her mind to such an extent that a physician was consulted. It should be stated that her mother and a maternal aunt were insane, the latter dying in an asylum. The physician did not recognize any form of mental aberration as being present, although she had for some time suffered from hallucinations and illusions, and delusions that her family did not treat her with sufficient kindness and consideration. Things went on without much change, though she was gradually getting worse, till in March, 1880, it became necessary to send her to an asylum. At this time she had well-marked delusions of persecution, and even conceived that her little daughter, a child scarcely six years old, had tried to poison her. While in the asylum she had two ribs broken, as she

[1] From Dr. Parsons's MS. " Reports of Cases in the New York City Lunatic Asylum, Blackwell's Island."

declared, by one of the physicians striking her, but, as investigation showed, by her falling over a chair while walking about the ward in the night. During her entire stay in the asylum she continued to hold the delusion that her daughter had tried to poison her. Then her husband concluded to remove her, and, as she was quiet and able to conduct herself outside of her delusion with reasonable decorum, he was hopeful that at home she would be more favorably situated than in the asylum for receiving the care which her condition still required. In a few days after her return, amendment began, and in a week or two she was, so far as her husband could determine, free from any evidence of mental aberration. There were no delusions of any kind, and the fixed one in regard to her daughter was only remembered as a subject for astonishment that she could ever seriously have entertained such an idea.

But in a very short time, her husband states in less than a week, she began to be wakeful at night, and to be tormented by horrible dreams. Twice he found her walking about the house with a lighted candle after everybody else was in bed, and she stated, on the first occasion, that she was looking for John the Baptist, and on the second that a celebrated preacher, whom she named, had got into the dining-room and was hid under the table.

Then she imagined that she was pregnant, and that another preacher, whose name she refused to give, but whom she designated as her "spiritual essence," had seduced her. This was followed the next day by another to the effect that during the night she had been delivered of a child, which had been murdered by her husband. All these things she spoke of with the utmost *sang froid*, and conversed with her husband about them without evincing any of the emotional disturbances which would doubtless have been exhibited if her erroneous beliefs had become firmly and indubitably established in her mind. It was quite evident that, though she accepted her delusions to such an extent as to express her belief in them, she yet did not absolutely credit them as facts admitting of no doubt. Indeed, she spoke of them with the manner of a person relating unpleasant dreams, which, though they had made an impression on the mind, were nevertheless known to be mere figments of the imagination. The subject of intellectual monomania, of either the exalted or depressant type, does not question the truth of his delusions. Arguments are of no avail with him, and he acts exactly as he would act were his false beliefs real convictions.

Every day, sometimes every hour, there was a new delusion, and each was almost invariably of such a character as to be entirely beyond the limit of possibility. Thus, at one time she thought she had been adopted by the Shah of Persia as his daughter, because, as she said, she was begotten by the sun, and the Shah worshipped the sun as his god. At another she imagined that her husband had become Pope, and that, in order to assume the duties of the papacy, it was necessary for him to be divorced from her. She therefore went about the house with a letter to the Governor, in which she asked that a divorce might be granted, and which she requested every one to sign. At times she was much depressed in spirits, and wished that she might die, but she never even hinted at suicide, and it was quite evident that her wish had no very great sincerity in it. Again she was all smiles and good nature ; no one was ever so happy as she, and she would not change places with the richest or most powerful person who ever lived. Even in her moments of deepest mental depression, as well as in those of greatest exaltation, she talked incessantly. But with all this she was entirely capable of accurate reasoning upon common every-day topics. She went to church, listened attentively to the services and sermons, and talked rationally upon the discourses she had heard. She attended to all her household duties as well as she ever had, going to market every day and purchasing with discrimination what was needed. On one occasion, however, she went shopping, and came home with forty yards of red and white ribbon, which she said she had bought to use for a flag she was going to make as a present to an eminent statesman she named. When I saw her for the first time she said that she had only come to please her husband, and that there was nothing the matter with her. She admitted, however, that she did not sleep well, and that she suffered from occasional pains in the head, and from almost constant dyspepsia. As to her mind, she expressed the conviction that it was as good as it had ever been, in fact, better, for that it had undergone great development in the direction of causality. She was engaged now, she said, in endeavoring to ascertain the causes of all the events that had ever taken place in the world. On my asking her if she really believed this, she said she did, that she was sure of it, for that several phrenologists had told her so, and that, moreover, she had read allusions which she was convinced were to her in Dr. Combes's *Phrenological Magazine*. But, a half hour afterward, on my repeating the question, she admitted that she did not believe it, that she had been mistaken, and that she was a poor ignorant woman who ought to be sent to school in order that she might be taught the rudiments of the English language. During her visit, which lasted about an hour, she enunciated six distinct delusions, not one of which she believed when she took her departure. If left to herself, she went on talking, her conversation consisting entirely of revelations of the various delusions which passed through her mind. At times she was incoherent both in words and ideas. It was always possible, however, by asking her questions, to get her away from her erroneous beliefs, and then she spoke coherently and rationally. Unless her mind was thus engaged, she immediately reverted to her own reflections, and became as loquacious as before. While talking about her delusions there was a good deal of muscular action; she gesticulated with animation, and alternately laughed and shed tears, in accordance with the character of the ideas evolved. But, in the very midst of her discourse, a question relating to any very different topic which might be addressed to her was sufficient to stop her volubility, to sober her, as it were, and to obtain a coherent and rational answer.

I regarded the case as one of chronic intellectual mania, secondary to the intellectual monomania with depression with which she had previously been affected, and different from the latter in its manifestations except in so far as both were mainly concerned with the intellect.

I saw her once subsequently, but her condition was essentially unchanged.

Chronic intellectual mania, whether a primary or secondary disorder, is of long duration. There is always a tendency to the passage into a still lower form of mental derangement—dementia—and this is, after two or three years, the usual termination.

d—REASONING MANIA.

Although it is scarcely possible that so well marked a mental disorder as that which forms the subject of the present consideration could have escaped the notice of the earlier observers, no distinct account of it appeared till Pinel,[1] in 1801, published the first edition of his remarkable work. Under the head of "Mania without Delirium," he gave excellent accounts of several cases, and then in a few words summed up his description of the affection:

"It may," he says, "be continuous, or characterized by the occurrence of periodical accessions. There is no marked change in the functions of the understanding, the judgment, the imagination, the memory, etc., but perversion of the emotional faculties, and blind impulsions to the perpetration of acts of violence, or even of sanguinary fury, without its being possible to recognize the existence of any dominant idea, or any illusion of the imagination, to which the acts in question can be ascribed."

In the second edition, published in 1809, he treats more fully of the subject:

"We know that one of the varieties of insanity, called in the asylums reasoning mania, is especially characterized by the most marked coherence of ideas and correctness of judgment. The lunatic reads, writes, and reflects as though he enjoyed his normal reason, and yet he is liable at any time to perpetrate some act of violence."

Farther on, he says, speaking of these cases:

"The lunatic makes the most correct answers to the questions addressed to him, without the least incoherence of ideas being noticed." He gives the following instance:

"A badly directed or neglected education, or rather a perverse and undisciplined nature, produces the first symptoms of this species of mental alienation. An only son of a weak and yielding mother was indulged in every whim and caprice which an irritable and ungovernable temper could suggest. The violence of his disposition increased with his years, and the unlimited amount of money with which he was supplied removed all obstacles to the gratification of his desires. If resisted, he became furiously angry, and attacked his adversary with ferocity. He was, therefore, continually

[1] "Traité médico philosophique sur l'aliénation mentales," Paris, t. ix, p. 155.

embroiled in disputes and quarrels. If a sheep, a dog, a
horse, or any other animal offended him, he immediately
killed it. If he went to any public meeting, he was certain
to come away bruised and bleeding from the blows he had
received in the brawls he had excited. On the other hand,
when he arrived at manhood he came into the possession of a
large property, which he managed with discretion, performing all his duties to society, and even indulging in some acts
of benevolence. Wounds, lawsuits, and heavy fines were generally the consequence of his numerous disputes. Finally
an act of especial violence put an end to his career. Enraged
at a woman who had used abusive language to him, he seized
her and threw her into a well. He was arrested and tried,
and, on the testimony of many persons acquainted with his
character and furious deportment, he was adjudged insane,
and was committed to the Bicêtre for life."

Yet, although Pinel had some idea of the affection under
notice, he did not have a very exact conception of it. He
seemed to be under the impression that a blind tendency to
the perpetration of unwarrantable acts of violence is its most
marked feature, whereas we know very well that such are
often done by its subjects after very thorough deliberation,
and from what are deemed ample motives. He certainly had
in his mind cases in which reasoning mania was combined
with some form of instinctive or emotional insanity, as the
instance just cited plainly shows.

Esquirol,[1] under the designation of ".Reasoning Monomania," describes the disorder more accurately. He says:

"In reasoning monomania the patients are active, continually in motion, speaking a good deal, and with vivacity.
They were good-tempered, frank, and generous, they have
become peevish, deceitful, and wicked; they were affectionate and kind to their relations and friends, they have become
discontented and abusive to those they once loved; from
having been economical they are changed to spendthrifts;
their actions were reasonable and right, they are now incon-
siderate, venturesome, and even reprehensible; their conduct, which once was in accordance with their social position,
has become incongruous, and at variance with their position
and their means. They are guided entirely by their own
wishes; but, by their bearing and their conversation, these

[1] "Des maladies mentales," etc., Paris, 1838, t. i, p. 355.

people impose upon those who have had no previous acquaintance with them, or who only see them occasionally, so well do they know how to restrain themselves, and to dissimulate their real feelings."

The younger Pinel [1] had a still clearer, though yet not an exact, idea of reasoning mania. "The subjects of it," he says, "are turbulent, indocile, quick to anger, committing outrageous acts, which they are always ready to justify by plausible reasons, and who are to their families, their kindred, and their friends, constant subjects of anxiety and grief. They are continually doing wrong, either by neglect, by malice, or by wickedness. Incapable of mental or physical application, they destroy and subvert, and unsettle everything with which they are brought into contact, and which they can injure."

Pinel calls the affection "Mania of Character," although he appears not to regard it as insanity properly so called. In this opinion he is very evidently inconsistent with himself.

Speaking of the subjects of the disorder in question, Morel [2] says :

"Some have great ambition and pride, and consider themselves as being destined to the performance of acts of momentous importance. No consequence, however absurd, to which their insanity leads them, shakes their confidence in themselves. Others are impelled by bad tendencies to the perpetration of the most extravagant or monstrous acts. They rebel against all family and social obligations and duties, and are constantly considering themselves the victims of misunderstanding or injustice. For the persecution of which they imagine themselves the subjects they seek to avenge themselves on their relations, their friends, and the world at large, by making a parade of their immoral conduct, thinking to compromise the interests of those who ought to be dear to them by the shameful exhibition of their depravity. They go into the streets and other public places in a filthy and ragged condition. They let their hair grow, and endeavor to attract attention by all kinds of ridiculous and improper acts. Others apply their brilliant intellectual faculties, notwithstanding they are marked by an irregularity and incoherence of action, to the production of literary works of which the ex-

---

[1] "Traité de pathologie cérébrale," Paris, 1844, p. 330.
[2] "Traité des maladies mentales," Paris, 1860, p. 546.

tent and the plan exceed the limit that it is possible for human power to reach. These works are often in their teachings contrary to public morality and feeling. They are dreamers, utopians, false guides, who, in their mental conceptions and in the results of their intelligence and imagination, exhibit the same eccentricity, the same shamelessness, as in their acts."

This, it appears to me, is a very exact description of the subjects of reasoning mania so far as it goes. There are several phases of the affection, however, upon which Morel has not touched.

Dagonet [1] less accurately says of them, under the head of "Reasoning Mania":

"Left to themselves, they are led by the most contradictory considerations. The first sudden impression, an idea occurring by chance, an accidental circumstance, influences them, and becomes the point of departure for their conduct. There is with them not only a considerable amount of irritability, and, thus to say, a furnace ready to be kindled, but, in addition, they are habitually dominated by impulses of various kinds. They follow blindly the passionate instincts which trivial circumstances are constantly provoking. Sexual desires, jealousy, ambition, vengeance, influence them at every moment of their lives, and, notwithstanding their wishes, prompt them to the commission of acts to be subsequently regretted. With the best intentions, the individual cannot subdue himself, or stop his headlong descent along the fatal declivity which leads to disorder.

"In the institutions to which they may be committed, they incite the patients against each other, and urge them to acts of insubordination. They take pleasure in worrying the attendants with their complaints, and never cease their animadversions on the directions or advice given them. The most various sentiments—suspicion, malevolence, and calumny— are the elements in which they live, and without which they could not exist."

I have quoted thus extensively from other authorities in order to present at the beginning some idea of the characteristics of reasoning mania, as well as to show that such a mental disorder is well recognized by medico-psychological

[1] "Nouveau traité élémentaire et pratique des maladies mentales," Paris, 1876, p. 202.

writers. I have confined my citations to French authors, for the reason that the affection was first differentiated by alienists of that country, and has been more thoroughly studied there than elsewhere, but I might have drawn fully as largely from English and German writers. Indeed, Prichard, Connolly, Bucknill, and Maudsley among the former, and Hoffbauer, Caspar, Griesinger, Liman, Kraft-Ebing, and others of the latter, have written quite as strongly in support of the actuality of the affection as those I have cited. In this country the most distinguished authority in the affirmative is Dr. Isaac Ray.

The most prominent characteristic of reasoning mania as it has come under my notice is an overbearing egotism, which shows itself on all, even the most unimportant, occasions. The individual is vain of his personal appearance ; he imagines that he is the subject of conversation of all whom he sees talking together, and that every one who glances toward him carries admiration on his countenance. Without social position, without wealth, without education, and without political influence, he conceives that he has only to make his wishes known to those in authority to have them granted. He hence does not hesitate to push himself forward as an applicant for a high office, and this when he has not a single qualification fitting him for the position he seeks ; refusals do not dismay him, the most pointed rebuffs do not abash him. He is sure that his application will be favorably considered, and any little act of common politeness that may be shown him is at once construed into a promise of assistance. He is invariably sure his appointment is about to be made, and when, as always happens, some other person is selected, his chagrin is of short duration. He has some plausible excuse for his failure, and at once proceeds to direct his energies toward obtaining another and perhaps still higher position.

It may be said that these are the characteristics of all office-seekers, who are generally gifted with vanity in excess of all other qualities, but this I emphatically deny. We have in this country ample opportunity to study the natural history of the class in question, constituting, as they do, a large proportion of the inhabitants of the land, and I think most observers will bear me out in the assertion that it is exceedingly rare to find a person applying for an office for which he is totally unfit, and for which he could not obtain the endorsement of any intelligent person.

Not long since, a young man was under my professional charge, who for several years had been the cause of great anxiety to his friends on account of his vagaries and general impracticability. His father had a large shoe factory, and the attempt was made to instruct him in the details of the business. It was found, however, impossible to make him give his attention to the subject. He was firmly convinced that nature intended him for something a great deal better than a shoemaker, and he destroyed a good deal of valuable property—leather, tools, etc.—in order to disgust his father, and induce him to abandon the project. Finally he succeeded.

He had received a tolerably good education in the branches usually taught in the public schools, and was, moreover, exceedingly quick in his perceptions of things which he desired to understand. As he told me the story of what he considered to be the wrong done him by his father in trying to make a shoemaker of him, he reasoned with great plausibility, and tears came into his eyes as he detailed the story of the indignity which had been attempted to be put upon him. "The fact is," said he, "that when I went to school I paid great attention to the study of languages. Now, if I had known I was going to be a shoemaker, I would have turned my attention to the human foot, and then I should have been qualified to make the best shoes this country has ever seen. I have thought over the matter, and to-morrow I am going to Washington to ask the President to appoint me a Commissioner of Emigration, and send me to all the nations of Europe to see after the emigrants and instruct them in their duties as American citizens. I shall give lectures on the subject in all the principal cities of Great Britain, France, and Germany."

"But," said I, "do you speak French?"

"Well, I studied French. I can't say I speak it, but I can learn it on the way over."

"You understand German?"

"No, but as soon as I am in Germany I shall go to a private family to board, and I will soon pick up that language."

"Do you know anything of political economy?"

"That is not essential; emigrants do not require a knowledge of that science."

"Now, won't you tell me your idea of the duties of an

American citizen, in which you are going to instruct these people?"

"I shall simply read to them the Constitution of the United States in their own language, and then distribute copies of it among them. That paper," he continued, "contains the germs of all that a citizen requires to know."

"But," I remarked, "there is not a word in the Constitution about the duties of citizens. It relates to quite different matters."

"Nothing about the duties of citizens in the Constitution! Well, then, I'll supply the omission; I'll make it all right; I know just what I'm about, and I'm just the man for the place."

He drew up his application, went around among prominent persons asking for letters of recommendation, and, though he did not get a single one, he proceeded to Washington and sought an interview with the President. His father, however, followed him, but could not bring him home without the assistance of the police. He was soon afterward an applicant for the command of an ocean steamship, but, meeting with no success in this direction, turned his attention to hunting up claims against the United States, out of which he expects to make a great fortune. He asserts that he has ascertained that, during the late war with Great Britain, a vast amount of property was taken for public use for which no compensation has ever been made. He declares that he has found one heir to whom the Government owes over two millions of dollars, and that he is to have half for getting it. He actually has such a person under his control—one whom he has doubtless impressed with his own ideas to such an extent as to make him believe himself to be justly entitled to the sum mentioned. For he is crafty, specious, and insinuating, and could readily make a weak-minded person his dupe.

The intense egotism of these people makes them utterly regardless of the feelings and rights of others. Everybody and everything must give way to them. Their comfort and convenience are to be secured though every one else is made unhappy, and sometimes they display positive cruelty in their treatment of persons who come in contact with them. This tendency is especially seen in their relations with the lower animals and with children.

Another manifestation of their intense personality is their

entire lack of appreciation of kindness done them, or benefits of which they have been the recipients. They look upon these as so many rights to which they are justly entitled, and which in the bestowal are more serviceable to the giver than to the receiver. They are hence ungrateful and abusive to those who have served them, and insolent, arrogant, and shamelessly hardened in their conduct toward them.

At the same time, if advantages are yet to be gained, they are sycophantic to nauseousness in their deportment toward those from whom the favors are to come.

They never evince the least trace of modesty in obtruding themselves and their assumed good qualities upon the public at every opportunity. They boast of their genius, their right-eousness, their goodness of heart, their high sense of honor, their learning, and other qualities and acquirements, and this when they are perfectly aware that they are commonplace, irreligious, cruel, and vindictive, utterly devoid of every chivalrous feeling, and saturated with ignorance. They know that in their rantings they are attempting to impose upon those whom they address, and will often, as I have personally experienced, brag of their success in deception.

It is no uncommon thing for the reasoning maniac, still influenced by his supreme egotism and desire for notoriety, to attempt the part of the reformer. Generally he selects a practice or custom in which there is really no abuse. His energy and the logical manner in which he presents his views, based, as they often are, on cases and statistics, impose on many worthy people, who eagerly adopt him as a genuine over-thrower of a vicious or degrading measure. But sensible persons soon perceive that there is no sincerity in his conduct, that he cares nothing whatever for the cause he is advocating, that his cases or statistics are forged or intentionally misconstrued for the distinct purpose of deceiving; in short, that his philanthropy or morality which he affects is assumed for the occasion. Even when his hypocrisy and falsehood are exposed, he continues his attempts at imposition, and even, when the strong arm of the law is laid upon him, prates of the ingratitude of those he has been endeavoring to assist, and of the disinterestedness and purity of his own motives.

Again, the reasoning maniac, as Campagne [1] remarks, may go still further in his career as a redresser of all kinds of pos-

---

[1] " Traité de la manie raisonnante," Paris, 1869, p. 98.

24

sible and impossible wrongs—past, present, and future. "He displays in the performance of his part a degree of energy, activity, and caution which would be really admirable if his mission had any foundation whatever. Unfortunately, his warfare is waged against windmills, and he takes for incontestable truth that which is only a figment of his imagination. Truth with him becomes error, from the exaggeration, the depreciation, or the distortion to which it is submitted. He regards virtue through the medium of his own degraded passions, and never as it ought to be seen. Thus estimated, it cannot direct him to any good purpose."

The subject of reasoning mania is always more influenced by the emotions than by the intellect; not, however, because these latter have become stronger or more active, but because, his intellect being deranged either qualitatively or quantitatively, he does not subject them to proper control. In fact, he rarely judges calmly or dispassionately on any matter brought before him. The slightest cause often produces in him an intense degree of excitement, and he manifests his emotional disturbance by loud exclamations, vehement gestures, and the most foul and abusive language against those who have incurred his resentment. But, even when apparently most inflamed, and in the very midst of his maledictions, he becomes, under the influence of some different circumstances, good-natured and smiling, and finishes his cursing with a joke or a hearty laugh. There is no depth or sincerity either in his imprecations or his blessings.

This facility for passing from one state of feeling to another, both of which may be manifested by all the characteristics of intense passionate perturbation, is a striking peculiarity of reasoning maniacs. Of all people in the world, they seem to be the most capable of "blowing hot and cold with the same breath." A patient of mine, a young man, would in my presence declaim in the most vehement manner against his father, accusing him of all the sins of the decalogue, and of many others not found in that code, and in the next instant would declare that he was only trying to test his father's patience and forbearance, and that in reality no one could be kinder or more virtuous than he. But, ere these latter opinions were fully expressed, I caught him making faces and shaking his fists at his father when his back was turned. It was impossible to get at his real feelings, not, however, because he wilfully concealed them, but because he expressed, with apparently equal sincerity, love and hatred in all their degrees.

All authors have observed this symptom. Campagne [1] says, of reasoning maniacs :

"Passing, without the slightest transition, from one extreme to the other, they felicitate themselves to-day of an event which they sneered at the night before. In the course of a single second they change their opinions of persons and things ; novelty captivates and wearies them almost at the same instant. They sell for insignificant sums things they have just bought, in order to buy others which in their turn will be subjected to like treatment ; and, strange to say, before possessing these objects, they covet them with a degree of ardor only equalled by the eagerness they exhibit to get rid of them as soon as they become their owners. To see, to desire, and to become indifferent, are the three stages which follow each other with astonishing rapidity."

Although reasoning maniacs are not subject to irresistible impulses to commit motiveless crimes, they are prone to acts of violence from slight exciting causes, and these may be perpetrated either in the heat of passion or after such deliberation as they are able to give to any subject. Generally they are directed against those whom they suppose have injured them, or against former friends with whom they have quarrelled. Again, they may be committed solely for the purpose of gratifying the morbid feelings of pleasure which they experience at the sufferings of others. In the first category are embraced the many cases of arson, maiming, homicide, and other crimes, in which the motive alleged has been so slight as to be ridiculous.

Thus, in the case of William Speirs,[2] who attempted to destroy by fire the State Lunatic Asylum at Utica, there was a motive, though a very insufficient one, for the act. On the 14th of July, 1857, the cupola of the institution was discovered to be on fire. The central building was almost entirely consumed before the flames were subdued. Four days afterward, in the afternoon, the store, barn, and stables were also seen in flames, and a man was noticed at the time going from them. This man was William Speirs, who had been a patient in the asylum from 1850 to 1856, and then, having been

[1] *Op. cit.*, p. 88.   [2] *American Journal of Insanity*, vol. xv, 1858-'59, p. 200.

discharged by an order of a Justice of the Supreme Court, had been employed up to the time of the fire as a messenger and otherwise. He had been committed to the asylum on the ground of insanity, after a trial for arson, so that he had perpetrated at least three separate acts of incendiarism. He confessed to both the attempts at Utica, and was committed for trial on the charge of arson.

At the trial it was shown by his own confession how and for what reason he had set fire to the asylum. His motives were the facts that one of the assistants, Dr. Chapin, had sent him away from where they were making balloons, and would not let him help, and that Dr. Gray, the superintendent, had taken away his keys. These acts made him angry.

It was also shown that Speirs had previously been a patient in the lunatic asylum on Blackwell's Island; that he had had a sunstroke; that after that he would go out and stay whole days and nights, on one occasion remaining absent from home eight days, sleeping in wagons. During this period he went into a house and got some things, and was going to set it on fire, when he was discovered. He was tried and sent to the Blackwell's Island Asylum. Then he came to the city and got some work in a saloon. "Did some depredations there," was tried, and sent to the asylum at Utica. A sister was also insane, and had been in an asylum. Drs. Day and Deming, of Utica, and Dr. H. M. Ranney, the superintendent of the Blackwell's Island Asylum, testified to the insanity of the prisoner. The latter, under whose care Speirs had been, was very positive as to his insanity.

"I discovered no delusion," he said; "think he has no uncontrollable impulse. I believe the act resulted from a perverted condition of the several moral faculties of the mind, with a propensity to burn buildings, and a feeble intellect. . . . Perhaps anything that would excite the prisoner would induce him to burn buildings, or even might stimulate him to commit an assault with intent to kill. I judge that he is a pyromaniac, because he has committed these acts and is insane."

Drs. Gray, Cook, and Bell, however, testified to the sanity of the prisoner. The former stated that he had never believed him to be insane. We have seen, however, that he was kept in the asylum, under the charge of lunacy, for six years. Speirs was convicted.

Joseph Brown, as stated by Dr. Harlow,[1] entered his own house on the morning of the 16th of April, 1856, shortly after breakfast, where his wife, Annie Brown, was engaged with her domestic duties. Their little daughter, aged twelve, was also present. Brown went to his daughter, and taking out his wallet containing twenty dollars, gave it to her. On turning toward his wife, she kindly said to him, " Joseph, I am afraid of you." On which he immediately seized a long sheath-knife with one hand, and with the other threw her upon the floor ; while in this position he cut her throat, severing the jugular vein, from which she died.

It is stated that Brown was at this time about forty years of age, a member of the church, taking a prominent part in the religious exercises, and speaking loudly and vehemently. It was noticed, however, that his outside conduct did not comport well with his teaching. He indulged more or less in the use of stimulants. He was irritable and quarrelsome. His bad temper was particularly exhibited toward his wife, who was a feeble woman. He had been known to strike her with his fist, and to kick her from a chair, and this though there had been no provocation. Subsequently, he again, without a cause, kicked her from the chair on which she was sitting, and struck her violently on the head with a pair of boots. On this occasion he left the house, but soon returned, and gave his little daughter a piece of money. He was not intoxicated, and there had been no exciting conversation. After this he frequently threatened his wife with assault, and she was obliged to flee from the house to escape him.

Immediately before the murder he had had a quarrel with his brother, and tried to choke him. On being prevented, he laughed heartily, and left the house. Shortly afterward he returned, and, breaking open the door, threatened the whole family with violence. After sufficiently alarming them, he ran away rapidly for several hundred feet.

He accused his wife of infidelity, but exhibited no indignation or excitement at the idea.

The day before the murder he went to Belfast, but before going placed the following inscription on paper upon the door of his house : "Farewell, house, wife, and blessed little children !" At Belfast he drank, as he said, a quart of gin. On Wednesday morning at two o'clock he left for home, and

[1] *American Journal of Insanity*, vol. xiii, 1856–'57, p. 249.

arrived there at about seven o'clock. Shortly afterward he committed the murder.

He then, after making two futile attempts to drown himself, was secured and lodged in prison.

Brown's grandfather was subject to fits of depression, and once nearly succeeded in cutting his throat. His grandmother lived to be over seventy, and during the latter period of her life was demented and under the care of legal guardians. His mother was passionate and excitable, and her peculiarities were the subject of remark by the neighbors. An uncle was found drowned, and was supposed to have committed suicide. A brother had an attack of fever which was followed by mental aberration.

At the trial, Dr. H. M. Harlow, superintendent of the insane asylum at Augusta, testified strongly in favor of the prisoner's insanity. He was, however, found guilty, and was sentenced to be hanged. Before the sentence could be executed he committed suicide by cutting his throat with a piece of glass, thus adding, as Dr. Harlow says, the capstone to the accumulated evidence of his insanity and irresponsibility.

Hélène Jégado, a Frenchwoman, between the years 1853 and 1857, killed twenty-eight persons by poison, besides making several unsuccessful attempts. In none of her murders was any cause alleged or discovered, though undoubtedly the pleasure derived from the perpetration of crime was the chief factor. Her victims were her masters and mistresses, her fellow-servants, her friends, and several nuns, for whom in their last moments she displayed the utmost tenderness and care. The plea of monomania was set up in her defence, but no evidence of insanity was brought forward by her counsel save the apparent want of motive for her crimes. It was shown, however, that she had begun her career, when only seventeen years old, by attempting to poison her confessor; that she had, while perpetrating her wholesale murders, affected the greatest piety, and was for a time an inmate of a convent ; that she had committed over thirty thefts ; that she had maliciously cut and burned various articles of clothing placed in her charge ; that, when asked why she had stolen things that were of no use to her, she had replied, "I always steal when I am angry" ; that she was subject to alternate periods of great mental depression and excessive and unreasonable gayety ; that she was affected with pains in the head and vertigo; that when she was angry she vomited blood; and that, while in prison awaiting trial, she was constantly laughing and joking about indifferent subjects. She was found guilty, and, on being asked if she had anything to say why sentence of death should not be pronounced, made answer, "No, your Honor, I am innocent. I am resigned to all that may happen. I would rather die innocent than live guilty. You have judged me, but God will judge you." Her last words on the scaffold were directed to accusing a woman as her instigator and accomplice, whose name was not even mentioned during the trial, and who, upon inquiry, was found to be an old paralytic, whose whole life had been of the most exemplary character.

The case of Dumollard is in some respects similar to that of Hélène Jégado. This man, a peasant, of a low order of intellect, but by no means an imbecile, was plunged in the lowest depths of ignorance and want. The moral sense appeared never to have been developed in him; he was a savage, pure and simple; he was out of place among civilized people. This monster had a *penchant* for murdering servant-girls whom he pretended to hire, and then, conducting them to unfrequented places, put them to death. Six thus disappeared, and nine others barely escaped. Indeed, it is probable that many more than these were murdered, for, on searching his premises, twelve hundred and fifty articles of women's apparel were found, of which only fifty were identified. Insanity was urged in his defence, but he was found guilty and executed. On the scaffold he behaved with the utmost insensibility. His last words were addressed to an officer, and were a request to tell his wife that a man, Berthet by name, owed him twenty-seven francs less a sou.

The most noted case of similar character occurring in this country is that of Jesse Pomeroy, the boy torturer and murderer of Massachusetts. In 1872 there was great excitement in Chelsea, near Boston, over a number of horrible instances of cruelty perpetrated on little children. The victims were tortured in various ways—sometimes by being cut with knives in various parts of their bodies, again by being tied to beams and beaten with ropes and sticks till their bones were broken or their teeth knocked out, and again by having pins and needles run into sensitive parts of their bodies, upon which salt water was afterward poured. Pomeroy, a boy fourteen years of age, and the son of a respectable widow, was ascertained to be the perpetrator after about a hundred other boys had been arrested on suspicion. When arraigned, he admitted his guilt, and could only plead in his defence that he "could not help it." He was convicted, and sent to the House of Refuge. After remaining there a year and five months, he was—at the earnest request of his mother, and, furthermore, in view of his good conduct while in confinement—pardoned, and on the 6th of February, 1874, he returned home. On the 22d of April, a little fellow named Horace Mullen, the son of a poor cabinet-maker, was found dead in the Dorchester marshes. The body was horribly mutilated, the head was nearly severed from the trunk, and about thirty stabs were found in different parts of the corpse. Jesse Pomeroy was at once suspected as the murderer. On examination, a knife spotted with blood was found on his person, another spot on the breast of his shirt, and his boots were covered with mud like that found in the marshes. Upon repairing to the place where the body had been found, the officers discovered footprints which corresponded with those made by Pomeroy's boots. When confronted with the body of the murdered child, Pomeroy trembled all over, and turned away his head.

"Did you know that little boy?" inquired the officer.

"Yes, sir, but I don't want to look at him any more."

"Did you kill him?"

"I suppose I did."

"How did you get the blood off the knife? Did you wash it?"

"No, sir, I stuck it in the mud."

He was found guilty, and sentenced to be hanged, but his punishment was commuted to imprisonment for life. He has made several ingenious but unsuccessful attempts to escape, and has proven to be altogether intractable.

These cases are sufficient to illustrate the relations of reasoning mania to crime. They show, also, how slight may be the extraneous motive which prompts to the perpetration of criminal acts, and how strong is the innate feeling of personal gratification, born as it is of intense selfishness, which leads in the same direction. Dr. Ray [1] has touched the exact point when he relates the following incident :

---

[1] "A Treatise on the Medical Jurisprudence of Insanity," fifth edition, Boston, 1871, p. 223.

"I once asked a patient, who was constantly saying or doing something to annoy or distress others, while his intellect was apparently as free from delusion or any other impairment as ever, whether, when committing his aggressive acts, he felt constrained by an irresistible impulse contrary to his convictions of right, or was not aware at the moment that he was doing wrong. His reply should sink deeply into the hearts of those who legislate for, or sit in judgment on, the insane. 'I never acted from an irresistible impulse nor upon the belief that I was doing right. I knew perfectly well I was doing wrong, and I might have refrained if I had pleased. I did thus and so because I loved to do it ; it gave me an indescribable pleasure to do wrong.'"

As Campagne says :

"The intellectual power of reasoning maniacs is not great. Loquacious or unusually taciturn, heedless or morbidly curious dreamers, wearisome to all brought in contact with them, capricious and unmitigated liars, their qualities are often, in a certain manner, brilliant, but are entirely without solidity or depth. Sharpness and cunning are not often wanting, especially for little things and insignificant intrigues ; ever armed with a lively imagination and quick comprehension, they readily appropriate the ideas of others, developing or transforming them, and giving them the stamp of their own individuality. But the creative force is not there, and they rarely possess enough mental vigor to get their own living."

As to derangement of the intellect, continual study of the subject and the careful examination of some recent striking cases convince me that, though the emotions and the will are involved, the intellectual faculties are those which chiefly suffer. In a superficial examination, the intellect may appear to be unaffected, as it very generally happens that there is an absence of marked delusion. But a morbid susceptibility to be impressed by slight exciting causes ; an unquestioning faith in their own powers when these are far below the average ; an entire disregard of their duties and obligations and of the ordinary proprieties of life ; an impossibility of mental application or concentration for any considerable period ; deficient powers of judgment in matters of the utmost simplicity ; a general wrong-headedness, which prevents them perceiving matters submitted to their understanding as the mass of mankind regard them—are certainly indications of intellectual derangement. Most authors who have described the affection appear to think that it invariably exists without the participation of the intellect, and I was myself at one time of the opinion that this part of the mind was not its chief seat. More complete investigation has, however, shown me that this view is wrong, and that it is as regards the intellect that the most striking manifestations of reasoning mania are exhibited. Again, others, perceiving that the intellect participates to some extent in all cases of mental derangement, refuse to admit the existence of reasoning mania as a distinct pathological entity.

Reasoning mania, or at least the proclivity to it, is usually a congenital affection, though there are cases in which it has been acquired either as the consequence of other diseases, or of injuries, or as the result of degenerating physical and mental factors. Occasionally it is only developed in either sex at the advent of puberty. Again, it is sometimes intermittent in its manifestations, being particularly liable to exhibit activity in times of great public excitement.

According to Campagne,[1] there is no tendency in reasoning mania to degenerate into dementia, but there is reason to believe that the peculiar mental and bodily conditions which exist in reasoning mania may develop into the characteristic of general paralysis of the insane. The one affection is, therefore, probably not infrequently the precursor of the other. Thus, Brierre de Boismont[2] has pointed out that in general paralysis of the insane there are sometimes perversions of the moral sense, great irritability, failure of memory, and defects of judgment, preceding by several years the development of the special symptoms of the disease. Guislain[3] also cites cases in which mental symptoms similar to those mentioned made their appearance several years before any derangement of motility was observed, and when there was reason to suspect that general paralysis of the insane was lurking in the background.

Relative to the bodily peculiarities of reasoning maniacs, Campagne[4] says:

1. That the head is smaller than that of persons of sound mind.

[1] *Op. cit.*, p. 200.   [2] *Annales médico psychologiques*, t. vii, 1861, p. 88.
[3] " Lecons orales sur les phrénopathies," Gund, Paris, 1880, t. i, p. 266, *et seq.*
[4] *Op. cit.*, p. 146.

2. That it is smaller than that of lunatics in general.

3. That, as regards size, it is almost equal to that of persons of weak minds.

4. That it is larger than that of idiots.

5. That the antero-posterior curve, and particularly the posterior curve of the cranium, are less than those of persons of sound mind, lunatics in general, the weak-minded, and even idiots. It may be said that reasoning maniacs have a congenital atrophy of the posterior lobes of the brain, and that the cranium has been diminished in size at the expense of the occipital region.

This would conclude what I have to say relative to reasoning mania but for the recent existence of a marked example of the affection in the person of Charles J. Guiteau, the assassin of President Garfield. On the hypothetical question proposed by the prosecution, it is sufficiently apparent that the prisoner was of unsound mind ; and that his mental aberration is properly to be regarded as reasoning mania is, I think, equally clear. That question contains the following statements, accepted by the prosecution as facts :

That he had several insane relatives ; that while at college he abandoned his studies and entered the Oneida Community ; that he left it, and subsequently returned ; that he again left it and went to New York to establish a newspaper devoted to the dissemination of peculiar religious ideas; that he abandoned this project; that he studied law, and was admitted to the bar ; that he was married, and then divorced by his own procurement; that he became interested in religion, and delivered lectures on the subject ; that while thus engaged he attempted to strike his sister with an axe ; that, though a physician could find neither illusion, hallucination, nor delusion, he pronounced him insane "because of exaltation of the motives and expressions of emotional feeling, also excessive egotism, and that he was the subject of pseudo-religious feelings," and advised his confinement in a lunatic asylum ; that he soon afterward gave up lecturing ; that he associated himself with the National Republican Committee, and prepared a speech, which, however, he only delivered once ; that after the election of General Garfield he asked by letter for the appointment of Minister to Austria ; that he went to Washington to urge his claims ; that, not getting the position he applied for—that of Consul at Paris—"he earnestly and persistently followed up his application by verbal and written requests, having no special claims for this place except his own idea of the value of his services," and having the recommendation of but one person ; that he unwarrantably inferred from a remark of the Secretary of State that he might be appointed ; that, in spite of rebuffs from the officials in authority, he continued to expect the appointment ; that he made inquiries about a pistol which he subsequently purchased, borrowing money to pay for it ; that he practiced with it by shooting at a mark ; that he followed the President on two occasions for the purpose of killing him, but was deterred once because his wife, who was sick, was with him ; that finally he lay in wait for him at the railroad station and shot at him twice, intending to kill him, and inflicting a mortal wound.

That after the shooting he attempted to get to the jail for protection ; that he was arrested, and that a letter to General Sherman, asking for troops to protect him, was found upon his person ; that, in two letters written several days before the shooting, he declares that the President's nomination was an act of God, that he has just shot the President, "that his election was an act of God, his removal an act of God" ; that in another document, addressed to the American people, and dated as early as June 16th, he used this language : " I conceived the idea of removing the President four weeks ago ; I conceived the idea myself, and kept it to myself," and other words of like character.

That he subsequently claimed that he was inspired by the Deity to kill the President, and that he had had previous inspirations ; that, for years before the shooting, he had procured a precarious living, not paying his board bills, borrowing money, evading the payment of his railway fares, retaining money collected by him as a lawyer, and being several times in prison on charges of fraud ; and that on the stand he stated that he felt remorse for his deed so far as his personal feelings were concerned, but that his duty to the Lord and the American people was paramount.

On such a statement of facts as the above, and with a knowledge of the manner in which the prisoner conducted himself while being tried for his life, his abuse of his friends who were endeavoring to save him, his praise of judge and jury and opposing counsel at one time, and his fierce denunciation of them at another, his speech in his defence, his entire lack of appreciation of the circumstances surrounding him, his evident misapprehension of the feelings of the people toward him, his belief in the intercession of prominent persons in his behalf, and of his eventual triumph, his conduct in court after sentence was pronounced, his behavior on the scaffold, and, finally, the indubitable evidences of brain disease found on *post-mortem* examination,[1] show that Guiteau was a reasoning maniac, and hence a lunatic. There is not an asylum under the charge of any one of the medical experts for the prosecution, or, in fact, any other large asylum in any part of the world, that does not contain patients less insane than he.

Like some other reasoning maniacs, Guiteau feigned a different form of insanity from that which he really possessed. It is extremely probable that all his talk about feeling himself called by God to "remove the President" was made for the purpose of causing the belief to prevail that he was insane, and that he never really had any delusion of the kind, or, in fact, any insane delusions of any kind, other than such as were the result of his overweening egotism, selfishness, and general impracticability. As Campagne [2] shows, the subjects of reasoning mania are not only capable of concealing their own mental aberration when they have a purpose to accomplish, but are also able to feign such symptoms as their experience teaches them are generally regarded as being more markedly characteristic of insanity than those peculiar to their real morbid condition.

e—INTELLECTUAL SUBJECTIVE MORBID IMPULSES.

1. By an intellectual subjective morbid impulse is to be understood, first, the occurrence and recurrence of an idea

---

[1] In addition to the fact that Guiteau's head had the shape peculiar to reasoning maniacs, it was ascertained, on *post-mortem* examination, that the membranes of the brain were in places strongly adherent to the skull, and that the arachnoid was studded with opalescent patches. Microscopically, it was found that there was "unquestionable evidence of decided chronic disease of the minute blood-vessels in numerous minute diffused areas, accompanied by alterations of the cellular elements." So far as I am aware, this is the first case of reasoning mania in which the brain has been examined. That the patho-anatomical condition was that of incipient general paralysis is admitted by some of the most competent alienists in this and other countries, and is especially interesting in view of the opinion I have expressed relative to the connection of this form of insanity with reasoning mania.　　　[2] *Op. cit.*, p. 393.

which is known to be false, and, therefore, is not a delusion, but which by its persistency causes more or less mental derangement, and the logical consequences of which are restricted to the individual in whom it exists.

In a very interesting communication made by Billod [1] to the *Société médico psychologique*, December, 1869, he describes the condition in question, and adduces several cases in illustration of his views :

"I know very well," said one of his patients to him as he was going through the asylum wards, " that it is all false, but it torments me just as much as though it were true. You know my two nieces ; they are excellent girls, with hearts of gold. I am sure of them, and of their loving feelings toward me, and yet I am continually haunted with the idea that they wish to poison me, in order to receive at once the property which will come to them at my death. It is absurd ; I know its falsity ; I am ashamed of having such thoughts, but I cannot prevent them, and they distress me just as much as though they were true."

A lady consulted me who, for several weeks, had been subject to intellectual derangement, characterized by the constant recurrence of the idea that she was followed by detectives for the purpose of discovering whether or not she visited improper places. She was fully aware of the utter groundlessness of the thought; it was not for a moment accepted as being true, and yet it annoyed her beyond expression by its very persistency. Do what she would, she could not escape from it, and she went to bed every night knowing that at the instant of awaking it would be present in her mind, and hoping that she might die in her sleep. "I am afraid," she said, "that eventually I will really believe it, and then I shall be actually insane." She had taken every possible means to assure herself of the falsity of the idea, but, although everything established this fact, she was still pursued by the notion. For days she would stay in her bedroom, and, locking the doors, would sit down in the vain attempt to read some book which she hoped might divert her thoughts, but immediately the idea arose, " He is under the bed ; he came in before you locked the doors." At first she would resist, but eventually she would have to look under the bed. Then

[1] " Des aliénés avec conscience de leur état," " Des maladies mentales," etc., Paris, 1882, t. i, p. 492.

for a few minutes there would be a little rest, but again it would come: "You did not look in the wardrobe ; he is there concealed behind your frocks." And again she would be obliged to search, and so it went on all day, and day after day, till her life was a burden to her, and she seriously contemplated suicide. Lately she had not been quite sure that there were not hallucinations of hearing. So distinct was the idea as it was formed in ideal words that it almost seemed to her as though she heard them plainly uttered.

In another case, that of a young lady, who had overworked herself at school in the endeavor to learn the higher mathematics, the thought constantly recurred that she was descended from insane ancestors, and that she was, therefore, in danger of becoming the subject of mental aberration. She knew at the time that there had not been an insane person in her family, so far back as records went, and that was two or three hundred years, and, therefore, the idea was not accepted as true. On the contrary, she took the matter very pleasantly, often laughing over it, and speaking of how she would amuse herself if she really should be committed to an asylum. But all this was mere badinage, as she did not, except occasionally for an instant, entertain the slightest fear of such a termination. With her the idea resolved itself into words which she felt obliged to repeat to herself, and sometimes even to utter aloud :

"My father and mother were both insane,
And I inherit the dreadful stain ;
My grandfathers, grandmothers, aunts, and uncles
Were lunatics all, and had carbuncles."

Night and day, while awake, this silly stanza was passing through her mind in all the variations of accent, time, and arrangement. Sometimes with the emphasis on one word, and then on another ; sometimes very fast, and again very slow, and with all possible combinations of the words and lines. Indeed, it was often a task which occupied several hours of the day to arrange the elements of the verse into new combinations.

Lately she had been mentally singing it to all the tunes she had ever heard, and this caused her more discomfort than any other manifestation, for she had a good musical ear and education, and, consequently, suffered from the incongruous and unmelodious refrain which was constantly in her mind.

But nothing interfered with her good temper, though at times she was fearful that, through the persistency of the idea, her mind might become weakened. "I know I am not insane," she said, "and I hope I shall never become so, and I know that all my relations were of sound mind, but I should like to get rid of the foolish notion, and the eternal verse. I might stand them a year longer, but not longer; no," she continued, gravely, after a slight pause, "I don't think I could endure them longer than a year."

2. Or the tendency may be to the recurrence of an idea, or a mental image, which, though true enough, and probably at some anterior period entertained with pleasure, now wearies with constant reiteration, and may give rise to secondary mental and physical disturbance.

In a previous chapter I have incidentally alluded to a like condition, but have now to consider it more specifically. A case or two will explain it more clearly than any mere description.

A young man, a salesman in a hardware store, had a good deal of additional labor put upon him at the close of the year in taking an account of the stock on hand. He reached his home every night for a week at not far from midnight, and then, after eating a hasty but hearty supper, went to bed. But not to sleep. All night long his mind was filled with ideas of screws, tacks, locks, shovels, carpenters' tools, etc.; and images of these objects, and hundreds of others, were passing in a confused medley before him. In addition, there was an arrangement of words representing the principal articles kept for sale, which he was obliged to repeat mentally, and which, of course, added to his uneasiness. Toward morning he fell asleep for an hour or two only, and during the day, though exhausted, he was free from his troubles. As soon, however, as he got to bed, the same sequence was resumed with undiminished force, and kept on as before, till near morning.

But in the course of a week the taking of stock was completed. Instead, however, of obtaining relief from his ideas and mental hallucinations, they were increased tenfold, appearing in the day as well as in the night, preventing anything like a proper degree of attention to his business, and almost driving him to despair. Indeed, on account of the cerebral hyperæmia which evidently existed in this case, and which was indicated by the pain in the head, vertigo, insomnia, *tinnitus aurium*, as well as by the mental condition, there was every reason for regarding the matter from a serious point of view.

Luys,[1] under the head of *Hyperæmia of the Specially Intellectual Regions*, cites a similar case :

A young professor of mathematics, whose duty it was to prepare pupils for examination at the Polytechnic, was obliged, in the course of the day, to repeat his demonstrations in a loud tone many times. In a short time the mental erethism developed was so intense that, even when out of the class-room and endeavoring to get rest, the geometrical figures he had been employing all day appeared to his imagination. He heard himself speak, and he was impelled to repeat mentally the same words, the same problems, the same demonstrations, which he had used in the morning with his pupils. If he went out for a walk in the country, the same images pursued him. With all this, there were pain in the head and persistent insomnia. The symptoms continued for several weeks, and then disappeared under rest and appropriate treatment.

I have had several cases under my charge in which unmeaning or almost meaningless phrases continued to be mentally repeated long after the idea which originally excited them had disappeared, if there ever had been any such origin. Thus, one gentleman had the words "Can't get over the fence in time " constantly occurring to him. This phrase had its origin in a vivid dream, in which the patient imagined himself pursued by a wild bull, and in which, to save himself, he had run toward a high fence. In the morning the impression was so strong that he found himself repeating the words which expressed the fear he had experienced in his sleep, and, for several weeks previous to my seeing him, they had been running through his mind in all kinds of ways— sometimes to mental music, and then in several languages with which he was acquainted.

But the first account of intellectual subjective morbid impulses was given by the author[2] in a monograph " On Sleep

---

[1] "Traité clinique et pratique des maladies mentales," Paris, 1881, p. 433.

[2] *New York Medical Journal*, May and June, 1865. Also in a separate publication, " On Wakefulness," etc., Philadelphia, 1865 ; and again in " Sleep and its Derangements," Philadelphia, 1869.

and Insomnia," published eighteen years ago. The following case I cite from that memoir :

A lady, aged about thirty-five, unmarried, and of rather delicate constitution, consulted me in regard to persistent wakefulness with which she had been affected for nearly a month. According to the account which she gave me, she had received a severe mental shock, which had not lost its influence when a subject causing great anxiety was forced upon her consideration. Her menstrual period, which had been due about ten days before she came under my notice, had been anticipated by a week, and the flow was prolonged much above the ordinary time. She had, therefore, lost a good deal of blood, and was, in consequence, reduced in strength. When I first saw her she was nervous and irritable, her hands trembled violently upon the slightest exertion of their muscles, her eyes were bloodshot, the pupils contracted, and the lids opened to the widest possible extent. There was a constant buzzing in the ears, and the sense of hearing was much more acute than was natural. There was also increased sensibility of all that portion of the surface of the body (the skin of the hands, arms, legs, back, and breast), which I submitted to examination with the æsthesiometer. Her pulse was 98, irritable, small, and weak.

At night all her symptoms were increased in violence. Her mind was filled with the most grotesque images which it was possible to conceive, and with trains of ideas of the most exaggerated and improbable character. These succeeded each other with a regularity so well marked that she was able to foresee the routine night after night. "No one," she said, "can imagine the weariness I feel, or the horror with which I look forward to the long rows of too familiar phantoms and thoughts which I know will visit me before morning. There is one set," she continued, " which always comes as the clock strikes two. No matter what may be passing through my mind, it is banished by this. It consists of a woman with very long hair, who sits on a rock by the sea-side, with her face buried in her hands. Presently a man, armed with a long sword, comes up behind her, and, clutching her by the hair, drags her to the ground. He puts his knee on her breast, and, still holding her hair, cuts it off and binds her with it, hand and foot. He then begins to pile stones on her, and continues to do so till she is entirely covered, notwithstanding her piercing shrieks, which I hear as distinctly as I do real sounds. Turning, then, to the sea, he cries out, 'Julia, you are avenged! My vow is accomplished; come, come!' He then draws a dagger and stabs himself to the heart. He falls over the hill of stones he has raised, and instantly hundreds of little devils not more than a foot high swarm around his body, and finally carry it off through the air. My horror at all this is extreme. For more than an hour the scene is passing before me, and though I know it is all purely imaginary, I cannot shake off the terror it induces."

I questioned this lady closely, and found that she was very intelligent and fully sensible of the unreality of all her visions. I regard her case as one of passive cerebral hyperæmia, and one that, if not relieved, would probably terminate in a more advanced form of mental derangement.

In this and other instances that have come under my notice, there were no actual hallucinations; that is, the patients did not imagine they saw with their eyes the images which appeared to be present, or heard with their ears the voices which disturbed them. The forms and the sounds were altogether mental, and were of the kind called by Baillarger psychical hallucinations, to which attention has already been given under the head of "Perceptional Insanities."

M. Ball,[1] in a recent communication, reports several interesting cases of the affection under notice, without, however, apparently being aware of those cited by other authors. He regards them as instances of ideas being imposed upon the mind, and controlling it in spite of itself. To these ideas he gives the name of "intellectual impulsions."

In one of these cases, a man of great intelligence, and who had acquired a well-deserved celebrity for his scientific works, could never speak in public, nor read a book in a loud-tone. Hardly would he begin to speak ere a host of thoughts absolutely foreign to the subject rushed upon him, he lost the thread of his voluntary ideas, became embarrassed, and could not continue his remarks. If he tried to read aloud, the same phenomenon was reproduced with mathematical precision. Absorbed in the ideas which oppressed him, and which were entirely without relation to the text, he read, not only monotonously and without expression, but incorrectly, stammeringly, and in a way like that of the most illiterate person.

[1] " Des impulsions intellectuales," *L'Encephale*, t. i, 1881, p. 26.

Notwithstanding all his efforts, he could never succeed in overcoming his trouble.

In another case, the patient, a young man of intelligence, of good education, and free from hereditary tendency to neurotic affections, was pursuing his studies at college, when one day he heard his companions talking of the mysterious fatality connected with the number thirteen. At the same instant an absurd idea took possession of his mind. "If the number thirteen is fatal," he thought to himself, it would be deplorable if God were thirteen. Without attaching any importance to this conception, he could not prevent himself from thinking of it continually, and at each instant he accomplished mentally an act which consisted in repeating to himself "God thirteen." He began to attach a certain cabalistic value to this formula, and attributed to it a preservative influence. "I know perfectly well," he said, "that it is ridiculous that I should think myself obliged to imagine 'God thirteen' every instant in order to save myself from being thirteen;" but, nevertheless, the intellectual act was repeated without ceasing. Very soon he thought he ought to apply the same principle to eternity, to the infinite, and to grand ideas in general; and then his life was passed in mentally saying, "God thirteen! The infinite thirteen! Eternity thirteen!"

In consequence of the incessant repetition of this psychical act, the young man found it impossible to pursue his studies, which, until then, had been marked with success. He therefore went home and placed himself under medical treatment. But the continual progress of the affection was not arrested, and three years subsequently he was still every moment repeating his mental prayer. Aside from the sadness legitimately resulting from this circumstance, there was no mental trouble.

A third case is still more interesting:

A pharmacist, thirty-six years old, an intelligent and hard-working man, but for a long period a hypochondriac, set out one day on a journey by railway, during which he lost his ticket. He endeavored to repair tHe accident by paying a second time for his seat, when he discovered that he had lost his pocket-book. The consequences of this misadventure were of such a character as to affect him very powerfully, so that he, little by little, began to look for his pocket-book at all times, and finally this became the chief occupation of his life. In the midst of an interesting conversation, during a delicate manipulation, or when he was serving his clients, the idea would flash through his mind, "I have lost my pocket-book." Instantly he was compelled to stop everything and look for the object in question, which he always found in its proper place.

This silly idea made him ridiculous to all with whom he came in contact, and ended by becoming a real calamity. He was obliged to renounce his business, to give up a lucrative profession, and to retire into the country, where, however, he found no relief from his tormenting idea.

A somewhat similar case is at the present time under my own charge. A gentleman, while driving a fast trotting-horse over a muddy road, was bespattered from head to foot. On his return to the city he changed his clothes, but the fact made such an impression on him that the idea constantly occurred to him in these words: "I am covered with mud;" and instantly he made the motion of brushing off the soiled spots with his hands. Several years have elapsed, and yet the idea "I am covered with mud" passes through his mind every moment, and he is continually making the motion of brushing his coat, or waistcoat, or trousers with his fingers. He knows he is not muddy, but the idea is there, and the motion follows automatically.

Dr. W. J. Morton has given me the particulars of a like case occurring in his experience.

In all these cases there is probably a very limited form of disease in some part of the cortex. The fact that the individual does not accept as true the idea forced upon him, sufficiently indicates the restricted seat of the lesion. That this is a localized hyperæmia is, I think, exceedingly probable, and the results of treatment based upon this hypothesis—and which will in a subsequent part of this treatise be fully considered—certainly tend to support this opinion.

f—INTELLECTUAL OBJECTIVE MORBID IMPULSES.

An intellectual objective morbid impulse consists of an idea occurring in the mind of an individual contrary to his sense of what is right and proper, and urging him to the perpetration of an act repugnant to his conscience and wishes. It differs from an intellectual subjective morbid impulse in the fact that it is directed toward the accomplishment of a distinct object, and that often its operation is not limited to the person by whom it is experienced. If yielded to, therefore, the circumstance is often of such a character as to demand the serious consideration of society, for it is generally the case that the impulse tends to the committal of a deed of crime or violence. As in the previously described form of morbid impulse, there is no delusion and no necessary emotional disturbance, except such as would naturally result in the average man from the existence in him of an irresistible impulse to commit crime. Neither does the individual who is the subject of an intellectual objective morbid impulse exhibit any deficiency of intellect. He is perfectly aware of the nature of the act he is prompted to commit, and perpetrates it only because he is impelled thereto by a force which he feels himself powerless to resist. Very often he acts with calmness and deliberation, and again manifests agitation and excitement. He does not for a moment lose consciousness, as does the epileptic, who may also commit acts of violence under the influence of a paroxysm ; and, when his impulse has been acted upon, or his purpose changed by any momentary but more powerful cause, he recollects distinctly all the circumstances of the occasion.

It frequently happens that the subject of an intellectual objective morbid impulse struggles successfully against the force which actuates him even when on the very point of yielding, or when he takes such means as experience has shown him are sufficient to direct him ; or the impulse disappears apparently spontaneously, or as a consequence of appropriate medical treatment.

I have in a previous chapter related the details of several cases of intellectual objective morbid impulse, but the following will tend still further to elucidate the subject.

Very slight causes are often sufficient to destroy or overcome the morbid impulse. Marc [1] cites the case of M. R., a distinguished chemist and an amiable man, who, feeling himself impelled to commit murder, and knowing his inability to resist, voluntarily placed himself in a *maison de santé* of the Faubourg St. Antoine. Tormented by the impulse to kill, he often prostrated himself before the altar, and implored the Almighty to deliver him from his atrocious impulse, the origin

[1] "Consultation médico-legale sur Harriette Cornier," etc.

of which he could not explain. When he felt that his will was yielding, he went to the superintendent of the asylum and had him tie his hands together with a ribbon. This weak band was sufficient to calm the unfortunate man for a time ; but eventually he attempted to kill one of his keepers, and finally died in a paroxysm of acute mania.

On the other hand, a man, whose case is cited by Brierre de Boismont, rather than yield to an impulse to kill his wife, which he felt was rapidly becoming irresistible, cut off his right arm. Honest human nature could not go much farther than this.

Again, all the efforts of the affected individual are apparently unsuccessful, and the deed to which he is impelled is committed. I say *apparently*, because we never can be quite sure that the patient has exercised all his will-power, or availed himself of all those means to prevent the accomplishment of his act which ordinary reason would suggest. When he effectually resists, there are not wanting those who will declare that the case is not one of morbid impulse, while, when he yields at once or eventually, these same persons will just as strongly affirm that the impulse was irresistible. Several cases have come under my observation in which patients have confessed to me that they have had impulses to commit various kinds of crimes which they have been barely able to resist. These people have passed through life attending faithfully to their several duties, and entirely unsuspected of contending with themselves in so terrible a manner.

I was once consulted by a young man for symptoms indicating the existence of cerebral hyperæmia. He had pain in his head, dizziness, and was unable to sleep. He informed me that he had been for several months constantly troubled by a force, which was inexplicable to him, to kill a friend who was employed in the same office with him. Upon one occasion he had gone so far as to secretly put strychnia into a mug of ale which he had invited the young man to drink ; but just as the intended victim was raising the vessel to his lips, he had, as if by accident, knocked it out of his hand. Every morning he had awakened with the impulse so strong upon him that he felt certain he would carry it out before the day closed ; but he had always been able to overcome it.

This young man reasoned perfectly well in regard to his impulse, and very candidly admitted, and I entirely agreed with him, that, if he had yielded and committed the murder, he ought to have been punished to the full extent of the law.

The following extract from a letter, received several years ago, is likewise to the point:

"In the New York *Sun*, of the 30th instant, I noticed the proceedings of the Medico-Legal Society, in the College of Physicians and Surgeons, on emotional insanity, etc., and I was impressed particularly with your remarks on 'Morbid Impulse.' Some two weeks since, I was at work in my garden with a spade, and one of my little girl children, just three years old, came in where I was, and I was suddenly seized with an impulse to kill the child with the spade that I was at work with, and, in order to prevent my doing so, I had to make her leave the garden. Now, I love this child better than I do the apple of my eye, and why I was seized with that impulse I can't say. Since that time I have been feeling strange, and I am afraid to trust myself with my own family, though I know perfectly well what I am doing, and only feel actuated by these impulses. I have consulted a physician, and he laughed at me. If you can suggest any remedy for these strange impulses, I will pay you what you charge, and will consider that you have done me a favor that will *cause me to bless your name forever*. I don't consider that I am in any danger of murdering any one just yet, but the idea of such a thing is horrible, and I fear it may grow on me unless remedied."

In my reply, I called his attention to the admitted fact that he had his impulse under control; that he was able to reason calmly and intelligently in regard to it; that he had applied to me for advice, and that I urged him without delay to place himself under the restraint of an asylum. I further told him that, if he disregarded this advice, and finally yielded to his impulse, he would be fully as guilty of murder as though he had killed his child through deliberate malice, and that he ought to be just as surely executed as any other murderer.

An instance of the slightness of the cause often sufficient to arrest the course of an impulse has already been given. Such cases are by no means rare, and some notable ones have been recorded. Thus:

On the 10th of November, 1854, as related by M. Devergie,[1] a young man, aged nineteen, the son of a prominent merchant of Bordeaux, dined with his father, to whom he was much attached, and his step-mother, whom he had regarded with gradually increasing aversion for several years.

The dinner passed without any unusual incidents till dessert, when Jules ——, the young man in question, left the table and repaired to the drawing-room to warm himself. Not finding a fire kindled, he went to his own chamber, took his fowling-piece, and started out for a stroll through the country, as was his custom. He had not left the house, however, before the idea of suicide, which had haunted his mind for several weeks, suddenly recurred to him, and was as suddenly changed into the thought of killing his step-mother.

Without stopping an instant, he threw aside his fowling-piece, and, going to his brother's room, took two pistols, which had been loaded three weeks. He had pistols of his own which he might have taken, and which had been charged only the day before.

He descended to the dining-room, approached his step-mother, who was still at the table with his father, and, pointing the pistol at her head, discharged it with instantly fatal effect.

Madame X. fell to the floor, and the young man, recoiling, rested motionless against the wall. His father rose to seize him, but, a temporary feeling of self-preservation being aroused in Jules, he fled across the kitchen through the midst of the terrified domestics, and escaped from the house, exclaiming, "I am a madman, an idiot! I have killed my step-mother!"

He soon, however, changed his mind, and surrendered himself to the commissary of police, to whom he related all the particulars of the crime.

Before and until the murder, the life of this young man had been exemplary. He had performed his duties in the counting-house of his father with assiduity, and was an excellent son and brother. Though rich, he had studiously avoided dissipation of every kind.

Such were the obvious features of the homicidal act. Jules was tried before the Imperial Court at Paris. Calmeil, Tardieu, and Devergie, the most eminent alienists in France, tes-

---

[1] "Où finit la raison? Où commence la folie?" "Mémoires de l'académie impériale de médecine," t. xxiii, p. 1, Paris, 1859.

tified in favor of the insanity of the prisoner, and he was acquitted on that ground.

In his own account of the act he said :

"When I ascended to my room on the day of the crime, I was not thinking of anything. I should not have gone upstairs if I had found a fire in the drawing-room. When I reached my room, having no evil intentions, the notion of suicide possessed me ; then, my thoughts taking another direction, I threw aside my fowling-piece, ran to my brother's chamber, armed myself with two pistols, and went back to the dining-room, actuated by I know not what force, which dragged me in spite of myself. *If my father had addressed to me one word when I entered the dining-room, whatever it might have been, I would not have killed my step-mother.*"

Five years subsequently, Jules, several of whose ancestors had been insane, committed suicide at his step-mother's grave.

A lady, several years ago, was brought to me by her husband for advice in regard to her mental condition. She told me her own story as nearly as possible in the following words, which I transcribe from my note-book :

"I had been feeling quite badly for several days, had not slept well, and was suffering from slight but continuous pain in the head, and vertigo. Moreover, I had some little confusion of mind, as shown by the fact that I could not collect my thoughts, and called things often by their wrong names. I was not depressed in spirits, though I felt uncomfortable enough. This morning I awoke after a particularly restless night. I went to the window, drew aside the curtains, and looked down into the street. A slight snow, followed by rain, had fallen, and the sidewalks were slushy and slippery. All at once, with a suddenness and force that were overwhelming, the idea came into my head to throw myself from the window. I opened it hastily, and was in the act of plunging down head foremost, when my attention was attracted by a boy, with a basket of bread on his arm, slipping on the pavement and falling in the street. I burst into a hearty laugh ; my impulse was gone. I closed the window, gave a cry, and fell to the floor in a fainting condition. I recovered consciousness in a moment or two, and found my husband bending over me. I recollected everything that had happened. The print of my hands was still in the snow on the window-sill, and the boy had really fallen as I had described. Since then I have been feeling much better, but I am afraid of myself, for I don't know what impulse may come upon me next."

It will be seen, therefore, that an impulse of the kind under consideration may be sudden, and may exhaust itself by a single occurrence, or it may be continuous, lasting, with more or less intensity, for weeks, months, or even years. It may then disappear without its ever having been fulfilled, or it may be acted upon, and may then either be repeated or vanish, or it may result in the patient passing into a more generalized type of insanity.

An intellectual objective morbid impulse is sometimes excited by a suggestion which the individual suddenly receives. The action of this principle is well shown in the following instances :

A young man, a member of a highly respectable family, consulted me for what he very properly thought was a kind of insanity. It appeared that a few weeks previously, while walking down Broadway, he had been struck with the appearance of a lady in front of him who wore a very rich black silk dress. Suddenly the impulse seized him to ruin this dress by throwing sulphuric acid on it. He, therefore, stopped at an apothecary's shop and purchased a small phial of oil of vitriol. Hastening his pace, he soon overtook the lady, and, walking by her side, he managed in the crowd to empty his phial over her dress without being perceived. He derived so much satisfaction from this act that he resolved to repeat it at once on some other woman. He, therefore, purchased another supply of vitriol, and, singling out a lady better dressed than others around her, poured the contents of the phial over her dress, and again escaped detection. He then went home, and, reflecting upon what he had done, determined to persevere in the practice ; but a night's rest put him in a healthier frame of mind, and he concluded to abandon the idea. Indeed, he was so distressed by what he had done that he wrote out an advertisement for the newspapers, in which he requested the ladies whose gowns he had spoiled to reply through the same channel, giving their residences, so that he might compensate them for the losses he had caused them to sustain. But on his way to the newspaper offices he again felt the impulse, at the sight of a handsome silk gown, to throw vitriol on it, and again he purchased a supply, and repeated the acts of the day before.

He now began to consider more fully than he had yet done the nature and consequences of his conduct, and the next morning came to me for advice. He stated very frankly his entire conviction that his acts were in the highest degree immoral and degrading, but expressed his utter inability to refrain from their perpetration.

"A handsome dress," he said, "acts upon me very much as I suppose a piece of red cloth does on an infuriated bull: I must attack it. The bull uses his horns, while I use vitriol. I do not know why the idea ever came into my head. I certainly never would have conceived of such a thing if I had been blind. I was altogether excited by the sight of that handsome silk dress the first day, and it was impossible for me to resist after the idea had once had a lodging in my mind. I have often seen fully as handsome dresses in the street before, but never previously was the sight followed by such an impulse."

After the most careful examination, I could discover no evidence of disease, except in the one point of wakefulness, with which he had suffered for several months past. I therefore prescribed bromide of calcium for him, and insisted on his removing himself from further temptation by taking a sea voyage on a sailing vessel upon which there were no women passengers. He went to sea in a fishing schooner, and returned in three or four months perfectly free from his morbid impulse.

A gentleman, who came about once a week to consult me for cerebral congestion, the result of excessive application to business, and who lived in a neighboring town, informed me that during his journeys by rail he invariably experienced an impulse to throw himself from the train. Finally he was so strongly impelled that he stated the case to an acquaintance in the car, and begged him to sit near him and restrain him if he made any such attempt. After that he never came without bringing a friend with him, who had instructions not to lose sight of him for an instant. In telling me of his impulse, he described it as almost overwhelming, and that it seemed to be excited by the rapid motion, and by the fact that he had heard of people throwing themselves from railway trains.

It is well known that many persons standing on great

heights experience an impulse to jump off. So many individuals committed suicide by leaping from the *Colonne Vendôme* and the *Arc de Triomphe* in Paris, and from the Duke of York's monument in London, that precautions had to be taken to prevent further acts of the kind.

Marc relates the case of a nurse who felt the impulse to murder the infant she took care of whenever she saw its naked skin. She threw herself on her knees before her mistress and begged to be discharged, declaring that the whiteness of the child's skin excited her to murder it, and that she could not longer resist the impulse.

Several years since, I had under my charge a lady who, whenever she saw the naked shoulders of a young child, felt an impulse, which she declared she could not resist, to bite the skin. She had thus inflicted very disagreeable wounds on the children of her friends, and was finally arrested on the charge of assault; but the matter was hushed up on her promise to abstain from such conduct in the future, and she kept her promise.

Morbid impulses to commit violent acts are often developed by the sight of a suitable weapon for the purpose. Persons have hanged themselves on the suggestion excited by the sight of a rope; others have committed murder or suicide from seeing knives, pistols, etc., lying in inviting situations. A lady, seeing a phial labelled "nitric acid" on a table in my consulting-room, seized it, and, putting it to her lips, would have swallowed the contents if I had not fortunately perceived her in time and knocked it from her hands. As it was, she only succeeded in spoiling an elegant gown.

Even a word spoken in jest may, under certain circumstances, be sufficient. Dr. Oppenheim, of Hamburg, having received for dissection the body of a man who had committed suicide by cutting his throat, but who had done this in such a manner that his death did not take place until after an interval of great suffering, jokingly remarked to his attendant: "If you have any fancy to cut your throat, don't do it in such a bungling way as this; a little more to the left here, and you will cut the carotid artery." The individual to whom this dangerous advice was given was a sober, steady man, with a family, and a comfortable subsistence. He had never manifested the slightest tendency to suicide, and had no motive to commit it. Yet, strange to say, the sight of the corpse and the observation made by Dr. Oppenheim suggested to his mind the idea of self-destruction, and this took such firm hold of him that he carried it into execution, fortunately, however, without profiting by the anatomical instruction he had received, for he did not cut the carotid artery.

Closely allied to suggestion, and perhaps a more powerful cause of morbid impulse of the species under notice, is *imitation*. Thus, many crimes have been committed by persons who have had the impulse excited by reading accounts of the trials of other persons, or the detailed recitals of all the particulars of offences which the age requires the public press to contain. Epidemics of murder, suicide, arson, and other crimes are thus produced.

"Some years ago," says Dr. Forbes Winslow,[1] "a man hung himself on the threshold of one of the doors of the *Hotel des Invalides*. No suicide had occurred in the establishment for two years previously; but in the succeeding fortnight five invalids hung themselves on the same cross-bar, and the governor was obliged to shut up the passage."

Epidemics of suicide spread, according to Plutarch, among the women of Miletus, and, as is well known, in later days, among the women of Marseilles.

A careful study of the cases of suicide recorded in the daily newspapers shows that they are to a great extent influenced in character by the principle of imitation. A case of suicide by Paris green is published, and straightway half a dozen others due to this poison are the result. Or a man or woman jumps from a ferry-boat while it is crossing the river, and then this mode becomes the fashion for a while, to be followed in its turn by some other method.

When I was a medical student, a young gentleman from Georgia was on one occasion dissecting the same body that I was. He had drawn one of the lower extremities as his part of the subject, and he was assiduous and careful in his work. So far as my observation extended, he did not differ essentially from other medical students. He was cheerful in disposition, and gave no evidence whatever of mental derangement, or even of excitement or depression of mind. One morning we were told that he had been found dead on the floor of his bedroom. An examination showed that he had divided his femoral artery, and had died of hæmorrhage. It was then ascertained

[1] "The Anatomy of Suicide," London, 1840, p. 120.

that he had the evening before received a letter which had apparently caused him much unhappiness.

Now, suicide by division of the femoral artery is certainly a very unusual mode of self-destruction. I doubt if any case of the kind had previously occurred in New York. Yet within a week there were two others, one of which was Horace Wells, the alleged discoverer of the anæsthetic properties of sulphuric ether.

Here we have the principle of suggestion acting on the first victim, and then that of imitation on the others.

Imitation is of more force when the intellect is less fully developed. Even in the normal condition we find it more strongly exercised in women and children than in adult men. In the latter, the influence may be so powerful that actual disease is acquired. Thus, a child imitates the movements of another affected with chorea, or with stammering, and immediately contracts the disorder. Even squinting has been produced in this manner.

A lady received such a vivid impression at seeing her maid throw herself down a well that she never passed a well without feeling a strong impulse to throw herself into it.

An idiot, having killed a pig, felt impelled to kill a man, and obeyed the impulse on the first one he met.

A melancholic person was present at the execution of a criminal, and was immediately seized with an impulse, of which he was fully conscious, and could scarcely resist, to murder some one.

A child six years old strangled its younger brother. The father and mother, entering the room the moment the act was in process of accomplishment, demanded the cause. The child threw itself weeping into their arms, and answered that it was imitating the devil, whom it had seen strangle Punchinello.

Such cases as these, though not all of them, examples of intellectual objective morbid impulse, are at least of value if they cause us to recognize the force of the principle of imitation, and to render less public than they are now the slaughter of animals and the executions of criminals.

Intellectual objective morbid impulses have, according to their character, been classified as homicidal mania, or the impulse to commit murder ; suicidal mania, or the impulse to perpetrate self-destruction ; pyromania, or the impulse to burn houses and other things ; kleptomania, or the impulse to steal, and so on. The mere object of the impulse should not, in my opinion, be sufficient to elevate the act to the dignity of a distinct species of insanity. The names, however, are useful, as explanatory of the main symptom exhibited by the patient.

Again, many of the cases of each of the varieties mentioned are not instances of intellectual, but of emotional or volitional morbid impulse, or of epileptic mania, examples of which will be subsequently brought to the notice of the reader. The distinction of the intellectual objective morbid impulse being that it arises in consequence of an idea the fulfilment of which is in direct relation with that idea, whereas the impulse due to deranged volition or emotion has no such starting-point, still less has that which arises from epilepsy.

Intellectual objective morbid impulse is more apt to occur in persons who possess what has been called the "insane temperament" than in those of equally balanced minds. It may develop into some more pronounced and obvious form of insanity, or it may become continuous in the individual. Generally it is unaccompanied by illusions or hallucinations, but there are cases in which one or the other of these conditions of perceptional derangement has been the exciting cause.

CHAPTER V.

III.

EMOTIONAL INSANITIES.

THE emotions are in most persons difficult of control, but they may acquire such an undue and morbid prominence as to dominate over the intellect and the will, and to assume the entire mastery of the actions in one or more respects. This effect may be produced suddenly, from the action of some cause capable of disturbing the normal balance which exists between the several parts of the mind, or it may result from influences which act slowly but with gradually increasing force. In neither case is there necessarily either delusion or error of judgment, but it very generally happens that the intellect sooner or later becomes involved.

Within certain limits, all persons are influenced in their thoughts and actions by the emotions they experience. But, as these are generally of very fleeting and changeable character, the individual who relies upon them for his guides is, of course, as fickle and unstable as the emotions themselves. But cases occur in which an emotion not only becomes intensified in power, but assumes a permanency altogether inconsistent with the normal condition. Such a state is embraced under the designation of emotional insanity.

The emotional insanities, therefore, are those forms of mental derangement in which the aberration of mind is chiefly exhibited by disturbance in the normal action of some one or more of the emotions.

a—EMOTIONAL MONOMANIA.

The number of forms of emotional monomania is only limited by the number of the emotions, though some are very much more liable to derangement than others. As the term implies, emotional monomania refers to aberration of a single emotion.

The subjects of emotional monomania, usually before the occurrence of the most pronounced symptoms of the affection, evince more or less disturbance of the emotional system, either as a whole or in part. Thus, it was observed of a young lady, who had, so far as was known, no hereditary tendency to insanity, but who was nevertheless very impressionable, that she became more than ordinarily scrupulous in her dress. She would spend hours in the arrangement of her hair, the care of her finger-nails, the tying of ribbons, fastening of brooches, etc. This conduct, though it attracted the attention of her mother and sisters, was rather the subject of joke than of any apprehension relative to the integrity of her mind. She was laughed at for wasting so much of her time in personal adornment, as previously she had not been especially noted for neatness either of person or attire. This continued for several months, and then she began to talk about her beauty and attractions, and of the looks of admiration which were cast at her as she walked down the street. There was one gentleman who she declared had followed her home, and for whom she expressed great admiration. On inquiry, it was ascertained that the person to whom she referred had not followed her home, but that she had spoken to him, and had requested him to accompany her to the door of her residence, as it was getting dark and she was afraid. This he had declined to do, taking her, from her appearance and manners, to be no better than she should be. This episode resulted in her being sent to live with an aunt who resided in the country several miles from any town, and where it was thought she would have no opportunity to indulge in what appeared to be newly developed proclivities. But in this her friends were mistaken. She began to write letters to the gentleman to whom she had spoken in the street, and whose name and address she had ascertained, and three or four times a day despatched, with the aid of a servant-maid, a note to him, in which she either lauded him to the skies, as her knight, her Chevalier Bayard, her Admirable Crichton, who would, she did not doubt, come to her rescue and make her his wife ; or she described her own devotion and the anguish she was enduring at being separated from him ; or she abused in very outrageous language the hyena—her father—the she-dragon—her aunt—who had conspired to take her away from her "best beloved."

Suddenly she ceased talking of the object of her infatuation, and discontinued writing him letters. It was fondly hoped that she had abandoned her fancy, and congratulatory messages were accordingly sent to her father. Her conduct in other respects seemed to have undergone an improvement. She requested her aunt to mark out a course of historical reading for her, and for several days was rarely seen without a book in her hand. But one morning it was ascertained that she had taken her departure. She had left her bedroom by a window, had walked along the roof of a veranda to the edge, and had then dropped upon a flower-bed immediately under. She had then walked to the railway-station, a distance of two miles, had gotten aboard of a "milk train," and had arrived in New York at four o'clock in the morning. She had then taken a cab, and had caused herself to be driven to the hotel of the gentleman on whom she had fastened her affections. Here she stated at the office that she was his sister, and had arrived with important information, which it was necessary he should at once receive. She waited for him in the public drawing-room, and, on his entering the apartment, threw herself at his feet, exclaiming: "See what I have done for you. I have left everything—house, riches, father, and all—for you !

Do you now doubt my love?" The gentleman, who was in reality worthy of the name, at once recognized her as the lady who had addressed him in the street and as his correspondent. She had signed her letters "Stella," and he had not even taken the trouble to ascertain her name. Now, however, perceiving the real state of the case, he determined to act promptly ; so sending for a lady friend, who lived near by, to accompany them, he took the young lady as fast as a cab could travel to her father's house. In a few minutes the situation was explained to the astonished parent, and a short time afterward a telegram from the aunt arrived with its superfluous information.

Recognizing the fact that his daughter's mind was deranged, the father brought her to me that same morning.

On entering my consulting-room, she began in the most voluble manner to explain her conduct. "I am in love with Mr. ——," she said. "He is the noblest and the best man there is in the world, and I have selected him as my husband. If he were here now, he would tell you how devotedly I am attached to him. If he does not love me now, he will love me as soon as he has had the opportunity of making my acquaintance. Of course, all this fuss, merely because I left my aunt's house last night, is calculated to prejudice him against my family ; but I can soon make that all right if I am allowed the opportunity of a few minutes' conversation with him. I don't understand why I am brought to see you. I have no need of a physician ; I am in perfect health. I am simply in love, and nothing, oh, nothing!" she continued, clasping her hands together and rolling her eyes to the ceiling, "will ever make me renounce my noble ——, my lord, my king, my pope and emperor."

"Take me to him at once," she resumed, addressing her father. "You have no right to separate us. I am of lawful age, and I have a right to marry whom I please. Do you know what I will do if you continue to keep us apart? I will kill myself ; I will take poison, and the death of your daughter will rest heavily on your heart." It is impossible to describe the tragic air with which she walked up and down the floor while speaking these words, and the emphasis and passion with which they were enunciated.

I endeavored to quiet her, and so far succeeded that in a few minutes I had obtained important information relative to her physical and mental condition. In fact, on her father leaving the room, she spoke with entire freedom on all the points upon which I questioned her.

I found that, though she had no pain in the head, she suffered almost constantly from a feeling of constriction, as though a tight band pressed upon her forehead. She had at times had flashes of light before the eyes, and there was *tinnitus aurium* to a disagreeable extent. She slept badly, and had frightful dreams, alternating with others in which she experienced the delights of a domestic life with the man she loved. Her menstruation was regular in every respect, and there was no suspicion of uterine or ovarian disease. During the whole of her conversation with me she did not give expression to a single libidinous thought, if she had such, and subsequent inquiry established the fact that at no time had there been any apparent exaltation of the sexual feeling, however much it may have been the basis of her emotional derangement. Neither did I detect the existence of any delusion or other aberration of the intellect. So far as her ideas were concerned, there seemed to be the most perfect integrity. She admitted unhesitatingly that her conduct had not been proper. " I know," she said, "that I ought not to have spoken to —— in the street; that I ought not to have written to him; that I ought not to have left my aunt's house in the night; that I ought not to have gone to his hotel; but this is not a question of right. I love him, and that is the end of it. There is no use talking about the matter, I love him."

Up to this time there had been no hallucinations; but while in conversation with me she suddenly stopped talking, and seemed to be listening attentively, as though she heard a sound. A pleased expression passed over her countenance, and she exclaimed: "I hear ——'s voice in the next room. He wishes to see me. Don't attempt to stop me, for I will go to him." She opened the door of the adjoining apartment. There was no one there but her father. "I thought I heard —— calling my name," she continued, "but I must have been mistaken."

I advised that a strong and sensible nurse should be procured, and that the patient should be treated at her own home. A suite of rooms in the upper part of the house was set apart for her and her attendant. She was taken out to drive every day. Her bowels, which had been obstinately constipated, were kept freely open with aloetic purges, and the bromide of sodium was administered in large doses. She soon became calmer, began to sleep well, lost the sense of tightness about her head, and gradually ceased to talk of Mr. —— and of her love for him. There was still, however, a certain exaltation of feeling, which would, I thought, require but a slight exciting cause to develop it into a higher state of excitement, and I therefore recommended foreign travel. She is now in Europe, and at last accounts was rapidly regaining her normal mental condition.

It often happens that the subjects of emotional monomania of the variety under consideration do not restrict their love to any one person. They adore the whole male sex, and will make advances to any man with whom they are brought into even the slightest association. If confined in an asylum, they simper and clasp their hands, and roll their eyes to the attendants, especially the physicians, and even the male patients are not below their affection. There is very little constancy in their love. They change from one man to another with the utmost facility and upon the slightest pretext. "I was very much in love with Dr. ——," said a woman to me in an asylum that I was visiting, "but he was late yesterday in coming to the ward, and now I love you. I will never love any one but you. You will come often to see me, won't you?" While she was speaking, the superintendent entered the ward. "Ah, here comes my first and only love," she exclaimed. "Why have you stayed so long away from your Eliza?"

It is quite commonly the case that prominent public characters—men and women—are annoyed by erotomaniacs, who follow them from town to town and make every effort, personally and by letters, to obtain interviews. There is scarcely a celebrated actor or actress who has not been the subject of the passion of one or more of these people. Sometimes it happens that failure to secure recognition causes a change in the character of the emotion, and attempts at murder or other acts of violence are committed.

On the 8th of November, 1816, while Miss Francis Kelly was performing the part of Nan in the farce of "Modern Antiques," at the Drury Lane Theatre, London, the audience and the lady were thrown into a state of alarm and consternation by the report of a pistol, fired at her by a man who sat in the front row of the pit. He was at once arrested, and gave his name as George Barnett.

When Miss Kelly was informed of his name, she immediately recollected him as a person who had addressed her several love-letters, which she had disregarded. Barnett was an attorney's clerk, and he had been for several months sending almost daily, to the object of his devotion, amatory epistles, sonnets, acrostics, and other professions of his love. As no attention was paid by the lady to these effusions, he took the resolution of killing her "upon," as the relator says, "the very altar where her charms had kindled his ardent flame; and that, if he was to be debarred the possession of her, she should never become the prize of a happier rival."

Barnett was tried at the Old Bailey, acquitted on the ground of insanity, and confined in Bethlehem Hospital for the Insane. While there he composed an ode to Miss Kelly, but finally lost his love for her, and spent his time in addressing amatory poems to every young lady whose name and residence he could discover.[1]

It is necessary to distinguish the condition under consideration from nymphomania or satyriasis. In emotional erotomania there is very little tendency to obtrude indecent acts or words into the conduct or language, whereas in the two other affections obscenity is the principal characteristic. Doubtless it is true, as already intimated, that the genesic instinct is at the bottom of erotomania, but it is so well kept in the background as rarely to become a prominent feature. Indeed, in most cases there is a kind of mystical exaltation of manner, action, and language present, that effectually conceals any lower sentiment that may exist. Some of the female subjects of erotomania who have come under my notice have evinced toward the objects of their passion the highest kind of devotional feeling, such as might be entertained by a mortal for an angel. But, even in these cases, the sexual instinct still exists and constitutes the foundation on which the exalted passion rests. It is well known that the fact of the sexual orgasms occurring during sleep to nuns in the middle ages led them to the belief that they had been visited in the night by heavenly beings, with whom they had had sexual

[1] "Sketches in Bedlam; or, Characteristic Traits of Insanity," by A Constant Observer, London, 1823, p. 64.

relations, and for whom they forever afterward entertained the most intense mystical though physical love.

The emotions of *pride* and *vanity* are often the subjects of derangement to such an extent as to constitute a marked type of mental derangement. It is usually the case with the subjects of emotional disturbance of the kind in question that there is very little or nothing in them which can justify even a moderate amount of pride or of vanity, and hence there is a condition present nearly approaching delusion, but still not in relation to a matter of fact. The individual who, for instance, is insane on the subject of his ancestry, and in regard to which he exhibits the most pronounced pride and ridiculous vanity, need not really believe that he is descended from a long line of kings or other notable people. He affects to believe it, and for the time being may half persuade himself that he actually is a great man, or ought to be. His derangement comes from the fact that his intense selfishness and egotism cause him to look with the utmost degree of partiality upon everything connected with himself, and he thinks, therefore, that if his ancestors were not great people, they ought to have been, and he tells those who will listen to him that they really were such.

Occasionally, however, the emotion of pride or vanity is developed upon an actual fact to such an abnormal extent as to constitute veritable insanity. I was once consulted in the case of a lady who was in such a condition. She was a German, and some service of her husband to a German potentate had resulted in his being created a baron, she becoming a baroness. This so affected the emotions of pride and vanity that she refused to sit at the same dinner-table with untitled people, or even to live in the same house with them. She insisted on her husband going to Germany to reside, where, as she said, "proper respect was paid to rank." She dressed herself on all occasions in the most elaborate style, and without the slightest regard to expense, and she strutted about with all the airs and graces of an *opera bouffe* princess. And yet with all this there was no marked derangement of the intellect. There were no delusions; she talked in a very rational manner on all subjects, and even on that of her newly acquired dignity betrayed only a moderate amount of exaltation so far as her speech went. I saw her but once, and then she was surrounded by books on heraldry, out of which she was endeavoring to construct a coat of arms ; and, though it was ten o'clock in the morning, she had diamonds as large as filberts in her ears and on her breast, and a sort of diadem on her head, which she gravely informed me was the coronet of a baroness.

As Alibert[1] says, man is vain of everything—of the father who has begotten him, of the country in which he was born, of the wealth he has inherited, of the clothes he wears, of the roof that shelters him, of the carriage he drives, of the woman he loves, of the God he worships, of the master he serves, of the friend with whom he associates, of the man who salutes him, of the one who speaks to him and the one who listens to him. However much we may laugh at the vain man, his vanity is not inconsistent with perfect sanity. It is only when the emotion runs away with him, so to speak, as it did with the baroness, that we can call him insane. And it is the sudden change, as a consequence of an insufficient cause, that forms the chief element in our diagnosis. In such cases, there is always, as there was with her, more or less mental weakness, and there is also present a tendency to a still further involvement of the intellect.

Descuret[2] gives the following case, illustrative of the extent to which morbid vanity may carry the individual. Emilie B., of a lymphatic temperament, was attacked during her infancy with *tinea capitis*, which denuded of their hair several places on her scalp. She had hardly passed her fifteenth year when she plunged into the world of fashion, where the emotions are constantly finding new excitations. Here she heard the praises that are bestowed on the graces and the beauty of women, and the advantages they receive from a fine toilet. She was herself not without some charms, and, to make them of the utmost value, she indulged her vanity to the fullest extent, in which she was encouraged by a mother who idolized her. Nevertheless, the small triumphs she obtained were poisoned by the remembrance of her infirmity, which, although she could by the devices of the hair-dresser conceal from others, was a torment to her even in the midst of her pleasures.

She had hardly arrived at the age of eighteen when her mother died. Being thus left to herself, she took to reading

[1] " Physiologie des passions," Paris, 1825, t. i, p. 47.
[2] " La médecine des passions," etc., Paris, 1860, t. ii, p. 212.

romances and other books, which led her on to the still further development of her vanity, and she made many efforts to make her hair grow on the places that were bald. All these being unsuccessful, she went to Paris to consult eminent dermatologists, but even there failure resulted. One day at dinner a gentleman was loud in his admiration of the magnificent hair of a lady of his acquaintance. She was much chagrined at this, but managed to conceal her emotion, and the next day assisted her sister-in-law—the lady with the splendid head of hair—in making her toilet. She insisted on dressing the hair, and handled it with as much *sang froid* as she could command. But soon she was overcome, and, being no longer able to refrain from tears, she escaped from the room, and, going to her own chamber, hanged herself to the bed-post, where she was soon afterward found dead.

The emotion of *avarice* is one which is frequently developed to a point sufficient to cause it to exercise a morbid power over the rest of the mental organism, and to constitute a state of insanity. The case of John Elwes is one in which avarice was carried to such an extent as to come within the bounds of mental alienation. This man was immensely rich for the period at which he lived, having a fortune of nearly a million pounds sterling. He owned a large part of London, and built many houses, thereby largely increasing his income. He lodged in the corner of one of his houses, which was so badly situated that he could not rent it, and his only furniture consisted of two broken-down chairs and a common deal table. He kept no servant, and often he was in danger of dying for want of nutritious food. His clothes were composed of old tattered garments which he found at second-hand clothing shops, and which he wore as long as they would hang together. His wig he had picked up out of a gutter into which a beggar had thrown it. He would not allow his shoes to be cleaned, because rubbing them, as he said, would make them wear out sooner. One day he was kicked by a horse, but he would not, on account of the expense, send for a surgeon. This piece of economy cost him dear, for he was in danger of losing his leg through gangrene, and many visits of a surgeon were required. He ate things which the lower animals would not have eaten. A piece of rotten meat delighted him, for he could buy it cheap or get it for nothing. He used neither fire nor candle, and, rather than hire a cab or buy an umbrella, he faced all kinds of weather. Elected a member of Parliament, he did not see fit to change his mode of living. A singular point about Elwes was that he was perfectly willing to risk large sums of money in speculation. He gambled almost ferociously, and on one occasion lost seven thousand pounds sterling at a game of piquet. He was scrupulously exact in all money matters, and was a man of his word in all things. His intellect was above the average.

The will of a lady is now being contested in the courts of this State, of whom it has been shown that, although worth several millions of dollars, she denied herself the common necessaries of life, both as regarded food and clothing.

Descuret [1] cites a case that occurred in his own experience: During the severe winter of 1829–'30 he was summoned by the commissary of police to visit an old beggar-woman who had been found dead in her bed. In a vast garret, dirty and otherwise repulsive, the corpse was found. The body was emaciated to an extreme degree, and was covered with vermin. It was that of a woman of about sixty-five years of age. There were no signs of violence or of any bodily disease. Death was attributed to cold, for the icy wind had free access through the badly glazed windows. And more thorough examination made this conjecture a certainty. There was no other bed-covering than a thin woollen blanket full of holes. The chimney was closed hermetically, and the fireplace, free from ashes, showed that there had been no fire since the beginning of the winter. Doubtless she had contemplated having a fire if the cold weather continued, for half of the garret was filled with wood piled up to the eaves.

Several days afterward he learned through the public journals that the *juge de paix* had found more than ten thousand francs concealed in the mattress of this miserable woman.

It would be easy to adduce other examples of avarice constituting, by its morbid development, as true a state of lunacy as is to be found in the annals of psychological medicine.

Jealousy, when it exists to an abnormal extent, may also overcome the reasoning powers of the individual. Maillet [2] admits this when he says that under the influence of this passion there is produced such an outburst of grief that the

---

[1] *Op. cit.*, t. ii, p. 293.

[2] " De l'essence des passions, étude psychologique et morale," Paris, 1877, p. 398.

mind is overthrown. Such was the jealousy of Othello. Many crimes are committed through the influence of this passion, and the plea of insanity is often set up in behalf of the offenders against the law. Some are probably insane, others have simply acted through heat of passion. The difference between these conditions will be pointed out when we come to the subject of diagnosis. It may, however, be said now that, to constitute insanity to such an extent as to render the individual irresponsible for his acts, it must be shown that the emotion had really become ungovernable, that he had endeavored to subjugate it to his intellect and will, and that he was not merely yielding to a vicious propensity which he might have controlled.

Among the emotional monomanias, *nostalgia*, or the morbid state of mind produced by the desire to return home, is worthy of some special consideration. It is more frequently met with among sailors and soldiers, who are more or less restrained in the ability to return home, than among others. Indeed, the consciousness that the individual can do so if he chooses is of itself sufficient to prevent any development of the condition in question, while, on the other hand, the conviction that he is separated from his home and friends, without the possibility of returning to them, is a powerful predisposing cause of the disorder.

During the recent civil war I had the opportunity of observing a great many cases of nostalgia. As a rule, they occurred in young soldiers who were drafted into service, but, owing to the facility with which after the development of severe symptoms sick furloughs were obtained, deaths from this cause were infrequent. I have, however, in my earlier military service, witnessed one case in which there was a fatal termination.

Although there is ordinarily in an active campaign sufficient diversion for the mind of such a character as to prevent the soldier fixing his thoughts for any great length of time on home and its associations, yet when winter comes, or when from other causes it is impossible to continue active operations, or when garrisoning posts, where but little variety marks the days as they drag slowly along, the mind of the soldier who has a home instinctively turns to the fireside he has left. Imagination pictures to him the events that are there occurring; at night he dreams of them, awaking in the morning to pass another weary day in pining for the companionship of those he loves, and the scenes amid which he was born and has lived. The continuation of such emotions eventually produces a morbid condition of the mind, and with it marked disorder in the functional operations of the organism. The most prominent physical state is a general emaciation from want of appetite, and defect in the process of digestion and assimilation. Obstinate constipation alternates with exhausting attacks of diarrhœa, and sometimes a typhoid condition is induced, and the patient quickly succumbs.

At first, the mental phenomena are those of intense apathy. Nothing rouses the patient from the hebetude which exists, and which is apparent in every expression of his face and every word he utters. He cares for nothing. He only wishes to be left alone to indulge in the thoughts of home which are constantly passing through his mind. At a later stage there may be delirium, characterized by incoherence of speech, and muscular agitation and illusions and hallucinations are not uncommon. In these the scenes of his native farm or village, the appearance of friends, their voices, play a prominent part. Finally, gastro-intestinal symptoms become fixed, the delirium is more pronounced, the stupor more profound, and death closes the scene.

It was in this way that I saw a young Alsacian, a recruit in the Second U. S. Dragoons, die, in the summer of 1849, on the plains between Fort Leavenworth and Santa Fe.

But, even when the affection is in its last stage, the prospect of a return to his home will often cause the patient to rally. The promise of a furlough is, as Delasiauve [1] says, a touchstone before which the symptoms speedily vanish.

On the other hand, the music of some familiar song aggravates the deplorable condition. So strong is the influence of music that it has often been found necessary to prohibit the regimental bands playing airs which could recall or freshen the memories of home.

Some nations afford more examples of nostalgia than others. As a general rule, the more mountainous and wild the country, the more prone are the natives to nostalgia when removed from it. The Swiss, the Savoyards, the Laplanders, are peculiarly the subjects of this affection. The American

[1] " Nostalgie," *Journal de médecine mentale*, t. v, 1865, p. 238.

Indian also readily dies of grief if separated from the scenes amid which he has lived. On the contrary, the negro is little liable to the affection, even when forcibly abducted from his home and sold into slavery. So far as my observation extends, the Anglo-Saxon race exhibits little proclivity to nostalgia. The cause of this immunity is doubtless to be found in the fact that this race is, above all others, especially the American branch of it, the least attached to localities.

Young persons are more subject to nostalgia than individuals of mature age. In the army this is particularly the case, almost all the examples of it occurring in soldiers who have not reached their twenty-first year.

The best means of preventing nostalgia is to provide occupation both for the mind and the body. Idleness is the great immediate cause, obviously for the reason that time and opportunity are afforded for the indulgence of the imagination. Thus it is that the affection is apt to occur among the inmates of hospitals, especially in those who are wounded and confined to their beds, though capable of fully exercising their minds. Soldiers placed in hospitals near their homes are always more liable to nostalgia than those who are inmates of hospitals situated in the midst of or in the vicinity of the army to which they belong. In the one case the reminiscences of home are more powerfully brought before the mind, while in the other the current of thought is more liable to run in another direction. Besides, being near one's home is always a stimulus to the hope of reaching it, which expectation not being realized, the nostalgic condition is developed, while, when it is certain that under no circumstances can a return to one's fireside take place, the mind accepts the terms so imperatively imposed, and ceases to hope for what is impossible of attainment. Baudens[1] very strongly insists upon the carrying out of this principle in the location of hospitals, and in the regulations which should prevail relative to sending men home when they are temporarily disabled. The recent civil war in this country likewise furnishes ample experience of the correctness of the views here laid down.

That nostalgia is a form of insanity has been recognized from the earliest periods of the scientific study of the subject.

[1] " La guerre en Crimée," Paris, 1858, p. 36.

Pinel[1] regarded it as a species of melancholia. Esquirol[2] cites it as one of the causes of suicide, the Swiss and Scotch soldiers being especially prone to kill themselves under the influence of the despair which constitutes one of its most prominent symptoms. Delasiauve[3] considers it as evidently belonging to the order of partial moral manias. Benoist de la Grandieu[4] speaks of it as a neurosis of the brain, characterized by the inability of the patient to overcome a depressing passion—remembrance. And Haspel,[5] while affirming that it is not insanity, says :

" There is with nostalgics a distraction which is not usual, which may even lead to a certain incoherence of ideas, but which only in exceptional cases passes to such a degree as to constitute mental alienation. The intelligence, doubtless, is weakened, depressed, but not abolished ; there is a paucity of ideas and a feebleness in their production, and of words with which to give them expression, but they are always logical. The course of the ideas is slower than is natural, and their circle is narrowed, but that is all. The will is subjugated and in a condition of inertia and impotence, but the reason is not dethroned. There is a complete consciousness of exciting circumstances ; and, though the subjects of nostalgia are tormented by ideas which are sad and strongly melancholic in character, they are yet not insane."

It may certainly be said of this last expression of opinion that it is not justified by the immediately preceding statements.

Rey,[6] in an elaborate article, expresses the opinion that nostalgia is a disease in which there is organic perturbation with corresponding functional trouble, due primarily to a psychic lesion of the passion of remembrance. I may anticipate here what I will have to say relative to the treatment of insanity in all its forms by stating that nostalgia is not an affection in which much is to be gained by the mere administration of medicines. The emotion of hope, when once aroused, will do more than the whole dispensary in dispelling all symp-

---

[1] " Nosographie philosophique," etc., 5ième édition, Paris, 1813, t. iii, p. 97.

[2] " Des maladies mentales," Paris, 1838, t. i, p. 268.   *Op. et loc. cit.*, p. 232.

[3] *Op. et loc. cit.*

[4] " De la nostalgie ou mal du pays," Paris, 1873.

[5] " De la nostalgie," " Mémoires de l'académie de médecine," Paris, 1874.

[6] Art. " Nostalgie," in *Nouveau dictionnaire de médecine et de chirurgie pratiques*, t. xxiv, Paris, 1877.

toms of the disease, and in some cases it may be necessary for the military surgeon to send the nostalgic soldier to his home in order to save his life. This, however, should be done with all possible precautions to prevent his comrades becoming acquainted with the fact. If it is impossible to separate him from the army, all means calculated to amuse, to interest, and to occupy the mind should be brought into requisition.

Anger, the love of gambling, ambition, and other emotions may likewise, through excess, become insanities, but there is nothing special to be said of them different from what has been brought forward in regard to love, pride, and vanity, avarice and jealousy.

The emotion of *fear* in its relations to mental derangement requires, however, a more extended consideration, and to this division of the subject the attention of the reader is now invited.

Passing over the subject of fear, in the presence of real or apparent danger, and which by its intensity may cause insanity or even death, we come to those morbid fears which are experienced by some persons without the existence of any external cause, but solely in consequence of a disordered state of the nervous system. They may be either general and ill-defined or special, being experienced in one direction only.

Panophobia.—By panophobia is to be understood a form of mental derangement in which there is an imperfectly defined sense of fear ; an apprehension that something is about to happen to the detriment of the individual without any clear perception of the nature of the impending evil.

Usually there are prodromatic symptoms, consisting both of mental and physical phenomena. The individual is restless, anxious, sleeps badly, has abnormal sensations, such as a feeling of constriction, weight, fulness, or pain in the head. There is often an uncomfortable feeling at the pit of the stomach, and something similar in the legs, constituting the condition known as *anxietas tibiarum.* These are not inspired by illusions, hallucinations, or delusions, though these may all be developed in the course of the disease.

The countenance of the patient expresses the state of the mind. The eyes glance wildly or furtively about the apartment, the senses seem to be on the alert and to be morbidly acute, and the movements are those of a person on the lookout for and fearful of an attack of some kind or other. The conversation is mostly on the subject that fills the mind of the individual. " I know something will happen to me," said a lady to me a few mornings since ; "it is useless to reassure me, for you do not feel what I feel. I cannot tell you what it will be, but something terrible is impending." Ere long the symptoms increase in intensity, but never in definiteness, and the subject weeps and wrings her hands over expectant troubles and dangers which she cannot explain.

Cases of this disorder are by no means rare. The citation of one or two of the most striking that have come under my observation will give a clearer idea of the phenomena than any abstract description :

Mrs. K. consulted me November 10, 1880. She had been married seven years, but had never been pregnant. She was about twenty-seven years of age. For several weeks she had been unable to sleep more than two or three hours each night. Lying in bed awake was extremely unpleasant to her. She could not read, for the effort to do so made her head ache, so she generally passed the greater part of the night walking the floor or sitting at the window looking at the heavens or into the street. Toward morning she became completely exhausted, and then was able to sleep, as I have said, two or three hours.

One cause of her wakefulness was the apprehension that something would happen to her in her sleep. The foundation of this fear she based upon the fact that during the past year her father and two aunts had met with serious accidents while asleep. Her father, nearly seventy years of age, had lost the use of his arm from having lain upon it all night, and thus producing paralysis. One aunt had died from cerebral hæmorrhage, and the other had fallen out of bed and broken her thigh. She herself had several times walked in her sleep.

During nearly the whole period that she was awake she was in a constant state of apprehension lest something would occur to injure her. What it was that was going to happen she could not imagine, and, if questioned in regard to any probable event, always answered in the negative. I ran through the whole list of fire, murderous attacks, buildings falling on her, horses running away, mad bulls, hydrophobic dogs, poisoning, etc., to all of which she replied that she did not think it would be any of those things, but that something would happen. At times she got relief from her fears, but the least excitement would renew them in all their violence. Coming to visit me had excited the fear that I would do something to her, or that I would tell her something unfavorable to her recovery, or that the excitement consequent on seeing a strange physician might prove injurious. Her friends said she had never been more specific in her declarations, but, when asked what I would do, or what I would tell her, or what the excitement would produce, she did not know.

While in my consulting-room she walked up and down the floor, looking wildly about her, and gulping as if affected with the *globus hystericus*. When I asked her what she was afraid of, she wrung her hands together and said, " Oh, I do not know, I do not know; but I am sure I will never get away safely ; something will happen to me, I am sure." Then she opened each door in turn, then looked out of the windows, and then began to sob and moan.

In a few minutes she became more composed, but she would not go into my examination-room, and it was only after great persuasion that I succeeded in getting an ophthalmoscopic examination. I found double optic neuritis, though she had never complained of any failure of sight.

I at once gave her two drachms of the bromide of sodium in a single dose, and directed that she should take for three days a drachm three times each day. At the end of that time she was very decidedly better, and, under the continued use of the bromide, in doses of fifteen grains three times a day, she was in less than a month entirely well. During that period the nape of the neck was cauterized with the white-hot platina disk four times, and her bowels were kept well open with aloetic purgatives.

In the case of a lady whom I saw only a few days ago, the symptoms, though not of so long a duration, were even more intense at times, though she enjoyed periods of almost complete relief from the morbid apprehensions with which she was affected. Her physical symptoms were similar to those of the patient whose clinical history has just been given—that is, pain in the head, insomnia, restlessness, noises in the ears, etc. But, when the mental phenomena were at their height, her face and ears became very red, the temporal arteries were

27

enlarged and pulsated strongly, and the pupils were contracted to mere points.

But she came to see me of her own accord, and was willing
to do anything or to submit to any treatment, however harsh,
if she could only be relieved of her terrible apprehensions.
She sobbed and cried and wrung her hands, at the same time
exclaiming that she "knew nothing would happen. How
could anything happen? and yet I am afraid! I am afraid!
Oh, what shall I do, what shall I do? You will cure me, won't
you?" and so on at intervals during her visit of nearly an
hour.

She is still under treatment, but, from the good results
thus far obtained, a favorable termination may, I think, be
confidently expected.

This patient was subject to hallucinations of sight and
hearing, especially of the latter. Thus, she often heard voices
telling her there was no hope for her, that she was about to
die, and that she could shorten her anguish of mind by taking
her life.

In both these patients there was gastric dyspepsia and
constipation, the former evidenced by enormous eructations
of gas and a feeling of weight in the stomach, beginning
shortly after eating, and lasting two or three hours. The
food, in fact, underwent fermentation instead of digestion, as
it does in other cases of nervous dyspepsia.

But in neither, nor in others of similar character that have
come under my observation, was there any derangement of
the intellect when the mind could be brought to look calmly
at the situation. The emotion of fear was, however, so intensely manifested that when it was at its height there was
some intellectual confusion, and perhaps some delusions.
These latter, however, had no permanency, and were of the
most undefined character. A few words of reassurance and
confidence sufficed to dissipate them.

Dagonet[1] states that patients suffering from the affection
in question, which he describes under the name of "anxious
lypemania" (lypemanie anxieuse), are very often tormented
by suicidal impulses, which have no other motive than the
desire to terminate for themselves an existence which for
the crimes they have committed would otherwise end on the

[1] "Nouveau traité élémentaire et pratique des maladies mentales," Paris, 1876,
p. 241.

scaffold. I have never seen this symptom in simple panophobia, nor can I believe that it exists in the affection unless it is complicated with delusions. On the contrary, the patients are afraid of death, and at times they are afraid, as they say, that they may become insane and commit suicide, but not even hallucinations of hearing of the most pointed character have ever in my experience suggested the idea of self-destruction. Neither do I agree with him in the opinion that the prognosis of panophobia is bad. One of my cases, that of a young woman from New London, terminated in chronic melancholia, but all the others, seven in number, made good recoveries. It is very much more frequent in women than in men, according to my experience, and appears to be sometimes connected with ovarian disorder.

Undoubtedly panophobia may pass into insanity of a more pronounced form, and I have already given a case in which this result ensued, intellectual monomania with depression being the sequel. It is, however, equally certain that there are cases in which there is no tendency to a change of type.

But, besides this condition of general and undefined fear, there are other affections in which the emotion is manifested in a special, determinate, and restricted way. One of the first of these, recognized and described as a distinct form of morbid fear, is the fear of being alone in a large place, or, as it was designated by Westphal,[1] who first systematically described it, *agoraphobia*. Gélineau,[2] with perhaps greater philological accuracy, calls it *kenophobia*, and Legrand du Saulle[3] describes it under the name of the *fear of spaces*. As all these terms imply, there is a morbid fear on the part of the individual to go into large places, or into the street, or the open country.

But cases of the affection, without any special significance being attached to them, were observed long before Westphal published his paper on the subject. Thus it is stated of Pascal[4] that, in 1654, while driving on the Pont de Neuilly in a carriage with four or six horses, the leaders took the bits in

---

[1] "Archiv. für Psychiatrie," Heft i, 1871.

[2] "De la kenophobie ou peur des espaces (agoraphobie des allemands)," Paris, 1880.

[3] "Étude clinique sur la peur des espaces (agoraphobie des allemands)," Paris, 1878.

[4] "Preface aux œuvres de Blaise Pascal," par Bossut, Paris, 1819, t. i, p. xxxii.

their mouths and plunged so violently that, breaking the traces, they were precipitated into the Seine. The danger to the inmates was very great, but, happily, they escaped without other injury than a great fright. The incident, however, made so powerful an impression on Pascal that he ever afterward imagined that there was an abyss at his left side, or, rather, he knew there was not, but he had the morbid fear of falling into a large space. It was in vain that arguments were used with him; he could not overcome the fear, and hence he kept a screen on the side at which he feared the chasm was situated, so that he might by the device reassure his mind.[1] Gélineau[2] thinks that the great man was the subject of agoraphobia.

Benedict reported a case of agoraphobia, but failed to regard it in its true light. He considered the phenomena as being due to visual troubles, overlooking altogether the centric character of the affection.

As soon as the subject of agoraphobia finds himself alone, for instance in the street, he is seized with the most intense fear. He cannot advance a step, he cannot go back; he can only stand and tremble, with the perspiration starting from every pore, and terror depicted on every feature of his countenance. His head seems to go round, the houses appear to be in motion, and he clutches for support at an area-railing, a lamp-post, the side of a house, or crouches in his fright on the pavement. As soon as some one comes to his relief and leads him into a house, his alarm disappears, and the physical manifestations of his fright also rapidly vanish.

Mr. X., a Cuban gentleman, was sent to me by my friend, Dr. Desvernine, of Havana, to be treated for an affection from which he had suffered for several years, and which had baffled all means of treatment. I found that he would not go out into the street unless he went in a carriage, and that, in passing from the vehicle to the door of a house, he required the support of two men—one on each side of him. In his apartments at the hotel he walked freely, and would go up and down stairs without difficulty. As soon, however, as he found himself out on the door-step his terror began. It seemed to him as if everything was in motion, and as though it would be impossible for him to live another minute unless assistance

---

[1] See, for a full discussion of the subject, "L'amulette de Pascal," par F. Lélut, Paris, 1846.   [2] *Op. cit.*, p. 4.

were given him. At the same time, his brain appeared to be in motion within his skull. A cold sweat broke out over his body, especially his forehead, his heart palpitated violently, his arms and legs trembled with the terror that inspired him, and every now and then a severe spasm would seize him, and his limbs would be strongly contracted and his body bent forward in the shape of a bow. At night his alarm was less strongly manifested, and he would walk out if some one took his arm. During the day, however, he could not be persuaded to do more than to take the few steps necessary from a carriage to the door, and then an attendant had to take his arm.

Under medical and moral treatment he improved so greatly that I succeeded in getting him to walk from his hotel to my residence daily, a friend walking by his side and a carriage following him closely. Then he walked several miles through the streets in the lower part of the city, a friend still by his side, and eventually he came to my house alone, but this last was a severe task for him. He repeated it, however, on several occasions, and, when he returned home at the end of about two months, he was almost entirely free from apprehension when out in the streets.[1] He was still, however, nervous, irritable, and disposed to be hypochondriacal.

In another case, that of a gentleman from Connecticut, sent to me by Dr. Hubbard, of Bridgeport, there were similar symptoms, although not manifested to the same extent. There was a like terror, a feeling of distention in the head, and more or less confusion of ideas if the attempt were made to go out of the house into the street. This patient is still under treatment, but at the end of a week there is very decided improvement. These are the only cases of agoraphobia that have come within the range of my personal experience.

Although agoraphobia may exist as a primary disease, it undoubtedly often owes its origin to some previously existing morbid condition. Thus, it may be grafted upon the hysterical state, upon dyspepsia, or gout. The vertiginous condition met with in certain epileptics, or patients suffering from cere-

---

[1] On the 12th of September, 1882, about a month after this gentleman's arrival in New York, I operated on him in presence of Dr. Rubino, of Naples, and Dr. Cisneros and Dr. G. M. Hammond, of New York, for abscess of the liver, removing about seven ounces of pus from the organ. A perfect recovery followed, and to this date, January 19, 1883, there has been no return.

bral syphilis, such as the case described by Webber,[1] and which Gélineau[2] mistakes for agoraphobia, is certainly not this affection. Indeed, Webber's case and it have very little in common. In one of my cases, the first, there was dyspepsia which had existed for several years ; in the other, there had been excessive emotional disturbance in business matters.

In neither of my patients was there any intellectual disturbance, nor were there illusions or hallucinations. They were capable of reasoning, with entire correctness, in regard to their unfortunate state. In both of them—and the same appears to be true of all instances—if there was a certainty in their minds that, if anything happened to them, relief was at hand, they had little or no difficulty in going out. It was curious to observe how, in the case of the Cuban patient, as the condition became alleviated, less and less security was required. At first two attendants, one on each side, were necessary, then one holding his arm, then one walking alongside of him but not touching him, then a carriage at the distance of a few feet behind him, and so on till he was able to walk in the street without reliance on external aid. Bourdin[3] reports a case in which a man would risk himself on steep rocks and jump from one to the other with daring, provided there was below him a projection or a spot of ground on which he could fix his eyes. Without this his terror was such that he could not take a step.

Cordes,[4] who himself suffered from agoraphobia, regards it as merely a symptom of certain depressed states of the nervous system. It begins, according to his personal experience, in a simple fear of some unknown danger, which goes on increasing in intensity, and which is accompanied with palpitations, præcordial anxiety, flashes of heat, tinnitus, vertigo, heaviness, and numbness of the extremities—all working upon him at once and producing the most unsurmountable terror. He assimilates it to the vertigo a stomacho læso of Trousseau, from which, however, it is very different.

Regarding it as being due to a hyperæmic condition of the brain, I have treated my cases with the bromides of sodium and ergot, and the moral agent of insisting on the patient at-

---

[1] *Boston Medical and Surgical Journal.*   [2] *Op. cit.*, p. 26.
[3] "De l'horreur du vide," Paris, 1878.
[4] " Archiv für Psychiatrie und Nervenkrankheiten," 1872, Heft iii.

tempting to rely on himself in open places. Arthius reports two cases cured by statical electricity, and this means seemed to be of service in the one case in which I employed it, as did also cups repeatedly applied to the nucha.

The name *claustrophobia* has been given, by Dr. Verga, of Milan, to a morbid fear the very opposite in its characteristics to that just described. It consists, as the name implies, of a terror of closed places, the phenomena in other respects not being essentially different from those of agoraphobia. Cases similar to those given by Verga have been reported by Dr. Raggi, of Bologna ; by Meschede, at the Congress of German Naturalists and Physicians, held at Cassel in 1878 ; and by Professor Ball,[1] of Paris. A single case has come under my own observation.

In one of Professor Ball's two cases, the patient, a married lady, whose father had been insane, and who was the mother of three children, two of whom were imbecile and one epileptic, had been in good physical and mental health till an attack of typhoid fever deranged both her mind and body. She had attacks of cerebral congestion, was affected with extreme sadness, and had thoughts of suicide. One day she went with some friends to visit the tower of Saint Jacques, and, while making the ascent, was suddenly seized with terror. The idea occurred to her that some one had shut the door below, and that she would not be able to get out. She could not go up another step, notwithstanding the assurances of those who were with her, and descended as rapidly as she could to the ground, overcome with fright. As soon as she was out in the open air, the feeling of alarm disappeared. From this time on she had similar feelings whenever she was alone in a closed room. Nothing, she said, would induce her to remain in such a place. If the attempt be made, she is seized with vertigo, her head becomes confused, her terrors reappear, and she no longer knows what she does. The opening of the doors and windows gives relief.

Professor Ball concludes that there is a special form of delirium characterized by the fear of closed places, and that it is a true psychosis and not a mere sensorial trouble.

In the single case which has occurred in my own experience, the patient, a gentleman engaged in manufacturing

[1] "De la claustrophobie," "Annales médico-psychologiques," November, 1879, p. 378.

cotton goods, had suffered for several weeks with the symptoms of cerebral hyperæmia, the principal of which was insomnia. The cause was probably to be found in excessive anxiety due to business troubles.

He first experienced the phenomena of claustrophobia while ascending in a hotel elevator to his room on the fifth floor. A sudden terror seized upon him; he clung to the man who had charge of the apparatus, his head swam, a whistling noise was heard in his ears, and a cold prespiration broke out over his body. As soon as he stepped out into the hall above, the symptoms disappeared. He went to his room, feeling a slight degree of nausea, but, on entering the apartment, the feelings reappeared, though with less intensity. He opened the windows and the door, and then felt more at ease. Since then he has been unable to enter any small apartment without experiencing similar feelings, unless there are other persons present, and even then at times, his terror gets the better of him. A railway car is especially alarming, and the small ones used on the street railways he cannot enter at all. He stands on the platform in all weathers. Even the idea of entering a carriage excites apprehension unless it is an open one, and then he can travel in it with ease. Nothing, however, would induce him to get into a close vehicle, such as an omnibus or stage. There is no intellectual aberration with this gentleman. He does not believe anything is going to happen; he simply fears that some indescribable occurrence will take place, and this fear excites such an ungovernable terror that he becomes powerless to move or even to speak.

The foregoing extract from my note-book is dated October 29, 1879. I attached no particular significance to the special phenomena of the condition till I read Professor Ball's paper on the subject. Since that date I have seen the patient several times. I treated him in a manner similar to that I had used in the cases of agoraphobia, with equally good results. He has remained free from the affection.

Dr. Beard[1] has described several kinds of these morbid fears, all of which have a marked resemblance to each other, differing only in the cause. Thus, there is an *astraphobia*, or the fear of lightning; an *anthropophobia*, or the fear of society; and a *monophobia*, or the fear of being alone.

[1] "A Practical Treatise on Nervous Exhaustion," etc., New York, 1880, p. 27, *et seq.*

Of these two latter, several instances have come under my notice.

One species, which appears to me to be more characteristic than any other, and of which several examples have occurred in my own experience and in that of other physicians, I propose to consider at some length. This is *mysophobia* (Μύσος, *defilement, pollution, contamination,* and φόβος, *fear*), the fear of pollution, and was described by me in a paper read before the New York Neurological Society, April 7, 1879.[1]

In all, fourteen cases up to the present time constitute the basis of my experience. Of the first seven cases my notes are not very complete. I was not particularly impressed with the fact of the distinctive character of the affection, although in all I find it stated that the subjects had morbid fears in regard to pollution. Of the other cases, I select the following as exhibiting the features of the disorder :

M. G., a lady, thirty years of age, and a widow for three years, consulted me February 20, 1877, for what was considered to be incipient insanity, and an affection in all probability requiring, it was feared, incarceration in a lunatic asylum. The patient was quiet and orderly in her demeanor, and, so far as her friends' accounts went, entirely sane except upon the one point of fear of contamination, which was exhibited by mental distress and the practice of repeatedly washing her hands without there being obvious cause for so doing. She was perfectly coherent in regard to her clinical history, and I obtained from her the following account of the origin and progress of the disease, which I transcribe in her own language :

"I was, about six months ago, reading a newspaper one evening, when I came across an account of a man who, it was believed, had contracted small-pox from handling bank-notes which had been a short time previously in the possession of a person suffering from that disease. The circumstance made a deep impression on my mind, and, as I had only a few moments before counted quite a number of notes, the idea struck me that perhaps they had been handled by some person with a contagious disease of some kind or other. I had washed my hands just after counting these notes, but, thinking that I had not possibly removed all the taint, I washed them again. I went to bed, feeling quite uncomfortable, and

[1] "Mysophobia," *Neurological Contributions*, No. 1, 1879.

the next morning paid more than usual attention to the washing of my hands. I then recollected that I had placed the notes in a drawer of my dressing-table, in contact with linen which I had proposed putting on that day. I changed my intention, however, and selected some from another drawer instead, sending the other to the laundry. I then put on a pair of gloves, took out the notes, placed them in a letter-envelope, and had the drawer thoroughly washed with soap and water.

"Reflection upon the matter brought to mind the fact that, after counting the notes, I had touched various things before washing my hands. I could not recall what these things were, and hence I was made very uncomfortable, for the idea occurred to me that I must have touched some of these things after washing my hands, and that, therefore, I was still in danger. The very dress that I wore then, was the same that I had on now, and my hands had been more less in contact with it all the morning. I felt myself, accordingly, forced to wash my hands, to take off the dress, and again to wash my hands.

"From that I went on from one thing to another. There was no end to the series. I washed everything I was in the habit of touching, and then washed my hands. Even the water was a medium for pollution, for, no matter how thoroughly I wiped my hands after washing in it, a portion still remained, and this had to be washed off, and then again the hands washed. There was no end to it. The soap became connected in my mind with contamination, and I never used the same piece twice.

"Now, I can touch nothing without feeling irresistibly impelled to wash my hands afterward. If I am prevented doing so, I experience the most horrible sense of fear. I am always looking at my hands to ascertain if I can see anything on them, and I have a lens which I use to aid my eyesight. I have no particular apprehension of contracting small-pox or any other disease that I can specify. It is an overpowering feeling that I shall be defiled in some mysterious way, that presses on me with a force that I cannot resist. As to shaking hands with any person, nothing would persuade me to do so unless I had on gloves at the time.

"And, lately, even gloves do not seem to afford me entire protection. I know they are porous, and that, therefore, the subtle influence, whatever it may be, is capable of passing through them to my hands."

On my asking this lady if she really believed in the theory she had constructed, she answered that at times she was convinced that she was in error, but only for a short period, as the original ideas returned in full force; that, when reasoned with in regard to the absurdity of her notions, she was persuaded for the moment that she was wrong, but as soon as she was left to herself she was back in the old train of thought.

The expression of the patient was one of anxiety. As she sat talking to me she was continually rubbing her hands together, and looking at them closely every moment. After I had felt her pulse, she took a handkerchief from her pocket, moistened it with a little cologne-water which she had in a phial, and wiped the spot which my fingers had touched.

To test the sensibility of the hands, I made use of the æsthesiometer, without, however, detecting any abnormal condition; but she at once took another handkerchief and wiped all the places touched, with cologne, as before. She had a pocket full of clean handkerchiefs, never using the same one twice, and putting the soiled ones in another pocket.

She had given up reading, because handling books or newspapers was, she was sure, a certain source of contamination. At first this idea was only applied to books from a library to which she was a subscriber, but latterly it had been extended to all printed matter.

Further examination showed that she was subject to almost continual headache, mainly at the vertex, and that she had occasional attacks of dizziness. She slept badly, frequently getting only one or two hours of disturbed slumber. Her pulse was 96, weak and irregular. The heart-sounds were normal, but the action of the heart was feeble, with an irregular rhythm and an occasional intermittence. The ophthalmoscope showed nothing abnormal beyond a possible slight increase in the red tinge of the disk.

Menstruation was regular in every respect, but there was decided gastric dyspepsia. The phosphates of the urine were in great excess; in other respects there was no derangement of this excretion. No hereditary tendency to insanity or other neurotic condition existed. Previous to the occurrence of the mental disorder in question, she had been of equable temperament, and not at all disposed to melancholy or depression of spirits. Now, however, her mind was filled with the most gloomy forebodings and apprehensions. Her life was one continued state of fear lest she had become contaminated by something she had touched, and had forgotten to wash her hands after the contact, or had imperfectly washed them.

So far as could be discovered, there was no existing source of trouble or anxiety. She was in affluent circumstances, and had lived happily with her husband, who had, however, died, a year after marriage, of phthisis, with which he had been affected for several years. There had been no pregnancy.

Another case was that of a young lady, aged eighteen, tall and slender, whom I first saw January 23, 1879. From herself and her mother I obtained the following history:

About eighteen months previously she had gone to stay in the country with some friends, and on one occasion slept in a farm-house. On her return home she at once took a bath, and had her head, the hair of which was very long and thick, thoroughly washed ; to her great surprise and disgust it was found to be full of lice. She had always been exceedingly cleanly as regarded her person, and the shock she experienced on learning of the presence of these parasites completely unnerved her. She insisted on repeated washings of the head with soap, carbolic acid, and other detergent and disinfectant substances, and even then was not convinced that all the vermin had been destroyed.

This was the starting-point of all the subsequent mental disturbance. Little by little the idea became rooted that she could not escape sources of contamination, that other persons might defile her in some way or other, and that the various articles about her might also possess a like power. She was particularly careful in regard to avoiding children, and would not on any account allow a child to touch or even to approach her closely. When she went out into the street she carefully gathered her skirts together on passing any person, for fear that she might by mere contact be contaminated. She spent hours every day in minutely examining and cleansing her combs and brushes, and was even then not satisfied that they were thoroughly purified.

As to her hands, she washed them, as her mother informed me she had ascertained by actual count, over two hundred times a day. She could touch nothing without feeling irresistibly impelled to scrub them with soap and water. Gradually the idea of lice had been lost sight of, and for several months previously to her coming to me the fear of pollution had had a much more extended source. She could not define with any exactness what the *materies pollutionis* was, though she imagined it to be something that was capable of doing her bodily injury in some subtle manner by being absorbed into her system through her hands or other parts.

Some little time before coming under my observation she had extended her fear of contamination to the soap with which she felt compelled to wash her hands, and then she was obliged to wash them again in pure water in order to remove all traces of the soap. Then, as the towel with which she wiped them dry had been washed with soap, she rinsed her hands in water, and allowed them to dry without the aid of a towel.

In removing her clothes at night preparatory to going to bed, she carefully avoided touching them with her hands, because then she would not have sufficient opportunity for washing. She, therefore, had some one else to loosen the fastenings, and then she allowed her garments to drop on the floor, where she left them. Nothing would have persuaded her to touch any of her under-clothing after it had been worn till it had been washed. A great source of anxiety with her was the fact that her clothes were washed in the laundry with the clothing of other people ; but she saw no practicable way of escape from this circumstance. It nevertheless made her very unhappy.

When not washing her hands or examining her combs and brushes, she spent nearly all the rest of the day in carefully inspecting every article of furniture and dusting it many times.

Thus, her whole life is one continued round of trouble, anxiety, and fear. Her whole character and disposition have changed. She is suspicious of every person and of every thing.

She is subject to insomnia, frequent headaches, and loss of appetite. There are noises in her ears and flashes of light before the eyes, and an utter impossibility of concentrating the attention upon any other subject than the one which has obtained so complete a mastery over her. Her menstruation is scanty and somewhat painful, though regular in other respects.

Ophthalmoscopic examination showed the retinal vessels to be increased in size, and the choroids to be of a deeper hue than is ordinarily met with.

In conversing with this young lady, I had no difficulty in getting her to admit the absurdity of her ideas. She stated that whenever she reflected upon the subject she was convinced of their erroneous character, but that, nevertheless, she could not avoid acting as she did ; for, as soon as she was exposed to any possible source of contamination, the ideas returned in full force. It was only when she had, as she thought, done her best to cleanse her hands that she doubted the correctness of her notions, which had so thoroughly become a part of her mentality.

These cases are sufficient to show the nature and characteristics of general mysophobia. Interesting cases of the affection have since been described by Seguin,[1] Russell,[2] and Shaw,[3] and I have heard of others of which I have not been able to obtain full particulars.

But there is another form of the disease—two examples of which have recently come under my notice—and this is a fear of contamination from some one particular source. In one of the instances the patient, a distinguished mining engineer, had a morbid fear that he would be polluted in some inexplicable way if he sat down on chairs or benches used by other people unless there was a metallic plate between his body and the seat. He, therefore, carried about with him a copper plate about twelve inches in diameter and covered with black cloth. Whenever he sat down he interposed this plate, and thus considered that he had secured his safety. He was particularly apprehensive in regard to the cushioned seats of railway-cars, carriages, omnibuses, churches, theatres, etc. A plain wooden chair did not cause him so very much terror, but the idea of the others excited the most uncomfortable sensations, both mental and physical—similar in general features to those experienced by the subjects of agoraphobia or claustrophobia.

In the other case, which was that of a lady of this city, there was a combination of a morbid fear and an impulse to expose herself to the action of the source of the fear. Thus,

[1] " A Case of Mysophobia," *Archives of Medicine*, August, 1880, p. 102.
[2] " Mysophobia," etc., *Alienist and Neurologist*, October, 1880, p. 529.
[3] " A Case of Mysophobia," *Archives of Medicine*, October, 1881, p. 199.

she had read in the newspapers that persons had contracted diseases in some way or other from moistening postage-stamps with the tongue, and the fear soon afterward was excited in her that she might become affected with some horrible disease by like means. Notwithstanding the terror with which she was inspired, she felt impelled to expose herself to the danger she feared, and could with difficulty refrain from licking not only the stamps she used, but those employed by other members of her family. She was hence in a continual state of mental inquietude from the action of two kinds of emotional disturbance, and suffered the greatest agony in consequence. Not being always able to restrain herself, she would ask any one she saw about to close a letter to allow her to affix the stamp, and having performed the act, would be seized with the most overpowering fear of the consequences of what she had done, during which she would weep and wring her hands, and utter the most poignant expressions of the anguish she was suffering. It finally became impossible to keep postage-stamps in the family ; but she would buy them and stick them on envelopes, and then experience a repetition of her terror at the thought that she had again rendered herself liable to disease. I saw this patient several times, but, before much progress was made toward her relief, she was summoned to Europe by the sudden illness of her husband, and I lost sight of her.

Dr. Willis P. King,[1] of Sedalia, Missouri, has described an interesting case of *pyrophobia*, or the fear of fire, occurring in a ten years' old boy. Among other symptoms of the condition in question, it is stated that he went repeatedly during the day from room to room and inspected the stoves and the flues about the house. He went to bed at night protesting against the building of fires, and in the morning, when the cook began the preparations for breakfast, at the first noise of poker or shovel he would bound out of bed, not taking time to put on his trousers, and would hurry down to the kitchen to prevent the fire being made. He had to be watched by his mother during the preparation of the meal, and, as soon as the work was done, the fire had to be extinguished to allay his fears. He would deliberately extinguish the fire in the sitting-room against his mother's orders. On one occasion,

---

[1] "Case of Morbid Juvenile Pyrophobia," etc., *Alienist and Neurologist*, July, 1880, p. 345.

when the morning was cool, he succeeded, after a contest with his mother, in opening the stove-door and pouring a bucket of water over the fire. These contests were of daily occurrence. On all other subjects but that of fire he conversed rationally and intelligently. He was cured by quinine, the bromides, and the use of evaporating applications—ether—to the head.

These special morbid fears are not unlike those which some persons acquire relative to certain diseases. Thus, there is a *syphilophobia*, or the fear of syphilis ; a *hydrophobophobia*, or the fear of hydrophobia ; a *spermatophobia*, or the fear of spermatorrhœa, etc., many cases of which have come under my notice, and which are, doubtless, familiar to most physicians in large cities. The subjects of all these conditions struggle energetically against their fears, but they are rarely successful in overcoming them by their own unaided efforts. Though the intellect is scarcely if at all involved, they are, nevertheless, as truly insane for the time being as the most raving maniac, though, of course, to a less extent. Indeed, there are few more miserable beings in the world than he who fears that he is affected with spermatorrhœa, and few who show more terror than the subjects of hydrophobophobia. They generally yield promptly to proper medical, moral, and hygienic treatment.

b—EMOTIONAL MORBID IMPULSES.

Emotional morbid impulses differ from intellectual morbid impulses in that they have an emotion as their factor instead of an idea. They constitute a large and important part of that form of mental derangement described several years ago by Dr. Prichard under the name of moral insanity, but which have been designated by certain government experts in a recent notable criminal trial under the general head of "wickedness." In thus defining them, the experts in question placed themselves on record against the opinions of those alienists in this country and in Europe who are most competent to form a scientific opinion on a question of psychological medicine. Indeed, the number of alienists who do not believe in the existence of emotional morbid impulses as a form of insanity is not much greater than the number of experts for the prosecution in the trial in question.

Among these impulses is that which prompts to theft—*kleptomania*, as it is generally called. It is not so much from an exaggeration of the emotion of cupidity that kleptomaniacs exist as it is from the pure love of stealing. It is the act of taking what does not belong to them which is generally the source of the pleasure derived, and not the acquirement of the things stolen, which often are of no use, and are cast aside as soon as obtained and their very existence forgotten. As an instance in point, I cite from a recent communication[1] the particulars of an interesting case which occurred in my own experience:

"A young man, a student of law, suffered from an attack of scarlet fever. During the stage of convalescence, as he was one day sitting at the window looking out on the street, his attention was attracted by two men, each of whom wore a very large watch-chain. They passed on, and he thought nothing more of the circumstance till that night, when he awoke suddenly from a sound sleep with the idea that he must have those chains. He tried to dismiss the matter from his mind, but in vain. Do what he would, it constantly recurred to him; so he got up and sat down to think of the strange desire with which he had so suddenly become possessed. Two or three hours were passed in this way, and then, it being daylight, he dressed himself and went out to walk, hoping that exercise in the morning air would rid him of his infatuation. But the effect was very different from what he had anticipated, and, before he returned home, he had made up his mind that no pleasure in this life would be comparable to that he would derive from having the two watch-chains in his possession.

"He was in good circumstances, a graduate of a well-known college, and in all the relations of life had borne himself creditably; moreover, he had a very fine watch and chain which had been given him by his father.

"Five or six days elapsed, during which time the desire to obtain the watch-chains was the most prominent emotion of his mind. Hour after hour was passed in forming plans to get them into his possession, but there seemed to be no way by which his wish could be gratified. He watched from his window, he walked the streets, looking all around him, in the hope of seeing the men. He even went to several large jewelry establishments and inspected the watch-chains, with the

[1] "A Problem for Sociologists," *North American Review*, November, 1882, p. 424.

object of ascertaining if there were others like those on which his mind was set. He visited a large theatre and carefully scrutinized the audience, but all was to no purpose. Finally, one afternoon, as he was returning home from the office in which he was a student, he suddenly came face to face with one of the men he had previously observed. A glance was sufficient to show him that the watch-chain was still in its place. He at once turned and followed the man several blocks, till he observed him enter a jeweller's shop. He went in also. The man was talking to a salesman, and the watch and chain lay on a counter between them. The object of his desire was now within his reach. He stood by as if waiting his turn to be served, trembling with excitement and joy, his eyes riveted on the chain. He determined not to leave the shop without getting the chain into his possession by some means or other. Suddenly he felt that the time had come, and, without a moment's hesitation, he seized the watch and chain and dashed out of the door. The street was crowded, and twilight was just beginning. The cry of "Stop, thief!" was at once raised, and he was hotly pursued; but, after running a short distance, he contrived to mingle with the crowd, and, retracing his steps quietly, actually had the boldness to pass the jeweller's shop again. He reached his house safely, exhausted with the excitement he had undergone, but happy in the consciousness of having successfully accomplished half his self-appointed task.

"The gratification he experienced encouraged him to persevere in his efforts to get the other chain, and he continued on the lookout for the man who wore it. In the mean time he contemplated his acquisition with mingled feelings of pleasure and disgust. He had done more than he had intended, for he had no desire for the watch which he had stolen along with the chain. On the contrary, it was a source of great discomfort to him. Besides, although he was intensely gratified at possessing the chain, he could not disguise from himself the fact that he was a thief, and eligible to imprisonment for the crime of grand larceny. It was necessary to his peace of mind to return the watch, so he inclosed it in a box and sent it, with many precautions for insuring his own safety, to the jeweller from whose shop he had taken it, with the request that it might be returned to the owner. As to the chain, not valuing it for any use it might be to him, he wrapped it in a piece of India-rubber cloth and buried it in a hole which he dug for the purpose in the cellar. But after a time, from frequently analyzing his feelings, he perceived that the possession of the chain gave him no pleasure ; it was the act of taking it which was the source of the satisfaction he had experienced. He therefore dug it up, and sent it, also, back to the jeweller. He never saw either of the two men again, and gradually the desire to possess or obtain the other chain faded out of his mind.

" But about a year afterward he was attacked with wakefulness, which proved to be of the most intractable kind, and with pain in the head, vertigo, noises in the ears, hallucinations of hearing, and other symptoms of a disordered brain. He then came under my observation, and, in the course of the examination to which he was subjected, told the story which has just been related. He also stated that he remembered very distinctly that, when the dream to obtain the watch-chains first occurred to him, he had experienced a severe attack of vertigo, and almost fell from the chair on which he was sitting. He was not quite sure that he did not for an instant lose consciousness. On inquiry being made of the jeweller to whom he said he had returned the watch and chain, it was ascertained that the account he had given of the robbery and the restoration was entirely correct."

In another case, the patient, a young lady, who had been very carefully brought up, and who had for several years been an inmate of a large school, without having committed the slightest act against good morals, was suddenly seized with the desire to possess herself of all the small things belonging to others upon which she could lay her hands. Jewelry, gloves, handkerchiefs, fans, books, and even money, were taken from shops and private houses which she visited. No use was made of the articles. They were all, money included, thrown into a large drawer in an old piece of furniture which stood in an unused room. Finally she was detected, and a scandal was with great difficulty prevented. All the articles were discovered and returned quietly to their respective owners, and one or two importunate and impracticable tradesmen were silenced by considerable sums of money. Her father, believing his daughter's mind to be deranged, brought her to me, and no lengthened examination was necessary to convince me that she was the subject of brain disease. I found that she was sleepless, that she had repeated attacks of vertigo daily, that she had pain in her head, and at times more or less mental confusion. She spoke freely of the pilfering propensity to which she was subject, and of the great mental distress which it caused her. It was not from any desire to possess the articles stolen which induced her to take them, but an overpowering love for the act of stealing. The things, when once she had them in her possession, lost all interest for her, and she would willingly have restored them but for the shame attendant on the discovery that would have resulted, and the fear of the consequences. She knew perfectly well that it was both a sin and a crime to steal, and was perfectly aware of the consequences should she be detected. The desire, however, to appropriate to herself articles which came in her way was, as she said, absolutely irresistible. At least it could not be resisted without causing an amount of mental suffering the very idea of which filled her with horror. Once or twice she had for a time refrained from secreting things which she handled in shops she had visited ; but the anguish she had endured was such that she had been forced to return, and, on pretext of wishing to examine something else, to hide the articles in question in her muff or under her cloak. Then she felt comfortable, and, carrying them home, tossed them into the drawer without even looking at them.

While she was describing her condition, and was sobbing with unsuppressed emotion, I saw her quietly take a book from the table near which she sat. She did not look at it, but very stealthily put it under a sealskin jacket she was wearing. I said nothing at the time, but before she left the room I remarked to her, " If you are thinking of studying medicine, I would recommend you to begin with a book in the English language and of a more elementary character than the one you have under your jacket." She took it from its hiding-place at once and replaced it on the table. " You see how it is with me," she said ; "I was obliged to take the book." It was a volume of Wernicke's " Lehrbuch der Gehirnkrankheiten," not a word of which could she have read. A few days afterward I received by mail a bulky package, which, on opening, I found to contain a pair of my gloves, which, notwithstanding my vigilance, she had succeeded in abstracting from under my very eyes, and which she now returned, with the expression of her contrition.

I may anticipate here and say that, under the use of nuchal cauterization and the bromide of sodium, this lady entirely lost her impulse in about six weeks, and that she has remained well to this time—some six or seven months afterward.

Sometimes the impulse to steal does not extend beyond a single class of objects, and it may, as in the instance of the young man whose case I have given, be limited to one article, dying out when that article is acquired.

A few years ago a young man was arrested in this city for assaulting a young lady in the street. He was identified as a person who had committed many previous offences of a like character. His plan was to rush up to a young lady, seize her, throw her down, and take off her shoes, which he carried away with him. He did not attempt otherwise to injure her, or to take away any other article from her. On searching his trunks and drawers, they were found full of women's shoes. He said he had no use for them, and was actuated by an irresistible impulse which it was pleasant for him to gratify.

In another case, in regard to which I was consulted, the patient, a young man, eighteen years of age, had a desire, which he declared he could not resist, to steal books of whatever kind came within his reach. With him it was the love for the objects themselves that prompted him to theft. There was in this instance, as perhaps there is to some extent in all analogous cases, a decided weakness of the intellect. The love for books rarely prompted him to read any one of his acquisitions—which were many and valuable. He told his mother, a widow, that a gentleman had taken a great fancy to him, and gave him books in order that his mind might be improved by reading them. Finally, one night he attacked, in the streets of the town in which he lived, a smaller boy, who was carrying a package of books to the house of a purchaser. He knocked the boy down, and, taking the parcel, made off with it. He was arrested, however, and then all his misdeeds in the way of thieving from booksellers, libraries, and acquaintances were exposed. Although there was sufficient evidence to show not only the boy's insanity, but the hereditary character of his disorder, he was sent to the House of Correction, where he now is.

Kleptomaniacs can sometimes be diverted from their love

of stealing by turning their attention to some other way of satisfying their cupidity. Thus, I once overcame in a wealthy lady a strong desire to steal whatever she could lay her hand on, by turning her attention to the subject of botany, and inducing her to make collections of plants. She gradually became so infatuated with her new pursuit that she lost all kleptomaniacal symptoms.

In another case, that of a gentleman who could not resist the gratification he experienced at stealing silver spoons or forks from the dinner-tables at which he was a guest, I pointed out the interest attached to the corks of wine-bottles, and suggested that, if some one would make a collection of the different kinds, it would be curious and suggestive. He at once took up the idea, and began to take bottle-corks instead of forks and spoons. Of course, no one cared how many corks he took, and he could gratify his acquisitive propensity without danger to his reputation. He has an interesting collection of corks, classified according to the wines for which they have been used, and arranged with system and taste. He allows no one to see it, but he has willed it, so he tells me, to a prominent art museum.

Another variety of emotional monomania is the love of setting fire to houses and other things, and which is designated *pyromania*. This is an abnormal manifestation of the love of destroying, with which most persons are born, and which is often shown at a very early age. Many instances of this kind of mental disturbance are on record, and there is no doubt that it exists as a distinct type of morbid emotional disorder. It appears to be decidedly more common with women and girls than with males.

"A lady came under my observation who was subject to no delusion, and who had never exhibited any evidence of mental alienation except in showing an impulse, which she declared she could not control, to throw valuable articles into the fire. At first, as she said in her confession to me, the impulse was excited by the satisfaction she derived from seeing an old pair of slippers curl up into fantastic shapes after she had thrown them into a blazing wood fire. She repeated the act the following day, but, not having a pair of old shoes to burn, she used instead a felt hat which was no longer fashionable. But this did not undergo contortions like the shoes, and, therefore, she had no pleasurable sensations like those of the day before, and thus, so far as any satisfaction was concerned, the experiment was a failure. On the ensuing day, however, she felt, to her great surprise, that it would be a pleasant thing to burn something. She was very clear that this pleasure consisted solely in the fulfilment of an impulse which, to a great extent, had become habitual. She, therefore, seized a handsomely bound prayer-book which lay on the table, and, throwing it into the fire, turned away her face and walked to another part of the room. It was very certain, therefore, that she was no longer gratified by the sight of the burning articles. She went on repeating these acts with her own things, and even with those which did not belong to her, until she became a nuisance to herself and to all those with whom she had any relations. Her destructive propensities stopped at nothing which was capable of being consumed. Books, bonnets, shawls, laces, handkerchiefs, and even table-cloths and bed-linen, helped to swell the list of her sacrifices. As soon as she had thrown the articles into the fire the impulse was satisfied. She did not care to see them burn ; on the contrary, the sight was rather disagreeable to her than otherwise. But the power which affected her in the way it did she represented as being imperative, and, if not immediately allowed to act, giving rise to the most irritable and painful sensations, which she could not describe otherwise than by saying that she felt as if she should have to fly, or jump, or run, and that there was a feeling under the skin all over the body as though the flesh were in motion. As soon as she had yielded to the impulse these sensations disappeared. She was eventually cured by being placed under restraint and subjected to medical treatment."[1]

This patient was subject to attacks of migraine, during which her head throbbed violently, and the vessels of the face were greatly injected. She also suffered from insomnia and vertigo, especially at her menstrual periods.

Esquirol[2] cites from Henke the case of a servant-girl who, returning from a dance at which she had become over-heated, was seized with an incendiary impulse. For three days she experienced anxious and otherwise uncomfortable feelings, and then she set fire to a building. She declared that when

---

[1] "A Problem for Sociologists," *North American Review*, November, 1882, p. 430.

[2] "Des maladies mentales," Paris, 1838, t. i, p. 374.

she saw the fire she experienced a greater degree of pleasure than she had ever felt before.

A wheelwright's apprentice, a countryman, eighteen years of age, made sixteen incendiary attempts in the space of four months. He always carried with him a sponge coated with sulphur. Although to satisfy his appetites he had often been guilty of theft, and though he was poor, he never stole anything from the houses he destroyed. He was not actuated by any other feeling than the pleasure of seeing the fire he kindled, and in hearing the bells ring, the lamentations of those who suffered the loss of their property, the noises in the street, etc.[1]

Marc,[2] in calling attention to the fact that pyromania is often met with in young persons, cites the following cases among others from Henke :

A girl, less than fifteen years of age, affected with nostalgia, twice set fire to the house in which she lived. She declared that from the first moment of entering her master's service she had been seized with the desire of destroying his house by fire. It seemed to her that a ghost standing before her constantly urged her on to the act. This girl had for a long time suffered from pain in the head and disordered menstruation.

Another, aged twenty-two years, committed incendiarism four times. She said she was tormented by a nervous feeling which forced her to set houses on fire.

A third, servant of a farmer, twice set fire to the house. She said she had never had any trouble with her master or mistress, but that she was actuated by an impulse arising from a voice within her, which urged her to burn the house and then to hang herself. On the first occasion she looked with calmness and pleasure at the fire she had kindled ; the second time she gave the alarm, and then tried to hang herself. No signs of intellectual derangement could be discovered, but her physical health was bad.

Livi,[3] in an exhaustive study of the subject, expresses the opinion that incendiarism is not only committed as a consequence of illusions and hallucinations, mania or lypemania,

---

[1] Esquirol, *Op. cit., loc. cit.*

[2] " Considérations médico-légales sur la monomanie et particulièrement sur la monomanie incendiaire," *Annales d'hygiène publique et de médecin légale,* t. x, 1833, p. 435.   [3] *Archivio Italiano,* February, 1867.

and intellectual monomania, but through the influence of instinctive monomania, which is only another name for the emotional monomania under consideration. With Henke, Marc, and others, he thinks that the function of menstruation makes pyromania more frequent in the female than in the male sex.

Flechner,[1] on the other hand, contends that these factors are without special influence in producing any form of pyromania, but he admits, by inference, at least, that it may be due to a special morbid impulse which forces the subject to destroy by fire.

Another form of the destructive propensity is seen in the emotional form of *homicidal mania*. In this variety of mental derangement there is an intense desire to kill, and the development of pleasurable feelings, as the result of yielding to the longing. Murders are, therefore, perpetrated by the subjects of this variety of emotional monomania, which are without malice, or cupidity, or any other emotion, save that of the gratification of their passion for killing. And they often resist, with every evidence of sincerity, the morbid impulse with which they are actuated. Occasionally the desire to kill a human being may be diverted by turning the attention to the idea of gratifying the emotion by killing the lower animals. Thus, Georget[2] relates, on the authority of Werbe, the following particulars of a case in point:

"At midnight a man presented himself at the country-seat of the celebrated Antoine Petit, and begged him to cure him of an invincible propensity to kill his master, whom he had served for fifteen years. He added that he had also a strong desire to kill himself. The idea had come to him very suddenly, and he could not overcome it. Petit received the man kindly, made him sit down, quieted his agitation, and gave him a glass of good wine. At early dawn, under the pretext of getting some remedies for him, he took him to Paris, and, conducting him to a slaughter-house, made him cut the throats of several sheep. The man showed great delight at the proceeding, but at the seventh victim he suddenly turned pale, and fell fainting to the ground. This man assumed the trade of a butcher, and, on the first day of every year, came to thank Petit for having saved him from the scaffold."

[1] " Psychiatrisches Centralblatt," 1874.
[2] " Discussion médico-légale sur la folie," etc., Paris, 1826, p. 68.

A hard-working gardener, residing in this city, came to consult me for relief from a longing which he experienced to kill his niece, who kept house for him. The desire had gradually grown upon him, and he was fearful that he would not long be able to resist. It had first occurred to him one morning at breakfast, when he had suddenly experienced the feeling that it would be a gratification to him if he could transfix her neck with a pitchfork. He rose in some agitation from the table, and went into his garden. He looked over all his pitchforks, and selected one with three prongs, which he thought would be the best one to use in case he should indulge his desire. However, he came to the conclusion that it would be a horrid thing to do, and an act for which he ought to be hanged without mercy. But every day as he met his niece at breakfast, the desire appeared, and was evidently growing upon him. One morning he placed his hands around her neck and said to her, in a playful way, that it would be "a good neck to stick a pitchfork through." Still, he had no serious idea that he would ever yield. He was much attached to his niece, and she to him, and they had always lived together harmoniously. However, the desire grew on him, and finally became so strong that he began to feel that, after all, he would eventually be obliged to perpetrate the deed. Finally the idea occurred to him that he would make an image which he would conceive for the moment to be his niece, and that he would plunge his pitchfork through its neck. He purchased a *papier maché* bust, and, attaching it to a trunk made of bagging stuffed with straw, stuck it up in his hothouse. The next morning, when the impulse came over him, he took his pitchfork and drove it through the neck of the counterfeit niece, with the effect of at once satisfying his desire. Every day thereafter, for a month or longer, he went through this performance, but gradually it lost its power, and he again began to feel that he would have to indulge his impulse to transfix his niece. One morning he went so far as to bring the pitchfork into the room and lay it on the floor by his side, so as to be ready for use, but by great effort he was enabled to restrain himself. The same day he consulted me, and gave me the foregoing particulars. I found that he was suffering from wakefulness, pain in the head, vertigo, noises in the ears, flashes of light before the eyes, and almost constant twitching of the facial muscles. Besides these symptoms of cerebral hyperæmia, there was obstinate constipation of the bowels and dyspepsia. I gave him a prescription containing bromide of sodium, and directed the application of a dozen cups to the nape of the neck. Recognizing, however, the fact that the niece was in considerable danger, I sent the uncle to the extreme lower part of the city to get his prescription, and to have the cups applied, and in the mean time sent word to the niece to come at once to my consulting-room. I knew that the uncle could not get back to his house under a couple of hours, and within that time I hoped to have the girl out of the city. She came at once, and, on learning of the danger to which she had been subjected, decided to go immediately to her mother, who lived in Canada. Before the uncle got home she was out of his house, and that evening left the city. I told him what I had done, and he expressed great gratification that I had probably saved him from committing a murder. With the disappearance of the niece the desire faded out, and, under the influence of the medical treatment, his cerebral disorder also disappeared. Four years have now passed, and, though he thinks he is entirely cured of his desire, he has not yet succeeded in persuading his niece to return. Indeed, I have advised her not to do so, as there is no predicting with any degree of assurance that his impulse would not return.

Dr. Carpenter[1] quotes from the Report of the Morningside Lunatic Asylum for 1850 a case which is so apposite, as showing some of the chief phenomena of homicidal mania of the emotional form, that I quote it in full :

" The case was that of a female who was not affected with any disorder of her intellectual powers, and who labored under no delusions or hallucinations, but who was tormented by a simple abstract desire to kill, or rather, for it took a specific form, to strangle. She made repeated attempts to effect her purpose, attacking all and sundry, even her own nieces and other relatives ; indeed, it seemed to be a matter of indifference to her *whom* she strangled, so that she succeeded in killing some one. She recovered, under strict discipline, so much self-control as to be permitted to work in the washing-house and laundry, but she still continued to assert that she 'must do it,' that she 'was certain she would do it some day,' that she could not help it ; 'surely no one had ever suffered as

---

[1] "Principles of Mental Philosophy," etc., London, 1874, p. 664.

she had done'; was not her's 'an awful case?' And, approaching any one, she would gently bring her hand near their throat and say, mildly and persuasively, 'I would just like to do it.' She frequently expressed a wish that all the men and women in the world had only one neck, that she might strangle it. Yet this female had kind and amiable dispositions, was beloved by her fellow-patients—so much so that one of them insisted on sleeping with her, although she herself declared that she was afraid she would not be able to resist the impulse to get up during the night and strangle her. She had been a very pious woman, exemplary in her conduct, very fond of attending prayer-meetings and of visiting the sick, praying with them and reading the Scriptures, or repeating to them the sermons she had heard. It was the second attack of insanity. During the former she had attempted suicide. The disease was hereditary, and it may be believed that she was strongly predisposed to morbid impulses of this character when it was stated that her mother and sister had committed suicide. There could be no doubt as to the sincerity of her morbid desires. She was brought to the institution under very severe restraint, and the parties who brought her were under great alarm upon the restraint being removed. After its removal she made repeated and very determined attacks upon the other patients, the attendants, and the officers of the asylum, and was only brought to exercise sufficient self-control by a system of rigid discipline. This female was perfectly aware that her impulses were wrong, and that, if she had committed any crime of violence under their influence, she would have been exposed to punishment. She deplored in piteous terms the horrible propensity under which she labored.

"In the report of the same institution for 1853, it is mentioned that this female had been readmitted after nearly succeeding in strangling her sister's child under the prompting of her homicidal impulse. 'She displays no delusion or perversion of ideas, but is urged on by an abstract and uncontrollable impulse to do what she knows to be wrong, and deeply deplores.'"

In the year 1881, a woman came to my clinique at the University of New York to be treated for, as she said, an insane desire to kill her two children, a boy and girl, aged, respectively, six and eight years. The desire had first occurred to

her at night, about a month previously, as she lay in bed trying to get to sleep. She felt as though she must do it. She
accordingly rose from the bed, lit a candle, and went to the
room where the two children lay. They were sound asleep.
As she looked on them, the desire grew upon her, and increased to such an extent that she seized a pillow, and was
about to smother the boy when her legs gave way beneath
her, a cold sweat broke out over her whole body, and her
arms became so weak that the pillow dropped from her hands,
and she fell to the floor in an almost unconscious state. As
soon as she was able, she hurried back to her own bed, terrified
and weeping at the thought of the deed she had so nearly
committed. She did not sleep all night, and the next morning got up with a splitting headache and with a feeling as
though her brain were on fire.

Her husband, who had been absent, returned that day,
but she was afraid to mention her temptation of the night
before, lest he might summon a physician, and she should be
thought insane and placed in a lunatic asylum.

Besides, the desire to kill the children was beginning to reappear, and she felt that she would have to yield in order to
satisfy the longing which existed. She did not wish to be interfered with, and she resolved to make the attempt as soon as
the children came home from school, and while her husband,
who was a railway engineer, was absent. But when the boy
and his sister entered the room they rushed up to her with
some flowers a florist had given them, and that, she said, entirely changed the current of her thoughts and desires. She
clasped them in her arms, kissed them, and hurried them out
of her sight. From that time on the desire, though constantly present, was kept in subjection by the emotion of
maternal love ; but, fearful that it might again get the ascendency, she had come for medical treatment.

I found that she did not sleep well, sometimes passing the
whole night without closing her eyes ; that she had a constant
rumbling sound in her ears, and at times a loud and abrupt
noise in the head like that produced by the discharge of a
pistol ; that there was a dull, heavy pain in the top of the
head, and a sensation as though an "animal of some kind
was gnawing the scalp." Frequently during the day first
one ear and then the other would burn till it became painful,
and then all the head symptoms were increased in violence.

Her bowels were obstinately constipated, and her menstruation was generally retarded several days.

I could detect no intellectual disorder; neither were there illusions or hallucinations. She appeared to be of a calm and equable temperament, and she conversed in the most rational manner in regard to the terrible passion for killing her own children with which she was afflicted. She said that she felt it was becoming stronger every day, and that, unless something were done for her, she should end by murdering them. She had not yet told her husband anything of the subject. I directed her to send the children at once to their grandmother—and it was done before she left the room—and to send her husband to me as soon as he returned to this city. I saw him the next morning, and it may well be believed that his surprise and horror were intense when he heard what I had to tell him about his wife. He was a very sensible man, however, and, through his aid and that of the medical treatment to which she was subjected, she was in a few weeks entirely cured of her insane desire. As soon as she began to get sound and refreshing sleep, the impulse became feeble, and finally disappeared altogether.

Closely allied to emotional homicidal impulse is that form of mental derangement which consists of an *emotional impulse to the perpetration of suicide*. It not infrequently happens that the two conditions coexist in the same person. Dagonet[1] cites the following case from Georget :

The wife of a coppersmith came to me, says Georget, to request my advice for a state of mind which drove her to despair. She was apparently in good health, slept well, had a good appetite, and her menstruation was regular. She had no pain, and the circulation presented no evidences of derangement. But the woman complained of having at times ideas of killing her four children, notwithstanding that, as she said, she loved them better than she did herself. At these periods she felt afraid that she would do them some fatal injury, and she at the same time experienced a desire to throw herself out of the window. When these impulses were on her she became red in the face, and she was seized with a general trem-

---

[1] "Des impulsions dans la folie et de la folie impulsive," Paris, 1870, p. 65. Dagonet refers this case to Georget's "Discussion médico-légale sur la folie," etc., p. 21. No such case is, however, reported on that page, nor, so far as I can discover, on any other page of the monograph in question.

bling of the whole body. She had no wish to injure other children, and when the impulse affected her she took care to keep out of the way of her children, and to hide all the knives and other sharp instruments in the house. There was no other mental lesion. This state had lasted about a month. The impulse in this woman was not very strong. Had it been, says Georget, a little more intense, she would have committed several horrible crimes.

In some cases of emotional morbid impulse to suicide, the contemplation of the act is attended with feelings of pleasure. A man kills himself because he wishes to do so, and because of the satisfaction to be derived from gratifying his impulse. There is no abhorrence of the deed, no contest with himself in which he is overpowered. His intellect is not necessarily deranged ; he acts with the full knowledge of what he is doing ; and, if the circumstances require it, he employs the most systematic and recondite stratagems in order to accomplish his purpose. He is neither governed by delusions nor by logical reasons. He is simply actuated by a passion which it is pleasant for him to gratify. When, however, the impulse has passed without having been realized, as is sometimes the case from accident or some more powerful influence, he looks back upon it with horror, and, shuddering at the escape he has made, perhaps seeks medical advice for what he feels is a disease likely ere long to prove fatal.

Thus, a lady, who had obtained a divorce from her husband on the ground of adultery, and who during the trial had suffered greatly both in mental and physical health, consulted me in regard to her condition. I found that she was entirely free from hallucinations, illusions, or any intellectual disorder, but that at times she was affected by an impulse to kill herself with poison. At the first appearance of this disturbance she had no poison in her possession, and when it had passed off she had, of course, no wish to obtain the means ; but the second occasion occurred while she was walking in the street, and she at once entered a pharmacy near by and asked for two grains of strychnine, for the purpose, as she said, of killing rats. As she had no prescription, the pharmacist declined to let her have the drug, so she was obliged to go without it. In a few minutes the impulse disappeared.

These attacks alarmed her, especially as the second was much stronger than the first ; so she resolved to consult a physician. But, before she did so, she was visited by the impulse for the third time, and this was far stronger than either of the others. It appeared to her that no act that she could commit would afford so much real satisfaction as that of taking her own life. There was no reason why she should desire to do so except this. Her affairs were in good order, she was possessed of ample means, and the sympathy of the public had been with her in her dispute with her husband. She felt, however, as though it was impossible to resist the desire which was on her. She must do it. But she had no satisfactory means at her command.

She reflected that, if she cut her throat or killed herself in any violent way, the fact would be known by the appearance of her dead body, and she shrank from the idea of the disgrace which would attach to her in consequence. She would, she thought, get the poison, take it, and then go to bed to enjoy the idea that she had at last gratified the impulse; she would almost imperceptibly pass into a stupor, and, when found dead in her bed next morning, every one would think that she had died of heart disease. To give additional color to this belief would be the fact that she had consulted several physicians, all of whom had told her that she had disease of the heart. It was then about eleven o'clock in the morning. She went out, and, purchasing a phial of McMunn's elixir of opium, returned, and, putting it to her lips, took the whole of it—about two ounces. She then lay down and began to think.

But the result was quite different from what she had anticipated. At first she experienced the most intense gratification at the success of her plan. Nothing, she said, had ever given her such unalloyed pleasure as the thought that she had obeyed the impulse to self-destruction. But this feeling lasted only for a few minutes. The impulse suddenly disappeared, and with its flight came a realization of the awful deed she had perpetrated. She sprang from the bed, and, though scarcely able to stand and with her mind already half stupefied by the opium, staggered into her sister's room, adjoining her own, and told what she had done. While in the act of speaking she was fortunately seized with a violent fit of vomiting, as the result of the excessively large dose she had taken, and her life was thus saved.

For several days she was confined to her bed, and then again the impulse to self-destruction returned. It was just subsequent to this fourth recurrence—which was slight, and which, as her friends were now aware of her tendency, she had no opportunity of gratifying—that she came under my observation. She conversed with entire calmness and lucidity relative to her desire to commit suicide, and which she now regarded with aversion and terror. She was regular in her menstrual functions, had no pain in her head, slept well, and was apparently in good health, except that at the times when her impulse came she had a feeling of heat in the right side of her face, her ear burned and was red, and a humming noise was heard on that side. These, however, were phenomena indicative of vaso-motor paralysis, which often exist in conjunction with the most perfect mental and physical health. I directed that she should be watched night and day, and I treated her with the bromide of sodium and ergot, with the effect of preventing any further return of her suicidal impulse.

Marc[1] states that he himself, in his youth, experienced a periodical impulse to commit suicide, which was clearly emotional in its character. Enjoying perfect health, he was attacked, for three years, every autumn with a feeling of anxiety, accompanied with an indefinable desire to take his own life, so that he was obliged to request one of his friends to watch him during the accession of the paroxysm, which, after lasting several days, ended with a nasal hæmorrhage. There was no other evidence of cerebral congestion, his complexion being rather pale and sallow than high-colored. The only consideration which antagonized the desire for suicide was the thought of the grief into which his family would be plunged.

Bertrand[2] cites the case of a man, in good circumstances, free from any source of anxiety or grief, and of apparently sound intellect, who was harassed by the desire to cut his throat whenever he shaved himself. He felt as though no pleasure in life would be comparable to that which he would derive from committing suicide in this way.

At other times there is a terrible contest in the mind of the individual. Various emotions contend for the mastery, and the intellect may combat the desire for self-destruction which exists. Sometimes the will is overcome, and at others it resists all arguments and all other emotions, and the attempt is made.

---

[1] "De la folie considerée dans ses rapports avec les questions médico-judiciaires," Paris, 1840, t. ii, p. 162. [2] "Traité du suicide," Paris, 1857, p. 265.

Schnopp[1] reports the following interesting case :

F. de Z., an officer, twenty-seven years of age, at the
termination of an attack of rheumatic fever became timid
and taciturn, but remained perfectly reasonable and lucid in
his speech and writing. One evening he asked his servant for
a pair of pistols, but, as the man refused to give them to him,
he requested him to throw him out of the window. This also
being refused, he, with no better success, asked for a sharp
knife, adding that he wished to kill himself. He slept well
that night, but the next morning made the same request of
the cook, and then inquired if the court-yard under his window was paved or not. Left alone for a moment, he threw
himself out of the second-story window. By good luck the
fall did not result seriously. Interrogated as to his reasons
for so insane an act, he owned that for some time he had been
possessed with the wish to kill himself—a wish of which he
could not get rid. Neither his religious principles nor his
reason, nor the sense of the shame that would attach to his
family, could conquer the impulse, and that his tears and his
prayers to God had been equally ineffectual. He was cured
by travel and other hygienic means.

It is by no means always the case that the emotional morbid impulse to commit suicide is permanently abolished after
an attempt has been made. Thus, Brierre de Boismont[2] refers to the cases of individuals, one of whom had made several
ineffectual efforts to asphyxiate himself, and who always kept
a vessel full of charcoal in his room, so as to be in readiness
for his next attempt ; and another constantly carried a rope
about with him. A woman set fire to her furniture in order
to destroy herself, first having tried to throw her child out of
the window. Prevented in both attempts, she repeated them,
still unsuccessfully. Finally, one morning, she strangled herself. A man had the fortitude to make two attempts to kill
himself by swallowing nitric acid ; next he cut his throat with
a razor, but did not succeed in inflicting a mortal wound. The
fourth attempt resulted according to his wish. He kindled
several charcoal furnaces in his room, and died, asphyxiated.

Another man started out to throw himself into the river,
but was prevented by two persons, who followed him, suspect-

---

[1] "Paradoxie des Willens," cited by Dagonet, *op. cit.*, p. 66, and *Annales
médico-psychologiques*, juillet et septembre, 1870.

[2] "Du suicide et de la folie suicide," Paris, 1856, p. 442, *et seq.*

ing his purpose. A second time he mounted the parapet of a bridge, in order to jump from it into the water, but was prevented by a sentinel calling to him. He then gave up the idea of drowning himself, and made preparations for throwing himself from the window, but was stopped by the unexpected entrance of his brother into the room. Finally he succeeded with charcoal.

In a former chapter I have referred to a striking case in which the attempt at suicide was repeatedly made, and finally with success. In another instance recently under my observation, the impulse was renewed periodically as many as nine times, and three separate attempts to carry it out were made. In this case, as in the others cited in this connection, there were no delusions, but at each recurrence of the emotional disturbance there were hallucinations of hearing, apparently, however, without any relation, so far as their character was concerned with the impulse, to self-destruction. The patient, twenty-eight years old, was the wife of a physician in a neighboring State, and had suffered from repeated attacks of intermittent fever. She had been sleeping badly for several nights, and had been greatly troubled with frightful dreams. One night she woke with the sound of musical instruments in her ears, and with a desire to kill herself with a pair of scissors which she knew lay on a table in an adjoining room. Without disturbing her husband, who was sleeping by her side, she got up, lit a candle, and went to get the scissors. She recollected distinctly that while going to this room she had heard voices singing the words of a popular song of the day to an accompaniment of musical instruments. She recognized the fact that this was a hallucination, but the thought struck her that she would die to sweet music—a desire she had always expressed when the subject of death was discussed in her presence. She found the scissors, and, opening them, said aloud : "Now I am going to be happy," and instantly plunged the sharp blade into her left breast. The point entered just above the nipple, penetrating the mammary gland, but not entering the chest. Before she could repeat the blow, her husband, who had been awakened by her exclamation, entered the room and disarmed her. The wound was of no great consequence ; her *embonpoint* had saved her life.

Instead of consulting another physician, the matter was kept quiet, especially as it was thought by those about her that she had been excited by a large dose of quinine she had taken that afternoon. The impulse had disappeared, and she expressed the utmost gratification at the failure of her attempt. But exactly two weeks subsequently, while engaged in sewing one afternoon, she experienced a renewal of the impulse. Again she felt that nothing could give her so much pleasure as the act of suicide, but, instead of a pair of scissors, a penknife was indicated as the weapon. Again she heard delightful music. She immediately opened a small penknife which she had in her work-basket, and, rolling up the sleeve of her dress, gave herself a deep gash across the bend of the elbow. She watched the blood flow in a stream from her arm, experiencing all the time the most intense satisfaction at what she had done. She thought she had lost about a quart, when she became insensible, and knew nothing more till she found herself in bed and her husband standing by her side. She made a good recovery, though she was very feeble, and for over a month was confined to her room. Of course, great care was taken to prevent any further attempts of the kind, and, as she passed over several periods of fourteen days without any recurrence of the impulse, it was hoped it would not again make its appearance. In this, however, there was disappointment, for on the seventeenth day from the second attempt the desire to kill herself returned. This time, however, she was not alone, and she was prevented sticking a two-pronged steel fork into her chest. The accession of this impulse was, like the others, attended with the hallucination of music. After this she had, at intervals of fourteen days, five other recurrences of the impulse to kill herself, but, as she was closely watched at the expected times, she was unable to effect her purpose. Each was marked by the existence of a pleasurable feeling, and by hallucinations of music. She felt as though she could with an effort overcome the impulse, and she often reasoned in regard to it before making an attempt upon her life. The emotion of pleasure, however, which she felt would reach its height with the perpetration of the act, swept everything before it. The desire became so intense that no influence but that of main force sufficed to prevent her accomplishing her purpose. As she said to her husband one day : "If God Almighty and all his angels were to beg me to refrain, I could not do it." In the intervals she thanked those who had interposed for their good offices in having saved her life, but always reminded them that she knew she would make the attempt again, and that they must be on the watch. The impulse lasted not more than fifteen minutes. During its existence she struggled to escape from those who held her, or from the bands which confined her hands.

The ninth attempt was partially successful, owing to the fact that when the desire appeared she dissembled by pretending that she was sure it was not going to come this time, and sending her sister out of the room to get a glass of cider for her. As soon as she was alone she rushed to the window and endeavored to open it, so that she might throw herself out. It was nailed fast, and she could not raise it. She looked hastily around the room in search of means for her purpose, but could find nothing suitable. It was but the work of a moment for her to hurry to the dining-room, and seizing a large carving-knife, to draw it across her throat. Fortunately it was dull, and she was obliged to make several attempts before she succeeded in inflicting a wound of any importance. As it was, before she could fully accomplish her purpose she was seized. She had made half a dozen cuts in her neck, one of which only had been deep enough to cause hæmorrhage. This had cut the external jugular vein on the left side. A week subsequently she was brought to me, and gave me the foregoing particulars. I recognized the fact that she had periodical attacks of cerebral congestion, and, while I advised the use of arsenic and the bromide of sodium, I insisted that the treatment should be carried out in a place of greater security than her own house. I recommended that she should be placed under the care of Dr. R. L. Parsons, at Sing Sing. Her husband promised to follow my advice in every particular. He declared, however, that he must first take his wife home in order to make proper arrangements for her departure. On her way back, however, to the town in which she lived, she took a violent cold. Pleuro-pneumonia ensued, and she died within ten days thereafter.

Drs. McLean and Brown report two cases of women who exhibited strong impulses to suicide without the implication of the intellect. Indeed, with the exception of slight nervous irritability, and the impulses in question, both subjects were in a state of the most complete mental health. They were good-tempered, of remarkable intelligence, and declared that they were perfectly happy, but they were overpowered with a violent desire to die. One of these was a young girl, cheerful, amiable, and as happy as could be. She had tried repeatedly to poison herself with laudanum, then to strangle herself, and then to open a vein with a darning-needle. Finally she refused food, and had to be nourished by means of a stomach-pump.

Closely allied to the emotional morbid impulse to commit suicide is the tendency sometimes evinced to perpetrate some act of mutilation on the body. Most cases of these acts are the result of delusions, and are effected during paroxysms of acute mania or of melancholia, but some are due to emotional impulses similar in general features to such as have first been considered. Further reference, therefore, to them in the present connection is not necessary.

c—SIMPLE MELANCHOLIA.

By simple melancholia is to be understood a condition characterized by mental depression without delusions or delirium. It is altogether an emotional disorder. The accession is generally gradual, and though it usually makes its appearance in those who are naturally grave and reserved, yet this is by no means always the case, and a radical change of disposition and character is hence effected.

Perhaps the earliest symptom of the disorder in question is a perverted and exaggerated degree of impressionability to all excitations from without and reflections from within. Not only do such factors, when naturally of a depressing character, exercise their logical influence to an extreme degree, but those, which to mankind in general are pleasing, produce also emotions of sadness or sensations of pain. The least thing, therefore, suffices to disturb the equanimity of the patient, and to excite melancholic trains of thought which haunt him long after the cause should have passed into oblivion. By strained processes of reasoning he misinterprets the most indifferent circumstances as having been specially contrived for his discomfort or unhappiness, and construes acts of kindness into insults or injuries. As those with whom he associates are not generally disposed to bear with his fretfulness, his reproaches, his accusations, he avoids them as far as he possibly can, and, withdrawing from society, even that of his own immediate family, broods in silence, and often in secret, over his own gloomy thoughts. Although in this uncomplicated form of melancholia the individual shows no tendency to imbibe actual delusions, he constantly exaggerates the nature and consequences of his own acts and of those of others. Thus, if he has been somewhat wild in his youth, he is now sure that the results of his early indiscretions are making their appearance, and that punishment awaits him both in this world and in the world to come. If he has committed errors in his business, though they may really have been of no great consequence, he brings himself to the belief, or at least the fear, that immediate financial ruin is staring him in the face. If he has money invested, or commercial or other transactions in hand, he is certain the one will be lost, and the others will result unfavorably. He is, therefore, supremely unhappy, and the state of his mind is exhibited in every feature of his countenance, and shown in every gesture that he makes. He weeps, sobs, wrings his hands, groans, sighs, and laments in the most sorrowful accents, the cruel fate which has come upon him. He wishes he were dead; the grave would be a relief; and yet he knows that beyond this life there are greater sorrows in store for him.

Occasionally there are tendencies to suicide, but these are the result of reflection, and formed after what to the patient is a thorough survey of all the circumstances of his case, and as a consequence of the conclusion that death would be a relief. If he does not attempt self-destruction, it is because of his doubts as to the future, because he lacks the physical courage necessary to the act, because of the sorrow that his family would feel, or of some other rational motive. He often wishes he could so arrange matters that he could at once end an existence that has become too burdensome to be longer borne, and will sit for hours with the means of instant death in his hands, trying to make up his mind to bring his life to an immediate termination.

The intense mental depression which exists in these cases cannot fail to influence, with more or less effect, the other categories of mental faculties, though it may not bring them to actual aberration. Thus, the force of the intellect and the power of the will are generally indubitably weakened. The individual may be able to reason acutely enough in regard to matters with which he is familiar, and may, with a sort of spasmodic energy, conduct himself with credit in a dispute or an argument of short duration, but he is incapable of long-sustained mental effort, and unequal to the task of investigating subjects new to him. Indeed, the mental concentration necessary to such pursuits is rendered impossible by the preoccupation of his mind. How, for instance, can a man study a new field in philosophy or work out an abstruse mathematical problem when his emotions excite in him thoughts of financial ruin, desertion by his wife and children, or the damnation of his eternal soul?

From a very early period in the course of the disease there are marked physical symptoms. The patient sleeps badly, both as regards quantity and quality; there are dreams often of a frightful character, and always unpleasantly vivid. There are pains in the head, and other sensations, which, if not amounting to actual pain, are such as to cause discomfort. There is a sense of fulness, or of tightness, or of weight, always induced during any particularly marked paroxysm of emotional disturbance or period of intellectual exertion. The mouth is dry, and is liable to have a bitter taste form in it when the patient is unusually troubled. The cutaneous perspiration is diminished. The urine is likewise lessened in quantity, and the bowels are ordinarily obstinately constipated. The appetite is almost entirely abolished, and not only that, but food of all kinds may excite the greatest degree of repugnance. Unusual persuasion is, therefore, often required to induce the individual to eat, and it may become necessary to resort to forcible means of feeding in order to ensure the proper nutrition of the patient.

The mental hebetude has its counterpart in the condition of the body. There is an indisposition to move, even in the presence of such circumstances as render motion necessary to the life of the subject. Thus, in a case the particulars of which I am familiar with, an old gentleman, who had been the subject of simple melancholia for several years, refused to get up from bed, though the house in which he was had taken fire. "Let it burn!" he exclaimed; "I am glad of it. I will go with it," and he persisted so obstinately in his determination that he had to be removed by force.

There seems to be in many subjects of simple melancholia a tendency to wasting of the body, even though they may be sufficiently well fed. In others, again, there is a decided disposition to the accumulation of fat.

In women, the menstrual function is generally deranged, either by its irregularity as regards periodicity or quantity or by its complete suppression.

Although the subjects of simple melancholia generally exhibit some degree of cutaneous hyperæsthesia, this is in most cases a phenomenon of the earliest stage of the affection. Later on there is a decided blunting of the sense of touch, of that of pain, and of other excitations made upon the skin. Christian[1] has pointed out this fact in a very thorough manner, and has shown, through his researches, that melancholics of all kinds are often insensible to impressions which in normally constituted persons would give rise to the most agonizing pain. "I have seen," he says, "a melancholic open his belly with a nail; another, with a dull knife, extirpate his testicles; and a third cut off his thumb with a hatchet. I have at this time under my care a man, thirty-three years of age, who has been deranged for seven years with lypemania, who crushed his left hand by placing it on a rock and pounding it with a big club. All the fingers have their bones broken. It was necessary to amputate several phalanges and to extract a great many pieces of bone, during which operations the patient did not seem to feel the slightest pain."[2]

At times, under the influence of the depressing emotions which crowd upon him, or as a consequence of the abuse to which he has put his organs, the subject of simple melancholia may commit some frightful act of self-mutilation. A man within my own experience, a carpenter and a good workman, got out of work and became melancholic. Reflecting upon his condition and his inability to get anything to do, he called to mind the fact that a former employer had reprimanded him for some mistake he had made. He brooded over this circumstance till he decided that, as he was not fit to do good work, and that as it was to that inability the loss of his situation was to be ascribed, he would cut off the hand to which he owed his misfortunes. Moreover, had not the Bible said, "If thine eye offend thee, pluck it out and cast it from thee?" He therefore awoke one morning—and it is in the morning, on awaking, that all depressing emotions are most powerful—and, going to the wood-shed in the yard at the back of the house, laid his right hand on a log, and with

---

[1] "Étude sur la mélancolie. Des troubles de la sensibilité générale chez les mélancoliques." Paris, 1876.　　　　　　　　　　[2] *Op. cit.*, p. 31.

an axe cut it off at a single blow. He was found shortly afterward nearly dead from the loss of blood.

M. Sourier[1] has reported the case of an old sergeant of the army who was found one morning lying in his tent bathed in blood, and in a state of extreme prostration. At one side lay his penis and testicles, which he had cut off with a sharp clasp-knife. Nothing very satisfactory could be got out of him by questioning. He did not get drunk, and he was highly esteemed by his officers. It was called to mind, however, that for several days previously he had been unusually taciturn, and had avoided his comrades. He seemed to be disturbed at the idea that his military life was drawing near its close. A light admonition of the sergeant-major had caused him to shed tears. M. Sourier conceived that the man, arriving at the conclusion that he was approaching that age at which he would have to leave the military service, had become melancholic, and had, in a spirit of exaggeration, cut off his genital organs, in order to make himself still more unworthy. As he says, quoting Lisfranc, "Man places his dignity in the virile organs."

It is not always the case that simple melancholia is of gradual accession. On the contrary, it may make its appearance with great suddenness, either as the direct consequence of some severe mental shock or as a sequence of some bodily disease or injury. Dr. Dickson[2] mentions the case of a lady who was expecting the return of her husband from India, and, anxiously watching for his arrival, was informed by a relative of his death. She uttered a loud scream, but never spoke again, and sank into a profound melancholy, from which she never recovered.

Dr. Conolly,[3] in calling attention to the fact that melancholia, though usually a disease of slow growth, may supervene suddenly, cites the following case:

"A young gentleman, who appeared to be in perfectly good health, dropped down dead while walking in his mother's garden. His mother became speechless and almost immovable, and long remained so ; and to this state succeeded in a few weeks a profound melancholy, which lasted many

---

[1] " Recueil des mémoires de médecine de chirurgie et de pharmacie militaires," Paris, août, 1869.
[2] " The Science and Practice of Medicine in Relation to Mind," New York, 1874, p. 179. [3] " The Croonian Lectures " for 1849, London, p. 23.

months, during which she accused herself of being unpardonably wicked and despairing of God's mercy, but never alluded to the death of her son."

In a recent case, in regard to which I was consulted, and in which the accession of the disease was extremely sudden, there was a like oblivion of the cause of the mental disturbance. In this instance, the patient, a gentleman advanced in years, was abruptly informed that his daughter, a married woman, had eloped, with a disreputable man, from her husband and children. A state of profound melancholy was at once induced, and for several days not a word was uttered ; neither did the patient stir from his chair, nor eat a mouthful of food. His mental faculties appeared to have been completely stunned. Gradually, however, he, in a great measure, recovered from this state of profound hebetude, but he remained all his life the subject of deep melancholia, weeping and wringing his hands, and pacing the floor of his apartment day and night, in a state of the most profound grief. He was apparently filled with remorse for his past life and with apprehensions for the future, but he never once alluded to his daughter or her conduct. He had, among other functional derangements, absolute anorexia, and would not eat unless under great persuasion, or preparations to force him were made.

Then, with the protest that it was "a shame to make a man eat who did not want to eat," he would gulp down his food without apparently tasting it, and, with a sigh of relief, express the hope that he would now be left alone to think over his wickedness.

It is almost invariably the case that the subjects of simple melancholia are worse early in the morning than at any other period of the day, and that there is a gradual alleviation as night approaches. This fact is one which exists even with individuals whose minds are free from disease. If there is any unpleasant circumstance which is causing mental distress, its action is always more powerful in that state in which the individual, as morning approaches, is half awake. Those melancholics who commit suicide are much more apt to do so in the morning, soon after they have risen from bed, than at any other time. The course of simple melancholia is often toward one of the other forms of the affection next to be described. It is not infrequently cured, or terminates spontaneously in recovery. Again, it may pass into a chronic condition, with or without an alleviation of the more marked symptoms. In the case of a woman affected with simple melancholia, unattended by delusions of any kind, the affection had lasted over twenty-five years without any notable change in the symptoms except in regard to the tendency to suicide, which she had at first exhibited, but which has been absent for many years. There was no obvious cause—not even heredity—for the intense melancholy with which she is affected, and which causes her to pass the greater part of the day crying and wringing her hands. She had twice attempted suicide before she came under my observation, not from any delusion, but solely in order that she might escape from her intense mental depression. She is perfectly conscious of her situation, knows how groundless is her grief, and constantly laments her inability to control her feelings. She is now about fifty years of age, is unmarried, and has never suffered from menstrual or uterine disorder. The menopause occurred in her forty-fourth year.

d—MELANCHOLIA WITH DELIRIUM.

Melancholia with delirium is that form of mental aberration in which there is emotional depression conjoined with illusions, hallucinations, and delusions, singly or combined, together with incoherence of words and ideas, and more or less increased motility. It is sometimes designated acute melancholia, and by the French alienists is known as *lypemanie avec delire* or *melancholie avec delire* (lypemania or melancholia with delirium). It is, from whatever point it is regarded, one of the most terrible of all the forms of mental aberration.

Generally, melancholia with delirium begins with well-marked prodromatic symptoms, which do not differ essentially from those met with in other varieties of insanity except in the circumstance that the mental depression is more pronounced. From a very early period the patient sleeps badly, and is troubled with unpleasant dreams. He usually suffers from pain or other feeling of discomfort in the head, his stomach is deranged, his breath offensive, his bowels constipated, and his urine scanty and high-colored.

At about the same time changes in his habits and modes of thought are observed; he becomes gloomy and taciturn, shuns those with whom he formerly associated with pleasure, and imbibes the idea that his friends and relatives are wanting in proper respect for him, or are positively maltreating him.

His countenance undergoes a change in accordance with the alterations which are being effected in his mind and body ; his expression is absent, as if the thoughts were engaged with subjects not in relation with passing events, while at the same time there is a disquietude and apprehension exhibited which are evidences of the feelings within. The forehead is wrinkled —a characteristic feature ; the head is slightly inclined forward, and the lips are firmly compressed. The movements of the body are sudden, and are often made without any apparent object, however much they may be in accordance with the thought. A patient of my own, for instance, walked continually from one corner of the room to the other diagonally. When asked why he did this, his only answer was a look expressive of contempt for the questioner. Evidently there were reasons in his own mind for his peculiar movements, which he disdained to reveal to those whom he thought were actuated by impertinent curiosity.

The tendency to silence is often very strongly marked, and perhaps as often alternates with periods of great loquacity. During a paroxysm of taciturnity the patient appears to be in a state of active thought, and will frequently, by his gestures, give expression to the ideas which are passing through his mind. If spoken to, however, he preserves an obstinate silence, though his face may show his anger at being interrupted in his process of thinking. When disposed to talk, he rambles from one subject to another, but all his words are expressive of the delusions which are beginning to find a lodgment in his mind. He talks of the combinations which are being formed against him, of the great sins he has committed, of the fatal diseases with which he is affected, of the losses he has sustained in his property, of the treachery of his friends, and so on—everything of which he speaks being an evil, a misfortune, a degradation, to which he has been subjected.

Illusions and hallucinations make their appearance. Real sounds and real images are misinterpreted, for instance, into the voices of demons summoning him to punishment, or the forms of the demons themselves coming to convey him to hell. Hallucinations of hearing and sight are still more common. He hears voices urging him to do some act of violence—

often murder or suicide, or reproaching him with the unpardonable character of his sins, and revealing the terrible nature of the punishment he is to undergo in the next world. A patient of mine, on going to bed, had the hallucination of a voice, apparently, as he said, just outside the house, calling to him to come : "Come to me! come to me! Do not wait! Come! come! you are mine! I claim you now! Come! come!" and this for over an hour, till, wearied with the importunity, and at last accepting the hallucination as a verity, he sprang from his bed and rushed from the house into the cold winter air.

Another heard a voice, apparently, close to his ear, urging him, by every holy and reverent name, to save his soul by thrusting his hand into the fire. "This," it said, "will make your peace with God. This will secure your salvation. It is better to go to heaven with one hand than to enter hell with two. It is a bad hand. You have committed numberless crimes with it. Burn it off, and be done with it forever!" For hours he resisted. "I will not burn my hand," he said. "God cannot demand such a sacrifice of me. No, no, I will not! You are a devil! O God, deliver me from this demon!" But hours passed, and still the voice was crying in his ear, "Burn your hand ; it is a wicked hand!" The night was far spent ; he had not closed his eyes in sleep ; wearied in mind and body, he little by little accepted his hallucination for reality, and, rising from bed with a prayer to God on his lips, he thrust his hand into the fire that burned upon the hearth, and held it there till the flesh was charred into a black and shapeless mass.

At first, hallucinations of *hearing* are present only at night, but, as the disease advances, they occur also in the daytime, and then are rarely absent. Not infrequently they are associated with real personages, who may or may not be present, but usually they appear to come from indeterminate beings—angels, demons, or personages coined altogether from the imagination of the patient. Thus, a young lady affected with the disease under consideration heard voices coming, apparently, from two persons, male and female, whom she designated "Busho" and "Quampa," and which told her that her mother wished to poison her, that her brother had hired a man to commit a rape upon her, and that, in order to escape a painful death and overwhelming dishonor, she ought to drown herself in the bath-tub. They even prescribed how the drowning was to be effected. "Fill your mouth full of cotton batting," said "Busho," "fasten the dumb-bell you use, about your neck, then turn on the water, and lie down in the tub." "Hot water, boiling water!" interrupted "Quampa." "It will do the work quicker, and will not be so painful." She resisted these commands, and was fortunately placed under restraint before she reached the stage of accepting them as real orders coming from persons with the right to be obeyed.

Hallucinations of *sight*, though not probably so common as those of hearing, often coexist with them. They may relate either to persons in a state of action or repose, or to things of a more or less terrifying character. There may be the image of a man approaching in a menacing attitude, with a murderous weapon in his hand, or representations of scenes of torment typical or anticipatory of the fate in store for the victim. As the night is often passed without sleep, it is then that hallucinations of sight, like those of hearing, are more common. Long rows of horrible characters pass in endless procession before the strained and wearied eyes ; pictures of a vividness scarcely ever realized in life are presented, in which the most horrible acts are being committed by personages of frightful mien. Again, the scenes may be of saints of the church who are being tormented by heathens, and who call in agonizing tones on God for strength to bear their tortures with fortitude.

Hallucinations of *touch*, though not so frequent as those of sight and hearing, are, nevertheless, not uncommon. A patient of my own, a lady, with strong hereditary tendency to insanity, and who was herself the subject of melancholia with delirium, frequently had the sensation of a hot blast of wind blowing over her face, and which she imagined, from its intense heat and sulphurous smell, came from the prince of darkness, who was bending over her. Again, there may be sensations as though the body were being packed in ice, plunged into boiling water, or torn with red-hot pincers. A man affected with the disease in question informed me that every night a devil came and broke all his bones with a crowbar, and that during the day "the chief physician of hell" set them all, so as to have them ready to be broken again at night. Sometimes the hallucination connects the pains with some particular person, when the patient has the false perceptions of seeing and of hearing.

Hallucinations of *taste* may give rise to the delusion that poisoning the food is being attempted, or that it is rotten or otherwise unfit for use, and hence there is an obstinate refusal to eat. In the patient whose case has just been cited there was often the hallucination of the taste of oil of bitter almonds in his tea or coffee, and even at times in the water he drank.

Hallucinations of *smell* are the least common of all. Occasionally, however, they are very persistent, and give rise to troublesome delusions. Thus, a patient, whose case I have mentioned in another chapter, had the hallucination, among others, that the masons met in their lodges all over the country, and, by means of pipes leading from their rooms to his own, sent out all kinds of poisonous vapors for him to inhale. Upon one occasion he sprang from the bed in the middle of the night, exclaiming that a glass bomb full of poisonous vapor had been thrown in at the window, that it had broken in its fall, and that he was dying of suffocation. He declared that the odor was that of rotten fish, and that phosphorus entered into its composition.

As already said, the subjects of melancholia with delirium are among the most dangerous of all lunatics; the delusions which they entertain are to them as real as though based on actual facts, and they are accordingly guided by them in the same degree as they would be were they the most irrefragable truths. When, therefore, for instance, a man suffering from melancholia with delirium thinks he hears the voice of God commanding him to kill his wife and children, he unhesitatingly obeys, thinking that he has received an order from a superior being, to disobey whom would be a heinous sin. It was thus that Freeman, two or three years ago, killed his child as a sacrifice to the Deity.

Again, the patient may have exhibited no very striking evidences of mental derangement—not striking, at least, to superficial or ignorant observers—when suddenly an exacerbation of intense delirium occurs, and some terrible crime is committed.

A few years ago a horrible crime was perpetrated on Bergen Heights, a part of Jersey City. A policeman, entering the house of a laboring man, found the dead bodies of three children lying on the floor with their throats cut. In the corner stood the mother, looking placidly at her murdered children. "I killed them," she said, in answer to the questions of the officer; "I cut their throats with a razor, because I wanted to send them to heaven. They were sick, and I was sick, and I wanted to die with them."

Subsequently the father told the full details of the horrible affair. "I saw my wife," he continued, after telling how he had found the dead bodies of his children, "standing near the crib with a razor in her hand. I said, 'Good God! Mary, what have you done with the children?' She answered, 'I killed them with your razor.' I asked, 'Why did you kill them?' and she said, 'Because everybody said they were little devils, and I wanted to send them to heaven.'"

In answer to the question of the reporter, the father said that for five years his wife had been sickly. She was about forty years of age, and had never drank liquor. Since her sickness she was at times peevish, and sometimes acted strangely, but not enough to justify him in suspecting that her mind was affected. A few years ago, he said, she often used to remark that she was going to die soon, but lately she had not used that expression.

In the early part of the present year a woman in Milwaukee killed her three children in a most brutal manner, literally hacking them to pieces. The attention of the neighbors was attracted to the scene by the woman's attempt to hang herself in an outhouse. They cut her down and brought her into the house, where the most horrible spectacle was discovered. The woman, Mrs. B., was at once arrested. She took her arrest very calmly, stating that she had read in the good book that it was right to sacrifice children. The children were all girls, and were aged respectively four years, twenty months, and four months. When a reporter reached the apartment in which the deed had been committed, he beheld a terrible sight. At the left of the door stood a large, low bed, and on the scanty, dirty bed-clothing lay the forms of three little girls. Their bodies were naked, and were cut in a ghastly manner. The eldest girl had a large number of gashes, made with a butcher's knife, all over her body. The arms of the second girl were cut off near the shoulders, and the legs hung to the body by thin shreds of skin and flesh; the body was completely disemboweled. The body of the babe

30

was cut up into six pieces, the head and extremities being completely severed from the trunk. Near the foot of the bed a young woman, only partially dressed, and with dishevelled hair, crouched on the floor, held down by two strong men. She was the murderess. Her hands were bloody, and the front of her dress was saturated with blood. An unnatural smile played about her mouth, and her whole appearance was that of an insane person.

When placed before the fire in the police station, she told her story in broken German. When asked how she murdered the children, she replied that she stabbed one of them in the breast and the other in the shoulder, and that they cried but little, as she made quick work of the butchery. She smiled as she pronounced these last words. She used a drawing-knife and two small carving-knives. With the former weapon she had shaved the children's bodies as a cooper would a stave, and with the latter disemboweled them. While the bodies were shockingly mutilated, the heads were untouched. When asked what had caused her to do the fearful deed, she replied, " I read it in the book." She thought she had made a great sacrifice. She kept smoothing her back hair with her bloody hands, and looked at the crimson stains and smiled. Her eyes had a wild look.

In answer to a question as to whether his wife had shown any symptoms of insanity before that morning, the husband answered that she had not. He then recollected that at about Christmas time she had read something in a paper that seemed to have a great effect upon her. Since then she had spent whole days in looking at a small prayer-book on her lap, cooking no food, and not even heating the room. She had worried a great deal because the sickness of the children had prevented her attending church.

The delusions of the subjects of melancholia with delirium are either variable or fixed. If the former, they change generally only within certain limited bounds, being of similar characteristics, though perhaps differing in details. In the early stages of the affection they are more apt to be varied than in the later periods.

A symptom to which Poterin du Motel [1] has called atten-

---

[1] " Études sur la mélancolie," etc., " Mémoire couronné par l'académie impériale de médecine, Mémoires de l'académie impériale de médecine," t. xxi, 1857, p. 510.

tion is intellectual obliteration, or micromania, as he proposes to designate it. It is a tendency to attach importance to insignificant circumstances; a disposition to be abnormally minute, puerile even, in all their mental operations and characteristics. The woman whose case has just been given exhibited this symptom when she brought herself to murder her three children because she had read in the "good book" that it was right to kill children. In others some trifling circumstance, as for instance the delivery by the baker of two loaves of bread on any one morning instead of one, is construed into a deep-laid plan on his part to poison the family. The occurrence of a particular word two or three times on a page was deemed by a patient of my own a sufficient reason for attempting suicide. When asked what connection there was between the word witch and the act of self-murder, she replied that she was a witch, and that the Bible had declared, "Thou shalt not suffer a witch to live."

In such cases there is no logical relation between the premise and the conclusion, and the former is altogether inadequate to justify the acts committed, even if they were logically connected.

Crimes are, as we have seen, often committed by the subjects of melancholia with delirium under the influence of supposed commands from the Deity, or through the misinterpretation of passages in the Bible. Such would appear to be performed from a high religious sense, and from a feeling of duty to the Creator of the universe. Occasionally, however, there is the incentive of fear, and orders to kill, imagined to emanate from the devil, are probably due to this cause. Thus, a patient in Bethlehem Hospital became deranged from unknown causes, and killed one of her children, seven months old, by severing its head from its body. She was tried for the fact at the Old Bailey, and acquitted on the ground of insanity. She believed that the devil had directed her to do the deed. She was sent to the lunatic asylum in a very violent and dangerous state. She made several attempts to commit suicide, tearing the sheets and blankets into strips with which to strangle herself. All strings had to be removed from her clothes. She attacked every one who came near, but frequently spoke of her dead child in an affectionate way, and cried bitterly night and day. Finally she stopped talking, with the exception of answering every question with the phrase, "Forever and a day, as the boy sold his top." [1]

In another case [2] of similar characteristics, the patient, a woman twenty-eight years of age, had been a servant in a family, but had "got religion," and in a little time lapsed into melancholy and despair. She had a constant habit of biting her nails and the ends of her fingers, and lacerating her flesh for the purpose of mortification.

She was so merged in despondency and utter hopelessness that she firmly believed the devil was to have her when she should die; that the evil spirit had all the power, and the Deity none; that, seeing it impossible to be saved, she had given herself up to live in wickedness and idleness, and that all this was occasioned by her not believing in God. That she was never more to be happy, but was to be tormented forever and ever. This was the constant tenor of her lamentations from morning till night. She could not be induced to repair any part of her clothes, nor even to mend a hole in her stocking, wash her skin, or do anything whatever that could contribute to her own health or comfort, not so much even as to change her linen, unless when forced to do so. This patient finally recovered, as the sequence of a severe bodily illness, the nature of which is not stated.

Melancholia with delirium is generally characterized by the presence of remissions in the violence of the symptoms, during which periods the patients are free from excitement, and, if not disturbed, appear to be greatly improved. Sometimes there are distinct intermissions, and at these times there is such manifest change, not only as regards the delirium and the delusions, but even in the matter of the mental depression, that anticipations of recovery are entertained. Patients will then speak of their own state, and are fully aware of the former existence of mental aberration. Occasionally there is a well-marked periodicity in the occurrence both of remissions and intermissions.

The present appears to be the proper place to speak of a remarkable symptom sometimes met with in melancholia with delirium, and in other forms of insanity, and that is *hæmatoma auris*, or bloody tumor of the ear. This may be described as an effusion of blood within the cartilage of the ear, or between the cartilage and the perichondrium. This extra-

---

[1] "Sketches in Bedlam," London, 1823, p. 287.   [2] *Op. cit.*, p. 278.

vasation becomes encysted, and may remain in this condition for a considerable period. Eventually it is generally absorbed, and with its disappearance the ear shrivels and becomes dry and hard. There is another species of tumor of the pavilion of the ear, first described by Fischer, which consists of an effusion of serum, and which is a mild affection compared to the other.

Bloody tumor of the ear is more frequently met with in insane men than women. It is more common in all the forms of melancholia, in general paralysis of the insane, and in acute mania, than in other varieties of mental derangement. It may occur only in one ear, or both may be affected, and the left ear is more liable than the right. Its appearance is regarded by some authorities as of bad augury, so far as relates to the prognosis.

The origin of hæmatoma auris has been a matter of animated discussion. The fact that the left ear is the one generally affected has led to the conclusion, on the part of some alienists, among them Griesinger, that it is the result of pinchings or blows from attendants, or by the patient knocking his head against the bed-posts or other hard substance. Griesinger,[1] indeed, asserts that the impression of the finger-nails is sometimes observed, and that the affection can, by care on the part of the attendants, be made entirely to disappear from well-regulated asylums.

Biaute,[2] in a memoir published in 1877, asserts that alienists—meaning by the term the medical officers of asylums—do not admit that these tumors are ever of traumatic origin. In a subsequent paper he[3] cites several cases of blows received by lunatics on the ears without the production of hæmatomas.

On the other hand, again, M. Bouteille,[4] in an elaborate memoir, in which the opposing views of many authors are given, shows that it is by no means a prognostic sign indicating a fatal termination, and that it is the result of traumatism. He says :

"To resume, bloody tumor of the ear in the cases of boxers

[1] "Mental Pathology and Therapeutics," *New Sydenham Society Translation*, p. 438.

[2] "Observations sur les tumeurs sanguines du pavillon de l'oreille," *Annales médico-psychologiques*, mai, 1877.

[3] "Note sur les traumatismes de l'oreille," *op. cit.*, juillet, 1882.

[4] "Tumeurs sanguines du pavillon de l'oreille," *op. cit.*, juillet, 1878.

and lunatics presents the same symptoms, the same clinical history, the same deformation of the ear, and the same therapeutic indications. In boxers it results from a traumatic cause, and the origin in lunatics is the same.

"Without wishing to reject absolutely the alleged predisposing causes, we think they have not the value which has been attributed to them, and that hæmatoma only appears as the consequence of injuries inflicted on the ear by the patients themselves or by others. The affection as regards its prognostic value is of no importance." [1]

The truth is probably to be found in the facts that the insane condition acts as a powerful predisposing cause, that traumatism of slight character is competent to produce hæmatoma auris, and that its origin is to be found in the blows and other injuries inflicted by the patients themselves, by other patients, or by attendants.

Reference has already been made to the circumstance that the subjects of melancholia with or without delirium are particularly prone to refuse food. This act may be based upon one of three causes : (1) The patient has a delusion that the food given him is poisoned, and that if he takes it he will die ; or (2) he refuses to eat because he desires to commit suicide, and finds in starvation a ready means ; or (3) he does not eat because he has no appetite. It is important as regards the treatment that the physician should ascertain which of these is the governing motive.

In an interesting essay, M. Mabille [2] shows that there is often present in melancholics a sensory paralysis, partial or total, of the alimentary canal, and that this paralysis appears after they refuse food. He attributes it to nervous exhaustion from emptiness of the stomach, and to the sudden distention which the organ undergoes through the process of forcible feeding to which sitophobics are usually subjected.

Melancholia with delirium may terminate in complete recovery, or it may pass into the condition next to be described, or into chronic mania, or death may take place from suicide, exhaustion, or from the supervention of some other acute

---

[1] M. Bouteille is the physician in chief of the insane asylum at Armentières, and professor (agrégé) of the faculty of medicine at Lisle. His opinions on the subject cannot be suspected of bias against the asylum interest.

[2] "Étude clinique sur quelques points de la lypemanie," *Ann. méd. psychol.*, mai, 1880, p. 345.

or chronic brain disease. The duration of the disease is, therefore, variable. I have known cases to be cured in less than three months, and others last, with but little diminution in the intensity of the symptoms, for several years. The duration and general course of the affection are greatly influenced according as the medical and hygienic management of the patient is good or bad, and the hereditary tendency weak or strong. Under advantageous circumstances, a short duration and a favorable termination may reasonably be expected, even in very violent cases. But under bad management, or with a marked heredity, slight cases do badly.

e—MELANCHOLIA WITH STUPOR.

Melancholia with stupor—the melancholia atonita of the ancients, and the acute dementia of English writers—owes its thorough study, like so many other mental diseases, to the alienists and psychologists of France.

Georget,[1] under the name of "stupidité," described the condition in question as one in which there was a suspension of the cerebral faculties, confusion of ideas, and an obtusion of the intelligence.

Etoc-Demazy,[2] in 1835, published a work on the subject, in which he refused to recognize "stupidity" as a distinct form of insanity, declaring that it was only a complication met with in certain cases of monomania and mania. According to him, it consists of a simple diminution of the sensory, intellectual, and moral faculties. He further expresses the opinion that the condition in question is due to an intracranial infiltration of serum, the flattening of the convolutions of the brain, and the tension of the dura mater.

But the views at present generally entertained relative to the nosological position of "stupidity" are based upon a work published by Baillarger[3] in 1843. The author describes "stupidity" as characterized by confusion of the ideas, perceptions, and sensations, and by the existence of general delirium of a melancholic type. It differs from simple melancholia or melancholia with delirium by the facts that there is a general transformation of impressions, a loss of the identity

---

[1] " Considérations sur la folie," Paris, 1820, p. 115.
[2] " De la stupidité considérée chez les aliénés," Paris, 1835.
[3] " De la mélancolie avec stupeur," *Ann. méd.-psychol.*, Paris, 1843.

of time, places, and persons, a suspension of the action of the will, and by the physical symptoms.

The subjects of melancholia with stupor are in the early stages less profoundly affected than at subsequent periods, the symptoms being of gradual development. It may arise as a primary disease, or it may be the sequence of some other form of insanity. The former is more generally the case. When a primary disorder, it often originates suddenly, in consequence of some powerful emotional disturbance affecting the patient. In other cases it is developed gradually, with or without any apparently exciting cause.

The individual affected with melancholia with stupor presents a very striking appearance. He sits motionless, his hands clasped before him, his head bent forward, his eyes closed or staring vacantly, or fixed upon the floor. His half-open mouth allows the viscid saliva to drop from his lips. If spoken to, he does not answer or even give any sign that he has heard, and he rarely speaks spontaneously. If he does, he is very apt to utter some irrelevant word or sentence, and may go on repeating it for hours at a time, day after day. His movements are torpid, and rarely spontaneous. If told to rise, he takes no notice of the direction, but, if pulled up from his chair, makes only passive resistance, or none at all. His cutaneous sensibility is greatly diminished, both to sensations of touch and of pain. His expression is either one of absolute apathy or vacancy, or is indicative of astonishment or terror. The pupils are, as a rule, widely dilated. Occasionally one is dilated and the other contracted, a circumstance which some authors regard as an unfavorable prognostic point.

At times tears flow from his eyes, and he exhibits all the evidences of grief ; and again he appears to be under the influence of extreme fear. As stated by patients who have recovered from their disease, these and other signs of intense emotional disturbance were due to terrible hallucinations of sight and of hearing, of events taking place from which they were powerless to escape.

But in the most intense form of the disease there are no external signs of the emotions which fill his mind. He may be the subject of the most vivid illusions and hallucinations, which he accepts as realities so far as he is capable of accepting anything without the active exercise of his intellectual powers, but he sits impassive, as if petrified.

Dagonet,[1] who has very thoroughly considered the affection under notice, thus graphically describes the patient suffering from this stage of melancholia with stupor:

"When the delirium is present in a marked degree, it is generally noticed that the individual, struck as he is with stupor, can be assimilated to the man who is the subject of a painful dream or nightmare, in which all impressions and sensations exercise a painful action, while he who is visited experiences an absolute impossibility of reacting against the terrors which fill his mind.

"The patient, being entirely passive, is essentially a true automaton. If the events passing around him are transformed into painful impressions, as they are in those suffering from the systematized delirium of lypemania or megalomania, he does not, like them, submit to his diseased mental faculties the acts he sees or the sounds he hears, in order to furnish new aliment to his false convictions. His mind remains in a state of inextricable chaos, as his sensations are themselves in a condition of the greatest composure. With him all is vague and indeterminate. Deprived of the power of attention, he is incapable of arranging his sensorial impressions into a harmonious system, and he neither endeavors to understand the painful illusions of which he is the sport, nor to explain to himself, in a more or less logical manner, the extravagant circumstances in the midst of which he thinks he is placed. He neither reasons affirmatively nor negatively, for that by which he is most distinctly characterized is the absence of all cerebral activity, and one cannot actually affirm that there is any exercise of the intellectual faculties, since these were entirely controlled by the accidental impressions which he experiences. With him inertia and impotence are carried to the highest degree—even to the point of indicating the absence of all thought; to the suspension of every faculty.

"The life of relation is in a great measure extinguished in the patient affected with stupor. He may have the most frightful visions, and, notwithstanding, he remains motionless, and in a degree impassible, in the presence of the scenes which cause his intense distress. He is surrounded by brigands, he

---

[1] " De la stupeur dans les maladies mentales et de l'affection designée sous le nomme de stupidité," Paris, 1872, p. 19. Also, *Annales médico-psychologiques*, 5ième série, t. vii, mars, 1872.

hears the clicking of many guns aimed at him, but he does nothing to avoid the dangers by which he is menaced. He sees the fire, hears the frightful voices attendant in the conflagration, but he does not stir from his place. Nothing betrays the emotion which troubles him; he is, as it were, changed into a statue."

In melancholia with stupor the pulse is generally slow and weak; again it may be frequent, but it rarely indicates fever. The temperature is more apt to be slightly reduced than increased. In women, menstruation is either entirely suppressed or disordered, both as regards periodicity and quantity.

Examined with the ophthalmoscope, the optic disk is seen to be paler than is natural, and the retinal vessels are straight and attenuated. Œdema of the disk is rarely observed in any but the most severe cases.

Dr. Aldridge,[1] who, however, regards melancholia atonita as a different affection from acute dementia, different at least in degree, confirms this statement relative to the ophthalmoscopic appearances in the two disorders. He finds in both, the optic disks pale, the retinal vessels small and shrunken, but in melancholia atonita there is no œdema, while in profound cases of acute dementia this condition may exist.

The saliva is often greatly increased in quantity. In a patient whom I saw quite recently the amount exceeded a pint in eight hours—a pint, that is, that flowed from the mouth in a vessel placed to receive it, without reckoning the quantity that was swallowed. The stomach sometimes rejects all food that may be swallowed, and the bowels are usually obstinately constipated.

Occasionally in the first stages of melancholia with stupor there is a tendency to the practice of masturbation, and this, in my experience, is especially the case with females. During the more advanced periods of the disease, however, this disposition disappears. In one case, that of a young woman brought to me by her mother, the patient did not hesitate to make attempts to perform the act in our presence.

Sauze[2] asserts that "stupidity" is more frequent with

---

[1] " Ophthalmoscopic Observations in Acute Dementia," " West Riding Lunatic Asylum Medical Reports," vol. iv, London, 1874, p. 296 et seq.

[2] "De la stupidité de sa nature psychologique et de son traitement," Thèse de Paris, 1852.

males than with females. It appears to be more common between the ages of twenty and thirty than at other periods of life. Its duration rarely exceeds a year, and the prognosis in uncomplicated cases is tolerably good. It should be stated, however, that instances of recovery after the disease has lasted much over a year are rare.

ƒ—HYPOCHONDRIACAL MANIA, OR MELANCHOLIA.

Hypochondriacal mania is not to be confounded with that much less grave affection known as hypochondria, and which may exist without any more serious implication of the mental faculties than a slight emotional depression. This latter is unaccompanied by illusions, hallucinations, or delusions, and is rather to be assimilated to the morbid fears already brought under consideration. By most authors, hypochondriacal mania is regarded as a form of melancholia, and such, undoubtedly, is its true nosological position.

Hypochondriacal mania is characterized by the existence of morbid fears relative to the health, mental or physical, by intense depression of mind, and by the presence of illusions, hallucinations, and delusions relative to the condition of the body, or of one or more of its organs.

It is usually of slow development. The individual at first, perhaps, begins by manifesting symptoms of disordered bodily health. He sleeps badly, and is troubled with morbid dreams, which make no inconsiderable impression on his mind. His bowels are obstinately constipated, and there appears to be a special proclivity to torpor of the colon and the impaction of fæces in that part of the alimentary canal. His stomach is inactive ; the food, instead of digesting in proper time, remains in the organ till fermentation begins, and he consequently suffers from flatulence. The liver is inactive, and the kidneys excrete a pale-colored urine in more than the normal quantity. He suffers from palpitations of the heart ; the respiratory act is insufficiently performed, and there is consequently frequent sighing.

The mind participates in the disturbance. The patient secludes himself, as far as possible, from observation, renounces those amusements which formerly gave him pleasure, is indisposed to mental exertion, neglects his business, restricts his conversation almost entirely to the subject of his health and the various sensations he experiences in different parts of his body, is irritable, and hyperæsthetic. The least pain causes him inordinate suffering, the weather never suits him ; if his affairs go wrong, he exaggerates the difficulty ; if they are prosperous, the prosperity is more apparent than real, and disaster is sure to come in a short time. Though he has no idea of persecution or injury from those with whom he associates, he is sure that they do not appreciate the serious condition of his health.

By degrees his conviction that he is the subject of profound disease becomes strengthened, though probably he has as yet no very definite notion of the nature or seat of his malady. Accident generally determines these points. He reads the details of a case of disease, he sees a person suffering from an extraordinary affection, or he has an unusual sensation in some part of his body, and the bent of his mind is at once settled. The moment his attention is concentrated upon the organ which he imagines is diseased, his symptoms become more pronounced. Every sensation he experiences in it is exaggerated and misinterpreted. He is constantly on the watch for the symptoms which he has ascertained are connected with the malady which he thinks he has. He measures his urine, examines it by all the tests at his command, inspects his fæces, scrutinizes his countenance in the glass, and, as one of my patients did who imagined himself to be impotent, may even take notes of the quantity, viscidity, or odor of his semen.

He goes from one physician to another, giving long accounts, often written out, of the symptoms he has, or imagines he has, and takes all the medicines that may be prescribed with a degree of punctuality that is itself an evidence of insanity. He buys medical books on his imaginary disease, and brings them with him to the physician under whose care he is for the time being, calling his attention to certain features which he thinks have been overlooked, and suggesting the use of remedial measures which he finds mentioned.

Up to this time his illusions and hallucinations have only been such as relate to visceral or cutaneous sensibility, but ere long the special senses show signs of perceptional derangement, sight being the one to be first, and perhaps most, profoundly affected. Any one or all of the others may become involved, and delusions soon follow. His life is now a perpetual source of misery to him. He thinks, talks, dreams of nothing but himself and his diseases. He experiments with the most extraordinary agents which he imagines may restore him to health, and, obtaining only failure, tries others still more fanciful. In his moments of despair he may talk of suicide, but it is generally only talk ; he rarely attempts it. Indeed, with the misery and sorrow which so strongly affect the patient, there is a predominating love of life which stands in the way of all tendency to self-destruction.

Dubois [1] divides the symptoms of hypochondria into the period of invasion and three periods of the fully developed disease, but he fails to make sufficient distinction between those cases which are simple hypochondria, and which never pass into a more fully developed stage, and those which very surely and rapidly tend to the further implication of the mind. He, however, recognizes the fact that there is a distinct form of mental aberration characterized by the existence of perceptional, intellectual, and emotional derangement. Of this he makes three varieties, named according to the part of the body associated with the physical and mental disturbance — hypochondriacal monomania, pneumo-cardiac monomania, and encephalic monomania; and three other forms, which would scarcely at the present day be considered hypochondriacal—the asthenic, the nostalgic, and the hydrophobiac. [2]

His division into periods is, however, better founded, and is a natural arrangement of the symptoms of hypochondriacal mania.

The *first period* is characterized by the existence of purely mental symptoms. There are no obvious physical derangements, and, if there are any such, they are entirely subjective.

In the *second period* there is the same mental condition, but there are functional troubles of various organs of the body.

And in the *third period* there is superadded to the foregoing categories of phenomena lesions of the organs, either in the nature of congestions, inflammations, or other more serious affections. Real disease is, therefore, induced, and the symptoms are such as are peculiar to the existing lesion.

The illusions, hallucinations, and delusions of hypochondriacal maniacs are among the most remarkable and prepos-

[1] " Histoire philosophique de l'hypochondrie et de l'hysterie," Paris, 1837.
[2] *Op. cit.*, p. 229.

terous to be met with in the whole range of psychological medicine, though, perhaps, in the earliest periods they may be not much more than suspicions or fears. Accepted not altogether with a certainty of their truth, they become more positive and abnormal as the disease advances, till eventually they reach the point of absolute impossibility of realization.

Thus it is related of Falret,[1] one of the most distinguished alienists that France has produced, that, while he was a pupil of medicine at Montpellier, he was present at a lecture on phthisis. Such was the impression produced upon him by the graphic description of the disease that he thought for a long time that he was affected, and was only relieved of his apprehensions by ridicule and more thorough knowledge.

Philip V, King of Spain, was constantly worried about his health. He was sometimes six months without leaving his bed. He would wear no shirts that had not been previously worn by the Queen, fearful that any others would poison him. He occasionally believed himself to be dead, and expressed astonishment that he was not buried. His insanity was so marked that he bit and scratched his wife, his confessor, and his physician.[2]

Joseph Frank speaks of a man in Vienna who only chewed his food, swallowing nothing but the juice. The residue he kept, and submitted it to his physician for examination. He mentions another who went every week to his physician, several miles distant, with vases full of the fæces he had passed; and a third, who, thinking himself affected with a liver disease, applied his tongue to his excrements in order to ascertain whether or not they were bitter. In this connection I may state that a patient of my own affected with hypochondriacal mania, and believing that the coats of his intestines were being expelled with his fæces, sent me once a large package of the paper he had used for several weeks in the water-closet, in order that I might examine it microscopically.

Louyer-Villermay[3] refers to the case of a man suffering from hypochondria who had a room in his house specially used to store the vases in which he kept his urine. He had a vase for each day in the week, and spent most of his time in their examination.

[1] Cited by Delasiauve in *Journal de médecine mentale*, t. v, 1865, p. 225.
[2] "Mémoires secrets," de Duclos, cited by Delasiauve, *op. cit.*, p. 226.
[3] Art. "Hypochondrie" in *Dictionnaire des sciences médicales*, t. xxiii, p. 127.

A young man, having read several medical books, contracted the delusion that his head was filled with water and pus, and insisted upon its being opened in order that the fluid might be evacuated and his life saved.[1]

"George Woods, from Lower Lincolnshire, was admitted in Bethlehem Hospital November 25, 1819. This unfortunate young man had been professionally brought up a surgeon, and the cause of his malady appeared to have been the persuasion that he had undergone the fate of Abélard, and this notion was the constant source of his lamentation; for his perpetual complaint was, 'Oh, what shall I do? what shall I do? They have taken away my ——! Gone, all gone! What shall I do? All gone! gone forever!' Convinced of this privation, he imagined the loss had caused a contraction of his limbs; and under this idea he had acquired habits of contraction extremely painful to himself and distressing to all who saw him. His elbows were pressed in as if screwed to his sides, his lower arms projecting outward on a line with his chest, and his hands continually clenched with such power that they could only be opened by force for the purpose of washing them; and then the palms were found to be so indented by the pressure of his finger-ends that they seemed almost to have grown together. But no sooner was he freed from restraint than they returned to their former position. He walked invariably on tiptoe, took very little exercise, and would stand for hours together in one spot without setting his heels to the ground, if not roused by the keepers and urged to walk about. At times he was without appetite, and very weakly; at other times his appetite was good, and he would sit down contentedly to dinner without any appearance of pain. But, as soon as he had finished his meal, he got up to the gallery and began his usual plaints: 'Gone! gone! all gone! What shall I do for my ——?'

"In May, 1820, a party of ladies of rank and distinction came to visit the hospital, and poor Woods was bewailing in his usual vein. 'Oh, my ——! What shall I do for my ——? They are all gone.' Then one of the ladies, a peeress, asked him what he complained of, but could get no reply but, 'Oh, my ——! What shall I do for my ——? Gone! gone! forever!' and this with a piteous look of tribulation.

[1] Michea, "Du siége, de la nature intime, etc., de l'hypochondrie," *Mém. de l'acad. royale de médecine*, t. x, 1843, p. 573.

"The lady, unable to comprehend his meaning, applied for explanation to a keeper, who with some discreet presence of mind told her ladyship that the poor patient was in the habit of collecting a quantity of pebbles, flints, and other rubbish about the airing-ground, which he fancied to be emeralds, rubies, diamonds, and other precious gems ; that it became necessary to take them away from him in order to prevent the accumulation of rubbish in the gallery ; and that a recent privation of this sort was now the subject of his lament. 'Oh, poor man!' said her ladyship, turning to the patient, 'never mind them. When his lordship comes here again he shall bring you some pretty ones which he has at home ; they will be much handsomer than those you have lost, so don't fret about them any more.' But poor Woods, not at all satisfied with the promised alternative, answered, with much displeasure, 'That won't do ! I will have none other but my own.' And thus they separated, each unconscious of the other's meaning." [1]

Probably next after false perceptions and delusions connected with the digestive system, those with the genito-urinary organs, similar to the case just quoted, are most numerous. A patient of my own, after great sexual excesses, took the idea that his penis and testicles were diminishing in size. He spent the greater part of each day in measuring them, and in recording the results in a book which he kept for the purpose. Finally he reached the conclusion that they had entirely disappeared, and, although he did not go about lamenting the fact, he was examining the region as often as he could get the opportunity, and making a record of the results of his examinations. As an interesting instance of the line of thought of a hypochondriacal maniac, I transcribe here a portion of his diary for one day :

"November 4th, 9 A. M. The event that I have been fearing has at length occurred. They have vanished, absolutely vanished, and I am ruined ! Oh, my God, how I am punished for my sins !

"9.30 A. M. Cold water does no good ; hot water is no better. Will try blistering.

"9.45 A. M. There is not even a vestige of either penis or testicles, not a vestige. I will consult a physician. No, I cannot exhibit my misfortune. Applied blister.

[1] "Sketches in Bedlam," by A Constant Observer, London, 1823, p. 113.

"10 A. M. Removed blister to see if they really had gone. Alas! it is too true. Blistering can be of no possible service. Removed it.

"10.15 A. M. Reflected that if they are really gone there ought to be something left to show where they had been. Find ample evidence. A vast cavity at the bottom of my belly. Will consult a surgeon; but how in heaven can he help me? Is there any medicine that can restore the organs when they have entirely gone, as have mine? It would be a mockery—a sinful mockery; and God knows I have sinned enough.

"10.25 A. M. There is no doubt of it! They have gone, and I am a ruined man! Man! I am no man. I am a eunuch; an unsexed man; a mere thing without purpose on the earth.

"11 A. M. I might sing in a choir if they are really gone; but, O God! for me, a man—a strong, lusty, vigorous, boastful man—to be reduced to singing in a church choir! It is horrible; but what else am I fit for? My mind is certain to become weaker. I shall grow to be fat and pulpy. I will be an oyster—a big, disgusting oyster.

"11.10 A. M. Have just urinated, and had the most singular experience. The urine oozed out from the place where the penis used to be, but, alas, where it no longer is!"

This will suffice. There were hundreds of pages of such stuff. He finally came to see me, and brought his diary with him for my information. He, with the utmost confidence in the correctness of his perceptions and judgment, attempted to demonstrate to me the complete absence of his penis and testicles. I could detect no deviation from the normal standard in either, but no arguments or tests that I could apply sufficed to undeceive him. He groaned and wept over his misfortunes, and walked up and down the room, cursing himself for his wickedness, and the science of medicine for its inability to aid him.

In another case the patient, a young lady, who had just left a school where her mental energies had been severely taxed, began to be troubled with insomnia and gastric and intestinal derangement. Her menstrual function, which had previously been normal, stopped altogether. One day she read in a newspaper an account of a so-called mysterious disease which had affected the people of a Western town, the chief symptom of which was a gradual blackening of the tongue. She talked about the matter for several days, and

31

expressed so much interest in the subject that her friends laughed at her, and one of them said, laughingly, "One would think you were afraid you will get this black-tongue disease." From that time on her anxiety increased. She not only talked about the disease in a general way, but she applied to herself the little information she had obtained on the subject, and was sure that the first symptoms were already present. She spent the greater part of each day in examining her tongue before a looking-glass, which she kept constantly about her. If anybody looked at her she at once conceived the idea that her tongue was the object of inspection. If two persons spoke together in her presence, she was certain they were talking of her. Finally, she was fully convinced that her tongue was really black, and that ere long it would drop off. No arguments, no appeals to her perceptions or intellect, had the least effect on this illusion and delusion. Her emotional system was even more disturbed. She wept almost constantly, and in piteous language spoke of the great misfortune to which she was subjected. "What have I done," she said to me, "that I should be made to suffer in this cruel way? I have tried to be good, and yet I am treated like a criminal. I would rather have my tongue taken out with red-hot pincers than see it, little by little, mortifying in this way. It might be a proper punishment for a slanderer, but I have never slandered any one."

I took a piece of very black paper, and held it by the side of her protruded tongue while she looked at both in the glass. "Yes!" she exclaimed, "my tongue is exactly like that; just as black, but shrivelled."

I found that tactile sensibility in the tongue, though not abolished, was greatly diminished. The points of the æsthesiometer could not be discriminated at a less distance than seven twelfths of an inch, instead of the twenty-fourth of an inch, the normal distance. The ability to feel pain did not appear to be sensibly impaired.

In the course of about two weeks I saw this patient again. She then conducted all communications with others by signs and by writing. Her tongue, she said, had dropped off. She had not seen it drop. It had disappeared in the night, during sleep, and she supposed she had swallowed it. In fact, she had, she declared, tasted something rotten in her mouth all the next day. She opened her mouth at my request, but when I asked her to put out her tongue she wrote, "How can I put out my tongue when I have no tongue?" When requested to open her mouth she did so, and when I pointed to her tongue and put my finger on it, and asked her what that was if it was not her tongue, she wrote, "It may look like a tongue to you, but it does not to me; it is simply the base of my mouth. The membrane there is very loose." When I asserted positively that it was her tongue, she wrote, "I am the best judge on that subject. I came here to see if a new tongue could be transplanted from some one else. I am willing to pay largely any woman who will sell me her tongue." I suggested an animal's tongue—that of a sheep, for instance. She quickly wrote, "I could not talk with a sheep's tongue. I should have to say 'ba, ba, ba' all my life. I would rather be mute."

I was considering the propriety of performing, with the consent of her friends, a piously fictitious operation on this patient, for the purpose of acting on her mind, when I determined first to treat her with aloetic purges, as recommended by Schroeder van der Kolk—a method that will be fully discussed under the head of "treatment." The effect was entirely satisfactory. Large quantities of hardened fecal matter were discharged, the menstrual function was restored, and, before thirty days had elapsed, she was entirely free from all perceptional, intellectual, or emotional derangement.

The late Colonel Charles May, of the United States Army, informed me that he had cured a brother officer of a delusion by a well-intentioned deception. The gentleman had the belief that he had swallowed a chicken-bone, which had stuck in his throat before reaching his stomach. He went about with his hands pressed over the place where he supposed the bone to be, refused to eat any but liquid food, and complained of a constant pain in the part. Examination by the medical officer, and exploration with a probang, settled the point definitely that there was no bone there. But the patient was not convinced; he felt it, and he knew it was sticking in his throat.

Colonel May then suggested to the doctor that an emetic should be given, and, while it was acting, he dropped a chicken-bone, unperceived by the patient, into the basin. The latter examined the vomited matter very carefully, found the bone, and, triumphantly exhibiting it as positive evidence of the correctness of his sensations and his idea, was at the same time permanently cured of his delusion.

The delirium of negation (*délire des négations*), as it is called by Cotard,[1] is only a variety of hypochondriacal mania. In it the patients think they have lost various parts of their bodies; their arms, legs, nose, eyes, head, stomach, womb, etc., have, they imagine, disappeared. I have already cited cases of this phase of the disease, but many others are on record still more pronounced. Indeed, it is by no means an uncommon manifestation of the affection in question.

There are many other categories of delusions exhibited by hypochondriacal maniacs. Thus, there is a delirium of little-ness (*délire micromaniaque*), in which the patients imagine that parts of their bodies have become reduced in size, or that the whole body has become smaller. A patient observed by Materne[2] desired to sleep in a cradle, "his legs being so small and his feet so narrow that he dared not sit up even for an instant."

The opposite condition may exist, in which there are illusions and delusions that things are larger than they really are. One man, for instance, conceived that he had grown to such an enormous size that he could not pass through a doorway, though in reality he was very thin. He apparently suffered the most exquisite torments, when some persons, thinking to cure him in that way of his delusion, dragged him forcibly through a doorway.

A gentleman, who came under my observation, had the delusion that his head was of enormous size. It was as large, he said, as a half-bushel measure, and was constantly growing larger. He insisted that no hat would fit him, and that the disease and exposure would soon end his life. The delusion had been excited by several friends, who, by way of a joke, conspired to tell him, when they saw him in town, that his head was growing bigger. At first he laughed at the idea, but one of them surreptitiously changed his hat for another much smaller, and that convinced him. He became terribly frightened, went home with the delusion firmly established, and was soon afterward, I believe, sent to a lunatic asylum.

[1] "Du délire des négations," *Archives de neurologie*, No. 11, 1882, p. 152 *et seq.*

[2] *Thèse de Paris*, 1874, obs. vii.

This form, which has received little notice from alienists, might properly be designated macromaniacal delirium.

Again, there are sensations of things of various kinds in the stomach and intestines, or the chest or brain. · One patient believes that there is a galvanic battery in his stomach, by means of which all his nerves and muscles are kept in a state of perpetual excitement. Another has the delusion that a steam engine is in his heart, and that boiling blood is being pumped to every part of his body. Another imagines that her womb contains every day a new fœtus, which is born in the night and carried away by her enemies. Another thinks his brain consists of snakes, which are constantly writhing and twisting within his skull; and others have demons, and fairies, and elfs, and giants located in various parts of their bodies, and annoying them with their jibes, curses, and commands. There is no end to the fancies of this kind, and they seem to be among the most persistent of all the delusions which the hypochondriacal maniac can entertain. It is probable that they are in the first place excited by various abnormal and real sensations, and that the peculiar character of the delusion in any one case is due to accident, or to the reading of stories of various kinds.

Hypochondriacal mania is not characterized by intermissions or by any marked remissions. There are times, as in all forms of insanity, in which the patient is more or less free from delirium, and does not obtrude his delusions on those around him, but questioning will show that they are still present, and that he is thinking of them with all the force of his mind.

The affection is much more common in men than in women, and in persons between the ages of twenty-five and forty than at other periods. Women are more apt to become the subjects at or about the menopause. It is one of the most obstinate of all the forms of mental derangement, though not by any means beyond the reach of remedial agents, unless it has, by lasting many years, become an integral part of the patient's mentality. In such a case a cure is not to be expected.

g—HYSTERICAL MANIA.

Hysterical mania has been considered by some authors as the analogue in the female of hypochondriacal mania in the male. The differences between the two affections are, however, so many and so great as not to warrant an assumption of their identity. Hypochondriacal mania is met with in women, and hysterical mania is sometimes seen in men. Moreover, in hysterical mania the delusions, though sometimes relating to the individual herself, differ altogether in character from those peculiar to hypochondriacal mania. The emotional disturbance has scarcely any affinities with that present in the latter disease, and it exhibits other phenomena, to which attention will be called, which hypochondriacal mania never presents. As hypochondria is not hypochondriacal mania, so hysteria is not hysterical mania. It may be, however, and often is, as in the former case, the pathological basis on which the mental aberration rests.

The disorder may arise suddenly, without any previous obvious symptoms, or, as is generally the case, it may be preceded by well-marked prodromata. These consist of the phenomena indicative of the hysterical diathesis, and have been well set forth by Georget.[1]

"Almost all these patients," he says, "are endowed with great physical activity. They are impressionable, possess a vivid imagination, are disturbed every instant of their lives, and by the most trivial causes; they are quick, impatient, irascible, self-willed, obstinate. Some exhibit great sensorial acuteness and irritability. The eyes cannot support a strong light; they hear the slightest sounds, and perceive the faintest odors. The least degree of cold or heat pains them, and a highly electric condition of the atmosphere is particularly unpleasant to them. Their sleep is rarely sound or continuous, and is often disturbed by painful dreams. Some are taciturn and disposed to court solitude; others, on the contrary, affect a gayety which is forced and unnatural. They laugh upon the slightest motive, and often without any apparent cause; others laugh and weep by turns without knowing why."

In addition, they suffer from headache, vertigo, and gastric and intestinal derangement. It may be, also, that they have experienced one or more pronounced hysterical attacks in their varied forms.

One of the most striking characteristics of hysterical mania is the complete perversion of the emotions which it exhibits. A young girl, for instance, brought up in the midst of the

[1] "De la physiologie du système nerveux," etc., Paris, 1821, t. ii, p. 270.

most refined and moral influences, suddenly or gradually exhibits a coarseness of manner and of language, and an immorality of ideas, shocking to all with whom she is in association. In the discussions which may take place in the family she defends the most atrocious criminals, and this in words never heard in polite society. Indeed, it is often a matter of astonishment where she could have obtained a knowledge of such expressions as she employs. If remonstrated with, she expresses her dislike, even hatred, of those who reprove her, be they ever so near relatives, and threatens to leave the house, and probably makes several attempts to escape from what she calls her jail and her jailers. A case reported by Chairau [1] is instructive in this relation :

"Mademoiselle B., aged twenty-eight years, of a decidedly lymphatic temperament, menstruated late, and always irregularly, and with pain. She had received a good education, and was very intelligent. When she was twenty-two years old her father's house was frequently visited by a young man to whom she became attached, and she persuaded herself that he was about to make a proposal of marriage. She spoke to her father on the subject, who said that, while he had no objection to the gentleman, there was nothing in his conduct to warrant the supposition that he contemplated marriage. He consequently insisted that his daughter should cease to concern herself with the matter. Several weeks afterward, the young man obtained a lucrative position in a foreign country, and left France without having shown the slightest desire to marry the lady. From this time Mademoiselle B. became depressed in mind. She ceased to occupy herself with those things which had given her pleasure, and shut herself up in her room. Her mental faculties, especially her memory, became weak, her appetite was lost, her menstruation became more irregular and painful, and attacks of hysteria were provoked on the least contradiction or obstruction of her wishes. At the same time, her digestion was deranged, she experienced sharp, epigastric pains, and her body was covered with acne. She began to be emaciated, and anæsthetic and hyperæsthetic zones appeared on various parts of her body.

"The moral faculties were altered in a marked degree, and she formed a fixed idea of running away. It was necessary

[1] "Études cliniques sur l'hystérie," etc., Paris, 1870, p. 57.

to bar the windows, to lock the doors, and to have an attendant constantly with her. She would have nothing to do with any member of her family. As she had persuaded herself that her clothes somehow or other were aids to her imprisonment, she was forever endeavoring to strip them off. If she was left for a few minutes alone in her room, she was found naked when the attendant returned. One day she was left for a short time alone in the garden. She profited by the circumstance to lock herself in the *cabinet d'aisance.* Neither prayers nor threats could induce her to come out. At last a mason was sent for to cut a hole in the wall. She was found entirely naked, and her clothes she had thrown down the hole.

"The maniacal symptoms were increased at her menstrual periods to such a degree that she struck furiously all those who attempted to arrest her in her movements toward flight."

But, as Legrand du Saulle [1] remarks, hysterical mania may make its appearance either as acute mania, melancholia, hallucinations, or irresistible impulses. Generally all these forms are combined. But with all these there is usually the distinguishing features to which I have alluded—the radical change in the character, mode of thought, expressions, and conduct of the subject, and this without apparent motive; solely, as it were, from a suddenly developed spirit of wickedness. It is no matter for astonishment, therefore, that in a period of the world's history when devils and demons were universally believed to exist, as they still are by ignorant or superstitious people, the idea that they could enter the system and misdirect the mind and body of an individual, should have existed. Holy women, saints and nuns, would all at once exhibit the most diabolical characteristics, and, influenced by the belief that existed, would proclaim aloud that the devil or some of his imps had taken possession of their bodies. The form of insanity has not changed since then; we merely explain it on a different hypothesis. Under the head of "epidemic insanity" this point will be more fully considered.

Morel,[2] in speaking of the spontaneity of hysterical mania, cites the following cases :

A young hysterical girl was dining with her parents. She left the table, and, her prolonged absence having alarmed the

[1] " Les hystériques ; état physique et état mental," etc., Paris, 1883, p. 293.
[2] " Traité des maladies mentales," Paris, 1860, p. 676 (*note*).

family, search was made for her. She was found in a neighboring wood, occupied in gathering stones with which to make an altar, before which she was going to be married. She was crowned with flowers, and had taken off all her clothes. Another left the arm of her father during a village fête, and threw herself into a stream of muddy water. In another case he diagnosticated the existence of hysterical mania in the case of a lady, twenty-four years of age, who was often seized with paroxysms, during which she would violently throw down any piece of work upon which she was engaged, rise from her chair, and break the glass or plates that might be in the room. One day she got up from the table, and, seizing a vessel of boiling water, emptied it, without the slightest manifestation of feeling, over the neck of her brother.

In the following case, also quoted from Morel, there was hereditary tendency to mental derangement, and the existence of the hysterical type of organization in a marked degree :

The young Eliza C., born of an intelligent mother, but whose father was of limited intellect and neurotic temperament, menstruated when twelve years old. Her disposition was always sullen, capricious, and eccentric, and she never exhibited the least feeling of tenderness toward either of her parents. She laughed and cried without cause, and committed, from an early period of her life, all kinds of singular and ridiculous acts. Placed among other girls to learn the trade of a seamstress, she could not be prevented from using insolent and obscene language. Soon she exhibited a series of spontaneous and delirious acts such as are met with in hysterical mania. One day, for instance, she crowned herself with flowers, took a guitar, and announced that she was going to travel through the world. She got up in the night and washed her clothes in the chamber-pot. Then she had convulsive seizures, mewed like a cat, tried to climb up the wall, was violent in her acts toward others, and finally fell into a state of stupor. These accessions were periodical, and it became necessary to send her to an asylum.

Though the conduct and language may often give evidence of the existence of erotic ideas, or even of the presence of nymphomania, it is rarely the case that there is any real exaltation of the sexual appetite. The acts and words in question appear rather to be the expression of a spirit of contrariety—a disposition to do something that will astonish or shock the friends—than of any actual desire for sexual intercourse. Indeed, women affected with hysterical mania have, upon several occasions, with great glee, while in a state of apparent libidinous excitement, informed me that they wanted to annoy such or such a member of the family. "You think that is bad?" said a girl who was suffering from a violent paroxysm of hysterical mania to her mother, who was shocked at some obscene words she had spoken; "well, what do you think of this?" and then she gave utterance to a series of ideas of so obscene a character, and in language so vile, that her poor mother rushed in despair and horror from the room. "I thought that would astonish the old lady," said the patient, with great satisfaction, "but that is nothing to what I could do if I really tried. Now bring me my Bible, for I want to read a chapter and say my prayers."

MM. Charcot,[1] Bourneville and Regnard,[2] Richer,[3] and others, have studied with great care certain manifestations of hysterical mania which had been noticed, with more or less thoroughness, by Brachet,[4] Dubois,[5] Landouzy,[6] Briquet,[7] Brigham,[8] and other writers, and by physicians generally. Into the full consideration of this variety of hysterical mania I do not propose to enter at present. A short description of it, and the citation of a case or two, will suffice to place the chief features of it before the reader.

In the beginning there is usually an epileptoid seizure, differing in no essential respect from a paroxysm of the *grand mal*, as ordinarily observed. This is succeeded, after a period of repose, by the "period of contortions and of great movements (clonism)."[9] It embraces two phases—that of illogical attitudes, or contortions, and that of great movements. Both of these categories require a suppleness of body and agility,

[1] "Leçons sur les maladies du système nerveux," Paris, 1876.

[2] "Iconographie photographique de la Salpêtrière," Paris, 1876, 1877.

[3] "Études cliniques sur l'hystéro-epilepsie," Paris, 1881.

[4] "Recherches sur la nature et le siége de l'hystérie et de l'hypocondrie," Paris, 1832; also, "Traité de l'hystérie," Paris, 1847.

[5] "Histoire philosophique de l'hypocondrie et de l'hystérie," Paris, 1837.

[6] "Traité complet de l'hystérie," Paris, 1846.

[7] "Traité clinique et thérapeutique de l'hystérie," Paris, 1859.

[8] "Observations on the Influence of Religion upon the Health and Physical Welfare of Mankind," Boston, 1835.

[9] In this description, I have abbreviated the very full account given by Richer in the work to which reference has been made.

and a muscular force well calculated to astonish the spectator, such as, at the time of the *convulsionnaires* of St. Médard, appeared to be above the resources of nature, and only to be explained on the hypothesis of divine intervention. Thus, the body may be bent into the form of a bow, more or less deeply arched, the heels and the head only touching the bed—a true opisthotonos being produced; or the limbs may be twisted into all kinds of fantastic attitudes, and the most remarkable flexions and extensions and leaps ensue, and cries of rage or fright are uttered. Then follows the third period, during which there are what M. Charcot has designated "passionate attitudes" (*attitudes passionelles*), in harmony with the hallucinations with which the subject is affected. She is, in fact, the prey of the false perceptions which govern her and carry her into an imaginary world. The expression of her countenance, as well as the motions of her body and limbs, reveals what is passing in her mind, and the words she utters still more forcibly express her thoughts. When the paroxysm has passed off, she remembers perfectly well all that has occurred and all she has experienced.

During this period of hallucinations the patient is entirely insensible to all external irritation. Pinching, pricking, touching the conjunctiva, the application of a bandage over the eyes, the inhalation of ammonia, loud noises near the ears, and other ordinary excitants, fail to interrupt the course of her delirium. There are only two means of stopping the paroxysm and restoring the patient to her senses. One of these is the excitation of the hystogenetic zones, and especially compression of the ovary, of which the effect is invariable and immediate; and the electric shock, which, without being always as prompt and as certain as the other, is, nevertheless, sufficiently evident.

Two phases of hallucinations are exhibited during the seizure, the sad and the gay; and these alternate, without interruption, during its continuance.

The following is one of the shortest of the cases reported by M. Richer, and will serve, though not one of the most striking, as a good example of the affection:

Juliette Dub., eighteen years old, tall, strong, and of good constitution, entered the Salpêtrière, in the service of M. Charcot, March 29, 1879. With the exception of an attack of typhoid fever when eleven years of age, Juliette enjoyed good health till her fifteenth year. At this time she had a paroxysm of epilepsy, and then others up to the time of her entering the hospital.

Six weeks after her arrival it was noticed that she had attacks of grand hysteria (hystero epilepsy). In addition to the more common symptoms, she was hemi-anæsthetic and achromatopic on the left side. Besides the ovarian hyper-æsthesia, she had the other hystogenetic zones — one over the vertebral column, between the shoulders, and one on each side of the sternum. Pressure over either ovary or over either of the other spots was sufficient to develop a paroxysm.

She exhibited the ordinary prodromatic signs of an attack —agitation, perversion of ideas and of feelings, ovarian pain, especially on the left side, thoracic pain below the breasts and on a line with the hystogenetic zones, a sensation of strangling, throbbings in the temples, and noises in the ears, principally on the left side. It was a noticeable fact that at the moment the convulsions were about to occur her sight became red.

On the 26th of September she had several attacks.

I. (a) At 10.36, epileptoid period, marked by rigidity of the whole body in extension, followed very soon by a general and violent trembling.

(b) The second period was characterized by five rapid and extreme " salutations," by irregular leaps or jumpings, a loud, prolonged cry, then the " arc of a circle," the patient resting on her side.

(c) The third period followed immediately ; was composed of passionate attitudes, varied with hallucinations, in the following order : Attitude of menace, wild expression ; expression calmer ; the patient puts a finger over her mouth, catches herself by the throat, and rolls about the bed as if suffocating. The face is congested. Another attitude of menace. Terror calmer ; appears to be preoccupied with a vision above and in front of her bed ; looks to the right and left, and changes her physiognomy every instant.

II. (a) At 10.40, another epileptoid period similar to the preceding.

(b) Several leaps ; attitude of "arc of circle," with the concavity in front ; the "arc of circle," with the concavity behind.

(c) Seated on her bed, the patient seems to question with

her expression an invisible person, the fingers of the right hand being pressed to her lips. Suddenly terror; attitude of defence, the elbow raised as if to ward off a blow, while her face assumes a furious look. Looks around her bed, touches it with her hand, lies down again, feels her pillow. Her eyes are again directed above; gesture of defiance. Bites her fingers; makes a sign with the hand as if to repulse some one.

III. (a) Suddenly her head is turned to the right. Body extended and rigid; then trembling.

(b) Five great leaps; cries varied; "arc of circle" anterior, posterior, lateral.

(c) At 10.48, movement of defence, look of defiance; crosses her arms, and seems to question some one. Pleasant vision above and to the left; makes signs of negation. Looks to the left on her bed, embraces her pillow, laughs, caresses it, embraces it again; attitude of terror, her look being directed above and to the right.

This is the record of three attacks. They are mild compared to others detailed in the same work, and in that of MM. Bourneville and Regnard.[1]

Though this form of hysterical mania is comparatively rare and of mild form in this country, several cases have come under my observation.[2] The following is of recent occurrence:

A young lady from a Western city was brought to me in the winter of 1881-'82. She had had repeated convulsive seizures, attended by delirium, which, from the description given, were easily recognizable as being attacks of hystero-epilepsy. I had the opportunity of seeing her in several of these at her hotel.

First, there was an epileptoid paroxysm, during which the body was rigid, the face purple, the respiration suspended. This was immediately followed by clonic convulsive movements lasting only about half a minute, and during which the patient foamed at the mouth.

Then ensued a state of opisthotonos, the head and heels only touching the bed, and this was followed by relaxation and various movements of an indeterminate character, and somewhat cataleptoid in appearance.

This stage was succeeded by another in which she became

---

[1] "Iconographie photographique de la Salpêtrière," Paris, 1876–'77.

[2] "A Treatise on the Diseases of the Nervous System," seventh edition, New York, 1881, p. 786, art. "Hystero-Epilepsy."

delirious and exhibited numerous passionate facial expressions and movements. At one time she leaped from her bed, rushed to the window, and would apparently have jumped out had she not been arrested. Then she struggled violently, at the same time crying out: "You shall not! I will not allow it! No, no! Oh, why is it so! Keep off, I say! Do you want me to kill you? Take him away; take him away!" Then, suddenly changing her demeanor and expression to one of intense pleasure, she went back quietly to bed, and soon fell asleep.

When she awoke, she had entire consciousness of all that took place after the epileptoid seizure. She said she had imagined that when she leaped from the bed some men were attacking her father in the court-yard below, and that he had called to her for help; that then the men had attacked her and had offered her various indignities, which she did not specify, but the character of which may readily be inferred; that finally some friends had come to her relief.

In one of her paroxysms she grasped a large knife that lay on the table, and would have killed her mother with it had she not been seized by her sister, who was present. She explained this subsequently by saying that she had thought her mother was a black man who was stealing her jewelry.[1]

In most cases of hysterical mania, hallucinations, especially of sight and hearing, are present. Generally those of sight relate to animals of various kinds, usually of such as are frightful. Thus, black pigs, serpents, lions, tigers, elephants, rats, and horrible bugs and birds are common spectra. Occasionally, but not so frequently as in a former period, devils, witches, sorcerers, etc., make their appearance. Angels and beautiful men with white flowing hair and rosy complexion are not infrequent. Hallucinations of hearing are generally of voices communicating pleasant or unpleasant information, or of music which is described as being "heavenly," or otherwise supernaturally melodious.

The other senses are rarely perceptionally deranged.

[1] I do not enter here into the consideration of the hypnotic, cataleptic, somnambulic, and other phenomena which hystero-epileptics sometimes exhibit. They are thoroughly discussed by M. Charcot and his pupils in the works to which reference has been made, and to some extent in a little book of my own, "On Certain Conditions of Nervous Derangement," New York, 1880. Some of them will be further considered in the remarks I shall have to make relative to epidemic insanity.

An important point connected with the manifestations of hysterical mania is the unreasonable and instinctive disposition to deceive which the subjects exhibit. There seems to be with the majority of the patients affected with the disease in question an inveterate tendency to practice the most unnecessary and illogical frauds, and to tell the most barefaced and improbable lies, without any apparent object in view, or any purpose to subserve, unless it may be the satisfaction of the desire for notoriety, which is so powerful a factor in determining the conduct of these people. Perhaps, in some cases, there may be the foundation of an illusion or a hallucination accepted as a fact, but I have never observed in my own experience any evidence in support of such a supposition. In the furtherance of these purposes of deception they often do not hesitate to accuse themselves and others of the most preposterous crimes. As Morel[1] says : " They envelop themselves in the most whimsical, false, ridiculous, and unjust ideas. The love of truth being no longer a dominant feature of their character, they never relate events as they actually occur, and they deceive with equal pleasure their husbands, parents, confessors, and physicians."

If they have any bodily disease, they exaggerate all the symptoms ; if they have none, they manufacture one for the purpose of deceiving their physicians, and show the utmost satisfaction when, through their lies and lamentations and expressions of fear, they have succeeded in their object. The distinguished French surgeon, Chomel, always avoided in his practice hysterical women, because he had often been deceived by them ; but he often told the following story :

A patient entered his service presenting neurotic phenomena, the singularity and eccentricity of which strongly interested him. He examined her with the utmost care, took notes of the more important and remarkable symptoms, and remained over an hour studying her case. Then, when he could think of no more questions to put, he asked her if there was anything more she wished to say. " Yes, sir," she answered, "it is that there is not one word of truth in what I have told you." [2]

---

[1] " Études cliniques sur les maladies mentales," Nancy, 1851–'52.

[2] Quoted by M. Huchard, " Caractère, moeurs état mental du hystériques," *Archives de neurologie*, mars, avril, 1882, p. 194.

Toulmouche[1] cites the case of a young girl, much given to devotional exercises, and subjecting herself to ascetic mortifications and violent flagellations, who one day seized a pair of scissors, and made with them more than six hundred cuts over her whole body. Then she asserted that the wounds had been made by a man who had endeavored to violate her person. Interrogated sharply by M. Toulmouche, she ended by confessing that she had herself made the wounds, and that she had done so a short time before one of the attacks of hysteria to which she was subject.

In 1873, says M. Huchard,[2] Mlle. de M., aged eighteen years, accused the vicar of the parish of having committed a rape upon her. She stated that on such a day and at such an hour, while she was saying her prayers in church, the vicar, after having shut all the doors, approached her and requested her to go with him into the sacristy. There he had made, she declared, indecent proposals to her, and, as she repelled him with indignation, he had pointed a dagger at her heart. She had fainted, and, when she recovered her senses, she discovered that she had been violated. During the trial of the accused priest the medical experts questioned her in regard to the *modus faciendi*, and, as she answered by giving childish details, she was submitted to physical examination, with the result of ascertaining that she was a virgin, and that there were no traces of violence.

Tardieu,[3] in calling special attention, in its medico-legal relations, to this tendency on the part of hysterical maniacs to lie, and to make charges against others which have all the appearance of being malicious, refers to a recent case, that of a young girl, an inmate of a convent in Gascony, who persuaded her father that she had been made the victim of all kinds of tortures and unheard-of outrages. He, believing what she said, went before the authorities and denounced the alleged perpetrators. Finding, however, that she had deceived him, not a word of her story being true, he took his life from chagrin and mortification.

In another case, a girl, by a lie of the same kind, had two young men imprisoned more than a year on the false charge,

[1] "Consultations médico-légales sur deux cas assez rare d'aberration mentale," *Annales d'hygiène publique*, etc., 1re série, t. i, p. 424, 1853.
[2] *Op. cit.*, p. 196.
[3] "Étude médico-légale sur la folie," Paris, 1880, p. 174.

as it afterward was proven, not only of having violated her person, but of having also, on many occasions, introduced into her rectum and vagina stones and pieces of wood and iron, that had to be extracted from her with great pain. At the end of the operation she had several convulsive seizures, followed by paralysis apparently of the whole body. She was taken into a hospital, in order that her case might be studied to better advantage. But there she again succeeded in counteracting the surveillance of which she was the object. In addition to the paralysis, she simulated a complete constipation. She did this by concealing the discharged fecal matters in the mattress, where they were subsequently found. Eventually her lies and frauds were exposed, and the two young men were released from their unjust confinement.

Such cases as these are interesting in their medical relations, and they are of vast importance in their bearings upon jurisprudence. Cases not infrequently occur in this country in which women laboring under hysterical mania falsely accuse others of crimes, sometimes making so full and detailed a confession of their own participation as to give the utmost similitude of truth to the story, and to lead many to believe that, however false the recital may be, it is accepted as true by the narrator. As already said, I do not think they are ever deceived. On the contrary, I am quite sure that they are fully aware at every moment that they are lying, and that it is this tendency to falsehood and fraud which constitutes a prominent feature of the disease. The following case, though no accusation of crime was made, is similar in all essential respects to those cited, and is additionally interesting by reason of the fact that the patient confessed that she had attempted deception.

Miss A. W., twenty-seven years old, unmarried, and in affluent circumstances, residing in a large Eastern city, accompanied by her aunt, consulted me, April 14, 1878, for an affection which she said was driving her mad. The most prominent symptoms were "nervousness," pain in the front of the head, inability to sleep, confusion of ideas, numbness of the arms and legs, tenderness over several parts of the spine, loss of appetite, dyspepsia, a fixed pain in the left groin, a constant gnawing sensation at the pit of the stomach, "like," as she said, "the pain that would be caused by some small animal biting and tearing me with its teeth," and, above all, by an ir-

32

resistible impulse to swallow pins and needles. Some eight months previously she had, as she informed me, accidentally swallowed a pin which, while dressing herself one afternoon, she had for a moment put between her lips. She thought very little of the circumstance at the time, and suffered no immediate inconvenience from it. In fact, it had passed out of her mind, till a few weeks afterward she had felt a sharp pain at a point on the inside of the left thigh, a little above the knee, and, on examination, had discovered the point of a pin protruding through the skin. With some little pain and trouble, she had extracted the foreign body, and then found it to be, to all appearance, the very pin she had swallowed.

The next day another pin slipped down her throat in precisely the same way as the other. She felt some pain in the region of the stomach very soon afterward, but experienced no other symptom from it till exactly one week subsequently she suffered a little smarting, just above the right knee, at a point corresponding to the place where the other pin had made its exit from the left thigh. On inspection, she discovered a sharp metallic body sticking out of the skin. She seized this with a pair of tweezers, and succeeded in removing a pin—doubtless, as she said, the identical one she had swallowed a week before.

She now began to feel, as she declared, a desire to swallow pins, and, yielding to it, allowed two or three every day to go down her throat. These subsequently made their appearance in various parts of her body. She had extracted them from the arms, breast, the neck, various points of the back and abdomen, the thighs and legs, and even as far down as the feet. One had come out of the eyeball, two from the ears, a dozen or more from the vagina, a great many had been passed from the bowels, and several from the bladder. In all, she thought she had swallowed over two hundred and fifty pins, and a number were, at the time she consulted me, making their exit from her body at various points of the surface.

She rather courted an examination than otherwise, and, on inspection, I discovered one pin protruding from the skin of the left forearm just below the elbow, another from the breast below the left mamma, another from the skin of the back on the right side, on a line with the first dorsal vertebra, two immediately below the umbilicus, and sixteen in the vagina.

I must say that I did not believe a single word of her story, and I was convinced, before examination, that all the pins that would be found would be only those that she had previously stuck under the skin. As a matter of fact, all protruded by the heads, and not by the points. Those in the vagina were in a bundle, with the heads toward the exterior.

Her chief object, she said, in consulting me was to be cured of her irresistible impulse to swallow pins and needles. I remarked to her that I had not found any needles, but she explained this by saying that she had that morning, before coming to me, taken out seven or eight, and that she had the previous morning swallowed as many as fifty, which would begin to make their appearance in the course of the week.

I refrained from taxing her with the fraud at this time. I saw that she was strongly hysterical, and I wished to subject her to medical treatment for a few days before accusing her of deception and thus losing her confidence.

But I had an interview with her mother, a very sensible lady, and told her my conviction that her daughter was practicing a deception for which she was not altogether responsible. She told me that no one had ever seen her daughter swallow either pins or needles, and at once agreed with me as to the falsity of the whole story.

At the daughter's subsequent visit to me, November 17th, she was, at my request, accompanied by her mother. She was feeling much better in every respect, but the pin and needle swallowing, she declared, still continued, and many were at that time sticking out of her body. I removed fifty-two pins and needles from various parts, including ten pins from the vagina—all with the heads and eyes pointing outward.

I then informed her that I was certain she had not swallowed a single pin or needle, and that all I had extracted had been previously put in the places where they had been found. She was at first very indignant, and pretended to be about to leave the room in a rage; but in a few minutes, after I had reasoned with her and informed her that it was the impulse to deceive of which she had to be cured, and not of one to swallow pins and needles, she began to sob and cry, and ended by a full confession that the whole story to me and her subsequent conduct were deceptions.

In this case the prime motive for the fraud attempted to be practiced appeared to be the desire to excite astonishment and sympathy, although the patient could give no very definite account of the matter. She said that the idea of the deception had not occurred to her till after she had left her own house to visit me. She was inclined to think that the governing incentive had been an idea that her real symptoms were not sufficiently striking to excite my interest, and that she would be more likely to obtain attention if she reported herself to be the subject of some unusual disorder. She went on improving, and is now, I believe, in very good health.

In another and still more interesting case, which has within a short time been under my care, the patient, a young lady of twenty years of age, carried on for several months a systematic course of deception which not only greatly injured an excellent young man, but damaged her own character to such an extent that her family were obliged to move away from the place in which they were living. In this instance the patient, by wearing pads over the abdomen and gradually increasing their thickness, led to inquiries from her mother as to the cause ; and, suspicious that an abdominal tumor existed, it was decided to consult an eminent gynæcologist of a neighboring city, when the girl, with tears and lamentations and self-reproaches, confessed that she was pregnant. Of course, the distress in the family was very great, and a great deal of anger was exhibited toward the supposed miscreant who had ruined a virtuous woman. For a long time she refused to reveal the name of the seducer ; but finally one morning she came down stairs with a letter she had written to her father, and in which a full but false revelation of all the circumstances was made. In this letter she declared that a gentleman they all knew and respected was the seducer.

Arrangements were made for her confinement in a distant city, and at the same time it was resolved to arrange, if possible, a marriage with the alleged destroyer of their daughter's honor. The father, accordingly, had an interview, at which the gentleman was offered the alternative of an immediate marriage or instant death from a pistol pointed at his head. Denials and protestations were useless; the father was obdurate, and the pistol, cocked, was very near his brain. He consented to the marriage, but only on the condition that he should at once be granted an interview with the lady in the presence of her parents. This was agreed to. A meeting took place at once, and the gentleman, who was a lawyer, succeeded, by his tact and the directness of his questions, in exposing the fraud and obtaining a full confession. It is, perhaps, scarcely necessary to add that the marriage did not occur.

As I have already said, the subjects of hysterical mania are not disposed to attempt suicide. Occasionally, however, a tendency in this direction is manifested, but it is often more apparent than real. It is an act of deception, like so many others perpetrated by hysterical maniacs. As Legrand du Saulle [1] says, when they attempt suicide they do not proceed as do other people : they try to hang themselves with the rose-colored ribbon of a box of bonbons, or they make a show of taking poison when others are present. In such instances they are generally actuated by a desire to accomplish some object they have in view, and which they think will be more readily secured by terrifying those in authority over them. Thus, a patient of my own, who for several years had suffered from attacks of hysterical mania, coming on at each menstrual period, and lasting for from six to ten days, made several attempts to kill herself with laudanum, but always took a dose so small that it produced no very marked result.

In another case, a lady, from a Western city, stopping at a hotel, terrified her friends and excited the greatest commotion by threatening to jump out of a fourth-story window. When I saw her she was fastened down to the bed by straps, which had been taken from her trunks, and her husband, mother, and half a dozen chambermaids were supplicating her with tears in their eyes not to kill herself. To all of which she was replying that she was determined to jump from the window, and begging them to let her end her life at once. Without saying a word of entreaty or condemnation, I loosened the straps, opened the window, and told her to jump out. I added that she was rendering her husband unhappy, disturbing the guests of the hotel, and that the sooner she put an end to the trouble she was causing the better. The strap around her waist trailed along the floor as she got up, went to the window, and looked down on the street below. I placed my foot on the strap as a measure of precaution, though I was sure such an act was not necessary. The result was just as I had anticipated, for, after a moment's contemplation of the pavement, and applying no very polite epithet to

[1] *Op. cit.*, p. 303.

me, she went back to bed, and I heard no more of her suicidal desires.

But at times the termination is not so fortunate, and, notwithstanding the publicity with which threats are made, and the obvious object of them, the act of self-destruction is really accomplished. Thus, the Marquise de Prie, mistress of the Duke de Bourbon, was exiled from court, and, of course, indifference and neglect followed her in her retreat. She, however, resolved to regain, by a *coup de théâtre*, the favor she had lost. She announced that on a certain day of the month, and at a certain hour, she would kill herself. Every one was amazed at the declaration that one so young, beautiful, and attached to life, contemplated suicide, and the news was received with derision. During the few days intervening, the Marquise gave several *fêtes*, at which she danced, played, and amused herself as in the days of her highest favor. No one had ever seen her gayer, more spirited, more adorable. The hour arrived. She called the new lover she had chosen to her side, and again announced her determination. The communication was received by him with a smile of incredulity. Believing it to be one of those mystifications to which she was accustomed, and that she was acting a part, he humored her so far as to give her, with his own hand, the draught she had prepared. It was in reality poison, and she died before assistance could be given.[1]

Although the vast majority of the cases of hysterical mania occur in women, it is by no means confined to the female sex, and many cases in men have been reported. Klein[2] has collected seventy-eight cases, and has added two others which have come under his own notice. The symptoms do not vary essentially from those met with in women, though, perhaps, they do not reach the same degree of intensity.

Two cases of well-marked hysterical mania, occurring in men who had for many years exhibited the ordinary phenomena of hysteria, have happened within my experience. In both of these there were paroxysms of delirium, characterized by the existence of illusions, hallucinations, and delusions, and by persistent and systematic lying, and other at-

[1] Taguet, " Du suicide dans l'hystérie," *Annales médico-psychologiques*, mai, 1877, p. 347.

[2] " De l'hystérie chez l'homme," Paris, 1880.

tempts to deceive in matters of no importance. In the intervals between the paroxysms both patients were in a measure free from mental symptoms, though there were twitchings of the facial muscles, the *globus hystericus*, insomnia, and a hyperexcitable condition of the nervous system generally.

The course of hysterical mania is rarely toward spontaneous cure, unless the conditions under which it exists are changed for the better. Thus, marriage and the cessation of the menstrual function are favorable therapeutic factors. Under the influence of proper medical and hygienic treatment the affection can generally be kept in check, and often effectually cured, though relapses may occur. The fact, however, must be recognized that, notwithstanding the generally beneficial influence of the menopause, there are cases in which this period is characterized by a recurrence of previously cured attacks, and others in which it is manifested for the first time.

h—EPIDEMIC INSANITY.

Closely allied to hysterical mania is the form next to be described, which, on account of the manner in which it has prevailed, is called *epidemic insanity*. I say *has* prevailed, for it is exceedingly probable that, with advancing civilization and intelligence, future epidemics of insanity will be exceedingly rare, if, indeed, the enlightened part of the world is ever visited by another. In a practical work, such as this is intended to be, this type of mental aberration need not long engage our attention. It is interesting mainly from a historical stand-point, and on account of the lessons it teaches relative to the forces by which the human mind is moved, and the depths of folly and ignorance which it can reach. The last epidemic of the kind occurred in France over twenty years ago, and has been well described by Dr. Constans.[1]

Several different types of epidemic insanity have existed. One of the most common was that in which the subjects were believed to be possessed by the devil—*demonomania*, as it is called. An epidemic of this form prevailed during the sixteenth and seventeenth centuries in many convents of Europe. It appears to have begun in a convent of the Ursulines at Aix, toward the end of 1609, by the confession of Madeline de Mandol, one of the nuns, that she was possessed by a great number of demons, and that she had been seduced by a sor-

[1] "Relation sur une épidémie d'hystéro-démonopathie in 1861," Paris, 1863.

cerer, through their agency, before she had arrived at her tenth year. At this time Madeline was nineteen years old. Very soon afterward another nun, named Louise Capel, declared that she was possessed by three devils.

At the time they made these confessions, these women were suffering from attacks of hystero-epilepsy, characterized, as they are at the present day, by illusions, hallucinations, delusions, violent convulsions, and cataleptic seizures, all of which they ascribed to the demons who had taken possession of their bodies, which demons, they alleged, were under the command of a priest, Louis Gaufridi, a man of cultivation and strict morality. At first the accused man denied the charges made against him, and endeavored, by arguments addressed to the reason of his judges, to show the true nature of the seizures. The effort, however, was in vain ; public opinion was against him. Nothing was more firmly believed than the doctrine that the devil and his demons had power to enter the bodies of human beings and the lower animals. The Bible, which was then appealed to to settle all questions in morals, ethics, and science—pathology included—as well as theology, supported the view. Witches and sorcerers—women and men—who had made compacts with the prince of darkness, were religiously believed to be living in the very midst of the people, and the Bible had said, "Thou shalt not suffer a witch to live."

From the excitement, from fear, and, perhaps, above all, by the force of the examples before him, Gaufridi became insane. He was affected with demonomania. He confessed all that was laid to his charge, and a great deal more that had not been imagined. He declared that he had worshipped the devil for fourteen years, and that he had engaged this demon to cause every woman on whom he breathed to become enamored of him ; that more than a thousand women had been poisoned by the irresistible power of his breath, and had been seduced by him ; and that Madame de la Pallude, the mother of Madeline, had been taken by him, in an unconscious condition, to the sabbath, and violated by him. Of course, Gaufridi was burned at the stake ; but it is stated that the two nuns continued to be delirious.

Among the convents visited was that of Sainte Brigitte at Lille. Several of the nuns had been present at the proceedings against Gaufridi, and had thus been subjected to influences readily capable of producing the disease. Among the sisters was one named Marie de Sains, who was remarkable for her many virtues, but who was now suspected of devoting herself to sorcery, and of being the cause of the possessions of the victims. She remained a year in prison without any formal proofs of her guilt being adduced, until at last she was positively accused by three of the sisters of having intercourse with the devil. At first the poor nun appeared to be surprised at this charge; but, as was generally the case, an accusation of intimacy with the devil was quite certain to induce demonomania in the accused person. It was not a surprising circumstance, therefore, that she should have recanted her denial and avowed herself the perpetrator of a series of such wicked and abominable acts that it was difficult to understand how the conception of them had ever entered her mind. Among them were numerous murders, stranglings of innocent children, ravaging of graves, feeding on human flesh, revelling in orgies of superhuman atrocity, unheard-of sacrileges, poisonings, and, in fact, every imaginable crime. In the presence of her accusers and exorcists she improvised sermons which she ascribed to Satan, discoursed learnedly on the apocalypse, and made long discourses on anti-Christ. She declared, also, that at a sabbath Gaufridi had invented a diabolical charm, with which the devil was so greatly pleased that he had given him the title of "prince of magicians." This charm was composed of the sacramental body and blood, of the powdered flesh of the male goat, of human bones, skulls of infants, hair, nails, human flesh, and the seminal fluid of the sorcerer, together with small portions of liver, spleen, and brain.

There are many other things confessed by this demonomaniac, and set forth with horrible accuracy of detail by Lenormand,[1] and to a sufficient extent by Calmeil.[2] The epidemic appears to have lasted in the Convent of Sainte Brigitte for about ten years.

A more noted example of diabolical possession is that afforded by the nuns of the Ursuline Convent at Loudun, in France, during the years 1632–'35, and which resulted in the death at the stake of Urban Grandier, after he had been sub-

[1] " Histoire de ce qui s'est passé sous l'exorcisme de trois filles possédées ès Flandres," etc., Paris, 1623.
[2] " De la folie," etc., Paris, 1845, t. i, p. 511.

mitted to the most atrocious tortures in order to make him confess to an alliance with the devil. These nuns presented all the symptoms of hystero-epilepsy in its worst form—that is, when modified by a bigoted and unhygienic religious life. During these paroxysms they accused their confessor, Urban Grandier, of having seduced them through the influence of the devil. Grandier, however, was made of stronger stuff than Gaufridi and Marie de Sains, and he died protesting his innocence to the last.[1]

Another noted outbreak was that which occurred in 1642 at the Convent of Sainte Elisabeth, at Louviers.

The following account of the symptoms exhibited by the possessed nuns is given by J. Lebreton,[2] a priest of that time, and who appears to have been an eye-witness of much that he relates.

Fifteen nuns out of fifty in the convent were affected. They were noted for their piety, their gentleness, and excellent conduct in every respect. During the intervals of their paroxysms they conducted themselves with the utmost propriety.

But when under the influence of the demons they exhibited a strange horror of the holy sacrament; they made grimaces and thrust out their tongues at it, spit on it, and blasphemed against it with horrible impiety. They denied and cursed God, more than a hundred times a day, with frightful boldness and impudence.

During these seizures they were affected with strange convulsions and contortions of their bodies, and among others was the bending of the body backward in the form of a bow, so that the body was supported on the forehead and feet without any other part of the body touching anything. They remained in this position a long time, and assumed it seven or eight times. After all these efforts and a thousand others, continued sometimes for four hours, they were as healthy, as fresh, as mild, the pulse as regular, as if nothing had happened.

---

[1] For a full account of this episode of conventual life, see " Cheats and Illusions of Romish Priests and Exorcists discovered in the History of the Devils of Loudun. Being an Account of the Pretended Possession of the Ursuline Nuns, and the Condemnation and Punishment of Urban Grandier, a Parson of that Same Town," Loudun, 1705.

[2] " La défense de la vérité touchant la possession des religieuses de Louviers," Evreux, 1643.

They accused their former confessor, Father Picard, and their actual one, Father Boullé, of having bewitched them through the agency of the devil ; and one of these, Madeline Bavan, made a detailed confession, not unlike those of Madeline de Mandol and Louise Capel against Gaufridi. Picard had been dead several years, but Boullé was arrested and put to the torture. He steadfastly denied all the charges made against him. He was condemned to be burnt alive, the body of the dead Picard to be burnt with him, and, with the corpse, or what remained of it, fastened to his body, he suffered death August 21, 1647.

The foregoing are a sufficient number of examples to show the horrible nature of those epidemics of demonomania as they occurred two or three hundred years ago in Europe. They were not confined to France. Italy, Spain, and Germany furnished fully as many and as notable instances.

The epidemic of 1861, at Morzine, France, if less shocking in its manifestations, is only so because the thought of the age is more enlightened. It is probably the last of its kind, though even here it was kept alive by the exorcisms of silly ecclesiastics, and would certainly have been much more extensive but for the good sense and firmness displayed by Dr. Constans. This gentleman was sent by the French government to put a stop to the epidemic, and he succeeded, notwithstanding the efforts made to thwart his plans.[1]

To dwell upon the epidemics of a similar character which have prevailed among Protestant sects, or those of *theomania* (among them are the Jansenists and others), though interesting, is not necessary to the elucidation of the subject. There is no essential point of difference between them.[2] A few words, however, in regard to a somewhat different type, *lycanthropy*, will probably not be out of place.

Lycanthropy is that form of mental derangement in which the individual believes that through the agency of the devil he is changed into a wolf at certain times. It is applied, also, to supposed transformations into other animals. It has prevailed epidemically, and isolated instances are even now occa-

---

[1] "Relation sur une épidémie d'hystero-démonopathie in 1861." Par le Docteur A. Constans, Paris, 1863.

[2] For a fuller consideration of these and analogous subjects, the reader is referred to the author's work on "Certain Conditions of Nervous Derangement," New York, 1881.

sionally met with, though not exactly presenting the same features as those of the sixteenth and seventeenth centuries.

The first epidemic of the kind appears to have occurred in the latter part of the sixteenth century among the mountains of the Jura, in a place which, taking its name from an abbey founded there in the fifth century, was called Saint Oyant, and finally Saint Claud.[1] The inhabitants of the region about this abbey were entirely subject to the abbots, and were plunged into the lowest depths of ignorance, poverty, and superstition.

Toward the end of the sixteenth century, lycanthropy appeared among these miserable people. Boguet, chief judge of the place, was charged with the duty of extirpating it, and he acquitted himself of his mission so faithfully that, according to Voltaire, he boasted, toward the end of his career, that he had strangled or burnt at the stake more than six hundred lycanthropes or demonolators.

Boguet's mode of procedure was to order the arrest of an accused person on the testimony of a single witness, to put him into a dark and narrow cell, to subject him to the most cruel privations, and finally to apply torture, if it should be necessary, as many as three times. Under this system the victim generally became insane, and confessed to all of which he was charged, and a great deal more. Boguet states in his work that the father testified against the son, the son against the father. Many took advantage of the fear and excitement that prevailed to accuse their enemies, and the depositions of little children were considered as being of especial importance.

As in all periods characterized by the existence of some cause capable of rousing the most intense emotions of the mind, many persons, from thinking of the subject, and terror at the idea of being acted upon by the devil, or of being accused of being in league with the powers of evil, became insane, and voluntarily came forward and made confession. They contracted the delusion that they were lycanthropes, that they ate children, destroyed sheep, and were in close relations with the devil and his demons.

Thus, a woman, Pernette Gaudillon, as we learn from Bo-

[1] The account of this epidemic is derived mainly from Calmeil's " Histoire de la folie," who quotes from Boguet, the judge who tried the cases and who wrote a " Discours des sorciers," published in 1603–'10 ; and from Voltaire, " Œuvres Complètes," t. xxxix, édit. de Baudouin.

guet, thought she was changed into a wolf, and, going on all fours through a field, seized a little girl, whose brother, aged fourteen, was engaged in gathering fruit. The boy defended his sister with courage, but Pernette, grasping a knife which he had in his hand, dealt him a blow in the throat, which speedily proved mortal. The people tore her to pieces.

Pierre Gaudillon, her brother, was arrested on the charge of sorcery. He had the delusion that he had devoted his two children to the devil's service, and had taken them to a meeting of sorcerers. One day when his scythe acted badly, Satan appeared to him and engaged him in his service. The demon was in the form of a black sheep, and spoke to him. He then went to the sabbath, where he met succubi and incubi.[1] He had often caused hail to fall. For magical purposes, he rubbed himself with an ointment which the devil gave him.

On dressing after having rubbed himself with this ointment, he felt himself transformed into a hare. Ordinarily, it was a wolf into which he was changed. When he was thus altered into a beast, his skin became covered with hair, and he took to running in the fields, attacking animals and even men when he was pressed by hunger. To change back into a man it was only necessary for him to rub himself with dew-covered grass.

George Gaudillon, son of Pierre, and his sister Antoinette, were also accused of sorcery.

George confessed that he went to the sabbath, and made use of an ointment to rub on his skin. He alleged that he had heard the devil speak, that he had seen succubi and incubi at the sabbath, and that he bore on his shoulder the mark of Satan. He declared that he had often been metamorphosed into a wolf, and had gone on four feet in the mountains. He had killed two she-goats during his nocturnal excursions. He rubbed himself in the dew-covered grass to become a man again. During the night of a holy Thursday he had re-

[1] A succubus was the name given to a female demon who, while the individual was asleep, had sexual intercourse with him. An incubus was a male demon, who had similar relations with women. The sexual orgasm, occurring during sleep in connection with lascivious dreams, was the origin of a belief which sent many a man and woman to the scaffold and the stake. At that period natural explanations were not sought. The tendency to look to what is called the supernatural is not yet extinguished in the minds of many otherwise enlightened persons.

mained three hours in bed as if dead; he came out of this stupor like a man awaking with a start from sleep.

Antoinette Gaudillon affirmed that she had made the hail fall on the harvest, and that she had gone to the sabbath with her father and brother. She there had sexual relations with a black ram, the devil having taken this form for the purpose.

All four of these maniacs were found guilty, were strangled, and then burned, their ashes being scattered to the winds.

The following brief confessions are taken by Calmeil from Boguet's work:

Thiévenne Paget. The devil appeared to me in full daylight, just as the loss of a cow had caused me great trouble. Hardly had I consented to give myself to him than he took me to a meadow where the sorcerers were accustomed to meet to celebrate the sabbath. There he had intercourse with me. Then he carried me through the air to the place whence he had taken me. The sexual organ of the devil is of the length and thickness of the finger; the suffering during coitus with him is like that of an ordinary childbirth. Three times since my arrest I have had intercourse with the devil. Very often before being put in prison I was transformed into a wolf. The devil went with me at night, when I ran in the mountains. I have killed many children; I dragged them through the ravines and over the rocks till they died. I have assisted at the meetings of the sorcerers. I have killed cows and horses by pronouncing impious words, or simply touching them with a switch.

Antoinette Tornier. I have been to the sabbath. I have there received the caresses of the devil; he had the form of a black man. His penis does not exceed the finger in size. I have danced with a demon disguised as a ram. His foot, which he offered me for a hand, was rough to the touch. I have made charms to change rain into hail, and have drank with sorcerers out of a wooden vessel.

Antide Colas said that the devil had come to her one evening under the guise of a tall man dressed in black, and muffled in a long beard. In an instant she felt herself going through the air, and was soon in the midst of the sabbath. Subsequently the devil came and took her, from time to time, from her bed, and transported her to great distances by taking her by the head and causing the sensation of a cold wind. This woman had a fistulous opening near the umbilicus, and surgeons had often probed it. She declared that it was into this opening that the devil was accustomed to introduce his genital organ, while marital connection was effected by the ordinary way.

This woman had impulsions to suicide, which were thought to be instigations of the devil.

Clauda Jean Prost declared that she had assisted as often as she could at the feasts of the demons. She had assisted at the dances of the sorcerers, and had transformed rain into hail. Often she had been changed into a wolf.

Clauda Jean Guillame possessed, she said, the art of changing herself into a wolf. She boasted that she had in an hour strangled two children in the mountains, and had also strangled a dog that had protected them.

Jacques Bocquet had been to the sabbath. He had resisted the importunities of the devil that he would give him his daughter, for whom he had conceived a violent passion. He accused himself, however, of having poisoned many persons. He had changed himself into a wolf and gone to the mountains after having rubbed himself with a certain ointment.

The three last named stated that they had more than once united in the work of killing children, and they gave the names of five of these that they had also partially eaten. They and the others avowed that they transformed themselves into wolves, and in this guise had killed many children, whose names they gave. Finally they confessed that, in 1597, they had met two children of Claude Baut; that they had killed the girl, but the boy had saved himself by flight. They generally ate parts of the children they killed, but never touched the right side. The fact of these murders was verified as well by the evidence of the fathers and mothers as by that of the villagers generally, who testified that the children named had been killed by wolves at such and such times. It is needless to say that all these lunatics were burned at the stake.

Calmeil says of these poor wretches:

"The singularity of the hallucinations of Thiévenne Paget and Toinette Tornier, who described the shape and size of the sexual organs of the devil, is surpassed by the strangeness of the sensations of Antide Colas, who imagined that the sexual congress between her and the devil was by means of the fistulous opening which she had in the linea alba. The astonishment of the judges when these women described their sensations is thus expressed by Boguet :

"'Ugliness and depravity are shown by Satan in his carnal knowledge of these sorceresses. To some he appeared in the form of a black man ; to others, as some beast or other —dog, cat, he-goat, or ram. He knew Thiévenne Paget and Antoinette Tornier as a black man, and when he had relations with Jacques Paget and Antoinette Gaudillon, he took the form of a black ram with horns. Françoise Sécretain has confessed that her demon sometimes appeared as a dog, sometimes as a cat, sometimes as a cock, when he wished to know her carnally.

"'It is necessary,' he continues, 'that I report a strange but well-established circumstance. Antide Colas de Bretoncourt, being a prisoner at Baume, for the crime of sorcery, and having been visited, was found to have a hole in the belly just below the navel, in addition to the natural opening. This was probed on the 11th of July, 1598, by Master Nicholas Milliere, surgeon, and its existence shown beyond doubt. And then the sorceress confessed that her devil, whom she named Lizabet, knew her carnally by this opening, and her husband by the natural one. But what will be thought of the fact that Satan knew these sorceresses in prison? Nevertheless, they have confessed to it, as has also Thiévenne Paget, who says that while she was a prisoner the devil approached her three times.'"

These are by no means all. Boguet is a faithful chronicler of the ravings of these lunatics, and of his own assiduity in ridding the world of witches, whom he religiously believed had sold themselves to the devil, and were enemies of the human race. He has, however, furnished the student of psychology with one of the most striking histories to be found in the whole range of the science.

Other places caught the infection, and lycanthropy became well known, engaging the utmost powers of the civil and ecclesiastical law to subdue the devil in the new field of operations he had selected. And it was not confined to France; it had its *foci* in Spain, Germany, Italy, and even in Scotland, but, as wolves were rare in this latter country, the maniacs believed that they took the forms of crows, hares, foxes, cats, dogs, and other animals. Doubtless, in some

cases, the subjects had abnormal sensations in various parts
of their bodies, especially of the skin, which originated the
delusion of their transformation.   Dr. Max Simon[1] cites from
De Vier a case in which such an origin apparently existed.
There was in Padua, in 1541, a man who thought himself a
wolf, and who ran about the country, attacking and putting
to death all whom he met.   After much trouble he was captured.   He then said, in confidence to those who had arrested
him, "I am truly a wolf, and if my skin does not look like
that of a wolf, it is because it is turned, and that, therefore,
the hair is inside."   To assure themselves of the fact, they
cut him in different parts of his body, and finally amputated
his legs and arms ; then, not finding the hair, they began to
think they were mistaken, and sent the poor wretch to a surgeon, who, however, notwithstanding all his skill, could not
save his life.

It would be interesting to consider the various epidemics
of *tarentism*, or *dancing mania*, and the other forms of
convulsive seizures, attended with mental aberration, which
have prevailed at different times, both in Europe and in this
country.   All of these were hysterical in character and existed
in times of great emotional excitement, which excitement
was almost invariably of a religious character.   As I have
said, however, no additional light could be thrown upon the
subject under consideration, and those interested in it can
readily study it from other sources.[2]

The *rationale* of the spreading of epidemics of insanity
is not difficult to understand.   Most of the cases occurred in
women, and hence the hysterical element was a notable feature in the affection.   In hysteria of all kinds the propensity
to imitation is great.   A single hysterical woman in a paroxysm will infect a whole ward of other women, as all hospital physicians know.   This was one factor in causing the
extension of the several manias that became epidemic.   A
second was the well-known fact, seen in our own day, that

[1] "Le monde des rêves," Paris, 1882, p. 172.
[2] Hecker's "Epidemics of the Middle Ages," *Sydenham Society Translation*.
Brigham's "Observations on the Influence of Religion upon the Health,"
etc., Boston, 1835.
Figuier's "Histoire du merveilleux," etc., Paris, 1860.
Mathieu's "Histoire des miracules et des convulsionnaires de Saint-Médard,"
Paris, 1864.
Hammond's "Certain Conditions of Nervous Derangement," New York, 1881.
33

when some remarkable event takes place—a great crime, for instance—there are always many persons whose minds, constantly trembling in the balance between reason and insanity, only need some such excitement to turn the scale against them. Hence they are apt, when the perpetrator is being sought for, to come forward and confess themselves guilty of the crime, and to court the punishment awarded to the offence.

A third was the ignorance and superstition which then prevailed in the world, and which induced the belief in the existence of devils and demons, whose business it was to entrap the souls of men and women by giving them worldly power in return for their eternal damnation hereafter. These influences were amply sufficient, as they would be now if they existed in like force, to cause the propagation, from one person to another, of any particular form of insanity.

And even now we see occasional instances of what example and the power of sympathy, much less powerful factors than those I have mentioned, but doubtless contributing somewhat to aid the work, will do in causing the spread of insanity. Upon two occasions within the last year instances of the kind have occurred in New York. In one of these a woman became insane in the street. Her two daughters were with her at the time, and they both became affected with a like form of mental aberration within an hour or two afterward, and all three were sent to an asylum the next day. The other case occurred during the present month—January, 1883. A woman suddenly became affected with what, from the account given in the public press, was probably hysterical mania. One after the other her five daughters, all of adult, or nearly adult, age, were similarly attacked, and it became necessary to send the whole family to an asylum. We have seen how, in the epidemic of lycanthropy, some of the particulars of which I have given, the victims were, many of them, members of the same family.

The *folie à deux*, or *folie communiquée* of the French, are names applied to insanity which is transmitted by one person to another with whom he is thrown in contact. In an interesting paper Dr. Brunet[1] gives several instances of this propagation, among them the following:

The woman, M., as a consequence of a great disappoint-

---

[1] "Contagion de la folie," *Annales médico-psychologiques*, November, 1875, p. 337.

ment, showed evidences of mental aberration. She was in a constant state of exaltation, thinking that she was pursued by powerful enemies with all kinds of terrible weapons. Living with her was her daughter, aged thirteen, a very quiet young person, who had never shown any disposition to mental disorders. At first she endeavored to soothe and reassure her mother, but ere long she herself became similarly affected. They uttered horrible cries of terror, and, in order to escape from their invisible enemies, rushed from the house, and went to sleep in the fields. MM. Lasègue and Falret,[1] after citing and commenting on seven cases of communicated insanity, arrive at the following among other conclusions:

One of the individuals is the active element, is more intelligent than the other. He creates the delusions, and imposes them little by little upon the second person, who is the passive element. Resisting at first, he ends by accepting the ideas submitted to him, but alters them more or less. He thus reacts on the first person, and thus the two eventually come to exhibit the same delusions in the same way.

In order that this end may be accomplished, it is necessary that the two persons should live together a long time, with the same interests, habits, feelings, fears, and hopes.

And, third, the delusion must possess the semblance of probability.

These conclusions will not account for the cases cited, nor for many others that have been reported. It is not, therefore, a matter of surprise to find that they are regarded by some alienists as being insufficient to explain facts in regard to the truth of which no doubt exists. Thus, M. Marandon de Montexel[2] arrives at conclusions more in consonance with the present state of the question. There are three varieties of transferred insanity.

1. *La folie imposée* (imposed insanity), in which a lunatic imposes his delirant conceptions on another intellectually and morally weaker than himself.

2. *La folie simultanée* (simultaneous insanity), in which two (or more) persons hereditarily predisposed contract at the same time the same delirium.

---

[1] "La folie à deux ou folie communiquée," *Annales médico-psychologiques*, November, 1877, p. 321.

[2] "Contribution à l'étude de la folie à deux,"*Annales médico-psychologiques*, janvier, 1881, p. 28.

3. *La folie communiquée*, in which a lunatic communicates his hallucinations and his false conceptions to another person hereditarily predisposed to insanity.

An interesting case of communicated insanity [1] is that of the Dubourques, father and son, the latter of whom is in confinement in a lunatic asylum for attacking women and killing one, and whose case has already been alluded to under another head. Here the father had imbibed the delusion that his brother had died in California, leaving him a large fortune, which had been appropriated by the government to its own use. Talking to his son, a weak-minded young man, he had gradually indoctrinated him with the truth of his false conceptions, and the two for several years were seen every day on Broadway carrying signs on their backs, stating that they had been defrauded out of a large fortune by the United States Government, and demanding the restitution of the money. There was no truth whatever in these statements, except that a brother of the old man had died in California. Neither he nor the son ever took the least pains to ascertain whether any money was left or not. At last the father died, and for a year or more the son walked alone. Finally, he committed the acts for which he is now in confinement.

Kiernan,[2] in an interesting communication on the subject, has adduced the case of a clergyman who, being insane, indoctrinated five other lunatics with his delusions. He also mentions the interesting fact that general paralytics very frequently enter into each other's delusions. To this point I shall return when the subject of general paralysis comes to be considered.

[1] The term *folie à deux* does not apply to all cases of the affection, as in some more than two persons are affected. It appears to me that, at any rate for English writers, the name " Communicated Insanity " is preferable.

[2] " Contributions to Psychiatry," *Journal of Nervous and Mental Disease,* October, 1880, p. 639.

CHAPTER VI.

IV.

VOLITIONAL INSANITIES.

THE forms of mental aberration comprised under the designation of volitional insanities are those in which the will is deranged, either in the way of exaltation or of excessive action, or in that of depression or of diminished action. By some authors it is contended that there can be no derangement of the will, for the reason that this faculty, if it ever is a faculty, is simply the result of ideation, and were there no ideas there would be no will. It is only sufficient, without going into the metaphysics of the question, to call to mind the fact that many of those persons who are strong of will are weak in ideas, both as regards their quantity and strength. An obstinate person, for instance, is by no means necessarily markedly intellectual.

Besides, experience teaches us that there are cases of mental aberration characterized by the features mentioned, and by very little disturbance of the other categories of mental faculties. It is these which I propose to bring to the notice of the reader, leaving to metaphysicians the task, if they desire it, to determine the exact nature of the will. That we have such a faculty every person who moves his finger knows.

a—VOLITIONAL MORBID IMPULSES.

By a volitional morbid impulse we understand those mental factors which cause the perpetration of acts which are neither dictated by an idea or an emotion. They are, therefore, motiveless, and are often perpetrated against the ideas and the desires of the subject.

Neither are they to be confounded with those acts performed by epileptics in a state of unconsciousness, and which resemble, in their external and more obvious characteristics, morbid volitional impulses. Very little observation is required to distinguish the one from the other.

The paroxysm may arise suddenly without any premonitory symptoms; and, when the act to which the individual is blindly impelled is committed, the normal balance between the several mental faculties is at once restored. A similar act, or any other from like excitation, may never again be performed. Usually, however, there is more or less tendency to a repetition of some kind.

Or there may be cerebral symptoms for a longer or shorter period before the culminating phenomenon occurs. These consist of pain, vertigo, heat, a sensation of fulness, of tightness, or of weight, and generally of insomnia.

It is related of Garrick, the celebrated comedian of the last century, that one day, while riding along the road in company with some friends, he suddenly descended from his horse, and, rushing toward a rider who was approaching, dragged him to the ground, and began applying his whip to him with a degree of vigor more astonishing than agreeable to the recipient. After he had administered a sound thrashing, the actor took off his hat, and was profuse in his apologies, both to the victim and his friends, who had looked on in amazement. "I could not help it," he said. "I never saw the gentleman before, and I beg ten thousand pardons for my outrageous conduct. I am willing to make any reparation in my power. Here is my whip; he may revenge himself on my hide; but I could no more have helped acting as I did than I could have flown." This is a good example of a volitional morbid impulse in which there was neither an idea to be executed nor an emotion to be gratified.

Marc [1] cites the following case:

K., aged eleven years and a half, was of backward mind, nervous, lazy, malicious, and obstinate. One day, when he refused to work, his mother permitted him to stay at home with her, and made him assist her in cleaning the house— moving the furniture, bringing hot water, etc. Finally, she told him to remain in the kitchen, and to keep the fire going in the stove. While thus occupied, he saw under the table a little hollow gourd used as a cup. Into this he put a live coal, and placed the whole in the thatch of the roof. "It came to me suddenly," he said, "and I was obliged to do it." A month subsequently he experienced an "infernal heaviness" in his head, and again he felt obliged to kindle a fire. On both occasions, as soon as the act was committed the impulse was satisfied, and he was the first to endeavor to extinguish the flames.

[1] "De la folie consideree dans ses rapports avec les questions medico-judiciaires," Paris, 1840, t. ii, p. 390.

Georget[1] gives a full account of the case of Pierre Joseph Delépine, a backward boy of sixteen. This youth had, without motive, attempted eight times to set fire to his father's house. He even, while in prison, put live coals in his bed, and then lay down on it while it was on fire.

Jacoby[2] quotes the case of Barbara Erkhow, a Russian peasant, who was delivered of a son, and was, two weeks afterward, left at home with her husband's mother. While Barbara was nursing her infant, the mother-in-law made a fire in the stove, and soon afterward left the room. In an instant Barbara seized her child and threw it into the stove. She then lay down on a bed which was in the chamber. Almost immediately afterward her mother-in-law re-entered the room, saw the infant in the fire, and snatched it from the flames. The child died in her arms. Barbara could not explain her conduct otherwise than by declaring that she had been seized with a sudden impulse to throw her infant into the stove, and that she had done so without thought or cause.

In 1828, a man, named Papavoine, killed in the forest of Vincennes two little boys, who were there on a holiday with their mother. He had never seen these children before, and, when seized with the impulse to kill them, went and bought a knife for the purpose, and, returning, murdered them before their mother's eyes, and made his escape. On being arrested and identified, he at first denied the charge, but subsequently admitted its truth. Confined in prison, he set fire to his bed, and attempted to murder a fellow-prisoner. When interrogated during his trial, he declared that at the time of the double murder he was in bad health, had been unable to sleep, and was nervous. He asserted that he had had no motive whatever to kill the two children. Inquiry into his antecedents showed that, though he had been quiet and taciturn in his habits, he had never exhibited any indications of insanity, but had discharged with fidelity the duties of an office he had held under the government, and had retired with a pension. The plea of insanity was put forward by his counsel, but it was disregarded by the jury, and he was found guilty and executed.

A few weeks since, a lady of this city brought her daughter to me, to be treated, as she said, for "nervousness." The

[1] "Discussion médico-légale sur la folie," Paris, 1826, p. 130.
[2] "Considérations sur les monomanies impulsives," Thèse de Berne, 1868, p. 12.

patient was eighteen years of age, in good general health, and suffered from no disorder of her menstrual function. While I was talking with her she suddenly rose, and, walking rapidly across the room, overturned a chair which stood against the wall. She then returned, and went on with her conversation. Her face was a little more flushed than it had been, but I noticed no other change.

After a few minutes I said to her: "Why did you throw over that chair?"

"I don't know," she answered.

"Do you know that you did throw it down?"

"Oh, yes; of course I know all about it."

"Then why did you do it?"

"I was obliged to. I cannot tell you any more."

"Did you want to do it?"

"No; I had no wish about it."

"Had you been thinking about the matter?"

"No; I had no thought about it; I felt compelled to do it."

"Have you ever done the like before?"

"Many times. I have torn books, broken plates and other things, and once I rushed out in the rain without any shoes."

"And you can't tell me why you do these things?"

"No, except that I am obliged to do them. As soon as I feel an impulse of the kind I do it, and then I am satisfied."

"Have you never tried to resist?"

"No, for there is nothing to resist. I don't think I could stop. I have no wish to do them, and no thought of doing them. I just do them, and that is all there is about it."

"But you might do serious injury some day."

"Yes, I have thought of that, and it gives me a great deal of trouble. But what can I do?"

In another case the patient, a gentleman who had received a serious wound of the head during the late civil war, consulted me for the cerebral symptoms that were developed, as well as for the irresistible impulses to which he was subject. I found on examination that the missile—a fragment of shell —had struck him in an oblique direction immediately over the external angle of the left eye, doing at the time apparently no greater damage than to plough a furrow in his skull, and to knock him senseless for a few minutes. The wound healed without trouble, and in a couple of weeks he was fit for duty.

He served as an officer of artillery all through the war, and then resumed the practice of the law. But, shortly after he had taken up his residence in a large western city, he began to suffer with his head. He had pain at the seat of the injury, repeated attacks of vertigo, and almost daily redness of the corresponding side of the face, attended with a roaring sound in the ear and a complete stoppage of the left nostril, so that it was impossible to force the air through it. These paroxysms lasted about two hours, and then gradually went off, there being at the same time a profuse discharge of nasal mucus.

But, in addition to these troubles, there was another, which gave him still greater anxiety. He was subject to occasional impulses, which came on without warning, which were unassociated with any idea, which were entirely purposeless, which were not prompted by any emotion, but of which he was thoroughly conscious, though unable to resist. Indeed, the question of resistance never arose in his mind any more than it did when he automatically took out his watch to see what time it was while he was busy writing or thinking of some business matter. As yet he had committed no very flagrant violation of the rules of propriety, the worst being that on the day previous to his visit to me he had thrown a heavy ink-stand through the window of his office. The deed was done in an instant, and without the least reflection or knowledge that he was about to do it. Other acts had consisted of breaking wine-glasses while at dinner, throwing water on the floor, and tearing leaves out of books. On one occasion he had broken a costly thermometer which stood on a table in a friend's library.

These acts were apparently instinctive and automatic. The epileptoid element was entirely absent. He was perfectly conscious both at the time they were perpetrated and afterward, and had full knowledge of all the steps of the performance. That they and others similar, to which attention has been directed, were due to lesions of the will, is, I think, perfectly clear.

And I think that authors generally have shown a disposition to confound all morbid impulses as being due to like factors. Undoubtedly, some which have been considered as volitional are ideational or emotional; but, making due allowance for these, there are others in which the will alone of all the mental faculties is deranged. Esquirol[1] saw this very clearly when he wrote: "There exists a species of homicidal monomania in which *neither intellectual nor moral disorder* is to be observed. The murderer is urged by an irresistible power, by a force which he cannot conquer, by a blind impulse, by an irreflective determination, without interest, without motive, without mental confusion, to an act which is both atrocious and contrary to the laws of nature." If the intelligence can be abolished or perverted, if the moral sensibility can be similarly affected, why cannot the will, the complement of the intellectual and moral being, also suffer in like manner? Why should not the will be influenced by troubles, by perturbation, by morbid weakness? What incomprehensibility is there in such an idea?

M. de Castelneau[2] speaks to a like effect when he says:

"Instantaneous, transitory, temporary mania is a mental disorder which is manifested suddenly at the instant of the seizure. The subject is forced by the action of his suddenly disordered will to the perpetration of automatic acts which have not been foreshadowed."

Kiernan[3] regards mania transitoria as simply a variety of acute mania. This is undoubtedly true as regards some cases, such, for instance, as those which have been designated as "fury"; but it is not, I think, correct of all cases, especially of those which are now under notice. Indeed, mania transitoria has, like morbid impulses, been made to embrace many different affections.

Billod,[4] in an elaborate memoir, discusses the question of lesions of the will very thoroughly, and adduces many examples of its derangement. Among them is the case of R., who, with a relatively fair integrity of the intellectual faculties, had almost constant irresistible impulses to travel and to steal. After a time the former ceased, but the latter not only continued, but were still more strongly developed with time. Nothing seemed to arrest his tendency to steal whatever he could lay his hands on. As soon as he saw anything, he en-

[1] "Des maladies mentales," Paris, 1838, t. ii, p. 341.

[2] "De la folie instantanée considerée au point de vue médico-judiciaire," *Ann. méd.-psychologiques*, 1857, p. 307.

[3] "Contributions to Psychiatry," *Journal of Nervous and Mental Disease*, October, 1880, p. 631.

[4] "Des maladies de la volonté," *Ann. méd.-psy.*, 1847; also, "Des maladies mentales et nerveuses," Paris, 1882, t. i, p. 144.

deavored to steal it. He would crawl up behind a person and try to seize with his teeth the hat held in the hands; at other times he would drag himself along the floor on his hands and knees in order to snatch something he felt impelled to steal. For more than a year he was in the asylum, and, notwithstanding the fact that he was kept most of the time restrained by a camisole, which prevented the free exercise of his hands, he managed to commit many thefts. It was not necessary for the objects stolen to possess any value; a stone, a blade of straw, a piece of paper, were fully as much the objects of his impulse as valuable articles. One day, as Dr. Billod passed, with some papers pertaining to a patient just arrived, R. rushed at him, forcibly seized the bundle between his wrists, and vainly endeavored to drag it away. R. was always calm, affectionate, reasonable, even, when there was nothing in sight that could excite his kleptomaniacal propensity. He greatly regretted and deplored his bad tendencies, and he had entire consciousness of his mental state. "I am wrong," said he; "I know it is madness, but what can I do? It is stronger than I. At the time the impulse to steal comes over me I am wild. I cannot compare my condition then to anything but drunkenness."

This patient presents features in some respects similar to those of the young lady affected with emotional kleptomania, but differing in the important element of there being a total absence of motive, a feature which characterizes all true volitional morbid impulses.

Esquirol[1] relates the case of a man, thirty-two years old, of a nervous temperament and quiet disposition, who had been well educated, and who was fond of the fine arts. He had suffered from a brain disorder, but had been several months cured. After being in Paris for about two months, during which time he led a perfectly regular life, he one day entered the Palais de Justice and attacked an advocate with great fury. The next morning, when seen by Esquirol, he was perfectly tranquil and composed, showed no anger whatever, and had slept well all night. The same day he designed a landscape. He recollected what he had done the previous day, and spoke of it with calmness. He declared that he had entertained no ill-will against the advocate, had never even seen him before, and had no business with him or any other

[1] " Des maladies mentales," Paris, 1838, t. i, p. 380.

lawyer. He could not understand, he said, what had actuated him to make the assault. Subsequently, he exhibited no indications whatever of being insane.

It often happens that with the performance of a single act, due to volitional morbid impulse, the tendency is exhausted and never reappears.

Volitional morbid impulses may be exhibited in many ways, constituting instances of homicidal mania, suicidal mania, kleptomania, pyromania, etc. Sometimes two or more of these forms exist in the same individual.

b—ABOULOMANIA (PARALYSIS OF THE WILL).

Under the designation of aboulomania (αβουλος, irresolute, and μανια, madness) I propose to describe a form of insanity characterized by an inertness, torpor, or paralysis of the will. So far as I am aware, Billod [1] was the first to call attention to this condition, in which, while there is an inability to exert the will, the other mental faculties are not necessarily affected.

The disorder, like other mental diseases, may arise suddenly, or it may, as is generally the case, be developed gradually after a more or less decidedly marked set of prodromatic symptoms. These latter may continue throughout the course of the affection, and consist of pain in the head, occasional sensations of vertigo, insomnia, noises in the ears, and other symptoms indicative of the existence of a hyperæmic condition of the brain, though they were present but in one of the cases—the fourth to be described—that have come under my notice. In the other cases there appeared to be rather passive congestion without other head symptoms than insomnia and occasional headache.

M. Billod details the particulars of the case of a patient, a notary, in whom the phenomena of the disorder in question were strongly shown. If he desired to go out, he could not exert his will to the extent of causing the proper actions to be performed, and so with many other movements. The derangement was, however, most strikingly shown when he attempted to execute a legal paper. He signed it, but when he came to affix his paraph [2]—his paraph, it is true, was of a very complicated character, but he had always been able to execute

---

[1] " Des maladies de volonté," op. cit., loc. cit.

[2] A flourish with the pen immediately under the signature, and which, in France, Spain, and Italy, is necessary to the validity of legal papers.

it with ease—it was in vain that he fought against the difficulty. A hundred times, at least, he tried to execute the movements necessary to the perfecting of his signature, but his hand refused to move. So long as he only made the motions in the air just above the paper there was no trouble, but as soon as the pen touched the paper he could not move. He strove with all his might to accomplish his object, till the sweat stood out in beads on his forehead. Then he rose with impatience and stamped upon the floor ; reseating himself, he tried again, but with no better success. The contest lasted three quarters of an hour, and then he succeeded in making the paraph, but a very imperfect one.

M. Billod was witness of another struggle, which was of much longer duration. The patient wished to go out shortly after dinner. He wished, he said, to get an idea of the appearance of the city. For five days he made many attempts to start. He would get up, take his hat, and get ready for his walk, but further than this he could not go ; his limbs could not be made to make the requisite movements. He could not will them to do so. "Would any one," he said to M. Billod, "believe in the existence of such an affection ? I am evidently my own prisoner. You do not hinder me from going out, since, on the contrary, you wish me to go. My legs are in good condition, they are not paralyzed, since, as you see, I walk well. What is it, then ? " He then complained of not being able to will, notwithstanding his wishes. Finally, at the end of five days, he succeeded in getting out, but returned in five minutes, covered with perspiration, and as much exhausted as though he had run several miles.

Instances of this impossibility of exerting his will occurred at every moment. If he wished to go to the theatre, he could not go ; if at dinner with congenial friends he wished to take part in the conversation, he could not say a word. There was always the powerlessness to do what he desired. It is true that often this want of power did not exist, but even then there was the fear of it, and generally his fears were realized.

A lady of this city, who had enjoyed good health up to the period of the cessation of the menstrual function, suffered, subsequently, in a way very similar to that of M. Billod's patient. She came under my observation in the spring of 1880, and I found the following-described condition to exist:

There were no cerebral symptoms of a somatic character

except an inability to sleep, with which she had suffered for several months, though not to any very great extent, as she usually obtained about five hours sleep every night. The circumstance, however, which gave her most concern was an inability to exert her will in accordance with her desires. If the thing to be done was of no consequence, and more of the nature of a routine act requiring no deliberation, there was rarely any trouble; but if it was a matter to be discussed, or which presented an alternative, or which required a determination to be made, then the difficulty of bringing the mind to bear upon it was of such a nature as to render the performance an impossibility. She thus transacted all her household duties which had become habitual to her without experiencing any inconvenience; but, if something out of the ordinary every-day run of events had to be done, there was sure to be an impossibility of her doing it. If, for instance, it was suggested that she should go to Saratoga, she at once assented and expressed pleasure at the idea; but when the time came she could not make the necessary preparations. If these were made for her, and the hour approached for her to go to the station, she became still more helpless: she could do nothing connected with the journey. The putting on of her bonnet was a task beyond her powers, and she had to be literally dragged to the door and placed in the carriage that was to convey her to the train. Arrived at the station, she could not get out of the carriage, and again aid was necessary. All this time she would utter lamentations over her inability to act for herself, while expressing her desire to make the journey.

The question of accepting or not accepting invitations always gave her a great deal of trouble. She would determine, perhaps, after much hesitation and many changes, that she would accept, and then the matter of writing the note came up to increase the difficulty. The getting the paper, the taking hold of the pen, the dipping of it in the ink, and writing the note, were all acts that she could not accomplish. She was not even able to ask some one else to write it for her. The consequence was that she rarely went into society, although naturally of a cheerful disposition and fond of gayety.

Her life was, therefore, not only a burden to herself, but to those around her; and lately her trouble had increased so much that, as she said, she saw no refuge but a lunatic asylum.

During her interview with me she exhibited no evidence

of her disorder till I asked her to put out her tongue. Probably she had not been requested to do so for many years, and it was, therefore, an act to which she was not accustomed. Evidently she tried very hard to show me her tongue, but she could not even open her mouth. The muscles of her face were contorted ; her eyes rolled, her mouth twitched, but it was not opened. At last she said, quite calmly, "I can open my mouth perfectly well, as you see now, but I cannot do it when you ask me. As soon as I feel the desire, the impossibility of exerting the will begins. I can do it very well if I do not think about it." It appeared to me at first that she labored under some defect of speech analogous to stammering. I had often seen people act in a similar manner when told to utter a word beginning with a labial consonant ; but her subsequent performances dismissed this idea. Desiring to examine her spine, I requested her to adjust her dress for the purpose. "I should like to oblige you," she said, "but I cannot begin. I cannot raise my hands for that object. I can move them about, but it is impossible for me to take off my cloak." I suggested that she should try hard to send a volitional impulse to her hands, so as to make them unbutton her cloak. She got red in the face, and the perspiration started out on her forehead, but her hands remained still on her lap. "No, I cannot do it," she said, "not if the salvation of the world depended on it." Eventually her daughter was obliged to remove her cloak for her, and otherwise arrange her clothing for the object I had in view. She dressed herself without the slightest difficulty.

When it came to leaving my consulting-room, she rose from her chair in haste and went toward the door, as if determined to overcome all resistance ; but as she approached it she began to hesitate, and finally stopped, unable to go a step farther. She then came back, and sat down as if in despair. But soon she made another effort, with no better result. She could not pass through the door, and it was necessary for her daughter and myself to take her, each by an arm, and lead her out to her carriage.

In another case, that of a gentleman from Massachusetts, there was an inability to exert the will solely in the matters of dressing and undressing himself. He would go to his bedroom, but as soon as he began to consider the subject of undressing, his indecision was shown. He would, after standing some time thinking of the subject, sit down and begin to unlace one of his shoes. Then the question would arise whether he had not better take off the other one first. After cogitating over this point for several minutes, he would begin with the other shoe, but then again doubts would arise, and he would stop. Perhaps, then, he would, rise and walk up and down the floor, deliberating over the question, when, looking toward the glass, he would see himself reflected, and his eyes would catch sight of his necktie. "Ah," he would say to himself, "of course that is the thing to take off first." But as soon as he took hold of it he hesitated, and the moment he hesitated he was powerless. And so it went on if he was left to himself, till it has frequently happened that daylight would find him still with every stitch of clothing on him. In the morning it was the same thing in putting on his clothes. He could never determine which stocking should go on first, or whether his shirt should be put on before his stockings, or even whether the right or left leg of his drawers or trousers should have the preference.

It is this phase of the disorder to which I think the term "aboulomania" is especially applicable.

This gentleman suffered severely from insomnia and occasional headache, but there was no mental aberration other than that of his will.

In another case, similar in all essential respects to the foregoing, so far as putting on and taking off the clothing were concerned, there was the additional phenomenon of an impossibility of determining which bed to sleep in. The patient, a gentleman of this city, had two beds in his room, and he could never will which one to occupy. Often, as he told me, he had passed the whole night vainly endeavoring to decide, and ending by thorough exhaustion and falling asleep in a chair, or on the floor. At one time he thought to avoid the difficulty by having one of the beds removed, but this caused him so much mental uneasiness that he was obliged to have it brought back. Finally he hit upon the device of having his mother decide for him by putting, every night, a placard on one of the beds with the words written on it, "This is the bed you are to sleep in to-night," and then he had no trouble. If by any chance the placard was forgotten, the old irresoluteness returned, and neither bed was occupied.

Cases similar to these have been reported by other authors.

Dr. Carpenter[1] quotes from Dr. J. H. Bennett's "Mesmeric Mania of 1851" the following instances :

"The first was that of a gentleman who frequently could not carry out what he *wished* to perform. Often, on endeavoring to undress, he was two hours before he could get off his coat, all his mental faculties, volition excepted, being perfect. On one occasion, having ordered a glass of water, it was presented to him on a tray, but he could not take it, though anxious to do so ; and he kept the servant standing before him half an hour, when the obstruction was overcome.

"In the other case the peculiarity was limited. If, when walking in the street, this individual came to a gap in the line of houses, his will suddenly became inoperative, and he could not proceed. An unbuilt-on space in the street was sure to stop him. Crossing a street, also, was very difficult ; and on going in or out of a door he was always arrested for some minutes. Both these gentlemen graphically described their feelings to be 'as if another person had taken possession of their will.'"

Under the designation of "Folie du doute (avec délire du toucher)" Dr. Legrand du Saulle has described a condition which, at first thought, appears to have some relations with that under consideration. Further examination, however, shows that the affection he has studied so thoroughly is in reality quite different. But M. Cabade,[2] under a similar title, has given the particulars of a case which is in many respects identical with those herein cited.

The patient, a man, thirty-four years old, was of a neurotic family, and had suffered from an attack of acute rheumatism with certain cerebral complications. The progress of the disease toward recovery was slow and painful, but eventually he seemed to have quite recovered. Hardly, however, was convalescence established when he began to experience symptoms of the affection I have called "mysophobia," and which has been fully described in a previous chapter of this treatise. Then came troubles of volition. He could not make up his mind to pass through a door ; before succeeding, he made many fruitless attempts, and often members of his

---

[1] "Principles of Mental Physiology," etc., London, 1874, p. 385.

[2] "Un cas de folie du doute," *L'encéphale, journal des maladies mentales et nerveuses,* October, 1882, p. 454.

34

family were obliged to encourage him by words, and even to aid him with their own hands to accomplish the act.

From this time on he could not perform the most simple acts of life without difficulty and hesitation, and, when he had at last succeeded, he repeated them many times. For instance, if he were seated and wished to change his place, he would rise, then sit down, then rise again, and so on, ten, fifteen, twenty times, before he could decide to take a step toward the point he desired to reach. If he were walking, and encountered a tree or a rock, he stopped before it, then retraced his steps, then resumed his original direction, stopped again, went back, returned, and so on, ten or twenty times, before he was able to pass the imaginary obstacle. Often, in order to pass the tree or stone which he came to in his walks, he was obliged to run. Often, after having succeeded, he would retrace his steps, and then the whole series of hesitations was gone over again. Thus, one day, entering the consulting-room of M. Ball, he went out again quickly, then returned, saying, "I was afraid I had come in badly."

In addition to this trouble with his will, the patient was also affected with intellectual subjective morbid impulses, a disorder to which I have already called attention. Thus, while suffering from hesitation, either in passing an object or in doing some other thing, he pronounced in a loud voice words which showed that he was possessed of an idea without relation to the act he was endeavoring to perform. At the beginning of his disease he repeated certain words which had struck him as being singular, or which had a special signification—for example, the word "corbillard." Later, he often repeated expressions of affirmation or denial, as if he were protesting against some imputation. "No, no; I am not this, I am not that. No, I am not guilty of such or such a thing." These words were accompanied with gestures of one or both hands, as if he were endeavoring to repulse some person or thing. From this it is evident that the case had its complications. Subsequently he had other attacks of rheumatism, and contracted syphilis. He also became the victim of morbid fears of various kinds; but, notwithstanding all these things, he married, and the account of the case ends with the mention of the difficulties he experienced in abstaining from cohabitation with his wife and continuing anti-syphilitic treatment.

Paralysis of the will or aboulomania may be produced by certain diseases and drugs. In hysteria, for instance, it is often the case that the patient takes to her bed, and remains there for months, or even years, without any other reason for so doing than that her power of volition is destroyed or greatly impaired, and that, therefore, she cannot get up and go about her work or duties. It is well known, too, that alcohol and opium have the effect of weakening the will to such an extent as to render the subject absolutely incapable of taking the initiative in any important undertaking, or of resisting influences brought to bear upon him, and which he knows he ought to resist. Wills are thus made, and property given away, which the individual knows he ought not to execute or part with, but with his diminished volitional power he yields, because he is not strong enough to successfully oppose.

De Quincey[1] sets out the volitional degradation of the opium-eater very forcibly when he says of him that he "loses none of his moral sensibilities or aspirations; he wishes and longs as earnestly as ever to realize what he believes possible and feels to be exacted by duty, but his intellectual apprehension of what is possible infinitely outruns his power, not of execution only, but of power to attempt. He lies under the weight of incubus and nightmare; he lies in sight of all he would fain perform, just as a man forcibly confined to his bed by the mortal languor of a relaxing disease, who is compelled to witness injury or outrage offered to some object of his tenderest love. He curses the spells which chain him down from motion; he would lay down his life if he might but get up and walk; but he is powerless as an infant, and cannot even attempt to rise."

It would appear, however, that in some cases of aboulomania there exists what has been called by Mr. Skey[2] the "latent force" of the will, which can be brought out, as in hysterical subjects, by some strong impression made upon the mind, or some exceedingly important object to be accomplished. This "latent force" exists to some extent with all persons, even in the healthy state. To use a simile suggested by Mr. Skey, let us suppose that a strong man has found by experience that he can barely lift two hundred and fifty

---

[1] " Confessions of an English Opium-Eater."

[2] " Six Lectures on Hysteria," etc., London, 1866.

pounds of sand with the utmost exertion of his will and muscles. Put two hundred and sixty pounds of gold before him, and tell him that, if he lifts it, it is his, and he will raise it without difficulty.

The ancients were fully aware of the existence of this "latent force." It is told of Alexander the Great that one day, while sitting in front of his tent, a soldier passed him staggering under the weight of a bag of gold he was carrying to the treasury. "My friend," said the King to him, "do not suffer so painfully. Carry the bag to your own tent, for it is all your own," and the soldier tripped off with the load as easily as though the sack had been changed for one of feathers.

The woman, also, who has been in bed for years, unable, as she thinks, to stand alone, and in whom the will power for certain acts is almost entirely abolished, jumps from her bed and runs nimbly down stairs if the house catches fire. Her latent will power, which only a strong impression can bring out, is at once developed, and she does what no ordinary excitation could possibly accomplish.

And the same is true of aboulomania occurring in persons unaffected with other diseases—a primary affection in fact; and the fact is well exemplified in the first case of the kind to which my attention has been directed, and to which I have alluded in another place.[1] In this instance a gentleman never could make up his mind how to invest his money, and every day he would go down town to Wall Street, thinking that at last he had found the investment to make, but always returning in the morning without having accomplished his purpose. Day after day this conduct was repeated, and several months elapsed without his money being invested.

I then lost sight of this patient, and did not see him again till the latter part of the year 1882, when he again came under my charge. In answer to my inquiries, he informed me that the trouble about the money had been settled, soon after I last saw him, by his wife taking it from his desk and purchasing some securities with it, but that soon afterward an extension of his hesitation had ensued, and that now there were many things he could not do. He had given up trying to invest his money, but he now had a like difficulty in buying anything, no matter how trifling, and this was a source of great disturbance to him. If, for instance, he went into

[1] "Cerebral Hyperæmia," etc., New York, 1879, p. 29.

a shop to get a pair of gloves, he could never determine for himself what kind to buy, or what colors ; and, when helped out in these matters by the salesman, he could not go through the movements necessary to getting out his pocket-book to pay for them. As a consequence, he either had to have some one with him to pay for the things he bought, or, as frequently happened, he would throw the articles down on the counter, and tell the people to send them home. At first, before he began to take some one with him to aid him in making purchases, he would often spend an hour or more in getting some commonplace article. But, upon one occasion, as he was walking along Broadway, the idea occurred to him that he would take a box of *bonbons* home to his daughter. He entered a shop which he thought was one he was in the habit of frequenting, purchased an expensive box, and had it filled with the finest sweetmeats in the shop. All this was only accomplished after a large expenditure of time, and after the display of much hesitation, which not only annoyed him, but caused many expressions of disgust from the shopkeeper. Finally, when he came to pay for the purchases, he found, as usual, all his difficulties increased, and this was a part of the procedure in which he would not be assisted by the dealer. After fumbling at his pocket for some time in the vain endeavor to get at his money, he requested that the things might be sent home. He had already found out that the shop was not the one he had intended to enter, and that he was unknown to the proprietor. He was not, therefore, surprised when that person informed him that the box could not leave his place till it was paid for ; but he was not prepared for the torrent of abuse which was rained upon him. The effect, however, was very different from what either of the contracting parties anticipated. In an instant my patient became entire master of the situation. He took out his *porte-monnaie* with as much decision as he had ever done anything in his life, laid the exact sum on the counter, and then, taking the box, threw it at the shopkeeper, and walked as composedly to the door as though nothing had happened. But the influence which had brought out his "latent force" was not yet lost. He stopped at the right shop, a few doors off, selected his *bonbons* without the slightest irresoluteness, and paid for them with as much ease as in the last purchase. The next day, however, he was as bad as ever.

It would appear from cases such as these that the general condition of cerebral excitement produced by certain factors carries with it an augmentation of the power of the will ; and it is not at all improbable that the pathological condition causing aboulomania is a state of passive congestion or anæmia. Carpenter,[1] referring to this state, says that " the strongest volitional effort may be inoperative through some defect of the apparatus by which the nerve-force is transmitted to the muscles which are to execute the behests of the will, as happens in paralysis. But there are states—and it is these which are now under consideration—of absolute incapacity for such effort, the mental *desire* existing, while the energy necessary to carry it into effect is deficient. That this incapacity arises from a deficient supply of blood to the ideational (cerebral) nerve-centre appears probable from the familiar fact that a general deficiency of volitional power over the muscles is a marked feature of the physical depression which betokens feebleness of the circulation, being especially noticeable in seasickness, while a defect in the distributive action of the vasomotor system of nerves (such as that of which we have evidence in many local congestions) might very well account for such cases as the two following."[2] . . .

CHAPTER VII.

v.

COMPOUND INSANITIES.

COMPOUND insanities are those forms of mental aberration in which two or more categories of the faculties of the mind are involved to a marked degree. In all the types to be considered under this heading there is, therefore, a general mental derangement, the perceptions, the intellect, the emotions, and the will participating in the disturbance ; and often with alternating predominance, or no special predominance, of one set over the other.

[1] *Op. cit.*, p. 385.   [2] These are the cases cited on page 529.

a—ACUTE MANIA.

By acute mania is to be understood a condition of mental derangement characterized by illusions, hallucinations, delusions, great mental and physical excitement, and often by a tendency to the perpetration of acts of violence and extravagance.

Pinel[1] defines acute mania as an affection in which there is a general and permanent hyperexcitability of the intellectual and moral faculties. It is exhibited by the most decided symptoms—alteration of the countenance, disorder of the clothing, acts of violence, and confusion of ideas, which succeed each other without order and without logical sequence. It is, moreover, characterized by intense nervous excitement, by extreme agitation, sometimes reaching the point of fury, by a general and more or less well-marked delirium, and often by a complete reversal of all the operations of the mind.

Broussais[2] says :

"Maniacs are agitated, vociferous ; they are irritated by the slightest cause, and even without provocation, but especially if they are spoken to. It is only sufficient to speak to them to excite them to the highest degree. Their ideas are incoherent, their eyes bright, their muscular strength prodigious. It is often necessary to restrain them, for they are actuated by the wish to break and destroy everything which comes within their reach, and they kill those who approach them unless they are kept in subjection. Some of them, when the accession has been sudden, had already murdered several persons before they could be confined. Many turn with fury against themselves, and stab or throw themselves from heights. The pulse is small and tense, and more or less quick. Sometimes there is scarcely any acceleration in the action of the heart. When they have not been bled, the face is red and swollen, the veins enlarged, the skin hot, the tongue red, the epigastrium tender to the touch, anorexia, and sometimes a yellowish tinge about the eyes. They can remain a long time in this deplorable state without food, without sleep, without feeling cold, yelling and blaspheming day and night, making

[1] "Traité médico-philosophique sur l'aliénation mentale," Paris, 1809, seconde édition, p. 139.
[2] "De l'irritation et de la folie," deuxième édition, Paris, 1839, t. ii, p. 352.

every effort to break the bonds which secure them, and always dangerous if they succeed in so doing."

This is a graphic picture of the acute maniac of fifty years ago. Fortunately, few such are now encountered. Acute mania is generally, but not always, preceded by a prodromatic stage, in which the symptoms are similar to those which precede the development of other forms of insanity. The period of incubation may last several days, or even weeks.

The most prominent symptoms which others observe in a person about to become the subject of acute mania are excessive irritability of temper from very slight causes, a general condition of unreasonableness, suspicions against those he has always esteemed and trusted, and marked changes in his modes of feeling and of expression. His subjective symptoms are pain or uneasiness in the head, vague fears, for which he cannot account, an indisposition to indulge in mental efforts, and often an impossibility of concentrating the attention on any matter requiring any considerable amount of thought, wakefulness, and sleep, when obtained, inquiet and disturbed by morbid dreams.

As the affection advances to fuller development, these symptoms are all increased in violence, and others make their appearance, going to establish a more or less radical change in the character of the individual. His dislike of friends and relations becomes pronounced, and he either treats them with unnatural indifference, or exhibits a degree of active hostility productive of ill feeling and quarrels. He does things in other ways, which excite the astonishment of those who have long known him. From having been economical, he becomes prodigal; from having been temperate and sedate in language, he becomes extravagant and profane; from having held the most moral sentiments, he expresses licentious and obscene views; his ideas are expressed in incoherent language, and often the ideas themselves are illogical and incomprehensible. His handwriting becomes more or less illegible, words are omitted, letters are dropped, he misplaces the date and signature, and introduces phrases which have no relation to the subject of which he is writing. His digestion becomes impaired, his tongue is coated, his breath is foul, his bowels are constipated, his appetite is at times extinguished, and again increased to the point of gluttony, his skin is hot and dry.

With all this he is entirely regardless of what others may

think and say of him. He bears no interference with his plans, which are often impossible of execution, and he becomes careless of his person and his dress.

This state may, as I have said, last several days or weeks, till, either gradually or through the action of some cause more than ordinarily exciting, it passes at once into the fully developed stage. Again, there may be no well-marked prodromatic stage, and the explosion occurs with startling suddenness.

And in some cases there may be a sudden accession of acute symptoms lasting only a few minutes, and followed by a period of comparative repose, during which the disease is permanently developed, or in which there is the establishment of a subacute form with frequent exacerbations of delirium.

The following case is an instance of this mode of accession and of the course of the type in question :

A gentleman, a widower, lived upon terms of great affection with his sister, who managed his establishment for him. For several years, they had occupied the same house together without anything occurring to disturb the sincere attachment which existed between them. He was as careful as possible to provide for all her wants, and exhibited a tenderness and love for her which were noticeable to all with whom they were thrown in contact.

One morning at breakfast, without any premonitory indications of a change in his conduct having been observed, he removed his boots, took off his coat, and seated himself at the table in this condition. His sister, surprised at these acts in one who had always been remarkably punctilious in all his social observances, inquired his reasons for such strange behavior, and made some laughing remark on the subject. He returned no answer, but, jumping up from his chair, began to swear and curse in the most violent manner. Becoming alarmed for her personal safety, she made her escape from the room and sent for the family physician. Gradually, however, her fears abated, and, approaching the door and hearing no noise within, she entered the room. To her great astonishment, she found her brother properly clothed, seated at the table as if nothing had happened, and waiting for her to pour out his coffee for him. At first he appeared to be in entire ignorance of his singular conduct, but at last he admitted that he believed he had taken off his coat and boots, and sworn a little. He excused himself by saying that his feet hurt him, and that he had felt very warm.

Nothing further evidencing any mental derangement took place till she began to notice a change in his demeanor toward her. He found fault with her personal appearance, said she arranged her hair badly, that her dresses were unbecoming, and that she was awkward in her movements. Then he accused her of neglecting the household, declared that she was ruining him with her extravagance, that her conduct toward him was disrespectful and insulting, and that if she did not amend her ways he should be forced to send her out of his house. She bore all his unkindness with great patience, and tried to convince him of the erroneous character of his impressions. But she might as well have attempted to change the course of the sun. His delusions had become fixed as a part of his mental being, and all efforts made to dissipate them only served to plant them deeper in his mind. Finally it became very obvious that he had acquired a decided aversion to her, and at last so hateful had the sight of her become that he ordered her to leave the house, giving her but three days in which to make her preparations for departure. Before she left his residence he had another attack of delirium which lasted several hours, and during which he attempted to cut his throat. Not till the occurrence of this second paroxysm did she have any idea that his conduct toward her was the result of insanity. After it passed off she spoke of his condition to other relatives, but no action was taken in regard to putting him in an asylum. The day subsequently to this attack he came home with a common woman whom he installed as housekeeper, and his sister took her departure.

After that I saw him frequently, and could discover no evidence of mental aberration, except that he had delusions relative to his sister, and that she and others had conspired to prevent him disposing of his property as he thought fit. He had, in fact, made a will, which, however, was never executed, giving all his property to his housekeeper. He appeared to transact his extensive mercantile business with as much thoroughness as ever.

But about ten days after his second attack of delirium he had a third, which was very severe, and which lasted about twelve hours. Up to this time he had never accused his sister of anything worse than disrespect, extravagant conduct, and neglect to provide for his comfort. After this last attack he informed me one morning, in a very confidential manner, that she had made two unsuccessful attempts to poison him.

Such cases as this are, however, rare. Ordinarily, there is a continuity of the delirium. Remissions there may be, but intermissions, except in the form known as periodical insanity, are very uncommon. In this latter variety of mental alienation the symptoms entirely disappear, and the patient is, to all intents and purposes, sane.

In the beginning of an attack of acute mania the mental symptom which is most prominent is the exaggeration of all the faculties of the mind. The *perceptions* are deranged, and there are both illusions and hallucinations, especially of the senses of sight and hearing. They may be of a pleasing, a frightful, or an indifferent character, and these several forms may alternate with surprising rapidity. At one moment the patient sees images which, to judge from the expression of his face, are causing him intense satisfaction, when instantly a change ensues in the nature of the forms or circumstances depicted, and he raves with terror or rage.

As regards hearing, he will stop in his walk, assume an attitude of listening intently, while a rapt smile passes over his face, and his hands are raised to command silence, when suddenly he utters expressions of fright or anger, places his hands over his ears, or puts his head between his knees, or under the bedclothes, in the vain attempt to shut out the sounds which madden him.

It is quite common for the acute maniac to mistake those persons who are about him for others; and even inanimate objects are, through his illusion, changed into men and women, or animals of various kinds. Again they appear to him as angels or devils, who either approach him with benevolent or evil intentions, as the case may be.

The sense of hearing is often exalted to a surprising degree, and very slight sounds are thus often heard at a distance which seems almost impossible. I have known a whispered conversation, conducted in a room on the first floor of a house, to be heard by a patient suffering from acute mania in bed in a room on the second floor, all the doors between being closed.

All the other senses may be the subjects of illusions and hallucinations, though not generally to the same extent as those of sight and hearing. The taste may be perverted to such an extent that substances taken as food have the flavor of noxious drugs, and odors generally regarded as pleasant may smell like some rotten substance. A patient of mine, to whose nostrils a nurse held a handkerchief sprinkled with cologne-water, exclaimed, "Take it away ; you are trying to poison me with small-pox. I know the smell ; take it away, I say !" and she closed her nostrils with her fingers and put her head under the bedclothes in her fright. Though illusions or hallucinations of the sense of touch are probably not common in acute mania, there is very generally a remarkable exaltation to tactile impressions, while the ability to feel pain is greatly lessened. Patients exhibit this first-named characteristic by taking off their clothing as fast as it is put on them, and keeping themselves as naked as possible. The contact of a single garment, or of the bedclothes, is irritating, and hence it is not surprising that they prefer to denude themselves of all clothing.

But while this condition exists there is, at the same time, an indifference to painful impressions which is astonishing. A man will hack himself with knives, inflict extensive mutilations on himself, and even plunge his head into the fire, and exhibit expressions of satisfaction while so doing. I have repeatedly asked patients after recovery whether or not, while they were in the act of perpetrating the most terrible wounds upon sensitive parts of their bodies, they had felt pain ; and the invariable answer has been in the negative. Either no pain was experienced, or the sensation was pleasurable. A lady, during an accession of acute mania, and while left alone in her room for a few minutes, cut off both nipples with pieces of glass which she obtained by breaking a lamp-shade. At the same time her fingers were, in several places, cut to the bone. Several months afterward, when she had recovered her sanity, she told me that she had mutilated herself in consequence of having a delusion that she would poison her baby (a year old) if she allowed him to take her breast, and that the best way to stop nursing him was to make the act impossible. So far from feeling any pain, the operation was pleasant, and, if she had not been prevented, she would have cut off both breasts as well. The sensation, she said, was an agreeable feeling of titillation.

In another case, the patient, a man suffering also with acute mania, had waked up in the night, and, while his attendant slept, had extirpated both testicles with a pair of dull scissors. After the operation, during which he had lost a good deal of blood, he woke the nurse, and, handing him the testicles, told him to give them to the ducks. I saw this patient several years afterward. He had then been sane for over two years, but had symptoms of an approaching recurrence. I inquired in regard to his former attack, and, among other points, asked why he had emasculated himself, and whether or not he had experienced any pain while so doing. He replied that he had felt a burning sensation in the testicles, that they seemed to him to be balls of fire, and that cutting them out had not only relieved him of his suffering, but had been attended with pleasurable feelings.

During the time when it was the custom to put to the torture and burn at the stake the maniacs who believed themselves witches or sorcerers, and who were supposed to be in league with the "powers of darkness," it was a subject of observation that the poor wretches, while being subjected to the action of agencies capable of causing the most acute pain, appeared to experience very little if any suffering. This immunity was ascribed to the fact that the devil looked after his own. In reality, however, it was due to the analgesic condition so frequently present in maniacs.

The illusions and hallucinations which afflict the subject of acute mania invariably involve the *intellect*, and are accepted as actual occurrences ; as a consequence, there are delusions in accordance with the character of the sensorial aberrations, and these are the mainsprings of the involvement of the emotions and the will, and of the conduct of the patient. His delusions have with him all the force of beliefs based upon the most undisputed facts.

At the same time, delusions may arise independently of illusions or hallucinations, being formed spontaneously or from the renewing by the mind of old beliefs and their reelaboration into abnormal conceptions.

A delusion having the same power with a maniac as a rational belief with a sane person, it is not surprising that acts of violence, extending even to murder and suicide, are committed. A maniac, for instance, imagines that the nurse coming toward him with a dose of medicine is an enemy approaching with an axe in a menacing attitude. The illusion is complete, and is accepted with unquestioning faith in its correctness. He consequently seizes a stool, or some other convenient weapon, and dashes out the nurse's brains. Or he constructs, without any sensorial basis other perhaps than his depraved sense of taste, the delusion that the medicine given him by the physician is poison ; he attributes whatever sense of physical discomfort he may have to its action ; he refuses to take it, and it is administered by the agency of a stomach-tube. Feeling himself the victim of a conspiracy to poison him, and experiencing the fear and the anger such a belief is calculated to inspire, he secretes a knife about his person, and, waylaying the physician, kills him not only without regret, but with the satisfaction a sane man would experience at killing a person who, he believed, was endeavoring to murder him. Or the delusion may be based upon such terrible hallucinations or illusions that, to escape from what he deems to be dangers that he cannot resist, seeing, as he imagines, the utter hopelessness of saving himself from frightful torments, he throws himself, in his terror and despair, from a window, or kills himself with some weapon that chances to be at hand.

Again, instead of being affected with delusions of a horrible or terrifying nature, the subject of acute mania is imbued with beliefs of the most enjoyable character. Every one he meets is a friend or a superior being, and his jolliness and good humor never desert him. Or, as is not uncommonly the case, the two varieties, with all intermediate grades, may alternate in the same individual.

Besides the matter of false beliefs or delusions, there are very often in the beginning of attacks of acute mania a sharpness and clearness of the intellect which are decidedly abnormal in character. He becomes cunning and adroit, is constantly on the *qui vive* against deception, and may even develop talents which no one ever suspected him of possessing. One, for instance, who has never shown the least mechanical skill or knowledge of ship-building, will construct a miniature vessel, perfect in all its parts ; another, who has never exhibited the slightest ability as an artist, will paint a very fair picture, or make a sketch with pencils, that in his sane state he would not think of attempting ; and a third, who has had no experience as a speaker, will deliver orations with a manner and a diction that evince a good deal of oratorical talent, if they are somewhat inflated and exaggerated in their language.

Relative to this division of the subject, Dr. Rush[1] says: "The records of the wit and cunning of madmen are numerous in every country. Talents for eloquence, poetry, music, painting, and uncommon ingenuity in several of the mechanical arts, are often evolved in this state of madness. A gentleman, whom I attended in our hospital in the year 1810, often delighted as well as astonished the patients and officers of our hospital by his displays of oratory in preaching from a table in the hospital yard every Sunday. A female patient of mine, who became insane, after parturition, in the year 1817, sang hymns and songs of her own composition, during the latter stage of her illness, with a tone of voice so soft and pleasant that I hung upon it with delight every time I visited her. She had never discovered a talent for poetry nor music in any previous part of her life. Two instances of a talent for drawing evolved by madness have occurred within my knowledge; and where is the hospital for mad people in which elegant and completely rigged ships and various pieces of machinery have not been exhibited by persons who never discovered the least turn for a mechanical art previously to their derangement ? Sometimes we observe in mad people an unexpected resuscitation of knowledge ; hence we hear them describe past events, and speak in ancient or modern languages, or repeat long and interesting passages from books, none of which, we are sure, they were capable of recollecting in the natural and healthy state of their mind."

It is reported that a lady, becoming delirious, spoke in a language which no one about her understood. At last a person heard her who recognized the fact that she was talking in the Breton tongue, and it was then recollected that she was born in Brittany, but had left that part of France when she was a young child, and had entirely forgotten the language.

Coleridge[2] cites the case of a young woman who could

---

[1] "Medical Inquiries and Observations upon the Diseases of the Mind," fourth edition, Philadelphia, 1830, p. 151.

[2] "Biographia Literaria," London, 1847, vol. i, p. 117.

neither read nor write, but who in her delirium talked Latin, Greek, and Hebrew. It was supposed by a priest that she was possessed of a devil, and preparations were made to exorcise him; but at last some one remembered that the girl had been a servant to an old Protestant pastor, whose habit it was to read aloud from his favorite authors within the hearing of the girl. The words and sentences spoken by the girl had, many of them, been written out, and, on being compared with the books, so many identifications were obtained that there was no reasonable doubt as to their source.

Of course, the *emotional system* is greatly disturbed in cases of acute mania. Indeed, some of the most striking evidences of the disorder of the mind which exists are exhibited through the emotions. With every false perception and every delusion there is a display of passional activity in accordance with its character, and which is as variable as the exciting cause. It is no uncommon event to see maniacs exhibiting love and hatred, benevolence and revenge, and many other antagonistic feelings, in the course of an hour, or even less time. At one moment the acute maniac is anxious to embrace all who come within his reach, or some particular person whom he mistakes for a woman he loves; while during the next instant he is cursing and reviling the whole world, uttering the most astonishing tissue of obscenity and abuse, shaking his fists at real and imaginary persons, making the most horrible grimaces, and ready to attack with fury any one upon whom he can lay his hands. The emotion of anger is particularly easy to be aroused in those affected with acute mania. The mere act of addressing a word or two to them is often sufficient to excite it. They take the most violent prejudices against some particular person, and will resort to all kinds of deceit and cunning in order to do their imaginary enemy an injury.

While the subject of acute mania may be laughing one moment, and shedding bitter tears the next, it is generally the case that there is a decided predominance of either the gay or sorrowful emotions, and hence a particular cast is given to the tone of the patient. Probably the latter category is more frequently in the ascendent. It is rare to see a patient affected with the disease in question whose illusions, hallucinations, and delusions, and, as a consequence, his emotions, are always of a cheerful or pleasurable character.

The *will* exhibits weakness from the very inception of the disorder, though at times there may be for a short period an exacerbation of volitional power. A sustained effort of the will is, however, impossible with the acute maniac. Occasionally he is seen to be evidently making an exertion to restrain the excitement of mind and body which exists, or even to conceal the fact that he has false perceptions or false beliefs ; but the power can only be exercised for a short time.

The physical symptoms of acute mania are equally as striking as the mental. In the first place, the *countenance* is perceived to have undergone a change. The face is generally, though not always, heightened in color ; the eyes are often bloodshot and preternaturally bright, and are in almost perpetual motion. The pupils are exceedingly sensitive to light and darkness, and are often perceived to contract and dilate, apparently under the influence of some thought or perception. Strong light appears to be painful. Ophthalmoscopic examination generally shows the vessels of the retina and choroid to be enlarged and tortuous, and the optic disk to be in a hyperæmic condition. The hair is in disorder, and often possesses a peculiar electrical quality, which causes it to stand erect like that of a person on the insulated stool of a statical electrical machine. The expression is variable, in accordance with the ideas and emotions which influence the patient ; but there are an exaggerated degree of motility in the muscles of the face and an increased power of causing them to respond to the thoughts and feelings which are not possessed by him in his normal state. To these phenomena must be added the disorder of dress which is so generally exhibited. The clothes are put on without any regard for appearances, and are misplaced, torn, and made dirty, with a thorough disregard of the proprieties of life. One patient will tie his hat over his shoulders ; another puts his coat on hind part before, or uses his trousers for a coat; and another puts her stockings over her hands, and struts about in them as if they were gloves.

The *muscular activity* of the patient never seems to be exhausted. Often, for day after day and night after night, he is in a continual state of excitement and motility. His arms are gesticulating violently ; he walks, runs, jumps, rolls over the floor, dances, and twists and turns his body into every possible shape. At the same time he is rarely silent ; he talks at the top of his voice one moment, whispers in a low

35

tone the next, and then shouts, yells, laughs, sings, prays, curses, and howls, till the room in which he is seems like a pandemonium. With all this, there is rarely any marked disturbance of the *pulse* or *respiration* other than what would be caused in any one indulging in the violent and incessant movements peculiar to acute maniacs. Neither is there any elevation of *temperature*. There may be subjective sensations of heat in the skin and other parts of the body, but there is certainly no increase of temperature determinate by the thermometer or by Lombard's thermo-electric calorimeter.

The *digestion* is almost invariably impaired throughout the whole course of the attack. The appetite is capricious, the tongue coated, the bowels obstinately constipated. The saliva is generally thick, viscid, and reduced in quantity.

The urine does not usually show any increase or diminution in the amount excreted, but there is almost always a large increase in the proportion of phosphates eliminated. In some cases the quantity of urea is increased.

Menstruation is deranged, either by becoming irregular or undergoing entire suppression.

Pregnancy, if existing at the time of an attack of acute mania, is rarely modified thereby, the process going on to full development. Of course, accidents, such as blows or falls, may produce miscarriage ; but even these factors do not seem to act with as much force as in sane women.

It sometimes happens that acute maniacs (though general paralytics are more liable to the condition), while in insane asylums, get their *ribs broken*, or, at least, are found with their bones fractured soon after their admission into such institutions. It is a question whether the condition is due to excessive fragility of the bones, rendering them liable to be broken on the application of very slight force, or whether it is the result of severe blows or pressure received previous to or after the admission into the hospital. It has been asserted that the injury is the result of pressure applied by the knees of hospital attendants to the lunatic while in a recumbent position, or to the blows received in his contests with other patients.

It is probable that the truth is to be found in all these alleged causes. Fractures of the ribs in the insane rarely attract the attention of the subject himself, and are not likely, in the absence of evidences of suffering, to be noticed by the physicians or attendants of asylums. Thus, Dr. Lauder Lindsay[1] states that he has known almost all the ribs of a young man's side to be broken without there being any outward indication or the exhibition of any kind of symptom. No complaint ever emanated from the patient. There was no bruise-mark, no lung symptom, no indication of the slightest suffering, from first to last; nor was it ever discovered how the injury was inflicted. The patient never could comprehend why he was confined to bed and swathed in flannel. Dr. Lindsay quotes Dr. Workman, of Toronto, to the effect that two cases of acute mania came under his observation in which five and seven ribs, respectively, were fractured. In these cases the fractures must have existed prior to admission, and they would not have been known without post-mortem examination.

At the same time, it cannot be successfully denied that these fractures often occur within the walls of asylums by violence applied by attendants or patients. Doubtless attendants are sometimes unjustly accused, but the discipline that admits of such an act on the part of a patient as that described by Dr. Rogers,[2] superintendent of the asylum at Rainhill, England, cannot be very strict. In this case a patient was found with broken ribs—"one or more." He accused an attendant of having knocked him down and kicked him, but afterward told a different story, and, on further inquiry, another patient said "he wanted to come into my ward to build a chimney six miles high, and I pushed him down stairs."

But in the same number of the journal from which this account is quoted is a statement from the editor, Dr. Maudsley,[3] which goes to show that the asylum attendants are not always the angelic creatures they are sometimes asserted to be. Speaking of fractured ribs in lunatics, he says:

"These injuries of patients are so uniform in character that it is clear they must arise from a uniform cause. In both these instances the commissioners were told of falls received by the deceased. We are not of those who believe that symmetrical fractures of three or four ribs on either side of the sternum can by any possibility arise from any fall which

---

[1] "Mollities Ossium in Relation to Rib-Fracture among the Insane," *Edinburgh Medical Journal*, November, 1870, p. 444.

[2] *Journal of Mental Science*, July, 1880, p. 253.   [3] *Op. cit.*, p. 252.

produces fracture of no other bones, and often no external bruises. How, then, are they caused? We cannot help thinking that they are sometimes due to the violence of attendants, and that they happen in this manner : A patient is refractory, or in some way or other comes into collision with an attendant or attendants. The latter resort to the expedient of 'downing' the offender—that is, throwing him down and holding him on his back till he promises to do what is required of him. If the patient resists, and the attendant is alone, the latter may have to exert great force to keep the other on his back. Possibly he may have heard of the great power of the chest to withstand pressure, of enormous stones being broken upon it with hammers, and so forth ; more frequently, however, in blind, stupid ignorance, he presses or kneels upon the front of the chest to prevent the patient rising. Now, so long as the latter can keep his lungs inflated, and his ribs expanded, he may, if not a very enfeebled person, withstand a very great pressure ; but there comes a time when he empties his chest, his lungs collapse, and the front of his thorax is stove in. Of course, this is more likely to happen as age advances and the ribs are less elastic and yielding, but we think the force applied must often have been sufficient to break the ribs of any person, old or young."

It appears to be probable that in some cases at least there is an abnormal degree of fragility of the ribs in insane persons. Dr. Hearder[1] found this condition to exist in eleven cases of twenty autopsies made at the Carmarthen County Asylum in 1870. He thinks that the fractures of those bones which occur in asylums are only rarely to be ascribed to ill treatment on the part of the attendants.

Professor Guddur,[2] of one hundred autopsies—fifty of men and fifty of women—found sixteen cases of broken ribs, of which only two were in women. These fractures are usually first discovered at the autopsy, and then in most cases they are old. He thinks they are caused by the patients running or falling against something—but none such have come under his observation—by the patients injuring each other, or by the ill treatment of attendants. And he says, in conclusion, that the more intelligent, attentive, and gentle the guardians, and

---

[1] *Journal of Mental Science,* January, 1871.

[2] " Archiv für Psychiatrie," Bd. ii, Heft 3 ; and " Psychiatrisches Central-blatt," February, 1871.

the more absolute their control and the less they resort to force, the fewer rib-fractures there will be.

Laudahn[1] has adduced the case of a maniac in whom there was a separation of several of the ribs from the cartilages, and who, after his cure, declared that he never received any injury ; but certainly one case proves very little, even if we admit the validity of the testimony. In the case cited, under the head of chronic intellectual mania, in which ribs were broken by the patient falling in the dark over a chair, there was no suspicion of any special fragility of these bones existing.

Among the subjects of acute mania no somatic symptom is more notable or of more importance than the obstinate *wakefulness* so generally present. It is the condition of all others which most effectually tends to produce exhaustion and death, and it is generally of so obstinate a character as to resist all ordinary means of relief. It is one of the chief phenomena to which the attention of the physician should be directed, for, if sound and refreshing sleep can be obtained, the prospect of an entirely favorable termination of the attack is very much increased. It is to be borne in mind that the same pathological condition of the brain which produces the maniacal paroxysm is that also which causes the insomnia.

The ordinary sleep of the acute maniac is seldom undisturbed by dreams. The muscular actions, the cries, the words spoken, the sudden awaking in terror—all go to show that his dreams are of a character with his illusions and hallucinations when awake. Such sleep as this can be of very little service in securing rest and the recuperation of the hardly-tasked nervous system of the patient.

The *habits* of acute maniacs as regards the care of their persons and attention to the ordinary rules of modesty and decency are often radically changed. In addition to the use of profane and obscene language, there is a proneness, even in those who have been remarkable during their sanity for a strict observance of all social requirements, to indulge in indecent conduct, and to be guilty of acts which are the very quintessence of filthiness. Exposing the person, lascivious gestures, urinating and defecating in presence of others without the slightest sense of shame, smearing themselves with urine and fæces, and even drinking the one and eating the

[1] " Archiv für Psychiatrie," Heft 1, 1872.

other, are acts from which they not only do not shrink, but which they commit with pleasure and bravado. I have known a refined and educated woman, in an accession of acute mania, to bedaub her face and hair with her own ordure. In this case, however, the act was committed under the illusion and delusion that she was anointing herself with a holy oil which was to save her soul from eternal punishment. In other instances such performances are the result of a spirit of mischief and opposition, the patient knowing perfectly well the nature of the act he is perpetrating, and taking exquisite delight in the trouble and disgust he is exciting. Coprophagy is more common with chronic dements than with other classes of lunatics, and will be considered further under another head.

Loquacity and *incoherence* are almost constant symptoms in cases of acute mania. The disposition to talk is unconquerable, and words are poured forth in a constant stream of incoherence. It seems to make no difference to the maniac what he says, or whether he is listened to. If there is no one to hear him, he talks to himself, or to the images his deranged perceptions have brought up before him.

There is both incoherence of words and of ideas. The thoughts follow each other so rapidly that the speech cannot express them before others, crowding in, stop the articulation in one direction to direct it to another.

Frenzy or *fury* is a condition liable to occur during attacks of acute mania, and consists in an exaltation of the excitement, both mental and physical, under which the patient labors. In this state the subject is especially dangerous, and is constantly making attempts to commit acts of violence. If unrestrained, several murders may be committed, either as a consequence of the ungovernable rage which exists, or as the result of some delusion which, for the time being, is in the ascendant.

A patient, for instance, will have been suffering for several days or weeks from an ordinary attack of acute mania of no very severe type, when suddenly, without previous warning of any kind, the paroxysm of fury occurs. The face becomes redder, the eyes glisten with excitement, the actions become more violent, and, if allowed, a murder, or a series of murders, may be committed, all of the most horrible description, and perpetrated with an astonishing degree of violence.

Such is a description of acute mania in its typical form. Of course, there are many cases which vary more or less from the category of symptoms presented, but the differences are in no respect essential. At the same time there may be present in the affected individual some pre-existing condition which modifies the course of the disease either by rendering it milder or severer, or by adding to it features of a specific character. Thus, sometimes there is a decided predominance of good humor and gayety. The patient is in a constant state of hilarity. He dances, sings, laughs, plays tricks of various kinds, brags of his strength, and other qualities, but rarely passes the bounds of probability, in this respect presenting a marked contrast with the general paralytic.

Or the attack may assume a religious, erotic, or other emotional type, and the actions, language, illusions, hallucinations, and delusions are in harmony therewith. These types of acute mania are very different from the emotional monomanias to which attention has been directed.

But there is a well-marked variety of acute mania which has been at times confounded with an emotional monomania, and that is the form known as *satyriasis* in the male, and *nymphomania* in the female, and which some authors have failed to distinguish from erotomania. In the latter disorder there is no obvious excitation of the sexual appetite, however much the instinct in question may be the *substratum* of the mental derangement. It is the *emotion* of love which is exalted, and not the genesic appetite, which, so far from being obtrusively manifested, is effectually kept in entire subjection to the intellect and the will.

But in satyriasis and nymphomania it is the sexual appetite that governs, and which puts its impress upon the character of the sensorial derangement, the delusions, the language, the acts, and other phenomena. There is in either sex an intense and irrepressible desire for sexual intercourse, and for indulgence in lascivious conduct. The speech is obscene, the gestures are suggestive of what is passing in the patient's mind, and indecent advances are shamefully made to all of the opposite sex who come within reach. With these symptoms there are heat and a sense of irritation in the genital organs, which of themselves prompt to frequent acts of masturbation.

In men the venereal excitement may run so high that

rape and murder are perpetrated, while in women there are spasmodic movements, followed by the sexual orgasm and ecstatic or epileptiform convulsions at the mere sight of a man. It is not at all uncommon for the act of masturbation to be performed by friction of the genital organs against the bed or some article of furniture, the clothes, or by voluntary contractions of certain muscles of the body. I have known a female patient, the subject of nymphomania, to bring on the sexual orgasm, in spite of all means to prevent it, by what appeared to be contractions of the gluteal, the constrictor-vaginæ, and the compressor-urethræ muscles.

Nymphomania, as a type of acute mania, is more common than satyriasis, for the reason, probably, that women have fewer opportunities than men for the gratification of their sexual desires.

There are other forms of genesic aberration still more degrading in their manifestations, entirely independent of acute mania, and which do not, therefore, now require our attention.

Acute mania exhibits a tendency to run a certain definite course, which, however, is not limited as to duration. Some cases last a few weeks, others a few months, and others perhaps a year. Rarely does the affection extend in its original form beyond this last-named period. Its average duration is about three months. In the course of the attack there are remissions in its violence, which are followed by periods of increased excitability. In favorable cases, after a time there is a gradual abatement in the intensity of the phenomena, the patient begins to sleep better, illusions and hallucinations become less frequent, and are not of so decided a character, and the delusions are not held with the same tenacity as formerly.

Again, the case may terminate in dementia, or in chronic intellectual mania, which in their turn may end in complete recovery ; or,

Again, the patient may die from acute inflammation of the brain or its membranes, from some other organic cerebral lesion, or from exhaustion of the system.

The prognosis in ordinary cases of acute mania is rather favorable than otherwise. The factors which militate against recovery are a feeble state of the system generally, the circumstance of the attack not being the first, and the existence of a strong hereditary tendency to insanity.

b—PERIODICAL INSANITY.

By periodical insanity, or recurrent insanity, as it has also been called, is to be understood mental derangement generally in the form of acute mania of a more or less severe type, occurring at stated periods, which are generally alike for each individual. It does not comprehend those cases of lunacy of any form in which there are remissions or even intermissions in the violence of the symptoms, some phenomena still remaining. It applies only to those instances in which all the manifestations of a disordered mind have disappeared, and in which, consequently, the patient is to all intents and purposes sane, able to attend to his affairs, and to conduct himself after his normal manner. In those cases in which the intervals of apparent sanity are very short, such as a few hours, close examination will almost always, if not invariably, show that some evidences of mental derangement still remain, and that the phenomenon is a remission only.

Periodical insanity is, therefore, a distinct variety of mental aberration, the characteristic feature of which is a disappearance of all the symptoms, their return in the same form at some subsequent period, and their continuance for the same length of time, as in the first instance. This sequence may be repeated for many years.

In a case of periodical insanity occurring in a lady of this city, the accessions, which are those of acute mania, last only eight days. On the ninth day she is entirely sane in every respect, with a somewhat indistinct remembrance of the symptoms she has experienced. In exactly three months from these cessations she is again attacked. The illusions, hallucinations, and delusions characteristic of each accession are by no means alike, though there is a degree of similarity in them all. Thus her sensorial aberrations, always relate to dead people, but not to the same persons. During one paroxysm she will see no other forms than those of little children which are laid out in their coffins, or being borne through the air by angels, or which entirely surround her in all positions as she walks the floor of her apartment, or lies down in her bed. Her conversation is entirely in regard to these infantile corpses, which she identifies as the Princes in the Tower, or the children of John Rogers the Smithfield martyr, or some other infants or young persons of whom she has read or heard.

Again, her hallucinations will consist of dead Indians. Powhatan, Pocahontas, King Philip, Tecumseh, Red Jacket, Black Hawk, Billy Bowlegs, Sitting Bull, and other defunct aborigines are grouped about and talk with her. Occasionally she will have illusions that persons about her are among the dead persons she sees and talks with, but these are not common, hallucinations greatly predominating.

Though she has been affected for about twelve years, and in that time has had nearly fifty recurrences, she has never had the same set of hallucinations more than once. The last that I have been informed of consisted of the dead Presidents of the United States.

All her dead visitants are not present at the same time. She talks with the utmost volubility, and expresses wonder why this or the other has not yet made his appearance. Some she lauds to the skies, others she abuses in very profane language, and on several occasions the images have not, so far as could be judged by her conversation, presented an entirely decorous appearance. Two or three times she has manifested slight sexual excitement in regard to some of her corpses.

There is no very great degree of motorial agitation. Her sleep would be bad if it were not systematically procured by the administration of morphia, chloral, or the bromides.

There is no derangement of the menstrual function ; neither do the attacks apparently have any connection with the menstrual periods.

Another case was that of a gentleman, aged thirty-five, who, about the first week in January of each year, was seized with a paroxysm of acute mania, during which there were strong suicidal tendencies. Knowing the certainty of the recurrence of the paroxysm, he was accustomed to place himself in the care of a medical friend till the seizure, which lasted about three weeks, had passed off. He was then perfectly sane in every respect—perceptionally, intellectually, emotionally, and volitionally — and able to transact with marked ability and success the very extensive mercantile operations which he carried on. This gentleman has been cured by the administration of the bromide of sodium continuously during the intervals of the attacks, having had no seizure now for several years.

The particulars of a case were given by Mr. G. P. Avery, at the February, 1883, meeting of the Society of Medical Jurisprudence, in which an individual of his acquaintance was affected with a paroxysm of acute mania at the time of each presidential election. The attacks were particularly characterized by the existence of the delusion that he was elected President of the United States. He proceeded to appoint his cabinet, and to assume other functions of the presidential office. Each attack lasted about a month, and then he was perfectly sane till the next election, four years afterward, when another paroxysm ensued.

Such cases cannot be regarded as lending any support to the doctrine of lucid intervals, and which has been discussed in a previous chapter of this work. During the so-called lucid interval, it may be repeated that the patient is not entirely free from symptoms of insanity. He is simply passing through a remission, and very slight causes may be sufficient to reawaken the phenomena in all their original intensity. But in periodical insanity the case is different. Here the attack runs its course and disappears, leaving the patient free from disease; and yet it seems a difficult matter for some alienists to distinguish between such a form of insanity and these very common occurrences in all varieties of mental aberration—remissions. This is the case with Koster,[1] who sees periodicity not only in every case of insanity, but in every other phenomenon of nature, and who attributes it to the influence of the sun and moon, acting in a manner similar to the exercise of their power over the water of the ocean, as well as to the magnetism of the earth. However efficient these and other factors may be in producing remissions and exacerbations in attacks of ordinary insanity, it is not at all probable that they have the slightest influence in periodical mania, in which the interval of sanity is sometimes several years.

Billod[2] makes the proper distinction between the two conditions, and clearly recognizes the existence of periodical insanity of the form now under notice. Thus, he says:

"I have, in the asylum of Sainte-Gemmes, several maniacs who, during the thirteen years that I have been at the head

---

[1] "Ueber die Gesetze der periodischen Irreseins und verwandter Nervenzustande," Bonn, 1882.

[2] "Considérations médico-légales sur les intervalles dits lucides chez les aliénés," Des maladies mentales et nerveuses, Paris, 1882, t. i, p. 416.

of the institution, have presented successions of paroxysms with intermissions of from one to two years. I can specially cite the case of a priest who, during his intermissions, is sufficiently lucid to perform the duties of the ministry and to fill the office of second chaplain without the fact of his successive paroxysms impairing in the least his ecclesiastical prestige. This is somewhat remarkable, for his audience are aware of his history, and have seen him stark naked during the height of his delirium. Now, when an individual remains a sufficiently long time without exhibiting the least sign of mental aberration, can it be said that he is in a lucid interval? No one, I think, can properly hold such an opinion. He is, during that period, no longer a lunatic, and the accession, when it returns, should be regarded as a recurrence. Its termination has all the characteristics of a cure, during the duration of which sequestration and isolation should, to a certain point, cease to be necessary ; and, that during which, also, the patient's acts should be regarded as rational—such, for instance, as making a valid will—seems to me to be unquestionable."

Distinct periodicity is seen, also, in many cases of emotional and volitional morbid impulses—such as suicidal and homicidal mania, pyromania, kleptomania, and the like, in which, in the intervals between the attacks, the subject is in his normal state of sanity.

c—HEBEPHRENIA.

Hebephrenia ("Ηβη, puberty, and φρὴν, φρηνιτῖς, the mind, frenzy) is the term applied to the insanity of pubescence, a form of mental derangement which presents many characteristic features, and which, as the name implies, is peculiar to that period in both sexes when the organism is undergoing the changes incident to its full development.

That there is such a type of insanity has long been known, but it is only within recent years that it has formed the subject of special study, and this has been heretofore to a very limited extent. The only monographs upon the affection with which I am acquainted are those of Hecker[1] and of Fink,[2] with whose description no inconsiderable experience enables me to agree in all essential particulars.

[1] "Die Hebephrenie," *Virchow's archiv*, B. lii, 1871, p. 394.
[2] "Beiträge zur Kenntniss der Hebephrenie," *Allegemeine Zeitschrift für Psychiatrie*, 1880.

The disease in the beginning is manifested chiefly in the emotional part of the mind. The subject becomes depressed in spirits, sometimes to such an extent as to cause more or less well-directed attempts at suicide. There appears to be a settled conviction that the efforts which are being made to perform the duties or tasks which have been assigned are not adequately appreciated, and that, no matter how faithfully labor may be performed, it will result in no personal advantage. The future, therefore, appears dark and forbidding, and the element of hope, of such vast importance as an incentive to youthful minds, is gradually eliminated from the mental organism of the boy or girl, as the case may be.

Of course, this is all morbid, but it is none the less real. Appearing at first as a mere apprehension or fear, it gradually increases till it becomes a predominating influence. The subjects feel that they are not understood, they misinterpret the actions of those around them, they become suspicious of those with whom they have heretofore associated, and whom they have regarded as their best friends, and they become not only the enemies of those with whom they have had direct associations, but of the whole human race.

It is not long before there is a marked deterioration in their moral qualities. Conceiving as they do that fair and honest dealing will avail them nothing, but, on the contrary, will be employed to their disadvantage, they do not hesitate to lie, to cheat, to steal, and to resort to all kinds of deceit and subterfuge to accomplish any object they may have in view. "It would have been no use," said a boy of fifteen to me, after he had run away from school with money and other things which did not belong to him, "for me to have asked the principal for money, and to let me go home, as I was ill. He would have refused, and have punished me besides. So I just took what I could lay my hands on and went off in the night when they were all asleep. You may send me back, but I'll run away again the first chance I get. Everybody is down on me there. If I learn all my lessons they find fault with me, and if I don't learn them it's no worse; so what's the use? Send me back, but the next time I run away I won't come home, and you won't find me either."

It is rarely the case that at this time the condition of the subject of hebephrenia is taken at its real value. The peculiarities of character and disposition which are being developed are generally regarded as so many evidences of wicked-ness, to be treated with severity, or perhaps to be let alone, as beyond cure by moral regimen. Schools get rid of such pupils as the one above referred to, and very properly, for their example is decidedly pernicious, and parents, not know-ing what to do with them, put them, if pecuniarily able, un-der the charge of a tutor, with instructions to eradicate, by some process which the tutor is supposed to know, the evil propensities which in some way or other have been con-tracted, or they send them to another school, from which they either soon elope or are expelled, or they are kept at home to do nothing, but to remain apt subjects for the future de-velopment of the disease.

In any event this development is sure to come. Delusions of various kinds begin to make their appearance, and these are formed not from illusions or hallucinations which are never present in the inception of the disorder, but out of the mor-bid thoughts of the subjects themselves, and are almost in-variably of an intensely selfish character. Thus, a young woman, seventeen years of age, who came to my clinique at the Bellevue Hospital Medical College, and who had several times run away from home, and been brought back by the police, had the idea that she had been specially endowed by the Virgin Mary with the ability to read the thoughts of people in any part of the world. Her father was a sailor, and was absent from home, and she was continually reminding her mother of what he was thinking at any particular mo-ment; and these thoughts were always of her, and of the deep pain he felt at the idea of the bad manner in which she was treated. On one occasion she went suddenly into the kitchen and threw the dinner into the fire, saying that her father thought it was not good enough for her to eat. Again she picked a mattress to pieces, because her father thought it was not soft enough for her to sleep on; and on still another occasion she threw all the crockery out of the window and broke the furniture, because, as she said, her father thought she ought to eat out of silver and use mahogany chairs and tables. Finally, intelligence was received of the death of her father, when she laughed, and said she had known all along he was not coming home, but that instead of being dead he had married another woman in Lisbon, and had taken her to the East Indies. Soon after this she went before a police magistrate and made oath that her mother had beaten her severely, showing some bruises which she had received by a fall on the ice, and returned home with a policeman armed with a warrant for her mother's arrest. In this case masturbation was verified. The disease went on unchecked, and the patient is now in a state of hopeless dementia.

In addition to the involvement of the intellect as regards false conceptions, there is always a marked deterioration of the force of the mind. The power of concentrating the attention is diminished, sustained thought upon any one subject becomes impossible, and the ability to comprehend is greatly impaired. The facial expression exhibits the mental weakness of the patient, and there are frequent paroxysms of silly laughing, the reason for which is never given. Accessions of acute mania are not at all uncommon at this period, and then illusions and hallucinations are formed. In a young gentleman, the subject of hebephrenia, whom I saw in consultation with Dr. Kittredge, of Fishkill, and who had several times run away from home, there were almost constant hallucinations of hearing and paroxysms of imbecile laughing. He had had several attacks of acute mania. In another, whom several years ago I committed to Dr. Kittredge's asylum, there were similar phenomena, conjoined with well-marked systematized delusions.

These symptoms may exist for several years before the passage of the affection into the stage of dementia ensues. Sooner or later, however, this is the termination.

Probably hebephrenia is equally common to the two sexes, although Fink[1] restricts it entirely to males. It appears to be induced by any cause capable of lessening the vital powers of the individual, among which masturbation and also the inception of the menstrual function are preëminent. One of the worst cases I ever saw occurred in a boy of sixteen, from South America, and was the result of excessive masturbation. I sent him to Dr. Parsons, at Sing Sing, and it was found necessary to watch him night and day without intermission, to prevent the act of onanism. The case was in all respects a typical one of hebephrenia. Several months had elapsed when the patient first came under my observation ; there were then illusions and hallucinations, there had been several acute

[1] "Beiträge sür Kenntniss der Hebephrenie," *Allegemeine Zeitschrift für Psychiatrie*, 1880.

maniacal attacks, and there was the characteristic tendency so frequently observed, to run away. The favorable result obtained by Dr. Parsons's care goes far to lessen the force of the gloomy prognosis usually expressed in regard to the affection.

Undoubtedly masturbation when practised to excess may modify to a greater or less extent the symptoms of hebephrenia, but the product is not entitled to be considered a separate form of mental derangement. The insanity of masturbation is simply hebephrenia, with the additional phenomena due to excessive onanism. Just as we meet with the peculiar condition produced by this vice without there being hebephrenia, so we encounter the latter affection when there is no reason to suspect masturbation. Nevertheless, the connection is an important one, and ought not to escape the attention of the physician. The influence of masturbation in causing insanity has been known from the earliest period, but the relation has never been so graphically set forth as by Dr. Luther Bell,[1] of the McLean Asylum in Massachusetts, who published his observations nearly forty years ago. It has also been described by Schroeder van der Kolk,[2] but many authors, as for instance Ellis,[3] fail to discriminate between cause and effect in their remarks on the relation of onanism with insanity. Nothing is more common than for lunatics of all types to practice masturbation, and doubtless the vice produces modifications in the physical and mental condition of the patient.

Hebephrenia is most apt to make its appearance, not at the very beginning of puberty, but a year or two afterward, when the system is experiencing to the utmost the demands made upon it. Hereditary influence is certainly a strong predisposing factor in its etiology.

d—CIRCULAR INSANITY.

By circular insanity (*folie circulaire*, Falret; *folie à double forme*, Baillarger) is to be understood a variety of mental alienation characterized by alternations of depression and ex-

---

[1] " Annual Report of the McLean Asylum," 1844.

[2] " The Physiology and Pathology of Mental Diseases," Rudall's translation, London, 1870, p. 139.

[3] " A Treatise on the Nature, Symptoms, Causes, and Treatment of Insanity," London, 1838.

citement, each period being entirely distinct one from the other.

Two forms of the affection are recognized. In the one, there are periods of sanity between the accessions; in the other, the stages of depression and excitement alternate continuously without intermission.

The fact that attacks of melancholia were sometimes succeeded by paroxysms of mania with mental exaltation has been noticed by many writers, but no one, before Baillarger[1] published his first memoir on the subject, gave it the attention it deserved. He was followed almost immediately and apparently independently, by Falret,[2] to whom we owe the term *folie circulaire*, or circular insanity. Since then the affection has been studied by alienists in all parts of the world, but by none so thoroughly as by those of France.

Baillarger's paper is based on six cases, and as the results of their study he arrives at the following conclusions :

" 1. Besides monomania, melancholia, and mania, there exists a special variety of insanity characterized by two regular periods, the one depression, the other excitation.

" 2. This species of insanity may appear, *a*, as an isolated accession ; *b*, the seizures following each other in an intermittent manner ; *c*, occurring without intervals between the paroxysms.

" 3. The duration of an accession varies from two days to a year.

" 4. When the accessions are short, the transition from the first to the second period is sudden, and ordinarily takes place during sleep. It is effected gradually, however, when the accessions are prolonged.

" 5. In this last case the patients seem to pass into a stage of convalescence at the end of the first period ; but if the return to health is not complete after fifteen days, a month, or six weeks at most, the second period is developed."

It is thus seen that Baillarger recognizes three varieties of circular insanity, while Falret[3] describes but one, the second

---

[1] "Note sur un genre de folie dont les accès sont caractérisés par deux périodes régulières, l'une de depression et l'autre de l'excitation," *Bulletin de l'académie impériale de médecin*, t. xix, p. 340, 1853-'54.

[2] "Leçons cliniques de médecin mentale," 1re partie, Paris, 1854, p. 219.

[3] "Mémoire sur la folie circulaire," etc., *Bulletin de l'académie impériale de médecin*, t. xix, 1853-'54, p. 382.

of Baillarger, in which there is a distinct interval between the accessions.

Among German authors, circular insanity has been recognized as a distinct affection of the periodical class by Kirn,[1] who designates it *die cyclysche Psychose;* Kraft-Ebing,[2] *das circuläre Irresein;* and Koster,[3] *periodischen Manie abwechselnd mit Melancholie.* In this country the only alienist who has alluded to it is Spitzka,[4] who has given a short but accurate description of the affection.

Period of Depression.—The period of depression by which the first stage of circular insanity is characterized may consist of *simple melancholia* without delirium or illusions, hallucinations or delusions. The patient is indisposed to either physical or mental exertion, he shuns the companionship of others, is averse to speaking, frequently remaining silent for hours, and if forced to respond to questions put to him does so in the fewest possible words, and without change of countenance. Again, he talks at times volubly enough, but his conversation is entirely in regard to himself, of his horrible feelings, his despair, his weariness of life, and the unhappy hours he passes, his mind filled with the most dreadful thoughts of the past, the present, and the future. His countenance is a fair reflection of the condition of his mind. His eyes are scarcely raised to look at those who address him, and the most exciting events do not engage his attention. The pupils are dilated, the brows contracted, the corners of the mouth drawn down, his whole aspect that of a person plunged in the deepest sorrow.

The sentiment of affection for relatives and friends is utterly extinguished. The only grief he is capable of experiencing is at the contemplation of his own real or imaginary sufferings, and yet this does not rise to the highest point, for nothing causes the flow of tears or any other violent expression of anguish.

The power of the will appears to be nearly abolished. His duties are neglected, for he has not the force to perform them, even if he felt the obligation to do so. His business affairs

---

[1] " Die periodischen Psychosen," Stuttgart, 1878.

[2] " Lehrbuch du Psychiatrie," Stuttgart, 1879-'80.

[3] " Ueber die Gesetze des periodischen Irresein," Bonn, 1882.

[4] *New York Medical Gazette,* May 9, 1880.

no longer interest him, and he views with equal indifference large gains or large losses.

At the same time, the intellect does not escape the general hebetude which has overwhelmed the other categories of mental faculties. The ability to think is markedly impaired. He no longer comprehends even simple matters with the quickness and exactness which formerly characterized him, and his ideas rarely extend beyond himself. His habits, which may formerly have been cleanly, are now the very reverse of neatness ; he neglects his person, and, though not actively filthy —for to be so would require a degree of physical exertion of which he is incapable—he is entirely regardless of those proprieties of life which are essential to the comfort of sane persons.

In addition to the somatic symptoms mentioned, there is very generally a decline in the bodily weight; the head feels full, or there is actual pain experienced in this part, and there are sometimes attacks of vertigo. The cutaneous sensibility is either diminished or augmented or perverted. The sight is sometimes indistinct ; there is intolerance of light, and the ophthalmoscope shows the optic disks and choroids to be abnormally pale, and the vessels of the former to be attenuated.

The bowels are usually constipated ; the appetite is abolished ; food is taken with reluctance, and only when the pangs of hunger become unbearable or actual force is used. There is stomachal dyspepsia, and large quantities of flatus are discharged from the stomach and the intestines.

The respiration is slow and labored, and the pulse, which becomes small and feeble, falls sometimes to fifty, forty, or even thirty beats in a minute. Ritti [1] has noticed a vasomotor disturbance, which has been observed in hysterical women, or as an independent affection, and that is a spasm of the arteries of the fingers producing the phenomenon known as *digiti mortui*, and which is characterized by coldness and bloodlessness of these members.

Menstruation is sometimes unaffected, and again ceases during the period of depression, to be resumed during the period of excitation.

The ophthalmoscope will show an anæmic state of the fundus of the eyes in almost every case. The optic disks are

---

[1] "Traité clinique de la folie à double forme," Paris, 1883, p. 166.

paler than in their natural condition, and the retinal vessels are smaller.

In other cases, the melancholia, instead of being of the simple form described, is marked by delirium, by sensorial aberrations, and by delusions, constituting essentially the form already brought to the attention of the reader, in the previous chapter, under the name of *melancholia with delirium*.

Ritti,[1] in his admirable work on the disease in question, makes four classes of the delirious ideas which are met with in this variety of melancholia.

In the first there is a *tædium vitæ*, which may reach such a degree of intensity as to lead to the development of suicidal ideas, and even to attempts at self-destruction.

In the second class there are conceptions of personal unworthiness, or guilt which is past all pardon, either in this world or in that to come. Morbid fears of all kinds may exist, mostly concerned with the idea of the "unpardonable sin" and eternal damnation. Again, the patients may conceive that they have committed sins of various kinds, and that officers of justice are in pursuit of them; or they may think that expiation is only to be made by self-inflicted suffering, and they may accordingly refuse to eat, or may even mutilate themselves in various ways. A patient of my own, who had for several years suffered with circular insanity, had, in one of his periods of depression, driven nails through his hands and feet, under the idea that he should try to become like Christ in everything. Sometimes they refuse to speak, and, when they do attempt to converse, their language is often incoherent, although few words are used. Indisposed as are the subjects of this form of melancholia to physical exertion, they sit in one place throughout the day, moving only when compelled by energetic commands or actual physical force. The patient to whom I have just alluded allowed, on one occasion, the water to flow into the bath-tub till it ran over the top and did a great deal of damage, rather than rise from his chair and turn it off.

The third class is characterized by the existence of the delirium of persecution, and by the presence of delusions and hallucinations in accordance with the delusions. Under the idea that the food is poisoned, patients thus affected refuse to eat, and forcible feeding has to be resorted to.

[1] *Op. cit.*, p. 62.

In the fourth class the melancholia assumes the hypochondriacal type, and the illusions, hallucinations, and delusions of the patients relate almost entirely to themselves.

It is rarely the case that any one of these several forms is met with uncombined with some one or more of the others.

In a third type, which is by no means as common as either of the other two, the mental depression is of the form previously described under the designation of *melancholia with stupor*. This may be of different degrees of intensity, from the simple suspension of some one or more of the faculties of the mind, to that in which, conjoined with the torpor of mind and body, there are terrifying illusions and hallucinations of sight and hearing, apparently threatening the patient with the most horrible torments from which he believes it impossible to escape.

In none of the cases of circular insanity which have come under my observation were there the cataleptic phenomena referred to by Ritti,[1] though I have in two cases witnessed symptoms in a measure approaching thereto.

Period of Excitement.—The period of excitement in cases of circular insanity may, like that of depression, be of three different but analogous varieties. There may be a state of simple mental exaltation in which there are neither sensorial nor intellectual perversions, but in which all the categories of mental faculties are in a more or less excited condition. The ideas flow with rapidity, the emotions which predominate are those of a gay character, the language is brilliant and often startling in the conceptions which are expressed, and which, though possessing these features, does not indicate the existence of delusion in the mind of the patient.

Conjoined with the excess of mental activity there is a corresponding condition of the muscular system. Patients thus affected are continually in motion. Rest is as painful to them as action is.to those who are passing through the stage of depression. They sleep but little, and yet do not appear to suffer from insomnia. They never complain. Obstacles are not heeded, and if engaged in business they are disposed to extend still further their operations, and to plunge into speculations which prudent persons would be apt to avoid.

Although there is rarely any incoherence in speech, there often is an incoherence of ideas. In fact, these frequently fol-

[1] *Op. cit.*, p. 87.

low each other with such rapidity that the speech cannot keep up with them, and the individual breaks off in the midst of a sentence, to begin another relating to quite a different subject.

Thus, although the memory participates in the general exaltation of all the mental faculties, and the individual recalls with vividness matters that occurred many years before, yet the ideas thus evoked come without logical sequence, and are thus blended into a confused mass, from which he finds it impossible to disassociate them. Events which happened, for instance, in his childhood, and which had been long since forgotten, are reçalled, but appear as though only a short time had elapsed since their occurrence ; while those which took place a few months ago appear to be contemporaneous with others of his infancy. This inability to obtain a correct idea of time in regard to past events is a marked feature of the condition under consideration.

Loquacity is certainly a very characteristic phenomenon of the simpler exaltation which often represents the stage of excitement. There is nothing about which the patient will not talk. He recalls whole chapters of the Bible which he learned when a boy, declaims the orations which he spoke at school, and, if he can recollect nothing, invents discourses for the occasion. The fact that he knows nothing about a subject is no bar to his conversing upon it. He assumes a knowledge, and will with the utmost seriousness advance views as being held by noted persons who have never expressed an opinion on the matter. Strongly impressed with the sense of his individuality, the subject of this variety of the period of excitement of circular insanity is not to be put down by those with whom he comes in conflict. He asserts himself vigorously on all occasions, and, if unable to carry his point by fair means, does not hesitate to lie and cheat to effect his purpose against those whom he imagines to be hostile to him, and even against his friends he often circulates the most infamous slanders, and takes a malicious pleasure in witnessing the pain and confusion he may have caused. He is, therefore, apt to be constantly in disputes, and not infrequently has condign punishment inflicted upon him by some one who will not tolerate his impertinences and his lies, or by the strong arm of the law.

Occasionally excitation or perversion of certain appetites

is observed in this class of patients, and excesses are committed which are beyond the limits of propriety or decency. Thus, a tendency to the inordinate use of alcoholic liquors, of opium, Indian hemp, and other stimulants and narcotics, may be developed in those who at other times do not touch these substances. Again, the sexual appetite is increased, and masturbation, venereal excesses, or unnatural practices, may be indulged in to a frightful extent.

The second form in which the period of excitement may be manifested is that of *acute mania.* Here there are illusions, hallucinations, delusions, incoherence, and intense mental and physical exaltation, the condition being such as has already been described in a previous section of the present chapter.

The third form is that of *mania with delirium of grandeur,* a state which recalls very forcibly the like condition which constitutes so marked a characteristic of general paralysis. The individual boasts of his great wealth, his immense physical strength, his skill in all the arts and sciences ; the great works he is about undertaking; his success in all affairs of the heart ; his influence with great men ; and so on through all possible conceptions of his active mind. There is no limit to the powers, the greatness, the proficiency which he claims for himself, and no end to the changes which his delusions may undergo.

The *physical symptoms* of the period of excitement are almost as striking as the mental, and are in marked contrast with those which were present in the stage of depression. The loss of weight, which was then a prominent feature, is now arrested, and the body begins to increase sensibly from day to day, till it reaches its normal standard. This result is due not only to the influence of the changed emotions, but also to the improved appetite and powers of digestion. There is no longer gastric or intestinal inertness.

The circulation becomes more active, the pulse not only rising in fulness and force, but also in rapidity, reaching sometimes to 120 beats a minute.

Attacks of cerebral congestion are common. They are evidenced by vertigo, slight loss of consciousness, and more or less severe convulsive twitchings of the limbs, or of individual muscles. These seizures are epileptiform in character, and occasionally may amount to a fully developed attack of *grand mal.* Periods of unconsciousness, but with the ability to perform voluntary acts, are sometimes met with. There may also be aphasia, temporary and localized paralysis, especially of the muscles of the eye and face, and sharp paroxysms of pain simulating neuralgia, or the fulgurant pains of locomotor ataxia.

The ophthalmoscope will almost invariably show a congested condition of the optic disks, enlargement of the retinal and choroidal vessels, and increased redness of the choroids.

These two periods of depression and excitement may follow each other immediately without intermission, or they may succeed each other with more or less regularity and with a distinct interval of insanity between them. These features, and others manifested in the disease, will be more strikingly shown by the detail of the particulars of a few cases than by description.

The case which, as Baillarger[1] says, was most in his mind when he wrote his account of the disease under notice, is the first given by him in his original memoir,[2] on the subject to which reference has already been made. It is manifestly proper to reproduce it here:

"Mademoiselle X., aged about twenty-eight years, has had since her sixteenth or eighteenth year several accessions of mania. After having been in good health for three years, there was a return, and since then the disease has never been absent. It appears in paroxysms, each one lasting about a month.

"During the first fifteen days there are present all the symptoms of a profound melancholia; then, suddenly, mania supervenes and lasts a like period.

"When the period of depression begins, Mademoiselle X. finds herself overwhelmed with a sadness which she cannot subdue. A kind of torpor, little by little, takes possession of her mind and body.

"The countenance assumes an expression of suffering, the voice is weak, the movements of the body are performed with extreme slowness; very soon the symptoms become more decided, the patient remains seated, motionless, and silent; the least excitation of any kind is painful to her; sunlight

---

[1] "De la folie à double forme," *Annales médico-psychologiques*, juillet, 1880, p. 5.

[2] *Bulletin de l'académie impériale de médecine*, t. xix, 1853–'54, p. 341.

fatigues and hurts her eyes. Mademoiselle X. understands very well all that is going on around her. She comprehends the questions which are addressed to her, but she answers very slowly in monosyllables, and in so low a voice that one understands her with difficulty. At the same time, in conjunction with these symptoms, there are insomnia, want of appetite, and obstinate constipation; the pulse is small and slow.

"At the end of three or four days the countenance has become profoundly affected; the eyes are surrounded with dark rings, are deep-set and without expression; the complexion is pale or yellowish.

"When this state has lasted fifteen days it ceases suddenly in the night, and the general torpor is replaced by a period of high excitement.

In the morning, the patient is found with her face animated, her expression bright, her speech quick, her movements sudden and quick. She cannot remain an instant in the same place, and runs here and there as if impelled by an irresistible force.

"Although her intelligence was weak, she is now bright and vivacious. She seizes with remarkable skill all the points in those around her which she can turn into ridicule. Her animation is inextinguishable, and is marked by continual epigrams on the persons and things about her. In this new state the wakefulness continues, but the appetite has returned.

"After fifteen days, calmness is reëstablished. She recollects all that has happened during this second period. She is a little sad and composed, but very soon she resumes her ordinary condition.

"The intermission is, unhappily, of but short duration; rarely does it extend to two or three months; generally, after fifteen or twenty days, another accession supervenes.

"The patient, who, during the period of depression, took but little food, emaciated very rapidly. At one time she lost twelve pounds in fifteen days. During the period of excitement, and during the intermission, the appetite was very great, and the return to stoutness took place rapidly."

As an instance of circular insanity, in which an interval occurs between the period of depression and that of excitation, I cite the following case from Baillarger: [1]

[1] *Op. et loc. cit.*, p. 345.

"Mademoiselle M., aged twenty-four years, had her mother and grandmother insane. She has herself been melancholic for four years. At the beginning there were sadness, idleness, and ideas of suicide. These symptoms, which were first noticed in the month of May, gradually became more marked, and the patient grew entirely stupid. She passed the whole day in her chair, motionless and silent. Her eyes were wide open, and her expression was that of stupor. The complexion was pale, the extremities cold, the appetite almost abolished, and the urine flowed involuntarily. This condition did not begin to improve till the month of October. The progress toward recovery was slow, and it was not till six weeks had elapsed that she was convalescent. Fifteen days had hardly elapsed when the symptoms of excitation appeared, and in a short time they were at their height. She made indecent propositions to those around her, and sometimes committed acts of violence. The period lasted about as long as the preceding one of stupor.

"Since then she has had three similar paroxysms."

There is no uniformity relative to the evolution of circular insanity. Sometimes the period of excitation follows at once that of depression, there being no intermission between them, and the transition taking place often in the night. Again, the symptoms of melancholia disappear gradually, and those of excitation supervene in the same way, so that the one step glides almost imperceptibly into the other. And again there is a distinct intermission of longer or shorter duration between the two periods. It is sometimes the case that the paroxysms follow each other without interruption, there being no intermissions at any time, but depression and excitation coming one on the other in an endless round. On the other hand, the intermissions between the paroxysms may extend to a year or longer.

It is also to be noted that there are all gradations in the intensity of the paroxysms, both as regards the periods of depression and excitation, from profound melancholia with stupor and intensely acute mania to simple depression of spirits and a little more than ordinary gayety. Geoffroy[1] gives the following case, the details of which were given to him by Baillarger, in which the phenomena were scarcely marked enough to be regarded as passing beyond the bounds of ec-

[1] *Thèse de Paris*, 1861, p. 96, cited by Ritti, *op. cit.*, p. 196.

centricity, but in which, nevertheless, they were very characteristic :

"There is a member of the Institute who, notwithstanding a *folie à double forme* with which he is affected, continues to take part in the meetings. To an attentive observer, however, he is a different man according as he is in the period of depression or that of excitation. When in the first-named state, he enters the room without saying a word to his colleagues, goes to his place, appears sad and cast down, indifferent to all that is said, and never speaking. When, on the contrary, he is in the stage of excitation, every one notices his entrance ; he talks to all, goes from place to place, speaks at each instant, constantly makes objections. After he has reached his home, his activity continues. He writes continuously, and dictates numerous memoirs to two or three secretaries whom he has under his orders."

The following cases, which occurred within my own experience, are sufficiently interesting to deserve citation :

H. S., a man twenty-seven years old, with hereditary tendency to insanity (his mother and two maternal aunts had been insane), consulted me, August 21, 1867. He informed me that he was subject to periodical attacks of melancholy, which were followed by paroxysms of great excitement, and that in the intervals, through one of which he was then passing, he was perfectly sane, and able to attend to his ordinary business, that of an importer of toys and fancy goods.

About seven years previously, as his wife informed me, he had met with considerable business reverses, and had in consequence become very much depressed in spirits, having suicidal tendencies, but no actual illusions, hallucinations, or delusions. This condition lasted about six months, and then suddenly disappeared, being succeeded almost immediately by a state of exhilaration that was noticed by all with whom he came in contact, and who had known his former state. By many the change was supposed to be due to the excessive use of alcoholic liquors. He himself ascribed it to a quack medicine which he had been taking for some time. The difference was so great that, although it was not supposed that he was insane, it was, nevertheless, very evident to his partners that he was in no better condition to transact business than he had been during his state of depression. When suffering from melancholia he took no interest in his affairs, but left everything to his partners to manage. It was impossible to rouse him sufficiently to get him to look into matters, and, when his advice was asked, he either gave the first reason that occurred to him, or declined to express an opinion. Now, however, everything was altered. He was meddling in all departments of the business, suggesting this thing and the other, making extensive purchases without consultation with the partners, and selling things at less than cost. He even rented an adjoining building, so as to be ready for an extension of the business, which he proposed to make in a short time.

At home there was fully as great a change noticed. Formerly, he had shown no disposition to converse, he took no interest in the household affairs, and, when a baby was born to him, refused to go to his wife's room to look at it. When it was brought to him, he said, "Take it away, I have seen as many of those things as I care to see," and immediately relapsed into silence. He did not see his wife till she was able to leave her room. His whole day was spent in sitting in a large arm-chair, with a book, from which he never read a line, in his hands. His appetite was bad, his bowels constipated, and he lost weight, his wife thought, to the extent of at least fifty pounds. He had in health weighed about two hundred and ten pounds.

Although he never attempted suicide, he several times remarked to his wife that he would like to die, and asked her what she thought would be the quickest and pleasantest mode of death. One day he remarked that, if the river were not so far off, he would go there and drown himself.

But suddenly all this disappeared, and the most extraordinary change in his mental and physical condition supervened. He talked incessantly, went to some place of amusement every night, proposed all sorts of schemes for the future, wanted to sell the house he lived in, and build a larger and finer one, talked of buying a country-seat, purchased a large quantity of jewelry for his wife, and bought stacks of new clothes for her, himself, and the children. Some of his purchases were of an incongruous character, but many were unnecessary, and some that he spoke of were beyond his means.

During this stage his appetite was enormous, and he rapidly regained his lost weight. Sleep was bad. Sometimes he would get up in the night and go out to take a " walk around the block," so as to be able to sleep better. He complained at times of a fulness of the head and of a pain in the forehead, but did not appear to attach much importance to these symptoms. Although fond of reading, he had never shown any literary ability ; but now he insisted that he was going to retire from business and devote himself to authorship, especially to the writing of novels. He purchased several reams of paper, a desk, a gross of pens, and numerous books of reference.

About this time, however, another change took place. He lost his excited manner, began to sleep well, ceased to speak of his many schemes, and became as sane in mind and as healthy and natural in body as he ever had been. The alteration was gradual, but was fully effected in a week or ten days. He spoke of his past conduct, both in his period of depression and of exaltation, with regret. He seemed to have a distinct recollection of all that had occurred, and of the thoughts he had had, and expressed his decided conviction that he had been insane.

He remained in perfect health, so far as could be observed, till February, 1862, when, without assignable cause, he suddenly became melancholic, and in almost precisely the same way as before. This state continued till the 11th of March of the same year, when it ceased—not at night in his sleep, but while he was sitting in his library, with the unread book in his hand. He had been in that position since early morning, when suddenly he threw the book on the floor, jumped to his feet, and exclaiming " By Heaven, there's been enough of this ! " rushed out of the house, his wife and other members of the family after him, screaming for help, under the apprehension that he was going to the river to drown himself. He was stopped by several persons, and brought back to his house, he laughing at the disturbance that had been created, and saying that he was the last man in the world to kill himself, as no one could be happier than he. The state of excitement, of which this was the beginning, was as nearly as possible like the preceding one of nearly two years before. He talked as he did then, bought clothes and jewelry, wanted to extend his business, and so on. It lasted till the 15th of April, when it disappeared in the night, while he was asleep, and he awoke perfectly sane.

He remained well till the 9th of the following September, when he was again attacked with melancholia. This lasted till the 12th of October, when he dropped his book as before with a like exclamation, and would have rushed out of the house, had he not been held by two friends who were present. This stage continued till the 14th of November, when it disappeared in the night.

Since that time, up to the period of his visit to me, he had paroxysms, of which the stage of depression and that of excitement were each of about a month's duration, with an intermission of about six months. All the periods of depression and all of exaltation had been as nearly as possible like others of their respective categories.

At the time of his visit I could detect no evidence of mental derangement, but he and his wife informed me that the stage of depression was expected in a few days, and might appear at any moment. In fact, it came the next day, and I saw him when it was at its height. It was, in all respects, similar to the previous seizures, and which have been sufficiently described.

This was on the 22d of August, 1867. On the 20th of September he suddenly exclaimed, "This has got to stop," and started at the top of his speed to get out of the house. He escaped, notwithstanding the efforts of people in the street to stop him—for he was in his shirt-sleeves and slippers, and without a hat, and all supposed something was wrong—and ran about half a mile ; he then walked back, and the stage of excitement such as has been described was initiated. It continued till the 24th of October, when it disappeared in the night. Since then he has continued to have the attacks, though they are not so long or severe as formerly, and the intervals are now over eight months.

During the period that he has been under my care, he has had very little physical pain in any part of his body. I have seen him over twenty times in each stage of the paroxysm, and have always found ophthalmoscopic evidence of cerebral anæmia during the period of depression, and of congestion during that of excitement. He is now in Europe.

In another case, the patient, a lady, aged thirty-six, married, with two children, and in good circumstances, having a slight hereditary tendency to insanity—a paternal uncle having died insane—became affected about the first of July, 1871, with melancholia, with delirium of a mild form. The attack lasted till August 18th, when it suddenly disappeared. She remained well till November 24th, when she had a sudden accession of acute mania, during which she fought and struck at those who approached her, sang, danced, swore, prayed, uttered the most obscene language, preached a sermon, made efforts at masturbation, and otherwise so conducted herself that she was sent to an asylum. She remained there till the first of March, when she was discharged as cured, though she had been free from delusion since the middle of January.

In July, 1872, she had another paroxysm of melancholia, with delirium much worse than the previous one, as she made several determined attempts at suicide. She was sent back to the asylum and was kept there till October 26th, though she had been sane since the latter part of August. A month after her discharge she had a second seizure of mania, and then, December 2, 1872, I saw her for the first time. She was then in a state of the greatest excitement, but, unlike the previous attacks, there was no disposition to violence. She had illusions and hallucinations, mostly of an erotic character ; was very loquacious, sang at the top of her voice, talked obscenely, and sang obscene songs ; was very desirous of taking off her clothes and showing her fine figure, etc. ; made repeated attempts at masturbation, but when stopped said, " All right, if you think it's wrong I won't do it," and burst into a hearty laugh.

The ophthalmoscopic appearances were always those of cerebral anæmia during the stage of depression, and of hyperæmia during that of excitement.

Under treatment this stage was kept within a condition of quietude when compared with the last seizure, and its duration was shortened to less than a month, for on the 28th of December she awoke apparently perfectly sane. She continued in good health, under treatment, till the 10th of March, a longer interval between the periods of depression and excitement than she had yet had. Then she experienced a return of the stage of melancholia with delirium, though in a much milder form. Under treatment the duration of this stage was shortened to two weeks, when she suddenly became sane, and has remained so ever since.

In this case there was an interval between the two periods which go to make up a whole paroxysm, in which there was neither depression nor excitement. Moreover, the accession of the stage of exaltation was of a more violent character than is generally met with in the affection.

In the description of the disease as given by Falret,[1] there is a gradual subsidence of one period and a gradual advance of the other ; then, again, a gradual disappearance until lucidity is reached. This period of remission is followed by the stage of excitement, for instance, and that by depression as before, and so on in an endless round for many years, or during the whole lifetime of the patient. It is to this form that Falret applies the term *folie circulaire*, while Baillarger employs that of *folie à double forme* to the type described by him. It is, however, preferable to embrace not only these, but all other forms, under one designation. There is certainly no good reason for regarding them as any more than varieties of one affection.

Falret considers the disease to be much more common with women than with men. Of seven well-marked cases that have come under my observation, five were in women. It is a disease of adult life, and is almost invariably developed in those in whom there exists a hereditary tendency to insanity.

It may terminate in recovery, in secondary dementia, in transformation into some other form of insanity, or in death.

e—KATATONIA.

By katatonia is to be understood a form of insanity first described by Kahlbaum[2] and characterized by alternate periods, supervening with more or less regularity, of acute mania, melancholia, and epileptoid and cataleptoid states, with delusions of an exalted character and a tendency to dramatism. The derivation of the word (κατατονος, *stretching down*) is taken by Kahlbaum to express the depressed mental and physical tension which is characteristic of the disease. From his monograph, and from that of Dr. J. G. Kiernan,[3] of Chicago, the only writer in the English language on the affection, I shall mainly take the description I am about to give.

---

[1] "Mémoire sur la folie circulaire," Bulletin de l'académie impériale de médecine, t. xix, 1853–'54, p. 382.

[2] "Klinische Abhandlungen über psychische Krankheiten," i. Heft, "Die Katatonie," Berlin, 1874.

[3] "Katatonia," *The Alienist and Neurologist*, October, 1882, p. 558. This paper was originally read before the New York Neurological Society, May, 1877, and was published in the *American Journal of Insanity* for July, 1877.

Katatonia may, like other varieties of insanity, be preceded by prodromatic symptoms similar in character to those which have been described in other parts of this work. There are pains or other abnormal sensations in the head, vertigo, insomnia, irritability of temper. Again, it may begin with an epileptiform convulsion, or the condition of melancholia or exaltation may be the first noticeable symptom. Then the cycle begins : Cataleptoid phenomena accompany or follow the melancholia, which is generally of the form described in this work as melancholia with stupor, and a period of excitement supervenes, during which the patient has sensorial derangements in the way of illusions and hallucinations as well as delusions. Again, the melancholia appears, perhaps, in a modified form, with cataleptoid and waxy conditions of the muscles, and a disposition to talk in an exalted or dramatic manner. At times, during the course of the affection, there may be convulsions or involuntary muscular actions, such as rolling on the floor or bending of the body. Masturbation is a common accompaniment, and during the stage of excitement acts of violence may be committed.

I cite the following case from Kiernan's memoir :

"T. R., aged thirty-six, policeman, single, common-school education, intemperate, as were also his parents. The patient had been a masturbator, and had indulged in sexual excess. He was at first melancholic, subsequently maniacal, but, recovering therefrom, became what his fellow-policeman called 'stuck up.' His temper changed from good-humor to irascibility, and asylum treatment was at length rendered necessary. He was admitted to the New York City Asylum for the Insane, March 17, 1873. A week previous he had gone to church, but soon returned, saying he had been followed by droves of dogs. He was a tall, powerful, good-looking man, and, though he had asserted that he would not commit suicide, he had cut off the tip of his ear in an attempt of this kind. He was somewhat subdued in manner, and had hallucinations of sight and hearing. The day previous to admission he was affected with spasm of the muscles of the extremities. Four days after admission he manifested the delusion that he had committed a great crime, and refused food, but said, 'This is not a penance for the crime.' He required artificial feeding for three days, took food voluntarily on the fourth, and again refused it on the fifth day. A period of excitement then occurred, and he became a subject of hallucinations differing from those he had on admission. After treatment a short time with opium and hyoscyamus, he grew quiet and took food voluntarily but very suspiciously. In about a week after, a spasm of the muscles of the neck, followed by slight unconsciousness and slumber, occurred, the pupils dilating widely, and so remaining for a few days. Two weeks after, he had very sluggish movements of the lower extremities, bearing a very suspicious resemblance to functional paraplegia, but this was really an incomplete cataleptoid condition, involving also the muscles of the neck and upper extremities. The patient opened his mouth, and performed other simple actions of that nature; these, however, were not ideational, but sensori-motor acts, as his attention to the subject was *nil*, and he was in a peculiar emotional state. That all the mental faculties were not in abeyance was shown by the fact that he involuntarily raised his hands, in an attitude of supplication, or as an acknowledgment of a favor just received. His pupils responded to light, and the organic functions were performed as usual. This condition continued for three days, with very little change, except that, when asked to perform a simple action, the request would be obeyed, and the action continued indefinitely in an automatic way.

"Five days after the beginning of the condition just mentioned, the patient had a rapid, feeble pulse, the beats of which ran into each other, and did not correspond with the heart's action, which, though rapid, was otherwise normal. His eyelids and lower extremities soon became œdematous, and the cataleptoid condition disappeared. The heart's action grew more irregular, the first sound being alone audible, and accompanied with a loud, blowing murmur, heard at the base. Pulse one hundred and thirty-two, and more rapid in the neck than at the wrist; respirations were increased, the lungs and temperature being normal. The heart's action soon returned to its normal condition, and the murmur disappeared. The treatment was directed to the alimentary canal only. The patient then became entirely unconscious as to his surroundings, though taking food and performing other actions involving only the organic functions normally, and so continued for about a week. He then began to have tonic contractions of the muscular system, followed by lessening of the œdema, which finally disappeared. The cataleptoid condition then returned, and was accompanied with considerable waxy mobility. Two days after, his muscles were extremely rigid, and he remained apparently unconscious for some time. One morning he suddenly spoke, and being asked his reason for not speaking before said, 'They told me not to,' and, when asked who told him not to, replied, 'God and the others,' and began to weep.

"The following day he had a return of the cataleptoid condition, in which he remained for some time. These alternations continued for three months, when he became suddenly violent, tore off a bar from the window, and tried to make his escape. This excitement continued three days, the patient then passing again into the cataleptoid condition, on emerging from which he was markedly dignified and very formal in conversation. This manner of speaking and acting continued for three months. He then had another cataleptoid relapse, succeeded by an attack of melancholia attonita (melancholia with stupor). Then followed a condition during which his pupils at first contracted and then dilated, his left hand contracted firmly, and from it a quivering motion extended over the left side, and gradually involved the entire body. The irregularities of circulation formerly observed once more appeared, and, as before, went away without special treatment.

"Melancholia atonita became the predominant condition, accompanied, however, by increased susceptibility to external influences. This remained four months, and was followed by a cataleptoid condition, with much waxy mobility. While in this state he was found to be developing phthisis. The disease ran a rapid, somewhat irregular course, terminating life, July 22, 1875, twenty-six months after his admission into the institution."

This is a fairly typical case of katatonia. Four others are reported in detail by Dr. Kiernan, though he states that forty-six cases were observed by him.

Before giving the particulars of the four cases that have come under my own observation, I desire to cite a well-marked instance which, though reported by its distinguished author as a case of circular insanity, or *folie à double forme*, is undoubtedly to be considered one of katatonia. No one, I think, reading the graphic description given by Dr. Kraft-

Ebing,[1] could fail to place the case in its proper nosological position, as an instance of the affection under consideration.

The patient was a man, twenty-two years old. His father, shortly before his death, had some kind of psychical troubles, and his mother suffered from habitual headaches. The patient was well, up to the period of puberty. At this time he got into bad health, suffering from general debility and palpitations, and on these accounts was excused from military service. This state was doubtless due to onanism, which the patient had long practiced to a great extent. In 1877, after a violent emotional disturbance, he passed suddenly into a state of stupor with intervals of maniacal excitement. Eight days afterward he was well. On the 28th of August, 1878, he became excited at a dance, drank to excess, and was subjected to mortifications by his mistress. On the 26th he appeared to be depressed and in bad humor. A few hours afterward, he fell into a profound stupor, without movement.

On the 28th he began to gesticulate, to speak by assonances, to discourse, and to be in continual motion. He upset everything, rolled on the floor, demanded that the curate should marry him, and talked in a manner altogether incoherent.

On the 30th he again became stupid, and was in this state when he arrived at the clinique. Aside from the fact that his pupils were dilated and not very active, nothing special was noted relative to his physical condition. He lay on the floor motionless, mute, and stupid.

On the 31st another period of excitation began, and again he spoke by assonances. He recited, in good German, some passages from the Bible, preached, and made tragic gestures, saying with great pathos all kinds of inanities; for example, "Twice six are twelve, eighteen is my brother," etc. When the attempt was made to undress him, he resisted with energy, cried out in a loud voice, grit his teeth, and contorted his face. As soon as he was let alone, he raised himself, and with a menacing tone said, "Come here!" For several hours he was quiet, and tolerably lucid up to the period of the visit. Sometimes also he had periods of stupor lasting several hours, during which there were theatrical poses and cataleptiform states, but in reality the patient remained until the 16th of September in a state of maniacal excitation, with insomnia,

[1] "Lehrbuch für Psychiatrie," Stuttgart, 1880, t. iii, p. 124.

great incoherence, recognition of what was going on about him, volubility, during which he discoursed in good German of God, the Virgin, and his mistress.

On the 16th of September, however, he fell again into a state of stupor, which continued till the 14th of November. During this condition he had no consciousness of his acts, passed his urine and fæces in the bed, assumed cataleptiform and other forced positions, and remained for a long time lying in one place, his eyes in a state of convergent strabismus, and fixed on vacancy. Generally he was mute, but when he talked he uttered all kinds of absurd expressions, and spoke by assonance, saying over and over again, "Flug, flüge, fleck," etc. By the 13th of November he was a little less stupid, said the blood was rushing to his head and gave him vertigo. In fact, there often was a redness of his face. It was observed that he masturbated during the stupor, and that the act increased the redness of his face.

On the 14th of November the period of excitation reappeared. He was wakeful, and again began in a pathetic manner to say things without sense, and spoke by assonances. There were great incoherence and a tendency to utter isolated words and phrases. He took those about him for the Pope and bishops, was in a state of continual agitation, rolled over and over in bed, and kept on uttering isolated words. Then, again, he assumed forced attitudes, and upon occasion showed anger.

On the 29th of November he was quiet, and in a stupor. This was characterized by symptoms similar to those of the preceding corresponding states, and lasted only a few days. By the middle of December he was quiet, and on the 10th of January he was discharged cured.

Certainly this was a typical case of katatonia.

A merchant engaged in the importation of Vienna goods consulted me March 11, 1880, or rather I was consulted in regard to him by his brother and one of his partners in business, and the patient, very much against his will, was brought to my consulting-room.

He entered the apartment with all the air of a prince, and sat down without deigning to address me. When I spoke to him he at first made no answer, but on my persistence with my questions of what his name was and where he lived, he looked at me for a moment in a supercilious way and finally said, "And the Lord spake unto Moses, saying." This he kept repeating, whether spoken to or not, during the whole of his visit, extending over an hour. Upon inquiry, I ascertained that without assignable cause he had, eight days previously, suddenly passed into a condition of melancholia with stupor, during which he was most of the time silent and in a state of almost complete immobility. It was also noticed that, when anybody took hold of his hand, the member remained for several minutes in the position in which it was left. On one occasion his neck had continued twisted, with his face as far as it could be turned over his left shoulder, for over half an hour, and had then slowly returned to its natural position. On my taking hold of his arm and extending it at right angles with his body, and leaving it there, it remained outstretched for thirteen minutes, and then slowly descended to his side. All the time that I was making this and other examinations of his muscular system, he was saying in a loud voice, "And the Lord spake unto Moses, saying."

The pupils were equal, were largely dilated, and did not react well to light.

I requested him to follow me into another room, in order that I might make an ophthalmoscopic examination. He took no notice of what I said to him, and, when his friend and I raised him from his chair to lead him into the apartment, he made himself as rigid as a bar of iron, so that we had to carry him. Arrived there, he would not sit down, but stood as erect as a statue. On feeling his muscles, it was easy to perceive that all were in a state of extreme tension. It was impossible, I found, to make the examination I desired ; so, after prescribing the bromide of sodium for him, in doses of twenty grains three times a day, I sent him away, with instructions to return in five days, and to continue the medicine till then.

On the 16th I saw him again. He was then in a state of high excitement. He entered the room without hesitation, and at once began an extemporary speech on the beauties of the solar system. Every sentence, however, he ended with the phrase, "And there shall be no night there." I wrote down from memory soon after his departure a portion of his address, as follows :

"And now, my friends, what is this solar system of which we have heard so much ? And there shall be no night there. Is it composed of homogeneous matter throughout its whole extent, or are some parts of it different from others? And there shall be no night there. Is it to be supposed that the sun, a light-giving orb, is of the same physical structure as the moon, a light-reflecting orb? And there shall be no night there. Is the earth, a light-receiving orb, like the sun, a light-giving orb, and the moon a light-reflecting orb? And there shall be no night there "—and so on for half an hour.

Since his last visit he had had several spasmodic seizures without loss of consciousness, coming on before the cessation of the period of melancholia, which took place on the 14th of March. Since that time he had done very little else than to declaim from Shakespeare and other poets, and deliver extemporaneous addresses. He was disposed to be very quarrelsome, and had knocked the hat off of a man's head on his way to my residence, because he thought the man had made a face at him as he passed. The convulsive seizures had consisted of movements of the head and of the muscles of the neck. The head, for half an hour or more, had on several occasions been kept in continued motion from side to side, while the face was undergoing contortions. One afternoon he had stood before an engraving of Washington and bowed for over an hour, and would have continued had he not been taken away by force.

On my asking him how he felt, he answered, "It's a wise child that knows its own father, but I feel quite well, I thank you." On my asking how he had slept the previous night, he replied, "It's a wise child that knows its own father, but I slept very well, I thank you." When I asked if he had any pain in his head, he said, "It's a wise child that knows its own father, but I have no pain in my head, I thank you." And so on, to every question I put to him.

Before he left, he began to speak in a staccato way : "I—think — I— shall—go—to—the—the—a—tre—to—night—to—see—Booth—in Ham—let."

I asked him why he spoke in that manner. He replied :

"Be—cause—I choose—to do—as—I choose to—do—and that—is—why—I speak—as—I—choose—to—speak."

"But," I said, "it is a silly way of talking."

"I—came — to you—for—med—i—cal—advice—and—not —for—a—les—son—in—el—o—cu—tion."

At this time there were the ophthalmoscopic appearances of cerebral congestion. The pupils were normal.

So far as I could ascertain, there had been no illusions or hallucinations, but there were delusions that he was to be made the director of the opera and manager of all the theatres, with a large salary from the State.

I directed the continuance of the bromide of sodium. On the 22d I saw him again. There was then a condition of catalepsy, without marked melancholia. Though indisposed to talk, he would answer if the question were repeated. The arms, legs, and head were in a waxy state, and at times he would take dramatic attitudes and keep them for several minutes. He stood in my consulting-room for seven minutes as "Ajax defying the lightning," and for the like time as the "Apollo Belvedere." "The dying Gladiator" he could only maintain for a few minutes.

At the time there was no mental aberration of any kind, but there was a slight degree of exhilaration present which was not natural to him, and a slight disposition toward dramatism. This, however, did not extend to speech, but only to the attitudes which he would assume without prompting.

Under the continued use of the bromide, this state passed away in a few days, and there were no further manifestations of the disorder.

The next case that came to my notice was that of a young German, living in St. Mark's Place in this city, whom I saw in consultation with Dr. Garrish. In this instance, the cataleptoid state and the tendency to utter high-flown language, and to assume histrionic attitudes, were strikingly exhibited. At the period of my examination the mental condition was that of excitement. The patient was talking volubly nearly all the time, walking the floor, gesticulating, grimacing, and occasionally speaking in alliterative verse. He had hallucinations of hearing, and would often stop and listen for an instant with a rapt expression of countenance. Then he would exclaim in pompous tones, "My lord, it shall be done!" This he repeated many times. He had passed through a stage of melancholy before I saw him. This had lasted a week or more, and during its continuance the patient mostly sat motionless in a chair, mute to all questions, and never taking the initiative in talking. Frequently, however, when spoken to, though he would not answer, tears would flow in profusion, and he would groan aloud. He afterward said that he had not spoken, because he had the idea that it had been decreed that, if he uttered a single word, his mother would at once die. I did not see this patient again, but was informed that he recovered under the bromide treatment advised. The pupils were contracted, and the optic disk and fundus of the eye congested.

The third case was that of a physician from a Southern city, who was brought to me by his friends, August 31, 1882. He was then in the stage of melancholia with stupor, attended with cataleptoid symptoms. He would not speak, but sat as long as allowed, motionless, with his eyes cast on the ground. If physical efforts were made to move him, his whole muscular system was thrown into a state of extreme tension. If the attempt were made to raise his arm from his side, for instance, the limb became rigid, and it was almost impossible to move it; at the same time there was no sign of any voluntary effort at resistance on his part. He sat as composedly as before on his chair, without a change of countenance, though the muscular strength brought to bear by him was certainly very great.

When I requested him to walk into an adjoining room, in order that I might make an ophthalmoscopic examination, he sat without moving a muscle. It was necessary to carry him, but, as soon as touched for that purpose, his body became perfectly rigid, and he could not even be made to sit down. He stood as erect as a statue. He appeared to be in a condition not unlike that of a person suffering from tetanus, in whom the slightest impression made upon the skin is sufficient to induce a spasm.

Previous to my seeing this patient, he had had repeated paroxysms of excitement, alternating with periods of melancholia, with stupor and cataleptoid phenomena.

After leaving New York, he improved to some extent, and would have improved still more, could he have been induced to take the mixture of bromide of sodium and fluid extract of ergot prescribed for him.

The only other case of katatonia that has come under my observation is that of a Swede, a man of about thirty years of age, who came to my clinique at the New York Post-Graduate Medical School February 15, 1883, and who formed the subject of a clinical lecture delivered to the class of medical practitioners in attendance. Twelve years previously, the man, while working in a stone-quarry, had a piece of timber fall upon his head. He was stunned for a few minutes, but the blow was not a serious one, and he recovered ; subsequently, however, he had some head-trouble, and did not speak for several weeks. All morbid symptoms disappeared, and he remained well till about twenty days before I saw him, when he became excited, thought people were going to kill him, that he had committed some crime, etc. This state only lasted a few days, when it was succeeded by a period of melancholy with stupor, during which he was mute, and sat nearly all day in one position. If his baby were put into his arms, he would hold it for hours without moving his hands or otherwise changing his position. He never asked for food or appeared to care about eating. If his meals were brought to him, cut up, and put to his lips, he would sometimes open his mouth and eat ; again, he would refuse. In my preliminary examination, I soon discovered the cataleptoid phenomena and the rigid state of his muscular system generally. Before the class, I stretched out one of his arms, and he kept it in a perfectly horizontal position for over ten minutes, when his brother, fearing he might be injured, put it down. Again, on trying to raise his arm, it was held so strongly against his side that it was impossible to move it. No answers could be obtained from him. He sat bolt upright, staring at vacancy without the least expression, unless it were one of slight astonishment, on his face. This attack was supposed by his father to be due to grief caused by the death of one of his children about a month before. I prescribed the bromide of sodium in doses of thirty grains three times a day, and directed him to return in a week for further observation. On his return at the time fixed upon, the cataleptoid phenomena had entirely disappeared, but there was still a tendency to dramatism. He came again on the 1st of March, and was discharged cured.

Many cases of unrecognized katatonia are to be found reported in writings on psychological medicine. One of the earliest is the following : [1]

James W. L., aged twenty-nine, was admitted into the hospital May 10, 1821. This young man had been a patient in the hospital before, and had remained for twelve months, when he was placed on the incurable list ; but, having got

---

[1] "Sketches in Bedlam," etc., London, 1823, p. 155.

much better, and continuing to improve for some time, six months' leave of absence was granted him, at the end of which time he came back completely well, and was discharged cured.

The character and symptoms of this patient's disorder, it is stated, were extremely curious. When the paroxysm came on, however he happened to be situated, his whole form from head to foot became stiff, as if all his joints and muscles were ossified. His eyes, though staring open, became fixed, and he foamed at the mouth. If sitting or walking, when his fit came on, he would instantly fall to the ground, completely extended at full length on his back with the same symptoms of rigid stiffness and insensibility; his eyes, open and inclined upward, were insensible to the touch of a hand passed over them, which did not produce the slightest wink. No symptom of animation remained, with the exception of breathing, and this so faintly as to be scarcely perceptible. His condition, in all other respects, resembled death, and in this state he would sometimes continue for one, two, three, and even four days, without any apparent change. He could not be induced on these occasions to eat or take any kind of sustenance, except under the direction of medical gentlemen, when rich broths were administered by injection. During the fits his whole person was literally as stiff as a plank, and he might have been raised to a perpendicular position and carried from place to place like a ladder without the least appearance of flexibility. Toward the termination of these paroxysms, when a hand was passed over the eyeballs, they would sometimes move, which was a prognostic of his recovery. On being roused from his stupor, he recollected nothing of what had passed, but he would speak of dreams, visions, heaven, hell, and the strange things he had seen. After these fits he always appeared weak and dejected.

Other cases of a similar character have been reported by Cullere,[1] Lagardelle,[2] and others, but without differentiating the affection now under notice, and without reference to Kahlbaum's monograph. The disease is more common in men than in women. Of twenty-six cases reported by Kahlbaum,

---

[1] " Observation de catalepsie chez un hypocondriaque persécuté," *Ann. méd.-psy.*, mars, 1877, p. 177.

[2] " Catalepsie consécutive à une manie aigue," *Ann. méd.-psy.*, janvier, 1878, p. 38.

twenty were in males. All of Kiernan's cases were in males, but this is explained by the fact that the asylum of which he was one of the medical officers had only male patients. All my cases were also in males.

f—PRIMARY DEMENTIA.

By primary dementia is to be understood a form of mental derangement characterized by the more or less complete weakness of the faculties of the mind, not secondary to any other form of insanity, but beginning as such in an individual previously sane.

The affection may be developed with great suddenness as the result of some moral shock, or it may supervene gradually. In the former case, the symptoms reach their highest degree of intensity with great rapidity ; in the latter, their progress is slower, and may be interrupted by periods of remission or intermission.

In instances of gradual progress the first symptoms may be of a very indistinct character. The patient evinces less concern than formerly in passing events, or in those things in which he would naturally be supposed to be interested, such as his family, his business, his food, etc. Perhaps he shows this first and most strikingly in regard to his dress and habits, for carelessness in the one and a disregard of the proprieties of life are among the earliest manifestations of primary dementia. Nevertheless, the changes from his normal characteristics are at first so very slight that they are not often attributed to their real cause, but are supposed to be due to mental preoccupation.

But little by little these phenomena become more intense, and there is also observed a weakness of the emotions, which is manifested by the display of excessive joy or grief at the occurrence of what to persons of normal mind would be slight disturbing causes. Tears are therefore shed over the veriest trifles, and violent laughter will be indulged in at circumstances which have little, if any, of the element of mirth about them. At times there may be an entire reversal of the ordinary evidences of feeling—the individual laughing when he would naturally cry, or at least feel sorrowful, and shedding profuse tears at some circumstance calculated to excite risibility in others. Thus, a young man, a patient of my own, laughed a whole morning over the intelligence that a railway accident had occurred by which a dozen or more persons were killed, one of them being his own mother ; and the next day cried like a child over an anecdote in the funny column of a newspaper.

The ability to comprehend matters submitted to the understanding is markedly impaired, and there is a difficulty in concentrating the attention sufficiently to get a correct idea of very simple subjects, while abstruse ones escape altogether. The faculty of observation, of directing the sensorial organs to the acquirement of information, is so greatly lessened that the most stirring events may occur in the presence of the subject of dementia, to which apparently his attention is fully directed, and yet, when asked immediately afterward in regard to them, he can scarcely state a single one of the details. The like failure is shown when he attempts to read aloud from a printed page: words are omitted or misplaced, without his being aware that mistakes are being committed. In writing, similar errors are perpetrated.

The memory soon begins to show signs of weakness, and this is at first mainly in regard to recent occurrences, though eventually even those of childhood are forgotten. A slight degree of amnesic aphasia is not infrequently developed, and the names of persons or things are forgotten. Many of my own patients have not been able to tell the cities in which they lived, or the names of their wives or children. As a rule, substantives are more readily forgotten than other words, and numbers, I think, are next in order.

The memory of events, as the disease advances, becomes so bad, that circumstances which occurred only a few minutes previously are forgotten. I entered the room of a patient who had become the subject of primary dementia very suddenly, in consequence of receiving intelligence of great losses in business, and in whom the memory was so far abolished that he could not tell whether or not he had dined, though the knife and fork were in his hands when I opened the door. This patient did not know his wife's name or the name of any one of his children, or the number of his house, or whether his father and mother were living or not, though he had only been affected eight days.

The will suffers with the other mental faculties, and often to a much greater extent. The patient is unable to rely on his own judgment, even in the simplest matters, or to arrive at a determination. Indeed, he does not make the attempt. If left entirely to himself, he would, in the extreme stage of the disease, do nothing whatever : if told to rise, he rises ; if to sit down, he sits down ; if to walk, he walks, and so on. He acts, as a matter of course, in accordance with the directions given him, provided they are commands which are to be obeyed at once. Otherwise, they are forgotten almost as soon as they are given. Probably no one symptom is more suggestive of the extreme condition of mental decay than the complete paralysis of the will, which so often exists in dementia.

Incoherence is generally exhibited by all dements after the condition is well established. It would seem as though there were not sufficient mental force to follow an idea out to its legitimate expression in words, and, as there is a forgetfulness of words, the language used consists of imperfect expressions, both as regards quantity and quality. The incoherence of a patient suffering from primary dementia is shown in the following letter, which he was told to write me as a statement of his condition at the time :

"You inform you I have in the health as you to you desired my head to-day yesterday is good and better as to you I hope. Sleep in my you to me good, and as before yesterday in the day and did walk to you as to you directed, my no more to-morrow and can more express. When see in next week my health still."

By this he intended to say about as follows :

"As you directed, I write to inform you of my health. To-day my head aches, but yesterday it was well, and I hope will be better. I sleep well, better than I did before. As you directed, I took a walk yesterday. My medicine will be all gone by to-morrow, but I can get more by express. I hope, when I see you next week, that my health will be still better."

Some of the subjects of dementia are affected with illusions, hallucinations, and delusions, but these are generally of a mild or puerile form, and are variable in character. The delirium which sometimes exists is of a low type, and the speech is not only incoherent, but is expressed in indistinct mutterings. Occasionally, however, there is a more exalted delirium present, and then acts of violence may be committed. These would, perhaps, be more frequent, but for the deficient intelligence and physical strength of the patient.

Destructive tendencies are more frequently manifested, and often appear to be of an automatic character. Buildings may be set on fire, articles of value destroyed, and animals killed or injured, from mere wantonness or deficiency of mind, just as similar acts are perpetrated by children. From like influences, homicides may be committed. In such cases the knowledge of right and wrong is lost, and in extreme cases the natural instincts appear to be abolished. Demented mothers kill their own children. Suicides of an intentional character are never committed by the demented, though self-destruction through ignorance is not uncommon.

A curious tendency in some dements is to the repetition of some act or phrase, and this indefinitely. Often, for many years, one patient will always turn round three or four times before sitting down, another makes profound salaams during certain periods of the day, another before speaking performs certain movements with his fingers, and so on. Again, some sentence is caught up and repeated thousands of times. A patient of mine, whenever spoken to, always first said, "Boscobel, boscobello, boscobellito, boscobellitito, boscobellititotito," before answering. It has appeared to me that, in some cases at least, there has been an idea that the acts or words were employed as a charm to assure good luck, but that, in the decay of the mind, the reason has been forgotten, while the movement or language has been continued automatically. I have observed dements who, in the beginning, could allege a motive for the performances in question, but who, at later stages of their disease, had lost all recollection of the original incentive, while persisting with the manœuvres or peculiar expressions.

A prominent feature in dementia is the loss of the sense of decency in patients who are its subjects. Obscene words are used to express their wants or appetites, and acts are performed in the presence of others for the doing of which even the most vulgar in a state of sanity seek seclusion. An educated and refined man or woman will, for instance, urinate in the public drawing-room of a hotel without apparently being aware that anything at all unusual is being done; and others, again, will make persistent public attempts at masturbation or sexual intercourse—not with the fury of the acute maniac, but automatically, and as if properly satisfying a natural appetite.

Coprophagy, or the eating of excrement, though not confined to the subjects of dementia, is more frequent with them than with other lunatics.

While the acute maniac and the melancholiac eat their excrements from illusions and delusions, the subjects of dementia are actuated by no particular motive other than such as would arise in the mind of an infant. Very young children put everything, even their excrement, into their mouths, impelled by what is with them the most powerful of all their instincts, if not the only one—the taking of food. Some dements act in the same way, and eat not only their own excrement, but that of others, and even of the lower animals. I have seen the subject of primary dementia playing with her excrement as a child would play with mud, and a few weeks subsequently, when the disease had advanced to a further point, eating it as a child would eat molasses. In the case of a patient, a lady, who became the subject of primary dementia from emotional causes, there appeared to be an active appetite for fecal matters. Not only would she, whenever the opportunity occurred, eat her own excrement, but she devoured with avidity that of an infant to which, occasionally, she could get access.

The subjects of dementia constitute the greater number of those patients in lunatic asylums to whom the term "wet and dirty" is sometimes applied. They obtain the name for the reason that they are in the habit of passing their urine and fæces in their clothes or in bed, and hence are almost always in the condition expressed by the words. To a great extent this tendency is under the control of the attendants, and is scarcely ever met with in well-regulated asylums.

The course of primary dementia, both as regards intensity and duration, is subject to great variation. Some cases reach their height in a few weeks or even days, while others advance so slowly that several years are required to arrive at the full development. In others, again, a certain stage is reached, and then further progress seems to be in a great measure arrested. But, whether slowly or rapidly, the course of primary dementia is always toward a further degradation of the mind. After a time, when the mental faculties are wellnigh entirely abolished, and the individual is, as Dagonet remarks, nothing more than a stomach, life may be prolonged for a long period.[1] In other cases, especially those which come on suddenly and advance rapidly, death generally takes place in a short time, and usually by exhaustion, or from the supervention of some intercurrent disease.

In the foregoing description of primary dementia I have attempted to present an account of the affection when it is fully established and is advancing with more or less rapidity toward complete development. But there are many gradations in the degree of intensity with which it appears. Some patients preserve for many years a tolerable amount of intelligence, and are able to extract considerable enjoyment from life, or to experience its pains. They do feel, even though they do not feel very acutely. In other cases some one or more of the mental faculties become impaired, while the others retain almost their original vigor. Thus, the memory may be the only part of the mind which suffers, or the emotions may be weak and easily affected, or the will alone shows any serious evidences of deterioration. But, although the affection may begin by involving a single category of faculties only, it is generally the case that the others, sooner or later, become involved. Physically the subjects of dementia are generally in good condition. The digestive powers are effective, there is little or no wear and tear of the body through mental influence, they sleep well, and they usually get fat.

g—SECONDARY DEMENTIA.

Secondary dementia is that variety of mental derangement in which there is a decay of the faculties of the mind as a consequence of some preëxisting form of insanity. In most of its features it does not differ essentially from primary dementia, but, originating as it does, gradually, and from the partial conversion of another species of mental aberration, it retains more or less sharply the characteristics of the disease from which it has been derived.

Thus, the subject of hypochondriacal melancholia, who has the delusion that a galvanic battery is in his stomach, continues to entertain the same erroneous belief through the whole course of the secondary dementia into which he may pass, so long as the mind is capable of believing anything; the acute maniac settles down into some one or two of the delusions he has entertained, and holds them till the mental

[1] *Op. cit.,* p. 358.

vigor is so greatly impaired that the intellect can no longer be concentrated upon an idea, or even an idea be formed ; and the patient with circular insanity continues to exhibit in a degraded way the alternations of excitement and depression which characterized his disorder when it was, so to say, a robust affection. Illusions, hallucinations, and delusions may therefore exist throughout the greater part of the course of secondary dementia, as may also morbid impulses, fears, and tendencies.

In other respects secondary dementia, as I have said, is similar to the primary form of the disease, and therefore requires no additional description.

h—SENILE DEMENTIA.

Senile dementia is that form of insanity which occurs as the result of old age, and which is characterized by the decay of the mental faculties. Spontaneously it rarely makes its appearance before the sixtieth year, and generally not till after the sixty-fifth or seventieth. It may, however, as a consequence of wounds or injuries, or of some exhausting disease, ensue at even the fiftieth year.

The first symptom noticed is almost always a weakness of the memory, and this is soon followed by other evidences of failing intelligence. The patient ceases to recognize persons whom he has known for many years, and even his own children are mistaken for other persons. He forgets where he lives, and can not.even find his way from one room to another in his own house. Owing to this failure of the recollection, he repeats over and over again such anecdotes as his intellect enables him to comprehend, forgetting that he has told them probably not ten minutes before.

It often happens that radical changes in the character and disposition are among the earliest phenomena. From having been liberal and generous in money matters, he becomes avaricious and penurious to an extreme degree, grudging every little item of household expense, and living, if left to himself, in a way scarcely befitting one of the lower animals. Occasionally there are periods of low delirium, marked by illusions and hallucinations, and by various morbid fears, or by delusions in regard to his personal safety. He is exacting in his demands, and readily imbibes ideas of neglect on the part of those about him, or of persecution or injury. At the same time he begins to show signs of lack of carefulness and tidiness in regard to dress and personal habits, and finally reaches a stage in which propriety and decency are entirely disregarded.

The failure of the power of the attention is another one of the evidences of diminished mental strength, it being often impossible for the patient to concentrate his perceptions or his intellect upon any matter to which they may be directed. As in the other forms of dementia, the emotions, especially those of an entirely selfish character, are sometimes unduly exhibited in a weak and childish manner. The speech is very frequently incoherent from an early period, and is always so in the latter stages of the disease.

The power of the will is generally greatly diminished, and sometimes utterly abolished, the patient relying altogether on those around him for guidance, or rather being perfectly passive in their hands. At times, however, a spirit of unreasonable determination or obstinacy is developed, in regard usually to some trifling matter, but again to a subject of great importance. I have known a patient in an early period of senile dementia when her ability to manage her affairs was still recognized, refuse to sign receipts for money paid her. She could allege no reason for this conduct, but simply declared that she would not sign them. On another occasion, she persistently refused to affix her signature to the deed of a piece of property she had sold a few days before. When asked if she desired to recall the sale, she said no, but that she would sign no papers; they must get along without her name; they might take the land, but she would sign nothing. She had no reason, except that she would not put her name to the paper in question.

In a few instances that have come under my observation, intense animosities have been engendered on the part of senile dements toward relatives and friends, and especially children. I have known a patient to deliberately inveigle a young child into approaching her closely, and then to seize her and pull her hair, pinch and scratch her. The like tendency to injure relatives and friends is sometimes shown in the disposition they make of their property by will. It is always a suspicious circumstance, indicating mental alienation of some kind, and in old people usually senile dementia, when such persons leave their estates away from those who have taken care of them, or with whom, up to recent dates, they have been on terms of affection, to missionary societies and other organizations of the kind.

In senile dementia there are occasionally periods of excitement approaching acute mania in their intensity, during which there are illusions, hallucinations, and delusions, with impulsions to the perpetration of acts of violence. Again, there is, especially in men, not infrequently a reawakening of the sexual appetite, and as the instinct is not controlled to a sufficient extent by the reason, and as the power is rarely restored to an extent commensurate with the desire, various indecent and immoral acts, coming under the head of what Tardieu[1] calls *attentats aux mœurs*, are committed. The records of the police courts abound with cases of the kind, in which old men are accused of obscene conduct with little girls and boys, and in which the existence of senile dementia can often be pleaded in extenuation.

The course of senile dementia, resulting as it does from regressive changes in the brain-tissues, is progressively onward to complete mental annihilation and eventually death.

i—GENERAL PARALYSIS.

The affection now known as general paralysis, general paralysis of the insane, general paresis, paralytic dementia, and other names, was first described, though imperfectly, by Delaye,[2] in 1822; then more thoroughly by Bayle,[3] in the same year; and finally, with much more completeness and exactness, by Calmeil,[4] in 1826. Although cases of insanity presenting the symptoms of general paralysis had been observed by several alienists, no one before the three writers whose names are here given had differentiated the affection from others, and raised it to the position of a distinct pathological entity. Since then it has been still more thoroughly studied, mainly as before by French alienists, who have in this, as in psychological medicine generally, occupied the first place, till now it is probably the best known in its symptoms, pathology, and

---

[1] " Étude médico-légale sur les attentats aux mœurs," 7ᵉ édition, Paris, 1878.

[2] " De la paralysie générale, incomplète," *Thèse de Paris*, 1822.

[3] " Recherches sur les maladies mentales," Paris, 1822, and " Traité des maladies du cerveau et de ses membranes," Paris, 1826.

[4] " De la paralysie considérée chez les aliénés," Paris, 1826.

especially its morbid anatomy, of all the forms of mental derangement.

General paralysis is a very common mental affection, the most common perhaps of all, and, aside from the implication of the mind, presents the very striking feature of a gradually advancing loss of motility. On account of the fact that the paralysis involves sooner or later nearly every muscle of the body, it is called "general." This paralysis may show itself at the same time that the insanity is manifested ; it may precede the mental derangement, or it may be subsequent thereto. The latter is much the more usual order. Although some of the more striking phenomena of general paralysis may appear with suddenness, there is nearly always a prodromatic period, during which there are symptoms, perhaps not very decided, of the morbid changes going on in the brain.

The most suspicious of all the circumstances, which may indicate the inception of general paralysis, is a gradual but obvious alteration in the mental characteristics of the individual. He does things which are not in accordance with his disposition or faculties of the mind as they have previously been manifested. He forms relations, often with women, which are matters of surprise to those who have long known him ; he contracts friendships with persons whom every one is certain he would have avoided but for the change which is coming over him ; he makes investments such as no prudent man would make ; he alters the details of his business, dismisses his best employees, who have been with him for years, and engages others whom he scarcely knows.

A weakening of the principles of morality, which the individual may previously have held, is also often among the prodromatic symptoms of the disease. He may, therefore, perpetrate frauds of various kinds—generally, however, of no very great extent—or commit obscene acts, under circumstances which are almost certain to result in detection ; or, what is perhaps still more common, he pilfers whatever he can lay his hands on, and without adopting the means of precaution which the common thief would use to prevent discovery. Moreover, the articles he steals are not in general of any use to him, and are thrown aside as soon as he has them in his possession. Many distressing instances of general paralytics, of the highest respectability, being arrested for petty thefts have been reported, and several such have come

under my own observation. In one of these, the patient, an
eminent lawyer, who had at one time been on the bench, was
detected in stealing engravings from a picture-dealer. He
was walking out of the shop with the prints rolled up under
his arm, and had got out of the door before it was discovered that he had stolen instead of having bought the pictures.
In another instance, a gentleman repeatedly stole the silver
forks and spoons from the tables at which he was invited to
dine, and was at length detected with a silver sugar-bowl in
his coat-pocket; and a third limited his depredations to
books, which he took from several libraries and shops of this
city. In all these persons, unmistakable symptoms of general paralysis were subsequently developed.

The relation between reasoning mania and general paralysis has been referred to when the first-named affection was
under consideration. That it not infrequently results in
general paralysis I am quite sure, and hence it may be regarded as sometimes the prodromatic stage of the more pronounced disease.

A general state of exhilaration, different from the patient's
ordinary manner and feeling, may exist for several months or
even years before any more obvious symptom makes its appearance. No one in his own opinion was ever in a better
state of health than he, no one more successful in business,
no one with better surroundings, or more intelligent or affectionate children. While this state is not exactly the delirium
of greatness, which forms so prominent a feature of general
paralysis at a later stage, it is, doubtless, the forerunner of
that symptom.

Among the physical prodromata are pain in the head, vertigo, insomnia, localized paralysis, and attacks of bodily
weakness. Ptosis is occasionally met with, as is also inequality of the pupils. I have known of two cases in which
the pupil of one eye was dilated for seven and six years
respectively, before there were any other notable symptoms
than the exhilaration to which reference has just been made.

Twitchings of the muscles of the face are frequently met
with in association with other prodromata.

It is usual with writers on general paralysis to divide the
phenomena of this disease into three, four, or even more
periods. It is difficult, if not impossible, to do this with any
degree of accuracy, as the several stages constantly run into

each other, and even alternate in the same patient. There is nothing either to be gained on the score of clearness of description by such a course, and I shall therefore disregard it and describe the disease as the symptoms ordinarily present themselves, pointing out at the same time the irregularities in the progress of the affection that are most apt to occur.

Occasionally there is no prodromatic stage, but the affection begins with an attack of congestion of the brain, during which there is delirium and the other phenomena, more or less modified, of an attack of acute mania ; or the first manifestation may be an epileptiform convulsion.

During both of these forms of seizure, there are often spasms and paralyses, the latter generally restricted to the muscles of the eye, the tongue, or the face.

Or these attacks may follow the prodromatic stage, and usher in the more pronounced symptoms of the disease.

They may be repeated several times, but are usually apparently completely recovered from, and the patient goes about his ordinary business, and transacts it with a marvellous degree of exactness in all its details.

Mental Symptoms.—Among the earliest of the mental symptoms generally noticed, when the disease is fully established, is an excessive anxiety in regard to matters which are really of no great importance, or which are of altogether imaginary importance. In one of the cases that have come under my care, this symptom was shown by a morbid apprehension on the part of the patient that he was not managing some trust funds in the best possible way ; in another, by the idea that he was constantly wounding the feelings of his friends ; another was continually changing his mind about the most trivial things, and apparently thinking that the world watched with great anxiety all his movements ; another thought that he had given syphilis to his wife, and that he saw the evidences of the disease on her person. He accordingly experienced the most poignant remorse, and spent the greater part of his time in self-reproaches and lamentations. He had had syphilis, but there was no reason to think that he had infected his wife ; and in another case the patient, who had all his life been a speculator in stocks, suddenly became impressed with a keen sense of the wrong of which he had frequently been guilty, and spent hours in devising impracticable schemes for making restitution.

In the beginning the general mental type is in most cases that of depression. The emotions are easily excited, and the delusions which soon make their appearance are of the melancholic form. The idea of propriety in the every-day affairs of life seems to be lost, and the patient will commit all kinds of indecent acts without appearing to be aware that he is doing anything unusual. He becomes regardless of his personal appearance, neglects to change his linen, appears in public half dressed, and indulges in other similar conduct, when previously he has been noted for scrupulous attention to all matters of cleanliness or etiquette. His memory fails rapidly, and his intellectual vigor is lessened from the first. At the same time he is often quarrelsome and disputatious, but, not being able to convince others of the truth of his ideas, he attacks with physical force those who venture to differ with him. His acts are in other respects eccentric and absurd. He spends money in things which are of no manner of use to him, and at the same time neglects to pay his small debts. A patient of mine sent home a wagon-load of snow-shovels, another bought a dozen sets of weights and measures, another sent out agents into the country and purchased all the turkeys' eggs he could get, and another drained the florists of tulip-bulbs. He harasses in every way those who are about him, gives them impossible orders, and then abuses them if they are not at once obeyed ; he is whimsical at his meals, his likes and dislikes are changed without adequate reason, and he either eats and drinks voraciously or declares that nothing is cooked to suit him, and leaves the table in a rage. At times he sheds tears over the veriest trifles, and often for no reason that he can allege.

This state of depression is not of very long duration, nor is it always well marked in its manifestations. So far as my experience goes, it is, however, almost invariably the earliest mental state of the fully established disease, either when there has or has not been a prodromatic stage. It is always accompanied by those physical symptoms so characteristic of general paralysis, and to which attention will presently be directed.

In some cases the depression becomes more profound, and a state of fixed melancholy, characterized by delirium, in which there are varied illusions, hallucinations, and delusions of a distressing or terrifying nature, is established. This may constitute the essential mental feature of the disease, but is

by no means so frequent a type as its opposite, that of exhilaration. It will be more fully considered further on, as one
of the irregular forms.

In the vast majority of cases the slight mental depression
which exists in the beginning of general paralysis disappears
either suddenly or gradually, and exaltation takes its place.
The patient becomes more cheerful, forms all kinds of impossible schemes for suddenly acquiring great wealth, and these
are quickly abandoned for others equally impracticable. One
man proposes to buy up all the water-power in the United
States, and let it out to applicants at high prices. He makes
a table showing, in his opinion, where the power is, its capacity, the price for which it can be obtained, and an estimate of
the sum for which it can be leased to manufacturers. The
profits by his exhibit amount to over a hundred millions of
dollars a month. Another is going into the ship-building
business, and intends to construct vessels capable of carrying
ten thousand cabin-passengers each, and of making the voyage to Europe in twenty-four hours ; and a third has printed
the prospectus of a company he is about organizing, to acquire from the principal governments of the world the exclusive right to manufacture India-rubber rattles. I cite from a
printed copy a few paragraphs from this document :

"Everybody, from the infant in arms to the decrepit old
man, likes to make a noise in the world. Those who object
are a few nervous individuals, who do not know what is good
for them. The noise that should be made is a gentle, undu-
lating, penetrating, but not irritating jingle. Experiments
have shown that such a noise properly applied has all the
soothing influence of opium and chloral without their dangers. I have established the fact, after the expenditure of
over ten millions of dollars, that the best rattles for the purpose of accomplishing the objects in view are made by a silver sleigh-bell enclosed in a hollow India-rubber sphere, to
which, for convenience, a handle of the same material is to
be affixed. Thus constructed, the rattle in the hands of either
infancy or old age, the youth or the adult, the maiden or her
lover, the old maid or the bachelor, the widow or the widower,
the barbarian or the civilized man, the king or the subject,
the gentleman or the ruffian, the honest man or the thief, the
Christian or the Jew, the saint or the sinner, the gentleman
or the blackguard, the moral man or the hardened wretch

who panders to the most depraved appetites of the scoundrels who fatten on the life-blood of the people—all, all, all must have the India-rubber, health-giving, and mind-soothing rattle.

"The undersigned has devoted over two hundred and fifty years, both in this world and in a former state of existence, to the investigation of the properties of India-rubber and silver. He has ascertained, after many failures in his experiments, and the expenditure of over twenty millions of dollars, that they exercise health and life giving properties to all men. Rattle and you will live, rattle and you will be happy, rattle and you will prosper, rattle and you will be successful, rattle and you will be able to procreate more children than the universe can contain.

"A company must be organized to carry out the beneficent objects which the undersigned has in view. No subscriptions in money are required, as he has taken all the stock, to the extent of one thousand millions of dollars. He is now making contracts for all the rubber the world can produce, and is about buying two hundred of the richest silvermines in the world. Every man, woman, and child on the face of the earth will require several rattles, for, by varying the tone of the bell, different properties are given to the rattle, and hence the same rattle will not do for every person or for every purpose. Come up, therefore, and aid in this grand undertaking in which profits of thousands of millions of dollars will be made every year, and the human race rendered happy."

There was a good deal more in the same strain. As will be perceived, the prospectus is written in good language, and is coherent. Later, this gentleman was unable to string together ten words in a logical manner, or to spell the simplest words correctly.

Thus, delusion after delusion rapidly succeed each other, and these in the great majority of cases relate to the grandeur, the wealth, the physical strength, or some other great quality of the patient, constituting the *délire de grandeurs* of the French. One will tell of his immense palaces, built of gold and inlaid with precious stones, and in the next breath will descant of his great wealth, or his extreme lightness, or of the number of children he has, or of the millions of operas he has composed. Another urges his great importance in the political world; tells us that he has elected all the members of Congress himself, that he has paid off the national debt, and that, in consequence, he is to be made Emperor of the United States, with a salary of a thousand millions a year; that he is going to have a thousand physicians, who are to be clothed in blue-velvet uniforms, embroidered in gold and diamonds; that he has chartered the Great Eastern for a pleasure-trip, and engaged ten thousand musicians, and a similar number of ballet-dancers, to go with him. The next day he has forgotten all these fancies, and is off on another series of absurd ideas. In no respect is he restrained in the extent of his delusions; impossibilities are not regarded. While scarcely able to drag one leg after the other, he will brag of his great fleetness of foot, and in the very death-gasp will mutter about his extreme strength and endurance.

But while the general paralytic is not confined to the limits of possibility in the delusions of grandeur which he entertains, and which, at this period of his disease, form its chief feature, it has appeared to me that he very rarely (never in my experience) imagines that he has assumed any supernatural or extra-mundane personality. He is never God, or Christ, or an angel, except so far as he, John Smith, for instance, may be God, or Christ, or an angel, without change of personality; indeed, it is scarcely ever the case that he assumes to be any other person than he really is. He will imagine himself to be a general, a king, an emperor, or as occupying some other great office, but he is always himself. It is he, in his own person, who is the grand personage, and this fact is made to appear in all that he says and does.

The following "proclamation" was issued by a general paralytic, and given to me by his brother, when the patient came under my charge. Nothing could be a better example of the exaltation of self to which I refer, or of several other points to which attention will presently be drawn:

"To all the People and Inhabitants of the United States and all the outlying Countries, Greeting:

"I, John Michler, King of the Tuskaroras, and of all the Islands of the Sea, and of the Mountains and Valleys and Deserts; Emperor of the Diamond Caverns, and Lord High General of the Armies thereof; First Archduke of the Beautiful Isles of the Emerald Sea, Lord High Priest of the Grand Lama, etc., etc., etc.: Do issue this my proclamation. Stand by and hear, for the Lord High Shepherd speaks. No sheep have I to lead me around, no man have I to till me the ground, but the sweet, little cottage is all of my store, and the room that I sleep in has ground for the floor. No chair have I to sit myself down, no meat have I to eat myself down, but the three-legged stool is the chief of my store, and my neat little cottage has ground for the floor. No children have I to play me around, no dog have I to bark me around, but the three-legged stool is the chief of my store, and my neat little cottage has ground for the floor.

"Yea, verily, I am the Mighty King, Lord Archduke, Pope, and Grand Sanhedrim, John Michler. None can with me compare, none fit to comb my hair, but the three-legged stool is the chief of my store, and my neat little cottage has ground for the floor. John Michler is my name. Selah!

"I am the Great Hell-Bending Rip-Roaring Chief of the Aborigines! Hear me and obey! My breath overthrows mountains; my mighty arms crush the everlasting forests into kindling-wood; I am the owner of the Ebony Plantations; I am the owner of all the mahogany groves and of all the satin-wood; I am the owner of all the granite; I am the owner of all the marble; I am the owner of all the owners of Everything. Hear me and obey! I, John Michler, stand forth in the presence of the Sun and of all the Lord Suns and Lord Planets of the Universe, and I say, Hear me and obey! I, John Michler, on this eighteenth day of August, 1880, do say, Hear me and obey! for with me none can equal, no, not one, for the three-legged stool is the chief of my store, and my neat little cottage has ground for the floor. Hear me and obey! Hear me and obey! John Michler is my name.

"John Michler, First Consul and Dictator of the World, Emperor, Pope, King, and Lord High Admiral, Grand Liconthropon forever!"

In addition to the exaltation exhibited by this production, it is also seen that there are several anti-climaxes in the assertions of the writer. This is a feature I have repeatedly noticed. Several of Dr. Mickle's[1] patients exhibited the like peculiarity. Thus, one said: "My father made all the clothing for the army; my mother was a lady in her own right, and took in washing." Another declared he could "speak two Indian languages, and had a dozen pairs of socks."

[1] "General Paralysis of the Insane," London, 1880, pp. 227, 235.

In a somewhat early stage of the disease, but yet one which exhibits the sensory and motorial phenomena characteristic of the disease, it is difficult to decide with certainty whether or not the ideas expressed by the patient are facts, delusions, or lies. They relate to his prowess in various fields, to his great influence and standing in society, and to the schemes which he has set on foot, but at the same time they do not pass the limits of possibility. For all that the examiner can tell by taking them only into consideration, they may be true, they may be false beliefs, or they may be deliberate lies, told either with the intention of deceiving or simply from a love of lying. Generally, however, but little difficulty will arise, for there are other circumstances which are sufficient to establish the point of sanity or insanity, and usually the stories themselves are of such a character that no sane man would relate them. Thus, in a case which I saw in conjunction with Dr. Meredith Clymer, the patient had inequality of the pupils, fibrillary contractions in the tongue, and a titubating gait. He had been violent on several occasions, had spent large sums of money in excess of his means, and for things of no use to him ; he had committed various offences against decency, and had previously been in a lunatic asylum. When, therefore, he informed us that, at eight years of age, he had seduced his cousin ; that his son, eleven years of age, had seduced the two daughters of one of the richest bankers in New York— being, therefore, as he said, "a chip off the old block"; that he was one of the editors of a prominent newspaper of this city ; that many ladies, some of them of the highest standing, had fallen in love with him, besides detailing with the utmost minuteness the particulars of various obscene acts which he and others had practiced—it did not much matter whether they were facts, lies, or delusions. They were all, perhaps, within the limits of possibility, but their improbability was such that the question of their truth was not worth considering. From any point of view they were equally good evidence of the person's insanity, for no sane person would have mentioned such things had they been true, or have lied in that style to two physicians who, he knew, were inquiring into his mental condition. Although pronounced sane by a sheriff's jury, composed of men supposed to be of more than the average juryman's intelligence, his subsequent conduct was of such a character as to prevent the judge confirming the finding.

A tendency to erotic delusions, almost reaching to the extent of satyriasis, and a marked increase in sexual appetite and power, are often witnessed, as in the case just cited. The whole conversation of the patient is of a libidinous character, and he may attempt acts of violence in accordance with his delusions and augmented venereal instincts, or form illicit relations with one woman after another, or descend to almost continual masturbation.

The whole manner and bearing of the patient are in accordance with the exaltation of which he is the subject. He is all good-nature and smiles, he makes friends with those around him, lets them into all his plans, and freely communicates his delusions. He bustles about noisily, whistles and sings—but wofully out of tune—inflates his lungs and slaps his chest, in the feeling of *bien être* which governs him. But there are periods when reaction occurs, when he shuns those with whom he has consorted, and quarrels with those about him, and when he is a prey to fits of mental depression almost attaining to melancholia. The patient whose case I have just given, only a few days after his discharge from the asylum, pointed a loaded pistol at and threatened to kill a man who did not do a piece of work according to his fancy. And instead of the great exaltation of the *ego* which I have described, there may be a more subdued condition, in which, while there is abundant evidence of the self-sufficiency which actuates the patient, there is not that swelling pride and vanity which lead him into the most preposterous delusions. His fancies are of a quieter kind. He is strong, in good health, "never felt better," can walk a dozen miles and feel no fatigue, has all the money he wants, is ready to lend to all who ask, is capable of filling the highest offices, can drink any quantity of champagne without getting intoxicated, can write better novels than Scott or better poetry than Byron, is going to write a play that will eclipse anything Shakespeare ever produced, is the best actor that ever trod the stage, and so on, *ad infinitum*. At times, however, there are apt to be paroxysms of a higher degree of exaltation, when there are delusions without limit, and the impossible is in the ascendant.

Billod[1] has described a form of mental derangement sometimes met with in general paralytics, in which, while the pa-

[1] "Recherches sur la paralysie générale des aliénés," *Ann. méd.-psychol.*, October, 1850; also, " Des maladies mentales," Paris, 1882, p. 300.

tient has the most correct ideas relative to his estate and social position, he has delusions only in regard to his capacity or some other personal trait. He relates an anecdote of an interview between M. Moreau, physician to the Bicêtre, and a general paralytic, which took place in his presence. The physician asked all the questions which could possibly elucidate the condition and the character of the delusion exhibited by the patient. The replies were modest, reasonable, and correct; he admitted that he was poor, of humble origin, without position, of little more than ordinary intelligence, and that he had no other resources than those which came from his trade of tailor. The able physician of the Bicêtre almost despaired of finding any defect in his reasoning processes, when the idea struck him to ask if he was well skilled in his art. "Oh, yes," he answered, with that emphasis peculiar to paralytics, "I am the greatest tailor in the world."

In a case under my own charge, the patient, who had all the prominent physical symptoms of general paralysis, exhibited no delusions except in regard to the one point that his eyes were of such extreme perfection that he could see the smallest objects at immense distances, could see through substances which to others were opaque, and that no microscope could equal them in the power to see minute bodies.

Another form, also described by Billod,[1] is characterized by the existence of apparent mental integrity, except in the fact that the subjects are abnormally vain of the qualities they possess or of the acts they have accomplished. They boast, but they boast of small things, which, though of no importance actually, are immense in their eyes. A physician, a general paralytic, exhibited this condition. After the most searching investigation, no delirious conception was discovered. He was modest, without fortune, of abilities which he took at their real value, and had no delusion of any kind. "But," said he very often, "the year 1844 was a great year for me; I made a great deal of money that year." "How much did you make?" "Eighteen hundred francs," he answered, with emphasis.

As I have said, the form may be continuously of the melancholic type, or there may be paroxysms of intense mental depression, in which there are illusions, hallucinations, and delusions occurring sporadically, as it were, or alternating

[1] *Op. cit.*, p. 301.

regularly with periods of excitement, as in circular insanity. Thus Calmeil[1] reports several cases of general paralysis, which were characterized by mental depression instead of by mental exaltation. Other writers, and especially Baillarger,[2] have described the melancholic variety. Lunier[3] attributes its more frequent existence at the present day than formerly to a change of type which the disease like others has undergone in consequence of different hygienic conditions and habits. Billod[4] describes it at length, and MM. Voisin and Burlureaux[5] have produced an exhaustive monograph on the subject. These latter go so far as to declare that depression is met with in a greater number of cases than is exaltation. Although this statement is not in accordance with the results of my own experience, and is probably not correct as regards this country, I am satisfied that the melancholic type is much more common than is generally supposed, or than insane asylum superintendents would have us believe.

The form in question may show itself as simple melancholia, with or without a tendency to suicide. Cases of this kind have been adduced by Calmeil,[6] Lunier,[7] Baillarger,[8] Voisin and Burlureaux,[9] and others. In this variety the intellect is not in the early stage markedly affected, though it has lost its strength, and ideas come slowly. It is as regards the emotions that aberration is chiefly to be observed. The patient is full of self-reproaches, avoids all companionship with others, thinks himself only fit to die, but is nevertheless full of apprehensions relative to the future life.

This, however, is only the first stage, for eventually delusions, often based on illusions and hallucinations, make their appearance, and the state is not essentially different

---

[1] "Paralysie considérée chez les aliénés," Paris, 1826, p. 243 et seq.

[2] "Nouvelles considérations sur la paralysie progressive incomplète," "De la melancholie avec stupeur," Paris, 1846, and Gazette des Hôpitaux, 1857.

[3] Annales médico-psychologiques, juillet, 1873.

[4] "Recherches sur la paralysie générale des aliénés," Ann. méd.-psy., October, 1850, and "Des maladies mentales," Paris, 1882, t. i, p. 308.

[5] "De la mélancolie dans ses rapports avec la paralysie générale," Paris, 1880.

[6] "Traité des maladies inflammatoires du cerveau," Paris, 1859, cases xx, xxii, and xxiv.

[7] "Recherches sur la paralysie générale progressive," Ann. méd.-psychol., t. i, p. 1, 1849.

[8] "Des symptômes de la paralysie générale," appendice au "Traité des maladies mentales," par Griesinger, Paris, 1865.

[9] Op. cit., p. 50 et seq.

from that of melancholia with delirium, already described, though perhaps never reaching the high degree of intensity attained in that affection.

Or the condition may be that of melancholia with stupor, the patient refusing to talk, and sitting or lying hour after hour with scarcely the motion of a limb. During either of these states there may be strong tendencies to suicide or to mutilation of the person.

Again, the type of melancholia is that of hypochondria, which, beginning from perverted sensations in various parts of the body, goes on with gradually increasing force till delusions of the most ridiculous character fill the mind of the patient. One imagines that his bowels are gone, another that his insides are passing away with his fæces, another that his anus is hermetically sealed, another that his tongue has disappeared, and so on through the whole range of impossibilities. Any one patient may in his own person be the subject of any number of delusions, following each other with a degree of rapidity so great that one is scarcely gone before the other has made its appearance. A patient of my own within the space of half an hour conceived that he was made of raw cotton, that his arms were absent, that he had no nose, that his penis had been turned inside out, and that he had perpetual spermatorrhœa. The delirium of negation,[1] to which reference has already been made when the subject of hypochondriacal melancholia was under consideration, is especially common in the hypochondriacal form of general paralysis, and the patients conceive that they have lost various parts of their bodies. A general paralytic affected in this manner will, in the course of a single day, conceive that he has lost every limb and organ. One of my own patients, a physician, thought that every part of him was gone except his tongue and the posterior part of the third frontal convolution. He was therefore able to talk, but could do nothing else, and lay all day with his eyes closed, perfectly motionless, but answering promptly every question put to him.

Again, there may be, especially in women, the micromaniacal delusion (*délire micromaniaque*), which has also been referred to under the head of hypochondriacal melancholia. In these cases, the patients think themselves much smaller than

---

[1] "Du délire des négations," par M. Cotard, *Archives de neurologie*, No. 11, 1882, p. 152.

they really are, like infants, dwarfs, or dolls.   Others imagine that their limbs have been reduced in size.

Moreau [1] (de Tours) refers to the case of a patient who felt his body get smaller and smaller till it did not exceed two feet in height.

A lady, the subject of general paralysis, in which the mental phenomena were of the depressant form, imagined that her mouth was so small that a spoon would not go into it. At last it reached, as she thought, such minute dimensions that no solid food could be taken, and she insisted on being fed through a small glass tube and with liquid food only. And in both forms, that of exaltation and depression, there is a notable impairment of the intellect, so far as its force, its majesty, and its ability to comprehend are concerned.   The patient affected with general paralysis passes, perhaps slowly, but with almost absolute certainty, to a condition of dementia. His memory, his judgment, his power of application, are weakened from the first.   Long-sustained thought on any one subject is impossible with him.   He is argumentative, but his arguments are feeble and illogical, and sometimes he has enough mind to perceive this fact, and to express chagrin at the circumstance.

Physical Symptoms.—In my experience, the first sign of loss of power—one which is sometimes observed before any evidence of mental derangement is perceived—is a slight defect of articulation, due to paralysis of the lips.   At first this is scarcely perceptible, there is merely a little trembling, an action such as is seen in persons who are endeavoring to restrain their emotions, but it is sufficient to give indistinctness to the utterance of those words which contain labial letters, and to impart a peculiar hesitancy or tremulousness to the speech.

The tongue is the next organ concerned with speech to be affected.   Examination shows that there are fibrillary contractions of its muscles, and that it is moved with less facility than in the healthy state.   The articulation is slow, words are slurred over, and there are both stammering and stuttering; owing to the weakness of the tongue, it cannot readily be

---

[1] " Du délire hypocondrique et de la paralysie générale des aliénés," *Bulletin de l'académie impériale de médecine*, t. xxvi, 1860–1861, p. 191. The extract from this memoir published in the Bulletin does not refer to this case, but it is cited by MM. Voisin and Burlureaux.

raised to the roof of the mouth or pressed with sufficient force against the upper teeth, and hence there is a peculiar difficulty in enunciating words containing what are known as the lingual letters. The words "National Intelligencer" are almost impracticable to the general paralytic, and in trying to pronounce them he concentrates his whole attention on the act. Generally, he notices his defective articulation, and in endeavoring to correct it makes matters worse. His inability to be correct contrasts strongly with his violent efforts. Gradually, the paralysis of the tongue becomes more complete, and at last this organ can only be moved with great difficulty and very imperfectly. The other facial muscles participate, and there is a blank, somewhat sorrowful expression always present.

At the same time, when the muscles of the face are in action, there is often an exaggerated degree of motility, a motility not in consonance with the emotions or the absence of all emotion, in logical accord with the thoughts as expressed by the speech. The patient appears to be aware that his facial muscles are deranged in their action. Instead, therefore, of allowing them to act automatically, as in the normal condition, without a thought as to their mode of action, he brings his will to bear upon them when he speaks, and as a consequence there is excessive motility. He does more with them than is necessary. I have seen the general paralytic, while expressing the most indifferent ideas, throw the muscles of his face into such extensive action that he had the appearance of a person laughing, so far as the countenance was concerned. He was like the child suffering with chorea, who attempts to pick up a pin. All the muscles of the body are thrown into action by the effort.

The muscles of deglutition are involved at an early stage of the disease, and hence there is difficulty of swallowing. The alimentary bolus is not grasped with firmness, and the paralysis of the tongue and of the temporal, masseter, pterygoid, and buccinator muscles prevent the due mastication of the food, and the propulsion of the mass toward the pharynx. In consequence of these troubles, choking is apt to occur, and this is rendered a still more probable circumstance by the fact that the sensibility of the lining membrane of the fauces is so diminished that no adequate idea of the quantity of food in the mouth is obtained. Hence more is taken in than can be swallowed, and a plugging up of the pharynx is the result, with suffocation, if relief be not afforded. I have known of several narrow escapes from death by this cause.

At a later period there are notable changes in the voice. It becomes nasal, like that of a person whose nostrils are stopped up, and, moreover, loses its inflections, degenerating into a kind of monotone. These changes are due to the paralysis of the palate and pharynx, and, as remarked by Luys,[1] are signs of great importance, as indicating the implication of the medulla oblongata in the morbid processes.

Another derangement of phonation is that which results from paralysis of the vocal cords, and which, though I have observed it in many cases, has not attracted the attention it deserves from writers on general paralysis. The voice becomes reedy, cracked, and this change is especially noticed if the patient can be induced to sing. It was observed to perfection in a general paralytic whose case, as it involved some medico-legal questions, I brought before the New York Medico-Legal Society some three years ago. This patient had, among his other delusions of exaltation, the idea that he could sing with wonderful sweetness and power. He ran through, one after the other, dozens of popular airs from operas, but his voice had the peculiar reedy quality referred to, and broke at notes in the middle register. Moreover, every note was about half a tone flat. I was informed that, before the accession of his disease, his voice was of good quality, and that he was especially noted for singing in tune.

As the results of numerous laryngoscopic examinations, Mr. Lennox Brown,[2] among other conclusions, established the facts that the reflex excitability of the pharynx is markedly diminished from the beginning of the disease, and that there is impairment of tension and of co-ordinate action in the vocal cords, unaccompanied by any distress of respiration. The first of these circumstances tends to make deglutition more difficult, as the act of swallowing does not receive its proper reflex excitation, and the second sufficiently accounts for the changes in the voice to which I have referred.

Closely connected with speech is writing, and here again there are notable deviations from the standard of correctness.

[1] "Traité clinique et pratique des maladies mentales," Paris, 1881, p. 564.

[2] "Laryngoscopic Observations in General Paralysis," *West Riding Lunatic Asylum Medical Reports* vol. v, 1875, p. 271, *et seq.*

The ability to write well, if previously possessed, is lost, and the patient not only exhibits a bad chirography, but omits letters from the words he uses, and words from the sentences, and in some instances appears to have forgotten how to spell. He seems to be guided in some cases by the sound of words, and hence spells them phonographically. In a letter which I recently received from a mercantile gentleman, affected with general paralysis, and who had been in an asylum, many words, of which it is quite certain he knew the proper orthography, were spelled apparently from the sound. "Pain in the knee" was "pane in the nee"; "I shall try to see you next week" became "I shal tri to see you next weke"; and "I take my medicine regularly every day" was "I take my medison regulaly every da"; and yet at this time there was a decided remission in the violence of his symptoms, so far as his mind was concerned.

The muscles of the eyes are also generally involved, producing ptosis from paralysis of the levator palpebræ superioris, diplopia from implication of the internal rectus, and dilatation of the pupil—all of these being due to lesion existing at the point of origin or in the course of the third nerve—or the external rectus may be involved, causing diplopia from the implication of the sixth nerve.

But the oculo-pupillary derangements are by no means restricted to a dilatation of the pupil on one side from the lesion of the third nerve. Both may be dilated; one may be dilated and the other contracted; both may be contracted; and one may be contracted while the other remains in a normal condition. Perhaps, of all the changes to which the pupils are subject, inequality, produced by the contraction of one pupil, is the most common, and this is due to paralysis of the sympathetic nerve. It is very rare that oculo-pupillary disturbances are not met with at some time in the course of general paralysis. The assertion of Austin,[1] that contraction or dilatation of the right pupil is associated with melancholic delusions, and contraction or dilatation of the left with elation, is not in accordance with my experience, or with that of any one else, so far as I know. With the change in the size of the pupil, whether this be constriction or enlargement, there is almost invariably a sluggish condition of the iris, so

[1] "A Practical Account of General Paralysis, its Mental and Physical Symptoms," etc., London, 1859, p. 34.

that it does not respond normally to increase or diminution of light. This may be a phenomenon even when the pupils are otherwise unaffected.

Luys [1] states that, under the influence of the emotions, and when the brain is in a state of increased activity, he has sometimes seen a sudden contraction of one pupil and a dilatation of the other.

Occasionally the outline of the pupil on one or both sides is irregular, but this is not a common phenomenon.

The gait of patients affected with general paralysis is very peculiar, and is of two different kinds. In the one it is similar to that of persons suffering with locomotor ataxia, and it is to this cause, as Westphal [2] has pointed out, that the derangement is due. The feet are lifted high, and are thrown down with a jerk, and with much force, the heel striking the ground first, and the sole coming down with a flop. As Westphal remarks, patients with this gait cannot stand with the eyes shut and the feet close together. The patellar tendon reflex is abolished. In fact, as Westphal [3] in a subsequent paper declares, the absence of this reflex is of itself sufficient to establish the existence of sclerosis of the columns of Burdach in conjunction with the cerebral lesions of general paralysis.

And, again, the disturbances of locomotion and the muscular derangements generally, point to the occasional existence of sclerosis of the lateral columns of the cord, and disseminated spinal sclerosis, as accompanying lesions of general paralysis. Cases of the kind have been observed by Claus,[4] Schultze,[5] and Zacker.[6] In the case of a patient affected with general paralysis, now under my charge, there are delusions of grandeur, inequality of the pupils, disturbances of speech, and other cerebral symptoms of the affection, conjoined with a spastic condition of the lower extremities and frequent contractions of their muscles. In cases with this combination, the feet are scarcely lifted from the ground, but are shuffled

---

[1] *Op. cit.*, p. 570.

[2] " Ueber den gegenwärtigen Standpunct der Kenntniss von der allgemeinen progressiven Paralysie der Irren," Griesinger's *Archiv*, Heft 1.

[3] *Berliner klinischer Wochenschrift*, i, 1881.

[4] *Allgemeine Zeitschrift für Psychiatrie*, 1878, p. 335.

[5] *Archiv für Psychiatrie*, Band xi, p. 216.

[6] *Archiv für Psychiatrie*, Band xiii, p. 155.

over it, the walk being serpentine in character, progression being effected by the body being swung forward on the femur as each lower extremity is alternately on the ground. Owing to the contraction of the adductors, the legs frequently get interlocked, and walking is impossible. This is the case with the patient referred to. In him—and I presume the same is true of other similar cases—the patellar tendon reflex is greatly exaggerated.

In other cases without accompanying spinal lesions, the gait is simply that of weakness. The patient staggers and stumbles and often falls, but there are no such disturbances as are met with in the forms just noticed. Hemi-paresis and hemiplegia, occurring in the course of general paralysis, are, as Mendel remarks, of temporary duration, unless they are the results of some organic associated condition, such as syphilis of the brain or cerebral hæmorrhage. They are quite certainly the consequences of the attacks of congestion of the brain to which general paralytics are liable.

As regards the upper extremities, the fingers lose their deftness and delicate co-ordinating power. The handwriting is shaky, and there is awkwardness in buttoning the clothing, tying the cravat, and doing other things requiring exact manipulations. The grip of the hand may still be strong, but there is an impossibility, as shown by the dynamograph, of maintaining a continuous muscular contraction for even a few seconds. The following is one of the tracings, made by a patient affected with the disease under consideration :

FIG. 6.

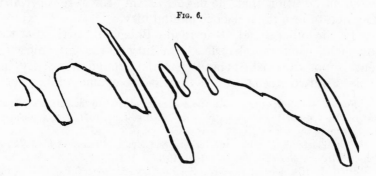

In analyzing this tracing, we see that it is not from feebleness of the muscles that the line is descending, for there are spasmodic elevations which show considerable force. It proves, however, that no matter at what point the pencil is placed, the patient cannot keep it there.

Tremor is almost constantly present, not only about the lips and tongue, as we have seen, but in the limbs also. It is most apparent when the patient attempts to perform a voluntary movement, such as that of raising a glass of water to the mouth. It is also perceived when the hands are outstretched, or when the attempt is made to bring the two index-fingers together from opposite sides.

Closely allied to tremor are the choreiform movements which occasionally occur in general paralytics, and which by some French and German writers have been supposed to be athetoic in character. As a matter of fact, they have no resemblance to those met with in athetosis. The motions in the latter affection are slow, apparently deliberate, and always result in increased muscular development, while the choreiform movements are quick, abrupt, do not lead to enlargement of the muscles, and are, in fact, only exaggerated tremors.[1]

The irritability of the muscles is, according to my experience, lessened, from the very inception of the disease, to all kinds of electric excitation. Lowe[2] ascertained that, to the faradaic current in the muscles of the face in the earlier stages of the disease, there was neither exalted nor diminished excitability, but that in the last stage not only these muscles, but especially those of the lower extremities, presented decided loss of excitability.

These results have been confirmed by Bevan Lewis,[3] who found in addition that the flexors of the foot were especially disposed to lose their electric excitability.

On the other hand, Brierre de Boismont[4] arrived at the conclusion that the electric excitability to the galvanic current is not diminished ; and Benedict[5] found it greatly increased in two cases that he submitted to examination.

[1] For a description of athetosis, the reader is referred to the author's "Treatise on Diseases of the Nervous System," first edition, 1871, and subsequent editions up to the seventh, 1881, New York.

[2] "On Electro-Excitability in Nervous and Mental Diseases," *West Riding Lunatic Asylum Medical Reports*, vol. iii, 1873, p. 204.

[3] "On the Histology of the Great Sciatic Nerve in General Paralysis of the Insane," *West Riding Lunatic Asylum Medical Reports*, vol. v, 1875, p. 95.

[4] "Du diagnostic différentiel des diverses espèces de paralysie générale à l'aide de la galvanisation localisée," *Annales médico-psychologiques*, 1850, p. 603.

[5] *Wagner's Archiv*, Band viii, 1867, p. 140.

I have tested the electric excitability with a great many general paralytics using the galvanic, the faradaic, and the franklinic currents, and in all stages of the disease. The muscles of the face do not often show any impairment to the galvanic current, or to sparks from the franklinic machine, but the electric excitability to the faradaic current is generally markedly diminished. The muscles of the upper and lower extremities give like results to all forms of electricity, and this is most distinctly shown in those muscles which are farthest from the nerve-centres.

Derangements of sensibility, general and special, are notable symptoms of general paralysis, and consist both of anæsthesia and of hyperæsthesia.

From the very earliest period anæsthesia is a phenomenon of general paralysis, and, according to De Crozant,[1] precedes all disorders of motility. It is general, but is not permanent, disappearing as soon as the disturbances of motility become well established. It is shown to all kinds of impressions— touch, pain, temperature—and patients often speak of the sensations of numbness which they experience, and which are those met with in other affections, "pins and needles," formication, and the feeling to which the term "asleep" is applied.

At a later stage of the disease, though perhaps not so general in its distribution, it is more distinctly evident in localities than it is in the beginning. Thus an arm or hand, one side of the face, and other parts may become its seat. Voisin and Burlureaux[2] cite the case of a general paralytic, in whom, in the first stage, but for two days only, they discovered crossed anæsthesia, the limbs on the left side, and the face on the right being affected. This condition coincided with a state of great excitability. The patient was afraid ; heard discharges of fire-arms, and saw the devil.

Hyperæsthesia is also often observed among the earliest phenomena. It takes the form of neuralgic pains, affecting the face, trunk, the limbs, or the viscera. Headache is generally a symptom from the very beginning, occurring with more or less persistency throughout the whole course of the disease. It may be of all degrees of intensity, from a dull,

---

[1] "Note sur l'anæsthésie transitoire de la peau dans la périodes prodromiques de la paralysie générale," *Ann. med.-psychol.*, 1847, t. i, p. 433.

[2] *Op. cit.*, p. 203.

boring pain, as if produced by a blow with a blunt instrument, to the sharp sensation compared by some to the feeling which they suppose might be caused by the driving of a red-hot dagger into the brain. With these pains there are sometimes vaso-motor disturbances, the face and head being flushed and hot, and the ears particularly red and burning. Facial and cervico-occipital neuralgiæ are not uncommon, and the electric-like or fulgurant pains, characteristic of locomotor ataxia, are met with in those cases complicated with this disease; visceral pains are also common. In regard to the special senses, the phenomena are usually of the greatest importance. Beginning with that of smell, we find Voisin[1] using this very emphatic language:

"The diminution of the sense of smell on one or both sides is a sign of the greatest importance, and this is especially the case as regards the prodromatic period. In fact, from the day that we establish the existence of a diminution of the sense of smell in a melancholic, all our doubts disappear, and we know that the patient not only will become a general paralytic, but that he already is one, when at the same time there may be no other somatic evidence of general paralysis."

Although not able to endorse this opinion in its entirety, I am very well satisfied that the loss or diminution of the sense of smell on one or both sides is an important symptom in the early stage of general paralysis, and one, therefore, of much diagnostic value. As Voisin further remarks, this deprivation is not met with in other forms of insanity save in exceptional cases, it being usually exaggerated if there be any change at all, and it exists from the very inception of the disease before there are derangements of speech, inequality of the pupils, or weakness of the memory.

It is a sign easy to evoke. Some substance, the odor of which is known—I generally use a small vial of powdered camphor—is held to each nostril alternately, the other being closed, and the patient not being allowed to see what the substance is. Ordinarily, in cases of general paralysis, no odor is perceived; in other cases it is mistaken for something else. During the remissions which take place in the course of the disease the sense of smell reappears.

While not willing to say, from the results of my own

[1] "Traité de la paralysie générale des aliénés," Paris, 1879, p. 39.

experience, that every case of melancholia, in which the sense in question is abolished or perverted, is one of general paralysis, I am satisfied that a large proportion of general paralytics—probably nine tenths—exhibit the phenomenon.

On the other hand, Jehn [1] attaches no importance to Voisin's view. Of twenty general paralytics, he found but three in whom the sense of smell was notably affected; in eleven, there was no change whatever. Mendel coincides with this opinion, not being able to find, even in the first stage of general paralysis, any confirmation of Voisin's doctrine. Obviously the matter requires further investigation.

Atrophy of the olfactory nerves has been found in many cases of general paralysis.

As regards sight, amaurosis and amblyopia are very common throughout the whole course of general paralysis. The retina is easily fatigued even in the prodromatic stage, and vision becomes blurred or otherwise imperfect. Double vision from paralysis of the internal or external rectus muscle is also common. In several cases I have observed color-blindness on testing patients with Galezowski's color-scale. The chief difficulty experienced was in distinguishing green from red. Sometimes it was impossible to do so; but, again, the patient could, by making an effort, arrive at a correct decision. In five cases there were various colored appearances —bluish-white, yellow, green, or red rings or disks, or halos of these colors—surrounding the objects looked at. In one case they completely filled the visual field. So far as I am aware, this condition of chromopsia has not been noticed by other writers on general paralysis.

The condition of the fundus of the eye, as revealed by the ophthalmoscope, is of such importance that I shall consider it at some length.

Bouchut [2] examined the fundus of the eye in all the general paralytics in the Salpêtrière hospital, and found no evident lesion which could account for the disease or for the inequality of the pupils. So far as I am aware, he was the first to apply the ophthalmoscope to the examination of the eyes in cases of general paralysis. The next statements on

[1] *Zeitschrift für Psychiatrie,* H. 30, p. 570.
[2] " Du diagnostic des maladies du système nerveux par l'ophthalmoscopie," Paris, 1866, p. 333.

the point are those made by myself [1] in 1871, and which were based on the results obtained from many examinations during the six preceding years. These were that, in general paralysis, "atrophy of the optic nerve causes amaurosis or amblyopia. Ophthalmoscopic examinations will generally detect this condition of the papilla at a very early stage of the disease, together with retinal and choroidal anæmia."

In the same year Dr. Clifford Allbutt [2] published the results of extensive observations with the ophthalmoscope in various nervous and mental diseases. He stated that, of fifty-three cases of general paralysis examined, changes in the optic nerve and retina were found in all but five. Of the remaining forty-eight he found atrophy of the optic disk in various stages in forty-one cases, the other seven being doubtful. He concludes:

"1. That atrophy of the optic nerves takes place in almost every case of general paralysis, and, I may add, of the olfactory nerves also.

"2. That it does not travel down from the optic centers and along the tracts, but attacks the optic nerve as an independent tract of sclerosis.

"3. It often becomes apparent as a hyperæmia of the nerve with slight exudation, but without much stasis—as a 'red softening,' in fact. It then whitens, generally from the outer edge inward, the nerve becoming white and staring, and its edge sharply defined."

Dr. Aldridge, [3] after premising that patients with general paralysis are rarely if ever seen in asylums till they have passed the first stage, gives the results of the ophthalmoscopic examination of forty-three cases, in nearly all of which great vascularity of the disk or atrophy was observed in one or both eyes. The left eye was more frequently affected than the right, especially in the female patients. Thus, of thirteen women examined, the left optic disk was more atrophic than the right in ten, while in the other three these changes were equally advanced in both eyes.

Gowers, [4] on the contrary, asserts that most of the cases of

---

[1] "A Treatise on Diseases of the Nervous System," New York, 1871.

[2] "On the Use of the Ophthalmoscope in Diseases of the Nervous System and of the Kidneys," London and New York, 1871, p. 393.

[3] "Ophthalmoscopic Observations in General Paralysis," etc., *West Riding Lunatic Asylum Medical Reports*, vol. ii, 1872, p. 223, *et seq.*

[4] "A Manual and Atlas of Medical Ophthalmoscopy," London, 1879, p. 163.

general paralysis which he has examined in various stages of the disease presented perfectly normal conditions. In one case only did he find the appearance of simple congestion of the disk.

Tebaldi,[1] of twenty cases of general paralysis, failed in one only to find abnormal ophthalmoscopic appearances. Klein[2] examined ophthalmoscopically forty-two general paralytics. Of these, two gave negative results and six were doubtful. Of the remaining thirty-four, nine had various special conditions, such as dilatation of the veins and the arteries, choroiditis, attenuation of the veins and arteries, etc.; five had retinitis; two atrophy of the optic nerve and the disk; one discoloration of the optic nerve; one hyperæmia of the nerve and disk; and sixteen retinitis paralytica.

Although Schüle[3] has very frequently remarked in the beginning of general paralysis an injected condition of the papilla with enlargement of the veins, he does not think that true atrophy of the optic nerve is an accompaniment of general paralysis.

Voisin[4] has little to say of disturbances of sight in general paralysis till he comes to the consideration of the second stage. Then he states that the sight is notably weakened; contours, colors, and objects become less distinct, and dyschromotopsia exists. Sometimes one of the eyes loses more quickly than the other its visual power.

Relative to the ophthalmoscope he says that it does not always explain the amblyopia. Of forty cases examined by him, in conjunction with Galezowski, in two only a partial atrophy was found; in two there was dilatation of the central artery of the retina; but in a large number of cases flexuosities and a congested condition of the arteries of the retina were met with—conditions which, as he declares, are to be accounted for by what we know to exist in the vessels of the meninges in general paralysis.

I have data of the ophthalmoscopic examination of forty-two general paralytics in the prodromatic stage, and of thirty-one after the disease was well established. Of these latter,

[1] "L'ottalmoscopia nelle alienazione mentale," Bologna, 1870.

[2] "Augenspielstudien bei Geisteskranken. Leisderdorf's psychiatrische Studien," Wien, 1877, p. 113.

[3] Cited by Mendel, "Die progressive Paralyse der Irren," Berlin, 1880, p. 141.

[4] "Traité de la paralysie générale des aliénés," Paris, 1879, p. 111.

seventeen belonged also to the prodromatic category, making fifty-six different patients. Of the forty-two exhibiting well-marked prodromatic symptoms, such as I have described in the beginning of this section, twenty-nine exhibited anæmia of the fundus. The arteries and veins were thin and straight, and the choroid was paler than in the normal condition. These appearances were almost invariably found in both eyes to the like extent. In four, the fundus appeared to be healthy, and in nine the vessels were enlarged and tortuous, and the disk was in a hyperæmic state.

Of the thirty-one other cases, twenty-one were examined while the patients were still in what is called the first stage. Of these, incipient atrophy, beginning on one edge of the disk, existed in seventeen ; in one there was choked disk ; in two hyperæmia of the disk, with enlarged and tortuous vessels ; and in one the fundus appeared to be normal. Eleven of these patients had been examined by me while they were in the prodromatic stage at anterior periods, ranging from two to ten months. All of them had atrophy of the disk.

The ten remaining patients were examined during the middle and closing periods of the disease, and all had atrophy of the optic nerves of both sides, though not to the same extent on each. Six of these patients I had examined at former periods.

The *hearing* I have found in some cases, during the early periods of the disease, to be decidedly intensified. This was notably the case in a general paralytic whom I examined in the City Prison some three years ago, who was discharged by the verdict of a jury from the custody of his relatives, on the ground that he was sane, and who is now in a lunatic asylum in Pennsylvania if he be not dead.[1]

Later, in some few cases, the hearing is markedly impaired, but in the majority of instances it is not perceived to be perceptibly lessened in intensity.

The *taste*, as might be expected in those patients who have suffered from diminution or loss of the sense of smell, is impaired in acuteness very generally. General paralytics, as Voisin remarks, eat with indifference everything that is put before them.

[1] "Remarks on General Paralysis, with Special Reference to the Case of Abraham Gosling," before the New York Medico-Legal Society, *Medical Gazette*, May 8, 1880.

Nutrition is not usually affected to any considerable extent during the early stages of general paralysis, but as the disease advances various derangements of the normal standard make their appearance. Sometimes, however, emaciation begins from the very inception of the disease. Later, atrophy of an active character may ensue in one or more of the limbs, and this is especially apt to be the case when the spinal cord is involved in the morbid process.

Bed-sores are often a painful and troublesome feature of the disease. They appear by preference on those parts which are subjected to pressure, in sitting or lying, such as the buttocks, the sacral region, the heels, the elbows, or the shoulders, though they are not always confined to these parts. When numerous or extensive, they cause a good deal of constitutional disturbance. The theory advanced by Charcot and his pupils, that the situation of the bed-sore is in anatomical relation with the nerve-centre which is the seat of the lesion, does not appear to hold good for general paralysis.

Hæmatoma auris, a condition which has already been described under the head of acute mania, is a not uncommon occurrence in general paralytics. Its appearance is said to be unfavorable from a prognostic point of view, but it is difficult to see how any event can add to the gloomy prognosis of so nearly uniformly a mortal disease as is general paralysis.

Fractures of the ribs and other bones are met with in general paralytics in asylum practice, and appear to be due to slight violence acting on bones which are in an abnormal state as regards nutrition. As the subject has already been sufficiently considered under the head of acute mania, it does not at present require further amplification.

The normal *temperature* of the body is subject to considerable variations during the course of general paralysis. Clouston[1] found it higher in the mean in patients with this disease than in any other form of insanity, and that the average evening temperature was always higher than the average morning temperature. He also found the temperature to be high in the first stage, low in the second, and highest in the third or last stage. These results were in the main confirmed by Mickle,[2] who has investigated the subject with great

[1] *Journal of Mental Science,* April, 1868.

[2] *Journal of Mental Science,* April, 1872 ; also " General Paralysis of the Insane," London, 1880, p. 43.

thoroughness, and ascertained several additional points. By means of Lombard's thermo-electrical apparatus, I have been able to establish the fact that after the disease has fairly entered upon the first stage, there is a decided elevation of the temperature of the head, amounting in some cases to as much as two degrees Fahr., and that the point of highest temperature is at the vertex.

Among other phenomena are those which relate to the *pulse* and the *bladder*, and other organs, the derangements of which do not require further consideration in a work devoted to the whole subject of insanity. As regards the pulse, Dr. George Thompson,[1] in an interesting memoir, shows that in general paralysis, the normal pulse-tracing, as obtained by the sphygmograph, is altered, so that the line of ascent becomes slanting and short, while that of descent is gradual and prolonged, and does not display the usual aortic notch, but instead presents a number of wavelets, which, if counted carefully, will be found to vary from six to ten in number. He ascribes this phenomenon to a persistent spasm of the vessels which exists as one of the earliest symptoms.

In the accompanying tracings, made by means of Pond's sphygmograph, from the same patient at different stages of the disease, the variation in the action of the heart and arteries is very distinctly shown.

The patient, a gentleman of forty-five years of age, was brought to me, July 20, 1882. He was then, I thought, and as the result showed, in the prodromatic stage of general paralysis. There was a slight degree of mental depression with excitement, inequality of pupils, and slight derangement of the articulation. These symptoms had been present for about two months.

The first tracing, No. 1, made July 20th, indicates vasomotor paralysis, and feebleness of the heart's action. There is no aortic notch. No. 2 was made September 3d, and is almost the opposite of No. 1 in all respects. It shows vasomotor spasm, and exhibits the wavelets, in numbers of from six to seven or eight, on each line of descent. The aortic notch is absent. The patient was at this time in a state of extreme *délire de grandeur*. He thought he had been commissioned by the President to build railroads in Mexico. He

---

[1] "The Sphygmograph in Lunatic Asylum Practice," *West Riding Lunatic Asylum Medical Reports*, vol. i, p. 58.

intended to make a "railroad gridiron" of that country; was going to buy up all the iron-furnaces in the country, and put them to work making rails; had bought, he said, over two hundred thousand engines and a million cars. Then he was going to tunnel all the mountains in Mexico, in search of gold and silver; and so on, with a dozen or more delusions, during the hour that I saw him.

FIG. 7.

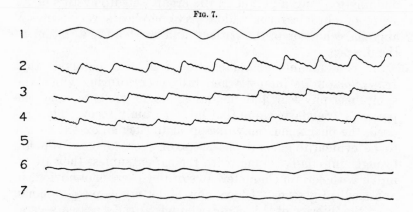

Nos. 3 and 4 were taken on September 29th and 30th, respectively. They show feebleness of the heart and increased arterial tension. The line of ascent is slanting; the line of descent has no aortic notch, and the number of wavelets reaches ten or more. Has delusions of immense wealth, and of high official position; owns all the brass-works in the world, and is governor of the Russo-Americo-Japano-Chinese Alliance for the buying of all the tea in the world.

Nos. 5, 6, and 7 were taken November 2d, 5th, and 10th, respectively. The patient was then in a state of dementia, was scarcely able to walk; had had two epileptic paroxysms since I last saw him, which was October 30th. These tracings show great cardiac and arterial debility, but the last two are better than the first. From that time on there was a decided improvement in the mental and physical symptoms, and a remission lasting till the early part of January ensued. He is now, however, in a relapsed condition, with mild delusions of greatness and marked ataxic symptoms.

The *bladder* is generally involved at some time or other in the course of general paralysis, and this is especially though not entirely noticeable in those cases characterized by the ex-

40

istence of ataxic symptoms. There may either be spasm or paralysis of the sphincter, producing ischuria or incontinence, or the bladder itself may be the seat of paralysis, in which case the urine dribbles instead of being passed with force and in a full stream ; or the sphincter and bladder may both be paralyzed, leading to involuntary dribbling. Again, in consequence of the paralysis of the bladder, the urine, remaining too long a period in the organ, sets up cystitis of an acute or chronic form, which may complicate very unfavorably the condition of the patient, and shorten the duration of the disease.

It is a notable characteristic of general paralysis that *remissions* in its intensity generally occur, during which the symptoms physical and mental abate in violence, and the patient's friends imagine that he is certainly recovering. Indeed, the phenomena may disappear to such an extent as not to be evident to general observers, or even to those who are brought into daily contact with the patient, unless they are familiar with certain characteristics of the disease not obvious to non-medical persons. I have now under my care a gentleman from the interior of this State, who has already passed several months in a lunatic asylum, on account of general paralysis. He has been out of the asylum about four months, and a month since I allowed him to resume his business, that of a merchant. When he first came to me, he had pain in his head, deranged articulation, trembling of the lips and tongue, inequality of the pupils, and a slightly titubating gait. There was no mental derangement, except a tendency to mental depression, and to shed tears upon slight occasion. After three months, every symptom, mental and physical, had disappeared, except the inequality of the pupils. He was cheerful, talked well, had no tremor, was strong and apparently healthy in every respect. When he had been back at his business for about a month, I saw him again. In the mean time he had done a great deal of work, and had travelled several thousand miles West and South, in the performance of his mercantile duties. There were still no symptoms that I could discern, except the inequality of the pupil. Even the hyperæmic condition of the optic disks had disappeared. I may mention incidentally that he was treated mainly with mercury, large doses of iodide of potassium, and counter-irritation to the vertex. Doubtless, if he were less prudent, accessions of mental disturbance would occur, but he is careful to avoid fatigue, excitement, and the use of alcoholic liquors; yet, notwithstanding all his care, the probability is that eventually his remission will come to an end.

In his original description of the disease, Calmeil[1] called attention to this peculiarity of general paralysis; and it has been subsequently, at different times, studied by Baillarger,[2] Sauze,[3] Doutrebente,[4] and others.

Sauze recognized three different kinds of remissions. In the first the somatic symptoms disappear, while the mental remain; in the second, the mind appears to return to its normal condition, while the somatic symptoms persist; and, in the third, the mental and physical symptoms are greatly ameliorated, but do not entirely disappear. There is never, therefore, according to him, a distinct, absolute remission of all the symptoms.

Doutrebente makes two classes of remissions, the incomplete and the complete, and each of them is divided into two kinds, the temporary and the durable.

The temporary incomplete remissions are the most frequent of all. Their duration is short, but variable, as is also their intensity. They are often reproduced a great many times in the same patient. In a case which I had before my class at the Post-Graduate Medical School, in February 14, 1883, a cursory examination revealed the existence of inequality of the pupils, tremor of the lips and tongue, defective articulation, and an exalted mental condition. As the hour had expired, I sent him away to return on the 21st, when I proposed to make him the subject of a clinical lecture. At that time, however, his pupils were equal, there was no tremor, his articulation was good, and his mind calm and equable, without the least sign of exhilaration. On the 24th, however, all the symptoms first observed had returned; and, so far as the mind was concerned, to an increased degree.

Incomplete durable remissions are not limited as to duration. They have been known, it is said, to last for ten, fifteen, or even twenty-five years, but one or more of the phe-

---

[1] "De la paralysie générale," Paris, 1826.

[2] *Union Médicale*, 1855; *Annales médico-psychologiques*, 1847, p. 335; and *Ibid.*, 1876 and 1879.

[3] *Annales médico-psychologiques*, 1858.

[4] *Annales médico-psychologiques*, mars–mai, 1878.

nomena persist, and the patients are generally subject to repeated congestive attacks, or epileptiform seizures.

Temporary complete remissions are more common in the beginning of general paralysis than at other periods. They are true intermissions of short duration, during which all the symptoms disappear. In my opinion, however, they are not instances of the entire disappearance of all the symptoms. It is true the symptoms almost vanish; delusions are no longer held, and the physical symptoms are so far mitigated as scarcely to be noticeable, but that is the most that can be said. Something—as the inequality of the pupils in the case detailed—remains, and soon the fire is in full blaze again.

A complete durable remission is in reality a cure. Many of these have been reported, and by authorities that cannot be questioned, and are cited in full by Doutrebente. Thus Billod reports a case in which there was an entire cessation of all the symptoms, and at the end of eight years they were still absent ; Lunier, one in which, after thirteen years, there was still complete absence of all symptoms ; Morel, one in which, after the disease had lasted eight months, it disappeared with the discharge of a large abcess of the liver, and three years afterward the patient was following his trade of a dyer in Paris without any derangement of his mind or body ; Delasiauve, one in which, after fifteen months' duration of the disease, it was cured, and eight years subsequently the patient was still in good health.

These are only a few of the cases adduced by Doutrebente, who also cites several which occurred in his own experience. I have never had the good fortune to witness a single case of the kind ; neither have I noticed one in which there was a complete disappearance of every symptom of the disease.

On this subject my opinion is in accordance with that of Baillarger and Luys,[1] which is that remissions are almost always the result of the disappearance of the acute maniacal or melancholic attacks which result from superadded congestion or anæmic conditions, and that the original substratum of the disease remains to produce its legitimate symptoms. If the focus or cortical lesion is small, the phenomena are restricted ; if it is large, they are more extensive.

Convulsive seizures have already been mentioned as occurring during the course of general paralysis. They are some-

---

[1] *Annales médico-psychologiques*, juillet, 1877, pp. 110, 111.

times characteristic features of the disease. Usually they are epileptiform, though occasionally they are of the nature of apoplexy. They vary greatly in character, sometimes consisting of attacks of *petit mal*, while at others they consist of strong convulsive seizures, not differing essentially from the *grand mal* of epilepsy. Voisin[1] cites several cases occurring in women in which the convulsive seizures were of the character of hystero-epilepsy. Accessions of coma are also met with. All these complications are doubtless due to sudden augmentations of the existing congestive state of the brain. Tetanic spasms have also been observed.

The *duration* of general paralysis is variable. Sometimes death results in a few months, and at others it may be deferred for five or six years. The average period is about three years.

As has already been intimated, general paralysis is almost invariably fatal. The cases of cure that have been reported, though amounting to perhaps a hundred all told, are scarcely to be considered when compared with the large number of cases that have gone on steadily to a fatal termination. Dr. Allbutt made his ophthalmoscopic examinations in general paralysis on fifty-one patients in the West Riding Lunatic Asylum. Four years afterward, when Dr. Aldridge came to make similar observations, not one of Dr. Allbutt's cases was alive.[2] About twenty per cent. of all the deaths occurring in lunatic asylums are from general paresis. Death may take place from a convulsive seizure, or during the coma resulting from congestion, from sheer exhaustion, from the gradual cessation of the respiratory process, or from the supervention of some intercurrent affection. But, before that event occurs, the patient, unless suddenly carried off by one of the causes referred to, passes with more or less rapidity into the stage of absolute mental and physical prostration. Bed-sores become a prominent feature, his urine and fæces are passed involuntarily, he is an extreme instance of the "wet and dirty" condition, which, perhaps, has existed with more or less intensity from an early period, but which now is his permanent state. Unable to speak, he mutters unintelligibly. But, if a word can be gathered here and there, it shows that he is still the victim of delusions, and often of those grand ideas of his

[1] *Op. cit.*, p. 221.
[2] *West Riding Lunatic Asylum Medical Reports*, vol. ii, 1872, p. 225.

strength and importance, his wealth and knowledge, which have played so striking a part in the clinical history of his disease. His life is almost reduced to the vegetative condition, so far, at least, as his relations with the external world are concerned. Swallowing is impossible, respiration is labored, the heart beats irregularly and feebly, and, when death comes, its approach is so gentle that those around scarcely notice that the patient is a corpse.

CHAPTER VIII.

VI.

CONSTITUTIONAL INSANITIES.

By constitutional insanities I do not intend to include those forms of mental derangement which simply owe their existence to a morbific influence acting as a cause only, and not giving a peculiar phase of its own to the aberration of mind. Thus, there is an insanity caused by malaria, another by alcohol, another by syphilis, another by gout, and so on for a dozen or more others. But I do refer to the insanities which are intimately related—not only etiologically but pathologically—with certain physical conditions which impress upon the mental disease something that makes it different from other insanities. To the most important of these the attention of the reader is requested.

a—EPILEPTIC INSANITY.

There is more or less mental derangement with every epileptic paroxysm, but there is a form of the seizure to which the term epileptic insanity or epileptic mania is especially applicable.

The relations of epilepsy to insanity were imperfectly known to medical writers of a hundred or more years ago, but they were first clearly formulated by Renaudin,[1] who showed that a paroxysm of insanity, temporary in duration, sometimes replaced the true epileptic seizure, or, if not altogether substituted for it, was violent in proportion to the feebleness of the usual attack.

[1] *Annales médico-psychologiques*, 1850, t. ii, p. 479.

Billod [1] regarded the maniacal and the ordinary epileptic paroxysm as two forms of one disease, and Falret [2] arrived at the conclusion that the paroxysms of insanity and of epilepsy occurring in an epileptic are only different manifestations of the same pathological condition, which can exist separately or together, or follow each other at longer or shorter intervals.

Morel [3] went still further, and showed that there was a form of insanity characterized by some of the most striking psychical manifestations of epilepsy, but in which there never had been any known association with true epileptic paroxysms. For a long time he had remarked that there was a certain class of patients in whom accessions of acute mania occurred with great suddenness, and then as suddenly disappeared. At first he had thought these cured, but the recurrence of the attacks, at more or less regular intervals, convinced him of his error. There were no prodromata other than an increased degree of activity and mental excitability, and they went on with their ordinary occupations up to the last moment. Then like a thunder-clap the seizure came, and in exactly the same form as previous attacks. Violence, extreme delirium, a tendency to the perpetration of acts of destruction or injury, irresistible impulsions, and then the subsidence of all the phenomena, and a return to the ordinary state of health. To this affection he gave the name of *épilepsie larvée*—concealed or masked epilepsy.

Since then Falret, Delasiauve, Legrand du Saulle, Spitzka, and many others have studied the subject in all its relations to medical and legal science. There are probably yet, notwithstanding all the labor which has been bestowed upon it, many points in its clinical history which have not been elucidated.

The ordinary form of an attack of epileptic insanity is characterized by a suddenness which has not its equal in the whole range of psychological medicine, and it is very often the case that an act of extreme violence marks the culmination of the paroxysm. The seizure then usually but not always ceases, and, after a short period of more or less mental disturbance, the patient regains his ordinary mental and phys-

---

[1] *Annales médico-psychologiques*, 1850, t. ii, p. 611.
[2] " Archives générales de médecine," t. xvi, 1860, p. 661.
[3] " Traité des maladies mentales," Paris, 1860, p. 480.

ical condition; sometimes the attack is prolonged through several hours, or even days.

The approach of the paroxysm may be indicated to the patient by sensations in various parts of his body, generally in the region of the solar plexus, or in the head, the former consisting of an anxious feeling, or such as is produced by hunger, and the latter ordinarily of vertigo. In the majority of cases there are no warnings or auræ.

The citation of a few cases, from the writings of others, and from my own experience, will tend to the elucidation of the symptomatology. Many of the instances that have been reported under the heads of morbid impulse, homicidal mania, mania transitoria, etc., are cases of epileptic insanity.

Legrand du Saulle [1] reports the following cases :

A young man of good intelligence, and belonging to a family of high rank, had at his command all the luxuries of life. Three or four times a year he experienced a particular sensation in the stomach, always of the same character, and in a few seconds afterward was overcome by a feeling which he could not describe, and he no longer possessed the consciousness of his acts. When he recovered his lucidity, at the end of a period lasting several hours, and sometimes one, two, or three days, he was surprised to find himself greatly fatigued, far from his home, on a railway or in a prison, his clothing in disorder, and himself without any recollection of what had passed. In his pockets there would be *porte-monnaies*, jewelry, cigar-cases, knives, laces, bank-notes, gold pieces, letters, medals, and many other articles. He had no idea how these things came into his possession, but would add that he must have had a paroxysm of his disease.

In May, 1867, Philibert V——, aged twenty-one, assassinated, at the corner of the Rue Princesse, at five o'clock in the morning, a peaceable old man, whom he had never seen before. He was arrested with the bloody knife with which he had done the deed in his possession. The fact of his insanity being recognized, he was sent to the Bicêtre, where he came under M. Legrand du Saulle's observation.

At first sight the young man appeared to be good-tempered, reasonable, and incapable of a criminal act. He knew nothing of what had happened, was surprised at being in arrest, and demanded to be sent back to his home. His mother

[1] " Étude médico-légale sur les épileptiques," Paris, 1877.

declared that he had never been affected with any serious disease, that he always behaved himself well, that he was sober, a good worker, but that from time to time he was singular, irritable, threatening, and that he had intentionally given himself several blows on the head. Then he would go out agitated, and return quite worn out at the end of twenty-four, thirty-six, or forty-eight hours ; and that, with the most honest purpose possible, he could not tell where he had been, or what he had done, or where he had slept, or what he had eaten. Then he went to work, and was as well as though nothing had happened.

The evening before the crime, Philibert had passed the whole day at the Exposition, and had brought back with him some Protestant books, which he had read during the night, notwithstanding the entreaties of his mother, who had begged him to take some rest. He had arisen in the morning very much excited, dressed himself hurriedly ; had abused his mother, possessed himself of a kitchen-knife, and had gone out in a furious state of mind. He was in this mental condition when he killed the first person he met.

M. Legrand du Saulle was convinced of the reality of his amnesic state. He called to mind the fact that the ordinary lunatic recollects the criminal act he may have committed, while the epileptic, on the contrary, does not, or does so very imperfectly. He did not, therefore, hesitate to give an opinion that the young man had committed the crime during a paroxysm of epilepsy.

Marc [1] relates the following instances :

A shoemaker, aged thirty-five, an industrious and sober man, rose early one morning and resumed his work. Shortly afterward his wife noticed that his speech was irrational and incoherent, and suddenly the unfortunate man seized his knife and rushed furiously upon her in order to kill her. His face was red, and his whole aspect was that of a maniac ; gradually he became quiet, but his pulse was full and frequent, his tongue dry, and the surface of his body covered with perspiration. In a few hours he was calm and asleep, and in the evening was perfectly rational. He had no recollection whatever of the events of the morning.

A Swabian peasant, who had for eighteen years been sub-

[1] "De la folie considérée dans ses rapports avec les questions judiciaires," Paris, t. ii, p. 510.

ject to epileptic paroxysms, experienced a change in the type of his disease, the fits being replaced by attacks of homicidal fury. The impulses to kill were preceded by somnolence and lassitude. When he felt them coming on, he would beg to be restrained, and would implore his mother and others to get out of his way. He had no subsequent recollection of his acts.

The following cases occurred in my own experience:

J. H. consulted me for epilepsy in the summer of 1869. His ordinary attacks were of the fully-developed form, but upon two occasions they were different from any with which he had previously been affected. In one of these, while over-looking some workmen, he was observed to put his hand to his head, and then suddenly to run toward a fence which he speedily climbed. Jumping down into the back-yard of an adjoining house, he seized a stick of wood near by, and made a furious onslaught on the doors and windows. He was, however, seized by several men, and forcibly held, notwith-standing his struggles. While thus being restrained, he re-covered his consciousness, but had no recollection of anything that had taken place after he had put his hand to his head, which action, he said, was due to severe pain and vertigo. The duration of the attack was not over three minutes.

On the other occasion, he was seized with pain and vertigo which engaged in paying a bill at a coal-yard. He rushed into the street and began to turn rapidly round. He was seized and held till he recovered his consciousness. This at-tack lasted about four minutes.

Subsequently he had a similar paroxysm in my consult-ing-room. His face became very pale, his eyes were fixed, and his pupils oscillated. Suddenly he rose from the chair, grasped the mantel-piece for an instant, and then rushed vio-lently around the room, throwing his arms about and utter-ing a peculiar inarticulate cry. I made no attempt to re-strain him, and in about two minutes he became calm. Dur-ing the whole paroxysm his face was pale, and at its close the pupils were dilated. He had no recollection of anything that had occurred after he rose from the chair, but was con-scious then of vertigo.

Another case is that of a girl brought to my clinique at the Bellevue Hospital Medical College during the summer of 1869. She had been severely injured in the skull by a fall against a mass of old scrap-iron. Necrosis subsequently ensued, and several large pieces of the external table were exfoliated. While before the class she started to her feet and walked several times around the enclosed area. She was unconscious, and to all appearance insensible. When the paroxysm was over, she returned to her seat. The duration did not exceed a minute, and there was no excitement or delirium.[1]

In this case there were no acts of violence, though there were probably hallucinations or illusions, for the girl went up to two or three of the gentlemen sitting on the front row of benches, and mumbled out some words to them, and it is possible there were delusions which influenced her conduct. In the two following cases there is still greater reason for supposing that the conduct of the patients was the result of erroneous mental conceptions.

A partner in an extensive mercantile establishment, who was subject to attacks of both the *grand* and the *petit mal*, left his office at about eleven o'clock for the purpose of getting a signature to a paper of some kind from a gentleman whose place of business was a few minutes' walk distant. Not returning by three o'clock, inquiry was made, and it was ascertained that he had visited the office, obtained the signature, and had left in apparently good health before half-past eleven. Since then nothing had been heard of him. He did not make his appearance at his own office till nearly five o'clock.

The last thing he recollected was passing St. Paul's Church, at the corner of Broadway and Vesey Street, just as the congregation was coming out after morning service. It was subsequently ascertained that he had gone to Brooklyn after getting the signature he wanted; had visited a newspaper office, and purchased a paper; had returned to New York, entered an omnibus at the Fulton Ferry, left it at the corner of Twenty-third Street and Fifth Avenue, entered the Fifth Avenue Hotel, and while there recovered his recollection.

But none of these cases, nor any of which I have seen the report, are equal in interest to one which occurred in my practice during the autumn of 1875. The patient, who was engaged in active business as a manufacturer, left his office at about 9 A. M., saying he was going to a florist's to purchase some bulbs. He remained absent eight days. He was tracked

---

[1] " A Treatise on the Diseases of the Nervous System," New York, seventh edition, p. 693.

all over the city, but the detectives and friends were always an hour or more behind him.   It was ascertained that he had been to theatres ; to hotels, where he slept ; to shops, where he had made purchases ; and that he had taken a journey of a hundred miles from New York, and losing his ticket, and not being able to give a satisfactory account of himself, was put off of the train at a way-station.   He had then returned to New York, passed the night at a hotel, and on the eighth day, at about ten o'clock, made his appearance at his office. He had no recollection of any one event which had taken place after leaving his office eight days previously, till he awoke on the morning after his return to the city, and found himself at a hotel at which he was a stranger.   It was ascertained beyond question that in all this time his actions had been entirely correct, to all appearance ; that his speech was coherent, and that he had acted in all respects as any man in the full possession of his faculties would have acted.   He had drunk nothing but a glass of ale, which he took with some oysters at a restaurant in Sixth Avenue.

It could not be ascertained that this patient had ever had an epileptic paroxysm ; but he had a year previously been under my charge for cerebral symptoms, indicating the existence of chronic basilar meningitis, and, only a week before his disappearance, I had discharged him cured after a month's treatment for severe pain in the head, vertigo, paralysis of the third nerve on the right side, and extreme insomnia. These were all indications of a specific cause, and I had treated him with large doses of the iodide of potassium, as on the former occasion.[1]

The following case, though differing in the most striking manifestations from the last two cited, is yet essentially the same in character.

I was consulted in the case of a young lady, an inmate of a fashionable school in this city, who, immediately before each menstrual period, was attacked with paroxysms of great and uncontrollable excitement, during which she attempted to destroy everything within her reach.   In one of these, which had occurred just before I saw her, she had broken a large drawing-room mirror, a mantel-clock, and several valuable vases and ornaments, before she could be restrained.   One morning she entered my consulting-room with her governess,

[1] *Op. cit.*, p. 694.

and, almost before I could speak to her, the fit seized her. Her face and neck became red, her eyes sparkled, she trembled from head to foot, and, ere I was able to prevent her, she seized a bronze, dagger-like paper-knife that lay on the table, and attempted to plunge it into her breast. Fortunately, it struck against the steel support of her corsets, and, before she could repeat the act, I caught her arm and took the weapon from her. In a few moments she was calm, and had no recollection of what she had done. The attack was clearly one of epileptic mania, and shortly afterward her seizures assumed the regular form of the *grand mal.*

A young man residing in Boston, and who was under my charge for epilepsy, of which he had attacks of both the *grand* and *petit mal* several times in the course of each month, one evening while eating supper with his mother, rose suddenly from the table, his face bearing a wild expression, and, rushing up-stairs to his bedroom, took a razor and drew it across his throat, before those who followed him could prevent the act. For several hours afterward he was in a state of exalted delirium. When this passed off, he had no recollection of anything that had occurred since he had sat down at the supper-table. A good portion of the meal, therefore, must have been eaten during the paroxysm, which in the beginning was of a quiet character.

The foregoing cases are sufficient to show the general characteristics of a paroxysm of epileptic insanity. It will be seen that there is not always a tendency to violence. During the seizure, it sometimes is very evident that the patient suffers from false sensorial impressions, for he utters words which show what is passing through his mind. Indeed, as is well known, the ordinary epileptic paroxysm is occasionally preceded by hallucination, and I have recently published a memoir on a form of epilepsy, in which hallucinations and unconsciousness are the only manifestations.[1] It would be a slight transition from this variety to that under consideration. The case, the particulars of which are given on page 318, is also an instance of the facility with which hallucinations can be produced in epilepsy. Moreover, there are certain cases in which the recollection of what has occurred during the seizure is not

[1] "On Thalamic Epilepsy," *Archives of Scientific Medicine*, August, 1880; also "A Treatise on Diseases of the Nervous System," seventh edition, New York, 1881, p. 695.

altogether lost, and in which, therefore, the patient is able to speak of the illusions or hallucinations that have occurred to him. Again, before losing consciousness, and passing into the paroxysm, he may have deranged sensorial perceptions, which he recollects very well, and which he can describe after the seizure has passed off. Many cases of either category are on record. The following occurred in my own experience:

A man, aged thirty-five, was subject to epileptic paroxysms, which were occasionally replaced by attacks of violent delirium, characterized by mental and physical agitation, and by efforts on his part to bite, scratch, strike, and kick those about him. He never inflicted any severe injury, and, having acted in the manner stated to those about him, would resume his walking, gesticulating, and speaking. His language showed that he thought the persons in the room with him were making fun of him, and ridiculing him by pointing their fingers at him, and calling him offensive names. The paroxysm lasted only a few minutes, and when it was over he had a distinct recollection of all that had occurred in connection with the illusions, but of nothing else.

In another case the seizure was always preceded by the appearance of red figures of various kinds—goats, sheep, oxen, horses, lions, tigers, and many others—which seemed to be running, skipping, and jumping before him. This continued for two or three minutes, and then the explosion took place, either into an epileptic paroxysm of the ordinary convulsive kind, or into an accession of epileptic insanity, in which there were all the phenomena of an attack of acute mania with tendency to acts of violence, concentrated into the space of less than ten minutes. In this case, only the hallucinations which occurred before the full development of the seizure were recollected, but the cries and actions of the patient during the continuance of the paroxysm left no room for doubt that there was intense sensorial aberration throughout the attack.

All these cases are of the kind to which Morel, as we have seen, applied the term "masked epilepsy" (*épilepsie larvée*). They take the place of the ordinary attacks. But there are others in which the paroxysm of insanity precedes, and others again in which it follows the epileptic seizure. All these varieties are especially interesting in their medico-legal relations, and have been very thoroughly studied from that stand-point by Lunier,[1] Kraft-Ebing,[2] and others.

Maniacal paroxysms occurring immediately before an epileptic attack are very rare ; and are probably not instances of epileptic mania, but of mania with epilepsy ; those following a seizure are common, and, according to Dr. Hughlings Jackson,[3] are the only forms of transitory mania accompanying epilepsy, or resulting from the existence of the epileptic predisposition in an individual. In this view, he is not, I think, supported by facts.

In cases of epileptic mania such as I have cited, there is in one sense a loss of consciousness, but in another sense the consciousness remains. There is a loss of the knowledge of the relations of the individual to the world and of his own identity, but he is conscious at the time of all that occurs during his paroxysms, although when this is over he has no recollection of his former state of consciousness. There are, in fact, two states of consciousness, in neither of which has he any recollection of the other. Several cases of prolonged states of double consciousness have been reported. In these the individuals led separate and distinct lives, knew different people, had different habits, and were possessed of different mental characteristics in each state. In each of the periods the individual was conscious, but he had no recollection in one state of consciousness of any circumstance which took place in the other.[4]

Epilepsy produces in many cases deterioration of the mental faculties and consequent dementia. In some instances this is only a temporary state of mental weakness, due to exhaustion of the brain by frequent discharges of nerve-force. It is, therefore, easily recovered from if the paroxysms are stopped. The other is secondary or terminal dementia, the result of organic lesion or want of cerebral development, and is incurable.

---

[1] "Zweifelhafte Geisteszustande vor Gericht," Berlin, 1869.

[2] "Die Lehre von der Mania transitoria," Stuttgart, 1865, and "Lehrbuch der gerichtlichen Psychopathologie," Stuttgart, 1875.

[3] "On Temporary Mental Disorders after Epileptic Paroxysms," *West Riding Lunatic Asylum Hospital Medical Reports*, vol. v, 1875, p. 105.

[4] See "Amnesie périodique, ou dédoublement de la vie," par M. Aznam, *Annales médico-psychologiques*, July, 1876 ; and paper by Dr. Mesnet, in *L'Union médicale*, July 21 and 23, 1874, translated in the *Chicago Journal of Nervous and Mental Disease*, August, 1880 ; also, *Neurological Contributions*, No. 3, New York, 1881.

b—PUERPERAL INSANITY.

The puerperal condition is something more than a cause of mental derangement. It imposes certain features of its own, and hence gives rise to a peculiar form of insanity, different in some respects from any other variety.

For the purposes of the present inquiry, the puerperal state may be divided into three distinct periods—the first beginning with conception and ending when labor begins ; the second beginning with labor and ending with the cessation of the lochial discharge ; and the third embracing the time during which the mother nurses her child. These last two overlap each other about a month. In these days, when mothers do not always nurse their offspring, this third period is often absent.

Period of Pregnancy.—During this period, although exalted forms of insanity are rarely met with, it is by no means uncommon to encounter various changes in the mental characteristics of the woman. These especially relate to the emotions and appetites. The likes and dislikes change ; unreasonable prejudices against relatives and intimate friends are especially apt to be engendered, and the husband is not infrequently singled out for particular aversion and hatred.

Morbid fears of various kinds take possession of the mind. In one case the patient acquired an unconquerable fear of water ; she would neither drink it nor use it for purposes of cleanliness ; the very sight of it caused her the most poignant distress.

In a case that came under my own observation many years ago, the patient, the wife of an officer of the army, during the second month of her pregnancy, became imbued with a fear of mice to such an extent that she adopted the most extraordinary precautions against them, and would not consent to be left alone even for a moment lest one of these animals should make its appearance. She always sat with her feet on another chair, and at night a fence was put up around the bed, as a means of restraint against her imaginary enemies.

Again, there are fears that the anticipated child will be deformed, or that it will be too large to admit of being born. These are not merely temporary apprehensions, but are so firmly implanted as to cause mental derangement while they last.

Sometimes an excessive erotism approaching satyriasis is developed. Again, there are "longings" for various articles of food or drink, or for things which are not eaten or imbibed by well-ordered individuals. A desire for alcoholic liquors may constitute one of the "longings," and, if indulged, may result in the formation of a habit which it is afterward difficult if not impossible to break. Earth, chalk, slate-pencils, paper, etc., are eaten with avidity. A patient of my own ate the ashes of the cigars smoked by her husband and brothers and left in the ash-holders, and another drank her own urine. These are, of course, perversions of the appetite for food, and rarely met with in other forms of insanity.

The general mental type is that of depression approaching melancholia, but occasionally there is an exalted condition present which is as unreasonable as that of depression, but certainly less disagreeable.

Illusions, hallucinations, or delusions are not especially liable to occur.

In a few instances there is, as I have said, a more decided state of mental derangement produced, and this may be either of the maniacal or melancholic type, without any special characteristics.

With the implication of the mind there are certain somatic symptoms of disordered cerebral action. These usually consist of headache, vertigo, and persistent wakefulness.

As the pregnancy advances, all the phenomena mentioned tend to disappear, and by the sixth or seventh month are generally no longer apparent.

Period of Labor.—It is at this time that puerperal insanity is most apt to be developed. It usually occurs during the first two weeks, sometimes during the process of delivery, again a few hours after the birth of the child, or it may be delayed for a month.

Two forms of puerperal insanity occurring at this time are recognized : that of acute mania, and that of some one of the varieties of melancholia. The former is much the more common type.

It would scarcely be worth while, in view of what has already been said when the subject of acute mania was under consideration, to enter at length into the description of all the features of an attack of puerperal mania of the acute

41

maniacal form. It will be sufficient if the peculiarities of the accession are brought to the notice of the reader.

The first of these is such a change in the natural instincts of the mother as to cause her to acquire a feeling of the most determined aversion to the child of which she has just been delivered. This disposition has been observed by all authors on the subject.

Esquirol,[1] in pointing out that the murderous tendencies of the puerperal maniac are not due to a desire which might exist of concealing the birth of a child, from shame or other like motive, refers to the case of a young woman who, being pregnant, made no secret of the fact, but got ready for her labor, and prepared the clothes for the child. The evening before her confinement she appeared in public. During the night she was delivered. The following morning she was found in her bed, but the infant was stuffed down the water-closet, and mutilated with twenty-one incisions and punctures with some sharp instrument, probably a pair of scissors. Shortly afterward she was arrested and carried on a stretcher a distance of two leagues from the house in which she was confined. During the journey she talked deliriously, and appeared not to know for what she was arrested. Several days subsequently she acknowledged her crime, but refused to eat.

Morel cites the case of a woman, twenty-one years old, who had been delivered eight days previously, and who, when she came under his observation, was in a high state of maniacal excitement, her eyes haggard, her hair dishevelled. "I am the devil!" she said, throwing herself furiously on those around her. It was necessary to take away her infant, for she wished to strangle it.

Fortunately, the opportunities for the subjects of puerperal insanity to murder their infants are not many, but in two cases that have come under my charge the attempt to do so was made. In one, a woman who had been delivered of a male child, nine days previously, suddenly exhibited signs of mental aberration. The infant was removed to an adjoining room in charge of a nurse, but the mother got up in the middle of the night, while her husband slept on a bed in another part of the room, and, going to where the child lay, seized it

---

[1] "De l'aliénation mentale des nouvelles accouchées et des nourrices," "Des maladies mentales," t. i, 1838, p. 115.

by the neck, and attempted to strangle it. In the effort she uttered a cry, "Die, you hateful thing!" and so loud that the nurse awoke in time to save the infant's life.

In the other, the patient had become insane four days after delivery; the child had been removed from her, but she expressed so urgent a desire to see it that it was brought to her. The instant she had it in her arms she dashed it toward an open window, about five feet distant. Fortunately, the infant struck against the sill, and fell back into the room.

But, in every other case, without exception—and they amount to fourteen in number—the patient has exhibited either active aversion to the infant or a passive indifference, fully as much at variance with the maternal instinct of love for her offspring manifested with more or less strength by the female of every species of the higher animals.

Another peculiarity of the condition in question is the proclivity, which very generally exists in a marked degree, to make use of obscene language. Women who have been brought up in the most careful and refined manner utter words which are only heard from the mouths of the lowest specimens of civilized humanity; and this not only occasionally, but in a continuous torrent, lasting for hours at a time. The wonder is, how they ever obtained the knowledge of the filthy expressions which flow with such fluency, and often without logical relation to each other.

Dr. James Macdonald,[1] writing thirty-five years ago, in giving the details of one of his cases, calls attention to the repeated use of indecent words as a symptom very common in puerperal mania, and further says: "In the acute form of the mania which succeeds parturition, we observe an intensity of mental excitement, an excessive incoherence, a degree of fever, and, above all, a disposition to mingle obscene words with the broken sentences—things which are rarely noted under other circumstances. It is true that in mania modest women use words which in health are never permitted to issue from their lips; but in puerperal insanity this is so common an occurrence, and is done in so gross a manner, that it early struck me as being characteristic. And is there no reason for it? Do not the disturbed uterine functions give rise to such

[1] "Puerperal Insanity," *American Journal of Insanity*, vol. iv, 1847-'48, p. 113.

ideas ? " Dr. Campbell [1] also remarks that the patient, though remarkably devout when sane, now launches out into such a torrent of obscene language that one is astonished that respectable females could have become acquainted with such expressions.

Dagonet, [2] while expressing the opinion that there is nothing special about the insanity of the puerperal condition, says : "It is, nevertheless, to be remarked that the disorder of ideas is most intense, that the general excitation is more violent than is observed in other cases of mania, and that it is often complicated with dangerous irresistible impulses and erotic ideas. The patients, readily absolving themselves from all regard for the child they have brought into the world, perpetrate acts which are due to a perversion of the maternal feeling. The language they use is obscene, they endeavor to strip off their clothing, and their gestures and conduct toward those around them are scandalous."

In addition, there is very often a strong disposition to suicide in the subjects of puerperal insanity, especially when it assumes the melancholic form.

As to this latter form, there are present in it equally strong perversions of the maternal instinct, and tendency to erotic ideas, and the use of obscene language, as are observed in the maniacal type.

Period of Lactation.—Insanity may be developed at any time during this period, or at a time soon after its cessation. It is not so common as the insanity of parturition, and presents no very characteristic phenomena. It may be of the maniacal, melancholic, or monomaniacal type. Strictly speaking, the insanity of lactation is not a puerperal insanity, but, as it is generally so considered, I have introduced it here in order to present the subject in a complete form.

Mental derangement from nursing may arise as a consequence of the increased weakness of the system, induced by the drain of milk in women of feeble constitutions. Again, it occurs at the time of weaning, apparently from the sudden stoppage of a function to which the organism has become habituated.

All the forms of puerperal insanity are of hopeful prog-

[1] *Journal of Psychological Medicine*, January, 1859, p. 14.
[2] " Nouveau traité élémentaire et pratique des maladies mentales," Paris, 1876, p. 500.

nosis, provided the patients can be submitted to proper medical treatment.

The subject of etiology is not now under consideration, but it may be stated that, though albuminuria is sometimes present, there is no reason for supposing, with Sir James Simpson,[1] that puerperal insanity, in any of its varieties of type or period, is due to uræmic poisoning.

c—PELLAGROUS INSANITY.

The disease which exists in Northern Italy and Southern France, known as pellagra, and which is an erythematous affection of the skin, is often accompanied by a peculiar form of insanity. The subject has been very thoroughly studied. Among many others by Strambio,[2] Brierre de Boismont,[3] Baillarger,[4] Billod,[5] Sacchi,[6] Gintrac,[7] and Lombroso,[8] from whose writings I shall mainly quote what little I have to say relative to pellagrous insanity.

There are many neurotic phenomena met with in individuals affected with pellagra, but the most important is mental derangement. According to Billod, three fifths of all the insane in the asylum of Astino were pellagrous; in that of Senarra, one third; and a like proportion in the asylum of San Servolo, at Venice.

Billod states that all the more typical forms of insanity are met with in pellagrous individuals. Thus, of two hundred and eighty cases in the asylum for women at Venice, there were of mania one hundred and eleven, of monomania six, of melancholia sixty-one, of stupidity ninety-seven, and of dementia five. This classification is, however, not very exact, and really gives us little information.

The character of the insanity of pellagra is, according to

---

[1] "Clinical Lectures on the Diseases of Women," New York, 1872, p. 561.

[2] "Due dissertazioni sulla pellagra," Milano, 1794.

[3] "De la pellagre et de la folie pellagreuse," Paris, 1834.

[4] "De la paralysie pellagreuse," *Mém. de l'académie de méd.*, Paris, 1848, t. xiii, p. 708.

[5] "Traité de la pellagre," Paris, 1870.

[6] "La pellagra nella provincia di Mantova," *Relazione della commissione provinciale*, Firenze, 1878.

[7] Art. "Pellagre," in *Nouveau dictionnaire de médecine et de chirurgie pratiques*, t. xxvi, Paris, 1878, p. 447.

[8] "Studi clinici ed esperimentali sulla natura, causa e terapeia della pellagra," Milano, 1870.

the majority of writers on the subject, of a melancholic form.
Gintrac thus describes it:

" The cerebro-spinal symptoms consist of an alteration of
the sensibility of the motility and of the intelligence. They
are vertigo, pain, or rather a feeling of heat, along the spine,
slight losses of consciousness, apathy, a great indisposition
to muscular exercise or any sort of work. These symptoms
gradually become more distinctly marked, the debility is
more intense, the gait is staggering, the lower extremities become the seat of numbness, and of weakness which sometimes
terminates in paralysis. At other times the pellagrous individuals are subject to tremors, and to a degree of ataxia which
renders their movements very uncertain and peculiar. They
have, besides, hallucinations of sight and of hearing, they remain obstinately silent, and preserve an immovable attitude.
They have a slowness of speech, an incoherence of ideas, a
sad delirium, a fixed idea of despair, and a degree of melancholia sometimes reaching to stupidity. In a word, they afford the sad spectacle of mental alienation, extending through
all degrees, from simple hebetude to mania and monomania,
and which often leads to suicide.

Strambio, observing that the subjects of pellagrous insanity
generally committed suicide by drowning, suggested the name
of hydromania for this form of mental derangement. The intense heat of the skin excites not only directly to immersion
in water, but also gives rise to delusions of fire, both in this
world and in the next, and the miserable victims plunge into
the water to extinguish at the same time the real and the
imaginary fire.

Gintrac adds that, in travelling through the districts in
which pellagra exists, he has been informed that every year
many pellagrous maniacs or melancholics are found drowned
in the ponds.

Baillarger finds in the phenomena of pellagrous insanity
so many similitudes to general paralysis, that he insists on
the existence of a striking analogy between the two diseases.
These, however, are mostly as regards the somatic symptoms—
the troubles of speech, the advancing paralysis.

Lombroso regards the emotional impressionability of the
subjects of pellagrous insanity as one of the most prominent
characteristics of the disease. The slightest untoward event
is sufficient to produce a degree of emotional disturbance

altogether out of proportion to the exciting cause. Thus, a woman missing mass is thrown into a condition of despair, because she thinks she is in consequence doomed to eternal damnation. A man becomes acutely maniacal because a friend to whom he has lent a pistol will not return it; and a woman becomes similarly affected because her husband, who is a fisherman, is a few minutes late in coming home. Sometimes the patients remain obstinately mute for long periods; refusal of food is common, as are various hallucinations. Derangements of speech are also met with. Hydromania is among the most characteristic symptoms: some crave water for the cooling and refreshing influence which it has on the skin, others simply desire to see it. One patient told Dr. Lombroso that nothing in the world gave him so much pleasure as the sight of water. Occasionally some patients have a strong dislike for water.

It appears to me, therefore, that pellagrous insanity should be regarded as a distinct pathological entity, the pathognomonic features of which are mental derangement, generally of the character of melancholia in some one of its forms, or of acute mania, and accompanied by the somatic phenomena of derangements of sensibility and motility, not unlike, in some respects, those which exist in general paralysis.

The prognosis of the affection is bad. Remissions may occur, but the symptoms are almost certain to return with increased violence.

d—CHOREIC INSANITY, ETC.

Chorea is quite often accompanied by mental derangement of a peculiar kind. Reference is not made to the various epidemics of so-called chorea, which in former times appeared in various parts of the civilized world, nor to those other forms of disorderly movements which are more or less contagious or epidemic in character, and which sometimes accompany great religious excitement. Some of them have been considered under the head of epidemic insanity. But by choreic insanity is to be understood solely the aberration of mind which is an accompaniment or a result of chorea, and which is due to the same cause which produces the convulsive disorder.

The first to study the subject systematically was Marcé,

and little has been added to our knowledge of the subject since the publication of his monograph over twenty years ago.[1]

Marcé distinguishes four categories of phenomena connected with the mind which may exist in conjunction with chorea—troubles of the emotions; of the memory and intellectual faculties generally; of the perceptions; and then maniacal delirium. The first three are, I think, observed with more or less completeness in all cases of chorea. In some instances they are slight, and may consist merely of defects of memory and weakness of the intellect in other respects; but in others there are great emotional disturbance and almost constant hallucinations of sight. Without dwelling on these symptoms to any great extent, it may be well to call attention to them in a few words before proceeding to consider the more pronounced type constituting choreic insanity.

The modifications of states of feeling which accompany chorea are in general well marked. The patient is irritable, impressionable, laughs in a silly way over circumstances not in the least risible, or sheds tears over events which are of the most inconsequential character. The tendency to deceive is developed to a surprising degree, and patients who have ordinarily been remarkable for their truth-telling quality and freedom from subterfuge and fraud, will lie with and without reason, and resort to altogether unnecessary tricks and cheats, actuated apparently by no other motive than a kind of automatic spirit of falsehood. It is possible that in some cases the stories that are concocted by choreic children have their origin in delusions which are mistaken by them for actual occurrences.

So far as the intellect is concerned, the principal aberrations are perceived as regards the memory and the power of concentrating the attention. Nothing seems to make any permanent impression on the understanding, though, as we have seen, the emotions are affected readily enough. Learning lessons at school becomes an impossibility. The child can neither apply itself nor retain the little it may acquire. These phenomena indicate a condition of mental weakness approaching dementia, and, indeed, the state of mind induced is in some cases as well-marked dementia as is ever seen.

[1] "De l'état mental dans la chorée," "Mémoires de l'académie impériale de médecine," t. xxiv, 1860, p. 1; also, "Traité pratique de maladies mentales," Paris, 1862, p. 576.

In some very severe cases of chorea the mental manifestations are very profound, and a state of stupor is induced, during which the patient is more or less insensible to what is
going on around him.

Indeed, it is almost invariably the case that the mental
aberration is in direct relation with the somatic symptoms.
When these latter are at their height the disturbance of mind
is always greatest, and, when they are diminished in violence,
the mind tends to the resumption of its normal condition.

Marcé states that it is not rare to meet with hallucinations
in chorea. Except in cases of fully developed choreic insanity, few cases of the kind have come under my observation,
and these, all except one, related to the sense of sight. In
this respect my experience is in accordance with that of
Marcé, who states that he has never seen the sense of taste
or of smell involved, and only one case in which the hearing,
and three in which the touch were affected. Hallucinations
in chorea are, as he states, more frequent between the ages of
fourteen and twenty-four years than at other times. In very
young patients they are never seen. Of forty patients examined by Marcé, eleven had hallucinations of sight. Of the
very many cases of chorea which have been under my observation and treatment in hospital and private practice, thirteen
only exhibited sensorial aberration unaccompanied by the
manifestations of acute mania.

As Marcé has pointed out, the peculiarity of choreic hallucinations is, that they are not present during the state of
wakefulness or when the eyes are open, but only appear in
that period between sleeping and waking, which occurs when
the patient is going to sleep or when he is about awaking.
The moment he shuts his eyes in the process of going to sleep,
they occur ; and again they may—but not with the same degree of frequency—make their appearance just as he is about
to open his eyes on awaking. Marcé had one case in which
hallucinations appeared during the day whenever the patient
shut his eyes.

The images are of all kinds—friends, relations, demons,
angels, all kinds of deformed persons, giants, dwarfs, and
every variety of animals. Sometimes when some person has
been vividly brought before the mind, the image of that person appears as a hallucination, and persists for a long time.

Occasionally the hallucinations appear before there are

any convulsive movements; in other cases they occur only when the paroxysms are most intense.

Of fully developed choreic insanity, only five cases have come under my observation. Three of these are referred to in another place,[1] and two have occurred in my experience during the past two years. It may make its appearance at any time during the course of the disease, and sometimes, as in one of my cases, before there are any convulsive movements. In most cases, however, it does not supervene till after the tenth day. So far as my observation extends, the essential points of difference between it and the ordinary form of acute mania are the occurrence of the hallucinations only at the time of going to sleep or awaking, and the existence of a peculiar species of incoherence characterized by the utterance of isolated words, which have no relation whatever to each other. Marcé alludes to this symptom. It appears to be due to the excessive rapidity with which hallucinations, illusions, and delusions succeed each other — a rapidity which is never in my experience equalled in acute mania of the usual type.

Thus, in a young lady of seventeen, who came to me from a neighboring city, mental derangement had supervened on the sixth day after the occurrence of choreic movements. These had gone on rapidly from the very beginning, augmenting in violence every hour till they involved her head, arms, legs, and trunk. On the sixth day she became violently excited in consequence of hallucinations of sight, which effectually prevented her sleeping. The moment she closed her eyes, old men and women, with black imps, appeared to be dancing round her, and pointing their fingers at her in derision. She could hear them laugh, as they capered around her in all possible combinations of dancing figures. After a night, during which she was entirely without sleep, delusions ensued, and her maniacal disturbance was still greater. Then she began to talk, but in such a way that no one could understand what she said. It seemed, as her mother said, as though she had taken a thousand pieces of paper with words on them, and, after shaking them all together, was naming them off one by one.

On the tenth day of the attack, I saw her at her hotel in

[1] " A Treatise on the Diseases of the Nervous System," seventh edition, New York, 1881, p. 732.

this city. She was then in a state of great exaltation, and the choreic movements were at their height. Two persons were necessary to keep her in bed, as, on the least relaxation of their vigilance, she would attempt to leave the room, and once had tried to get out of the window. She was talking at the top of her voice, but this was not high, as exhaustion was rapidly advancing, and she was then very weak, but, though she spoke distinctly enough, there was nothing but a string of disconnected words without the slightest relation to each other. At times she would close her eyes, as if about to sleep, but instantly would start up, frightened, and would begin to talk apparently with the object of saying something in regard to her hallucinations, but with the same utterance of unrelated words.

Conceiving the case to be one requiring prompt treatment, I put her under the anæsthetic influence of ether, with the effect of quieting both her mental and physical manifestations, and procuring for her the first good sleep she had had for several days. By means of the hypodermic administration of morphia and arsenic, she made a good recovery in about three weeks.

In another case, occurring in a young lady of this city, whom I saw in consultation with the late Dr. Henschel, violent chorea, with maniacal manifestations similar to those of the case just cited, was developed by the excitement consequent on a visit to the dentist. In this instance, a like means was successful in immediately quieting the patient, who ultimately recovered under the use of arsenic and bromide of sodium.

In connection with choreic insanity, there are very generally pain in the head, frequent attacks of vertigo, acceleration of pulse, and increased bodily temperature.

There are other alleged constitutional forms of insanity, but they are not included here, for the reason given on page 292. It is very well to speak of alcoholic insanity, malarial insanity, syphilitic insanity, and so on for a dozen or so more, but all these are simply instances of insanity of different types produced by alcohol, malaria, etc. It would be just as proper to regard traumatic insanity as a separate form of mental alienation, though it is well known that any of the varieties of insanity may have wounds and injuries for its exciting causes.

CHAPTER IX.

THE CAUSES OF INSANITY.

PREDISPOSING CAUSES.—The causes of insanity have been to a great extent considered in the earlier chapters of this work, so that it will not be necessary to do more in the present connection than to apply the principles there laid down, and to bring forward such other factors as are proper in illustration of the subject. Thus, under the heads of *Habit, Temperament, Idiosyncrasy, Constitution, Sex, Race, Age,* the influence of these agencies in producing mental derangement have been sufficiently dwelt upon, but there are a few others of what may be called the predisposing causes that require some consideration at this time.

Civil Condition.—The civil condition, as regards marriage or celibacy, is important in its etiological relations to insanity. The statistics of all civilized countries show a larger proportion of lunatics among those who are unmarried than among those who are married. In France, according to Dagonet,[1] there is one insane person to every 528 celibates over the age of fifteen, while among those who are married the proportion falls to one in 1,523. In large cities, the proportion of single women who become lunatics is greater than in single men. In the widowed, the proportion is one to 942.

Of 1,426 patients admitted into the Colney Hatch Asylum, England, during four years, the proportion was about equal,[2] but then, as the married persons in England and Wales, according to the census of 1871, are more than twice as numerous as the single persons, it follows that the proportion of lunatics existing among single persons is about double that among the married.

Most of the asylum reports of this country show like results. Taking one of the latest, that of the Illinois Eastern Hospital for the Insane at Kankakee, we find that of 424 patients admitted during the years 1881–'83, 209 were single, 152 married, 29 were widowed, 17 divorced or separated, and of 17 the civil condition was unknown.

Upon this point there is a general accord among writers on psychological medicine.

[1] *Op. cit.,* p. 473.
[2] Bucknill and Tukes's "Manual of Psychological Medicine," London, 1879, p. 88.

Civilization.—It is the generally received opinion that insanity is much more common among civilized nations than among those who are lower in the scale of enlightenment. It is difficult to arrive at any very exact conclusion in regard to this point. In the first place, as nations advance in intelligence and refinement, the insane are more readily recognized than they are among barbarous and savage peoples, or even than they were among ourselves a few years ago. Not long since no one was regarded as insane who was not either a jabbering idiot or a raving maniac. The individual who, under the influence of a morbid impulse which he could not resist, killed some one, was held to be responsible, and was punished accordingly. Such forms as morbid impulses, and many others, were not known. The individual who acted in accordance with them was supposed to have been " moved and instigated by the devil," and in all probability went to the stake for allowing himself to be subdued by satanic power. To say, therefore, that the number of the insane has increased with the advance of civilization is in reality only alleging that more insane are known to exist than formerly ; and another factor in adding to the number is the increased facility for discovering instances of mental derangement, owing to the development of the means for intercommunication.

Again, though additional influences capable of causing insanity are probably furnished by a higher state of civilization, it must not be forgotten, on the other hand, that many influences due to a low degree of civilization have been eliminated. People are better fed, clothed, and housed than they were two or three hundred years ago. And, again, among barbarous or savage nations, or those persons among civilized peoples whose minds are not developed up to a high standard, slight causes which would be of no effect in persons of educated minds are often influential in causing insanity. An ignorant person will, therefore, become insane from the action of a cause that would scarcely ruffle the equanimity of an educated individual.

But, whatever value is to be attached to these suggestions, the fact remains undisputed that there are more known cases of insanity at the present day than there were, for instance, fifty years ago. According to Marcé, the proportion of lunatics to the population was in Europe, in 1836, one to 3,080, while, in 1851, fifteen years later, it was one to 1,676, not far from double. Lunier states that the rate has in France progressively advanced. A part of this increase is undoubtedly due to increase of population, but, making all reasonable allowance for this circumstance, there is still a large margin left.

It has been stated, but I do not know whether or not on satisfactory evidence, that since the abolition of slavery in the United States the number of the insane among the negroes has very greatly increased.

Cities.—Large collections of people in one place certainly tend to the increase in the number of the insane. The larger the city, and the more the inhabitants are crowded together, the greater, other things being equal, will be the number of the insane.

EXCITING CAUSES.—The exciting causes are those which stand to the disease as its immediate producers. They are very numerous, and the influence of some that are generally considered to be strong factors in giving rise to insanity is very questionable.

Emotional Causes.—These are undoubtedly the most efficient of all the exciting causes of insanity. Their action is generally prompt and easily recognizable. Chief among them is *anxiety*, which, however, is more frequently a secondary emotion than one of primary action. A person, for instance, becomes insane, it is supposed, from love, but it in reality is not *love* that is the causative emotion, but anxiety lest the passion felt is not reciprocated. As soon as all doubt on this point is removed, whether by a favorable or an unfavorable termination, the anxiety disappears, and the condition of the patient becomes much more tolerable.

Again, a man engaged in business, and having constant need for large sums of money to meet his engagements, suffers the keenest anxiety day after day, to a greater or less extent, throughout his life. He is never quite sure that he will obtain the funds he requires, and hence the strain upon his mind is so great that it is not at all singular that it often gives way and that insanity is the result. On the other hand, if he does not get the money he needs, and bankruptcy follows, there is at once a relief from the strain, and comparative mental repose follows. The uncertainty and anxiety are far more apt to lead to mental alienation than the assurance of disaster.

Almost all the *domestic chagrins* to which Esquirol attributes so great an influence in the causation of insanity are only forms of anxiety. The father of a family, feeling the responsibility that rests upon him, is anxious relative to his ability to clothe, feed, and house his wife and children. A son or a daughter gives evidence of vicious inclinations, and again anxiety to one or both parents is the result. I am acquainted with the particulars of a case in which both the father and mother became insane in consequence of the anxiety felt in regard to the guilt or innocence of a son accused of highway robbery, but upon whom the crime was never proved. They neither of them believed in his culpability, but the anxiety as to the result of his trial, the doubt and uncertainty, were more than their minds could endure.

Anxiety in regard to political success is in this country not an infrequent cause of mental derangement. The tenure by which fortunes are held is often so slight, the ways by which they are obtained are often so uncertain, the risks are so great, the profits so large, that those who plunge into the vortex of "business," as it is called, often come out perhaps with a million or more of money, but with a mind shattered past recovery.

Chagrin, or active corroding grief, is also a prolific cause of mental derangement scarcely second to anxiety in power. Here, again, family and business affairs stand pre-eminent as the producers of the emotion. With some people, those in whom the hereditary tendency is strong, very slight causes are sufficient to produce intense grief, and consequent insanity. The case of a lady is within my own experience in which intellectual subjective morbid impulses were produced by the grief resulting from a leak in the bath-room, which ruined a finely-painted ceiling. She became wakeful, had pains in her head, and kept constantly repeating the words she had uttered when she saw the wreck that had been caused: "My God, it will cost a thousand dollars to repair it!" Night and day these words were passing through her mind, as in the cases mentioned under their proper head.

In another case, from the chagrin and disappointment resulting from failure to receive an office from the Government, for which he had been an applicant, a gentleman became affected with acute mania. In another instance, from a like cause, the resultant form of insanity was melancholia with stupor.

Fright and *terror* are also powerful emotional causes of mental aberration, and cases due to their action are common enough. Probably the forms most apt to be produced by them are the several varieties of melancholia, hysterical insanity, epileptic insanity, and acute mania.

Love.—Whatever may have been the power of this emotion, primarily acting, to cause insanity, its influence is being gradually extinguished. Forty-five years ago Esquirol[1] said that, however frequently love might be the cause of erotomania, or even of nymphomania, in warm climates, its empire in France is lost. The indifference of the sexes to each other, and the fact that amorous passions have neither the exaltation nor the purity requisite to the engendering of erotomania, have extinguished the influence it once had. Though things are not so bad as this in the United States, it is very certain that love is no longer the romantic feeling which it was fifty or even a less number of years ago. Marriage is now generally a business venture, into the arrangements for which love, as a passion, very rarely enters. This is even more true of men than of women, many of whom yet have some degree of sentiment in their organizations. The facilities which men have for gratifying the passions in an illicit manner, without assuming the responsibilities and expense of an establishment with a wife and children, are factors which are continually tending to lessen the power of virtuous love, and to reduce the number of marriages. I have never seen a case of mental or physical disturbance reaching the point of disease in a man from the effect of love, or of any disappointment consequent thereon.

It is scarcely necessary to specify particularly each emotion which is competent to produce insanity. There is not one which has not this power. There is no uniform manner of acting. An emotion of one kind may produce acute mania in one person, melancholia in another, intellectual monomania with exaltation in a third, katatonia in a fourth, general paralysis in a fifth, and so on. Indeed, the same emotion may at different times, in the same individual, produce different varieties of insanity.

Intellectual Causes.—The only intellectual factor in the pro-

[1] "Des maladies mentales," Paris, 1838, t. i, p. 31.

duction of insanity requiring consideration is that of *excessive mental exertion.* Doubtless it is true that, under certain circumstances, the undue concentration of the mind upon any particular line of thought will lead to mental aberration; but such cases are rare, mainly for the reason that there are comparatively few persons who use the intellect to excess in an abnormal way. The brain, like the rest of the body, is meant for work, and it is capable of enduring a great deal of labor without suffering. It is only when this is carried on regardless of the laws of health, relative to physical exercise, food, sleep, etc., that disease is liable to ensue. The person who works with his brain in overheated or badly ventilated apartments, who encroaches on the hours that should be given to sleep, and who attempts to do his work on an improper or insufficient diet, will run great risks of mental derangement. By depriving himself of sleep, he is giving the brain no sufficient opportunity to rest, and to repair the waste produced by his mental labor; and, by keeping his brain in action up to the very moment of going to bed, he induces a hyperæmia of the organ, which renders sleep impossible. Then he begins to suffer, and then it is that the danger of insanity is incurred.[1] But the employment of the brain in any congenial work for eight or ten hours a day, with sufficient opportunities for relaxation, will very rarely lead to mental disease. There is more danger in the case of children, whose nervous systems are undeveloped, whose whole surplus strength is required for growth, and who are often unduly tasked at school with subjects above their comprehension, and with a variety of studies which keep the brain in a continual state of erethism. In them, therefore, it is no matter for astonishment to find headache, insomnia, vertigo, even when they are at rest, and an aggravation of all the symptoms on the least attempt at mental concentration. Most physicians in the larger cities meet with such cases in large numbers, and with not a few in which positive insanity is the ultimate result.

Physical Causes.—The physical causes of insanity are very numerous. They embrace those which are *external* to and those which are *inherent* in the individual. Among the first are the following:

Certain *ingesta*, either taken as *food* or as *medicine*, are

---

[1] This subject is discussed with sufficient fulness in the chapters on sleep, to which the reader is referred.

exceedingly potential in the causation of insanity. Chief among these is *alcohol*.

It is not the intention here to speak of the influence of alcohol as it affects the brain immediately after its ingestion, or of the blood-poisoning which it produces in a more chronic form. These states are known as acute and chronic alcoholic intoxication, and are described in works devoted to the consideration of diseases of the nervous system, or to the general practice of medicine.[1] But it is the purpose to consider briefly the influence of alcohol in causing insanity independently of its immediate toxic influence due to the circulation of poisoned blood through the system, especially the brain.

That alcoholic liquors when taken to excess have this power is so well known that it is not a matter to be substantiated by the citation of authorities. Almost every form of insanity, from simple sensorial aberrations to general paralysis and epileptic insanity, may result from the inordinate use of alcoholic liquors. At one time I was disposed to think that they gave rise to a special form of mental derangement, to which the term *alcoholic insanity* could properly be applied; but continued observation and study of the subject have convinced me that there is nothing peculiar in the mania, melancholia, general paralysis, or any other form of aberration of mind caused by these agents, and that such a disease as *alcoholic insanity*, with special characteristics, does not exist. Marfaing,[2] among others, has described such an affection, and has given many interesting particulars of the disorder which he thinks he has differentiated. Thus, he contends that the hallucinations and delusions are almost always of a painful character. The patient sees frightful or repulsive objects, armed men, or horrible animals; he sees persons lying in wait for him, or a thousand obstacles are interposed between him and his desires; he hears menacing voices, and the supplications of his friends from dangers which encompass them.

Occasionally, however, the imaginings are of a more pleasant character. He is surrounded with flowers and fountains,

[1] See chapter on "Alcoholism" in the author's "Treatise on Diseases of the Nervous System," seventh edition, New York, 1881, p. 894; also, "Effects of Alcohol on the Nervous System," *Neurological Contributions*, No. 2, 1880, p. 29.

[2] "De l'alcoolisme considéré dans ses rapports avec l'aliénation mentale," Paris, 1875.

THE CAUSES OF INSANITY.

beautiful women are his companions, and, though his generative powers may be entirely extinct, he brags of his conquests, and of the favors which are showered upon him.

Another characteristic, according to Marfaing, of the hallucinations and delusions of the mania of alcoholism, is their changeability. Scarcely has he expressed one delirious conception than another is uttered, and so on for days at a time.

Now there is nothing at all characteristic in these phenomena. They are met with in melancholia with delirium, and in acute mania, no matter by what factor they are produced.

I have witnessed many cases of so-called alcoholic insanity, and I am forced to say that, after a full consideration of its symptoms, I have seen nothing typical in it. The acute mania, or melancholia, or general paralysis, or whatever it may be, presents no distinguishing features. For instance, various morbid fears, not distinguishable from those considered under the head of "emotional monomania" as resulting from other causes, are produced by alcohol. Thus, a gentleman whose case came under my charge, becoming addicted to the excessive use of alcoholic liquors, gradually contracted the fear that he would say something profane or obscene if he ventured into the presence of ladies, and hence he shut himself off from female society. Upon one occasion, he found himself accidentally in the company of a lady of his acquaintance, when he threw up his hands in horror, exclaiming: "For God's sake, go away, or I shall be compelled to insult you in the grossest manner! Go, go, go!" advancing toward her at the same time, and actually turning her out of the room.

Again, there is intense melancholia without the existence of delusions, and differing in no essential respect from the simple melancholia already described, during which the individual may attempt suicide or self-mutilation. Or there may be indefinable fear, despair, terror, shame, or some other form of emotional monomania, leading to the perpetration of self-destruction. "Intellectual monomania with depression," attended with delirium of persecution, is also a common result of excessive alcoholic indulgence.

But perhaps the most common of all the forms of insanity caused by alcohol is general paralysis. All authors recognize its influence in this direction. Drs. Bucknill and Tuke [1]

---

[1] "A Manual of Psychological Medicine," fourth edition, London, 1879.

place it in the front rank. "Drink causing poverty and poverty leading to drink (the former in by far the larger proportion of cases) are the familiar antecedents of an attack of general paralysis."

Mickle [1] names "alcoholic excesses" first in the list of causes. In my own experience it takes precedence of all other known causes, fully twenty per cent of the cases that have come under my observation being due to alcoholic liquors used to excess.

A somewhat peculiar variety of insanity is, however, produced by the drinking of absinthe, a habit which prevails to a great extent in France, and one that has many votaries in this country.

The condition in question has been well studied by M. Magnan, by experiments on the lower animals as well as by observations in man. The main fact appears to be that absinthe has an especial proclivity to produce epileptic convulsions, in addition to causing the other phenomena of insanity, due to the highly concentrated alcohol it contains.

Certain fungous growths, which affect grain used as food, are apparently productive of insanity. Thus, in those countries in which ergotized rye is eaten for long periods by the inhabitants, a peculiar condition, characterized by physical and mental phenomena, is produced. The forms of insanity have nothing special about them. In the beginning there may be several epileptiform paroxysms, followed by coma; or, without these, the patient passes into a condition of dementia, or of more or less permanent insanity. Sometimes it is acute mania, again, melancholia in some one of its forms, especially that with stupor, which is developed. [2]

For a long time it was supposed that Indian corn, or maize, was the chief if not the only agent in the causation of pellagra. The fact that millions of people in the United States eat no other bread than that made from Indian corn, and that they ingest this substance in some form or other in large quantities several times a day, not only without contracting pellagra or any other disease, but with the most evident signs of resultant good health, appears to have been overlooked.

[1] "General Paralysis of the Insane," London, 1880, pp. 101, 103.
[2] Schleger, "Versuchen mit dem Mutterkorn," "Memoir of the Medical Faculty of Marburg," Cassel, 1770; also, Hursinger, "Studien über den Ergotismus," Marburg, 1856.

More recently, however, it was ascertained, with a tolerable degree of certainty, that the Indian corn used in Northern Italy and Southern France is subject to the growth of a fungus. This liability appears to be due to the climate, and to the peculiar method employed in storing the grain. Gubler,[1] in a report made to the French Academy of Medicine on Fua's work on the hygienic and therapeutical properties of maize, states that when the grain is of good quality it produces no deleterious result, and that it is as absurd to charge it with causing pellagra as it would be to ascribe ergotism to healthy rye. He declares, however, that, when the grain is changed either by the products of decomposition or by the growth of low organisms upon it, it acquires poisonous properties, and may then be productive of pellagra and pellagrous insanity.

Nevertheless, there are many authors who do not consider maize in either its healthy or diseased state as responsible for pellagra. The fungus supposed to give rise to pellagra is known to botanists as the *sporisorium mayais*.

Certain medicines, such as *morphia, chloral*, the *bromides, belladonna*, and other substances, give rise to mental derangement when taken in excessive or long-continued quantities ; but it appears to me scarcely advisable to consider the delirium, dementia, or other phenomena of the derangement of mind from their use as separate and distinct forms of insanity. There is hardly a medicine in the whole materia medica that is not capable of influencing the mind in an abnormal manner ; indeed, some of the most bland and nutritious articles of food will, under certain circumstances, do the same thing. I have had many opportunities of witnessing instances of mental derangement due to the use of morphia, chloral, and the bromides, and have never seen anything sufficiently characteristic to warrant the creation of a morphia, chloral, or bromide insanity, any more than there is for the creation of the insanity due to alcohol, into a distinct form. Either of these substances may produce any variety of mental aberration.

Several years ago I[2] reported a number of cases in which large quantities of the bromide of potassium had caused in-

---

[1] "Bulletin de l'académie de médecine," avril 9, 1878.

[2] "On some of the Effects of the Bromide of Potassium when administered in Large Doses," *Quarterly Journal of Psychological Medicine*, New York, January, 1869, p. 46.

sanity. In one of these the patient for several days, at his own suggestion, took an ounce a day. "He was now decidedly insane; had delusions that lewd women had got into his mother's house; that he was pursued by the police; that his life was threatened by members of the family; that he had thousands of dollars in gold sewed up in his clothing, etc. . . . His manner was excited and rambling, and his hands either busy in fumbling in his pockets, picking threads from his clothing, or in searching for the gold which he believed was concealed in the lining of his coat. His character had also undergone a radical change. From having been very frank and brave, he had become excessively timid and suspicious of every trifling circumstance. . . . His symptoms were in many respects so much like those of an ordinary attack of acute mania, and his antecedents were of such a character, that I had reason to doubt the influence of the bromide in causing them. It was found, however, that he had secreted large quantities of it in various out-of-the-way places about the house.

"His mental symptoms had now become so prominent and constant, that his friends became alarmed for their own and his safety. He had several times attempted to throw himself from the window, and had battered down a door with an axe in order to escape from some imaginary danger. Under these circumstances I recommended his committal to a lunatic asylum, and he was accordingly removed to Sanford Hall, at Flushing. Here his symptoms gradually disappeared, and in a month he returned to his home well."

In another case, a lady, melancholia with delirium was the result. The memory was destroyed; she would burst into tears without cause, thought that she was deserted by her friends, that her child was dead, etc. In another case, of a lady, similar symptoms resulted, as they did also in the instance of a gentleman. In all these cases the remedy was given in medicinal doses.

Nothing characteristic was observed in any of these cases. Since they were reported, several others have come under my notice, and, while the prevailing type of insanity has been melancholia, it has been in no respect different from forms due to very different causes.

Again, the *appetite* for stimulants or narcotics has been called, according to its character, *methomania* or *dipsomania,*

THE CAUSES OF INSANITY.

morphiomania, chloralmania, and so on. I do not regard these disturbances of the appetites as insanity, and therefore they have not been considered in this work.

Wounds and Injuries of the Head are common causes of insanity, and very slight blows may, even after long periods, result in mental derangement. Esquirol,[1] in considering this subject, says:

"Falls on the head, even during the first years of infancy, predispose to insanity, and are sometimes its exciting cause. These falls or blows on the head may precede by many years the explosion of the insanity. A child of three years fell on its head; from that time there was headache, which at puberty became more pronounced, and at the age of seventeen mania occurred. A lady riding on horseback was thrown; some months afterward she became insane. In three months she was cured, but she died two years subsequently of brain-disease."

Dr. Rush[2] says:

"A young man died in the Pennsylvania Hospital in the year 1809, who became deranged at twenty-one in consequence of a contusion on his head by a fall from a horse in the fifteenth year of his age. A Mr. —— died of madness in the same place, from an injury done to his brain, by being thrown out of his chair, between two and three years before he discovered any signs of derangement. It is remarkable that injuries show themselves more slowly in the brain than in other parts of the body. Dr. Lettsom mentions a case, in the 'Memoirs of the London Medical Society,' of a disease of the brain induced by a fall from a horse, which did not discover itself until two-and-twenty years after its occurrence."

The subject of traumatism, as a cause of insanity, has been well studied in recent times. Kafft-Ebing[3] insists with much force upon the fact that, in those cases in which the insanity is delayed in making its appearance, the injury has only acted as a predisposing cause, which requires some other factor to further develop. Schläger,[4] however, who bases his observations on forty-nine cases of traumatic insanity in five

[1] *Op. cit.*, p. 33.
[2] "Medical Inquiries and Observations upon the Diseases of the Mind," Philadelphia, 1830, p. 28.
[3] "Lehrbuch der Psychiatrie."
[4] "Zeitschrift der k. k. Gesellschaft der Aerzte zu Wien," B. xiii, 1857, p. 454.

hundred lunatics, states that, in general, the patients exhibited from the time of the injury a tendency to cerebral congestion. In my own experience, I think, I can go further and say, that not only was a tendency exhibited, but that cerebral congestion was actually present from the time the injury was received.

In an interesting paper, Dr. Kiernan,[1] of Chicago, considers the influence of traumatism in causing insanity. He arrives at the conclusions from the consideration of forty-five cases occurring in his own experience, as well as of many reported by other authors:

"First, that traumatism produces certain psychoses.

"Second, that the majority of these are unaccompanied by epilepsy.

"Third, that the majority have a tendency to end in progressive paresis.

"Fourth, that a large proportion are accompanied by depressing delusions.

"Fifth, that the majority of these latter do not exhibit any hereditary taint.

"Sixth, that, with certain modifications, Krafft-Ebing's conclusions respecting the traumatic psychoses are correct.

"Seventh, that injuries received before the age of forty are probably of more effect in producing insanity than those received subsequently.

"Eighth, that slight injuries, from the insidious nature of the changes they set up, are as much to be dreaded as, if not more than, the grave injuries.

"Ninth, that traumatic causes did not have as much influence in the production of insanity as intimated by Schläger, he finding that over eight per cent of the cases were caused by traumatism, while at the New York City Asylum for the Insane but two per cent were so caused.

"Tenth, that certain cases of insanity caused by traumatism have been well-marked, systematized delusions.

"Eleventh, that in all cases of insanity caused by traumatism a guarded prognosis should be given."

Dr. Uritz,[2] of Chicago, reports an interesting case in which, soon after a severe blow on the head received by a man of about fifty years of age, a radical change of character super-

[1] *Journal of Nervous and Mental Disease*, July, 1881, p. 445.
[2] *American Journal of Neurology and Psychiatry*, May, 1882, p. 196.

vened, which was followed by hallucinations, delirium of an exalted character, and acts of violence. Shortly afterward he committed suicide. On *post-mortem* examination, the membranes were found to be adherent to each other, to the cortex, and to the skull.

In a case, in my own experience, a boy at the age of twelve fell from a tree and struck his head. He was taken up senseless, but recovered. For a year or more, he suffered from headache, but he passed the period of puberty safely. At twenty-five, thirteen years after the injury, he became acutely maniacal, and died before the end of the third month. On *post-mortem* examination, adhesions of the membranes to the skull and to the brain were found to exist at the seat of injury, and there were other indications of inflammation and congestion.

In 1868 I examined a boy of about seven years of age, at Metuchen, in New Jersey, in consultation with Dr. Hunt, of that place. He had periodical attacks of acute mania, in which he was extremely violent and destructive. During early infancy—four years previously—he had had a severe fall, and upon consideration it was decided to trephine at the supposed seat of the injury. I performed the operation, but no fracture was found. There was, however, an abnormal degree of thickness of the skull at that place. The boy made a good recovery, and the paroxysms ceased.

In the case of a boy, aged eighteen, who had received a blow on the skull by the fall of a heavy mallet upon it eleven years previously, by which an extensive fracture, involving both the parietal and the occipital bones, epilepsy and epileptic insanity were developed. I trephined him, removing with the assistance of Professor J. T. Darby about four square inches of the skull. The paroxysms, both of convulsions and mania, ceased, but they returned six months subsequently, and he is now in a state of hopeless dementia.

A boy, eleven years of age, was brought to my clinique at the Post-Graduate Medical School, who was subject to paroxysms of acute mania, coming on at intervals of a week or ten days, during which he was extremely violent and destructive. Upon inquiry and examination it was ascertained that, when he was about five years of age, he had fallen downstairs and had struck his head severely. The scar in the scalp was still visible, being situated immediately over the left frontal eminence. He had occasionally had temporary right hemiplegia. I decided to trephine him, and on the 28th of February, 1882, I performed the operation before the class. There was no fracture, but the dura mater was thickened at that spot. The result of the operation, as regards the insanity, is yet to be seen. At this date (March 2d) he is doing well, and is quiet.

Sunstroke, though not so common a cause of insanity as is popularly supposed, produces nevertheless a tolerably large number of cases during every summer season, especially in this country. Of four hundred and twenty four cases admitted into the Illinois Eastern Hospital for the Insane during the years 1881 to 1883, thirteen were from this cause ; like traumatism, the full action of the factor may be postponed for several years. Such, at least, has been my experience. I constantly see cases in which pain in the head, inability to exert the mind, vertigo, insomnia, and disturbances of the sight exist as the consequences of sunstroke or of heat-fever for several years, and in which insanity is the ultimate result. The form in which it generally appears is that of acute mania. Occasionally it ensues immediately on the reception of the injury.

Cerebral Hæmorrhage and *other diseases* of the brain are also occasional causes. The influence of *epilepsy* and *chorea* has already been sufficiently considered.

Of other diseases, a long list might be made out, each of which is recognized as having an occasional causative relation to insanity. Among them are *phthisis, gout, rheumatism,* the various *fevers, diseases of the heart, intestinal worms,* and other *causes of reflex irritations from the abdominal organs, uterine* and *ovarian disorders,* and *syphilis.* In regard to this latter, the attempt has been made to make a distinct form of mental derangement under the designation of *syphilitic insanity,* but, as I think, without sufficient reason. I have never seen anything sufficiently characteristic in the insanity following syphilis to warrant such a differentiation. It is true that, as regards treatment, there are characterizations ; but, if we are to classify the forms of insanity according to the manner in which they should be treated, we would do very little toward a scientific nosology, and would, moreover, be acting in regard to mental diseases in a way not followed with other affections.

Masturbation and *sexual excesses* are also to be placed among the etiological factors of insanity. In young persons, their influence is often decidedly manifested. Persons of mature age do not appear to incur, except as regards paralysis, any noticeable liability to mental derangement, unless they are practiced to an inordinate extent, and then they are prob ably the symptoms of an already existing mental disease. In youth, acute mania, melancholia with stupor, or more generally hebephrenia, are produced. Sexual excesses are, however, among the most common causes of general paralysis. On this point there is no difference of opinion among writers. In my own experience I have abundant evidence of its power as a factor in producing this disease.

The occupation followed by the individual may be an exciting cause of insanity, but it is exceedingly difficult to arrive at any conclusion on this point from an examination of the tables given in the lunatic asylum reports. The mere fact that a greater number of the members of one profession than of another are reported is of no value, unless the numbers following each profession in the district from which the insane come are also given. This is an almost impossible task.

For instance, the following table is given in the report of the Illinois Eastern Hospital for the Insane for 1882 :

OCCUPATION OF THOSE ADMITTED.

OCCUPATION.	Males.	Females.	Total.
Agriculture (proprietors).............................	41	25	66
Commerce (owners)........	9	12	21
Professions (learned)...............................	14	11	25
Professions (miscellaneous)	5	6	11
Day-laborers (unskilled)..............................	90	7	97
Domestic service	..	33	33
Needlework..	..	8	8
Trades and handicrafts	59	18	77
Disreputable..........................		1	1
No occupation.......................................	16	3	19
Unknown...	9	40	49
Totals..	256	168	424

If we judged solely from these data without regard to the point referred to, we should be forced to arrive at the conclusion that "disreputable" occupations are less conducive to insanity than any other, for there is no male patient who owes his insanity to such a factor, and only one female patient.

The influence, however, of certain occupations which are in themselves of a specially unsanitary character is more distinctly recognized. Thus, workers in *lead* are liable to insanity from the absorption of the metal into the system. The forms of insanity most apt to be produced are acute mania, or some one of the varieties of melancholia. In either case there are illusions, hallucinations, and delusions, or the toxic influence may result in epileptic seizures ; or these may be combined with either of the forms of insanity mentioned.

Workers in *mercury* are very apt to suffer from insanity as a consequence of the absorption of mercury into the body. Several cases of the kind have come under my observation, occurring in manufacturers of looking-glasses and workers in fire-gilding. The mental symptoms are generally well marked. There are hallucinations and delusions, accompanied with a high degree of maniacal excitement. As in lead-insanity, epileptic convulsions may be associated with the mental derangement. Other occupations, which require exposure to the direct rays of the sun, and consequently induce a liability to sunstroke, are also exciting causes of insanity.

Exposure to morbific emanations from the earth, such as *malaria*, may also conduce to the promotion of insanity. For reasons given I cannot admit the existence of any distinctive features about the mental derangement caused by malaria, but that it does produce aberration of mind is beyond question.

The influence of malarial poisoning as a cause of insanity was pointed out by Sydenham, who refers to a particular kind of mania, which, so far from yielding to purgatives and blood-letting, is rendered worse by those agencies. It is consequent upon intermittent fevers which have lasted some time, especially those of a quartan type.

Baillarger[1] cites several cases in which intermittent fever was followed by insanity, and in which cures were accomplished by the use of antiperiodic remedies.

Griesinger,[2] in speaking of this cause of insanity, and stat-

---

[1] "Sur la folie à la suite des fievres intermittentes," *Annales médico-psychologiques*, 1843, t. iii, p. 372.

[2] "Mental Pathology and Therapeutics," *New Sydenham Society Translation*, p. 183.

ing that it is not the intermittent fever which induces the mental disorder, but the endemic cause of the fever, says that the attacks of insanity may take the place of the paroxysm of fever. These consist of violent accessions of mania, with delirium, and there may be impulses to suicide. Eventually these forms may become chronic.

Again, the insanity may not be developed till after the cessation of the paroxysms of intermittent fever, and this he says is the most common mode of origin. As he declares:

"The mental disease frequently continues as a uniform persistent chronic affection, and the symptoms of the intermittent fever are no longer observed."

Other writers on psychological medicine, and perhaps the majority, entirely ignore the relation of cause and effect existing between the malarial poison and insanity, and some of them, as for instance Dagonet, express the opinion that there is no such connection.

Extensive experience in highly malarial regions in the Western and Southern parts of the United States have proved to me in the most indubitable manner that malaria is productive of insanity. Sometimes the form is that of acute mania; sometimes morbid impulses of various kinds are excited, and, again, morbid fears; or there may be melancholia, simple, with delirium or with stupor, or hypochondriacal or hysterical mania, and these may run into dementia. I reported two or three years since an interesting case of acute mania passing into melancholia, which occurred in my experience in this city.[1]

Emanations from *sewers, dissecting - rooms, slaughter-houses*, and other places where animal and vegetable decomposition is going on, are said to be among the causes of insanity.

CHAPTER X.

THE PROGNOSIS OF INSANITY.

Two chief questions are to be considered in the discussion of the subject of the prognosis of insanity. The first of

---

[1] "Insanity of Malarial Origin," *Neurological Contributions*, No. 1, 1879, p. 55.

these relates to the life of the patient, the second to his mind.

In regard to the preservation of the life of the subject of mental alienation, the prognosis varies, other things being equal, according to the type of insanity from which the patient suffers.

Thus, uncomplicated **perceptional insanities,** whether consisting of illusions or hallucinations, are very seldom of fatal augury. If, however, they are accompanied by physical symptoms, indicating profound lesion of the optic thalamus, or other parts of the brain, such as paralysis, tremors, destruction or marked impairment of the sight, hearing, or other sense, severe pains in the head, vertigo, etc., the prognosis is much more unfavorable. But, in those cases so frequently met with, which depend upon temporary variations in the blood-supply of the perceptional ganglia, the prognosis is exceedingly favorable, provided that the patient is promptly submitted to proper medical treatment.

Intellectual Insanities.—None of these are of bad prognosis, so far as relates to the life of the affected individual. Relative to megalomania, under which name he describes intellectual monomania with exaltation, Dagonet[1] says: "Of all the forms of mental alienation, this is perhaps the one most compatible with the prolongation of existence. Examples of longevity in monomaniacs are not rare in lunatic asylums. It appears that the tranquil life which they lead there, removed as they are from every cause of excitation, and the perfect content which they have with themselves, are circumstances which favor the regular action of the organic functions."

Though of the opinion that this is too sweeping a statement, it is undeniably true that the form of insanity in question is entirely compatible with long life. *Intellectual monomania, with depression,* and the depressed form of *chronic intellectual mania* are of more unfavorable prognosis. The asthenic effect of the constant terrifying delusions under which the patient labors is prejudicial to the normal action of the organs of the body. The digestive system is very apt to suffer, and hence the basis for intercurrent diseases of the stomach, intestines, and liver is laid. Moreover, a depressed condition of the mind is not favorable to long life, the powers

[1] *Op. cit.,* p. 276.

of resistance to morbific influences being much lessened by its action.

In addition, it must be borne in mind that the tendency to suicide, which sometimes exists in these varieties of insanity, as well as in intellectual objective morbid impulses, is an element in the prognosis not to be disregarded.

Reasoning mania and *intellectual subjective morbid impulses* are without special significance as regards the life of the patient.

The **emotional insanities** vary greatly in their tendency to a fatal termination, according to the peculiar form of mental derangement which exists. Some cases of *emotional monomania* tend to suicide, as do also certain instances of *emotional morbid impulses*. Others, again, of both these varieties, have no such tendency. Aside from the suicidal factor, there is nothing in either of these species incompatible with long life.

Simple melancholia is usually not a fatal disorder. Still, as in other depressed states of the mind, the influence upon the system generally is bad.

Melancholia with delirium is a far less hopeful disease. Death may take place from exhaustion, from the supervention of some other brain-disease, from an intercurrent affection, or from suicide.

Melancholia with stupor, though scarcely having as bad a prognosis as the delirious form of melancholia, is, nevertheless, a disease which tends to shorten life, either directly or by gradually leading to secondary diseases. The same is true of *hypochondriacal melancholia*.

In *hysterical mania* the prognosis as regards life is good.

There is nothing about epidemic insanity which specially tends to death, unless the form be one in which great mental depression or suicidal tendencies prevail.

Volitional insanities, except in regard to the act of suicide, which may be perpetrated as a *volitional morbid impulse*, are entirely compatible with long life.

Of the **compound insanities**, the prognosis as regards life in acute mania is fairly good. Death, however, may take place from exhaustion, from the supervention of some other disease, or from suicide. *Periodical insanity* may also result fatally from like causes, as may likewise *circular insanity*, but the prognosis in both these forms is better than in acute mania. *Hebephrenia* and *katatonia* are of still better prognosis, but occasionally they terminate fatally from exhaustion or from some intercurrent affection.

None of the *dementias* of this group are of themselves specially detrimental to life. The condition of mere vegetative existence to which some dements reach, in which the "wear and tear" of the body is at its minimum, allows of long life. Death, when it does come, often arrives with suddenness, and life is abolished during the night, without any one being the wiser, till morning reveals a corpse instead of a living body.

The remaining affection of this group, *general paralysis*, is the most uniformly fatal of all forms of insanity. I have never known a case to recover. A few instances of apparent recovery have been reported, but many authors doubt their authenticity. Death usually occurs within three years, and frequently within a few months. Occasionally life is prolonged to five or six years, or even, in very rare instances, to double this period.

Of the **constitutional insanities**, *puerperal* and *choreic insanity* are of very favorable prognosis. If death occurs in either of these, it is from secondary causes. As to *epileptic insanity*, the prognosis is not so good, though life may be prolonged for a considerable period. *Pellagrous insanity* is of bad prognosis as regards the life of the affected person. The constitutional disease is rarely if ever cured, and eventually the patient succumbs to it. In addition, the strong tendency to suicide, which is so prominent a feature of the mental derangement accompanying pellagra, adds greatly to the liability to a fatal termination.

The second question in regard to the prognosis of insanity relates to the restoration of the insane person to a normal condition of mind.

In **perceptional insanities** the prognosis is usually good if there are no disturbing complications, such as those referred to in the early part of this chapter, and if they have arisen as the consequence of some temporary variation in the normal amount of the intra-cranial blood. The readiness with which they yield to treatment, whether medicinal or hygienic, under these circumstances, or even spontaneously disappear, are matters with which most physicians are acquainted.

Of the **intellectual insanities** the prognosis in *intellectual* *monomania with exaltation* is fairly good : about half the cases recover under suitable treatment, the remainder dying, or, what is much more likely to be the termination, degenerating into dementia. Occasionally the original symptoms continue unchanged for many years.

In *intellectual monomania, with depression*, the prognosis is not so good, about one third only recovering their normal reasoning powers. Many cases are transformed into some form of melancholia, while others again terminate in dementia. The prognosis is better when the affected individuals are young, of good constitutions, and of temperate modes of life.

In both these forms the existence of a strong hereditary tendency to insanity renders the prognosis more grave.

Chronic intellectual mania rarely terminates in the recovery of 'the normal mental condition of the patient, the tendency being toward dementia as the patient advances in years.

Reasoning mania is quite a hopeless condition. In this affection there are original defects of cerebral organization which cannot be overcome. Under the most favorable circumstances there may be for a time some improvement in the mental condition of the individual, but this is only temporary, as relapses are very certain to occur.

Intellectual subjective morbid impulses are not ordinarily of serious import, unless there is a marked degree of hereditary tendency to insanity. Under proper medical and hygienic treatment they usually disappear.

Intellectual objective morbid impulses, though not of so favorable a prognosis as the last-mentioned form, do not generally resist suitable treatment.

The **emotional insanities** are very often the result of inheritance or of a strong development of what has been called the "insane temperament." The prognosis is, therefore, in several of the forms unfavorable. In *emotional monomania* and *emotional morbid impulses* the patient, if young and favorably circumstanced, not infrequently recovers under medical and hygienic treatment. All forms of *melancholia*, especially the hypochondriacal variety, are of rather unfavorable though not hopeless prognosis. As regards *simple melancholia*, however, the prognosis is somewhat better than that of the others, but the liability to relapses is great. *Hysterical mania* is of good prognosis, so far as any individual attack is

43

concerned, but here again the tendency to recurrences is strong. *Epidemic insanity*, such as is met with at the present day, is generally curable by sound moral and hygienic treatment.

The **volitional insanities** are often the results of original defects of organization, and in such cases are quite incurable. Some instances, however, are acquired through remediable causes, and such are of hopeful augury.

Of the **compound insanities,** *acute mania* terminates in recovery in about one third of the cases, the remainder either dying or passing into secondary dementia. *Periodical insanity* often terminates in recovery, if advantage be taken of the intermission to improve the mental hygiene of the patient. It rarely terminates in spontaneous cure. *Hebephrenia* is generally of quite hopeless prognosis, and that of *circular insanity*—I have seen one case recover—is not much better. On the other hand, in *katatonia*, recovery may often be expected if there be no unfavorable complications.

Primary dementia is not, unless there is a strong hereditary tendency to insanity, a disease of a very bad prognosis. *Secondary dementia* and *senile dementia* are scarcely curable. In senile dementia, however, it is sometimes the case that the disease is produced in a comparatively young person by some external cause, in which case a cure may occasionally be effected.

In *general paralysis* the remissions which occur are sometimes so long as to excite the idea of a cure, but such cases are exceedingly rare, and death is, as we have seen, the termination to be expected.

Of the **constitutional insanities,** *epileptic insanity* and *pellagrous insanity* are quite incurable in the great majority of cases. On the other hand, *puerperal* and *choreic insanity* usually terminate in recovery. A few general observations relative to the prognosis in insanity may well conclude this chapter.

In all cases of insanity there is a certain liability to relapses, and hence the mere fact of recovery in any individual attack affords no security against the recurrence of the disease, either in its original or in some other form. Thus it is stated by Dr. Ray,[1] in a paper read before the Philadelphia

---

[1] "Recoveries from Mental Disease," *The Alienist and Neurologist,* April, 1880, p. 136.

College of Physicians, that at the Pennsylvania Hospital for the Insane, "one man was admitted on the twenty-second attack, and one woman on the thirty-third ; six men and six women on the tenth attack ; ninety-four persons on the fifth attack, and one hundred and seventy-two on the fourth." Dr. Ray then quotes Dr. Kirkbride as follows :

" When an individual suffering from insanity is relieved from all indications of mental unsoundness, returns to his home and family without any developed eccentricity, resumes his ordinary relations to society, attends to his business with his usual ability and intelligence for a year, or even a much less period, we have no hesitation in recording such a case as 'cured,' without any reference to the future, about which we can know nothing. We have no power to insure any case, or to say that there will never be another attack. We have no right to assert that a combination of circumstances like that which produced the first may not cause another ; that ill-health, and commercial revolutions, and family sorrows, and the many other causes that may have originally developed the disorder, may not again bring on a return of the same symptoms, just as they may produce them in one who has never had an attack of the kind. Five thousand six hundred and ninety-five of those received here never had an attack before. Whatever induced the disease in them certainly may induce it in those who have already suffered from the same malady, for we cannot expect one attack of insanity to act as a prophylactic, and, like measles or small-pox, to give immunity for the future. But this new attack is no evidence that the patient was not cured of the previous one. If the patient, then, is well in the sense in which he is considered well from an attack of typhoid fever, or dysentery, or rheumatism, or a score of other maladies, when another attack is developed, it is as much a new case, and the recovery is a cure, as much as it would be if he suffered from any other form of illness, and it ought to be so recorded."

But, with all due respect for the eminent Superintendent of the Pennsylvania Hospital for the Insane, it appears to me that this is not the proper way of putting the question. No one contends that insanity acts as a prophylactic against a second attack, but it is asserted that the existence of one attack renders the individual more prone to another than he would be if he had never had the first. Would Dr. Kirkbride hold that his "five thousand six hundred and ninety-five" virgin cases, if all cured and discharged from the asylum, are not more liable to become insane than "five thousand six hundred and ninety-five" persons who have never been insane? Is it not true that these "five thousand six hundred and ninety-five" cured lunatics are more liable to second attacks of mental derangement than the same number of persons who have had "typhoid fever, or dysentery, or rheumatism, or a score of other maladies"? Was there ever a man who had twenty-two attacks of typhoid fever, or a woman thirty-three attacks of dysentery?

The fact is, that one attack of insanity predisposes the patient to another. The predisposition may never be required to act, but the subject of it is always in danger. In some forms this predisposition is not great; in others it probably will be influential in producing another accession, either from the operation of strong exciting causes or of others scarcely perceptible—factors which a person with a flawless clinical history would be able to resist.

But there is another point. The statistics of insanity are almost entirely derived from the records of lunatic asylums. For the future, owing to the growing disposition among physicians to treat at home many cases of insanity which formerly would have been sent to the asylum, this state of things is likely to be changed. The fact, however, has led to a curious result.

Dr. Pliny Earle,[1] Superintendent of the Northampton (Massachusetts) Hospital for the Insane, perceiving that the proportion of cured cases of insanity is less now than it was fifty years ago, inquired into the personal histories of twenty-five cases that were discharged as cured from the Worcester Asylum in Massachusetts. Each case was sought out, and the history before and after the discharge as "cured" was ascertained with all desirable minuteness. The conclusions established were as follow:

"1. The twenty-five persons were discharged *recovered* from the hospital forty-eight times, contributing forty-eight recoveries to the statistics of insanity.

"2. The five persons who died in the hospital had been

---

[1] "Subsequent History of Twenty-five Persons reported recovered from Insanity in 1843," and "The Curability of Insanity *vs.* Recoveries from Mental Disease," *The Alienist and Neurologist*, January, 1880, pp. 64, 82.

discharged *recovered* fifteen times, an average of three recoveries to each person.

"3. Of all the hitherto published representations of the curability of insanity, the most unfavorable are those of Dr. Thurnan, who based a general formula upon the actual results in 244 persons (treated at the York, England, retreat) whose history he had traced until death.

"'In round numbers, then,' said he, 'of ten persons attacked with insanity, five recover and five die sooner or later during the attack. Of the five who recover, not more than two remain well during the rest of their lives ; the other three sustain subsequent attacks, during which at least two of them die.'"

Dr. Earle states other points of interest, for which I must refer the reader to the original paper. He then says :

"As so many [fifteen] are still living, it is impossible to say what will be the final result in regard to the number dying insane. But already five have died insane at the hospitals, and two have died insane at home, making a total of seven. Two others are at almshouses, both having for a long period been incurably insane (they will undoubtedly die so), and one has died at home, 'who was never well (sane) but a few months at a time.'"

And Dr. Earle adds, "Can our statisticians, philanthropists, and statesmen, longer be surprised that the hospitals do not put a stop to insanity ?"

But, in the second paper in the same journal to which I have referred, Dr. Earle gives some data which are still more remarkable, and which are as follow :

"The total recoveries of the five persons at Frankford are *fifty-two*.

"At the Hartford Retreat, five persons have been reported recovered, as follow : one, fourteen times ; another, thirteen ; a third, nine ; a fourth, nine ; and a fifth, nine. Total recoveries of the five persons, *fifty-four*.

"At the Bloomingdale Asylum, as long ago as the year 1845, five men had been reported as recovered : one of them, seventeen times ; another, thirteen ; a third, twelve ; a fourth, eleven ; and a fifth, ten. Total recoveries of the five, *fifty-nine*.

"At the same institution, at the same time, five women have been reported recovered : one, twenty times [in a note it is stated that this woman has since increased her recoveries to forty-six]; another, nineteen; the third, seventeen; the fourth, thirteen; and the fifth, twelve. Total recoveries of the five, *eighty-one* [*one hundred and seven*].

"At the Worcester Hospital, five men have been discharged recovered: one of them, fourteen times; another, fourteen; the third, twelve; the fourth, nine; and the fifth, nine. Total recoveries of the five, *fifty-eight*.

"At the same institution, five women have been discharged recovered: one of them, twenty-two times; another, sixteen; the third, fifteen; the fourth, fourteen; and the fifth, eleven. Total recoveries of the five, *seventy-eight*.

"Uniting these two sex-groups of Worcester patients, and taking the highest five of them, one recovered twenty-two times; another, sixteen; the third, fifteen; the fourth, fourteen; and the fifth, fourteen. Total recoveries of the five, *eighty-one.*

"At the New Hampshire Asylum at Concord, even among the twenty-seven patients discharged recovered in the official year 1878-'79, there were five the number of whose recoveries has been: one of them, thirty-six times; another, ten; the third, nine; the fourth, five; and the fifth, three. Total recoveries of the five, *sixty-three.* The number of recoveries of these five persons is larger by eleven than that at Frankford. But, of all the patients ever treated at Concord, the highest *five* were as follow: one recovered thirty-seven times; another, sixteen; the third, eleven; the fourth, ten; and the fifth, ten. Total recoveries of the five, *eighty-four.*"

Dr. Earle then goes on to point out that, at the Concord Asylum, *ten* persons recovered a total of one hundred and twenty times, or an average of twelve recoveries to each. At Bloomingdale ten patients recovered one hundred and twenty-two times, and at Worcester one hundred and thirty-six times, an average of over thirteen recoveries to each patient.

These data, by an alienist who confessedly stands at the very head of the insane asylum superintendents, are sufficient to destroy the little vestige of confidence existing in regard to asylum statistics. Well might a member of the New England Psychological Association, at the meeting before which Dr. Earle's paper [1] was read, say that "he thought something

[1] *The Alienist and Neurologist*, April, 1880, p. 258.

should be said to counteract the evil effect which such a showing would have upon the public."

But what can be said ? Dr. Ray, who, in previous papers published originally many years ago,[1] had investigated some of the points connected with asylum statistics, in a paper[2] from which I have already quoted, and which was intended as in some measure an answer to Dr. Earle, concludes:

" I. Those qualities of temperament which lead men to unduly magnify their achievements are as common at one time as another.

" II. The practice of reporting cases instead of persons has not been confined to any particular period, and, therefore, while it may vitiate our estimate of the curability of insanity, it cannot make the proportion of recoveries larger or smaller at one period than at another.

" III. Cases marked by high excitement entered our hospitals in a larger proportion to those of an opposite character fifty years ago than they do now.

" IV. Under the influence of highly civilized life, the conservative powers of the constitution have somewhat depreciated, and to that extent have impaired the curability of insanity.

" V. During the last fifty years, cerebral affections, in which insanity is only an incident, have been steadily increasing, and thus diminishing the proportion of recoveries."

This does not make it any better for the statistics, which, according to Dr. Ray, are as bad now as they have ever been.

It really looks as though cases of circular insanity and of periodical mania are reported as cured every time the patient has an intermission. Just as though a person with a tertian ague should be reported as cured fifteen times in one month, although he has had fifteen paroxysms.

But there is one factor to which in the body of his paper Dr. Ray alludes, and that is the appearance of general paralysis within little more than the last thirty years. Previous to that time this fatal disease was unknown to American physicians. It did not exist in the country, for " Dr. Bell, who first observed it in Europe in 1845 [and who certainly was ac-

---

[1] "Statistics of Insanity," and "Doubtful Recoveries," "Contributions to Mental Pathology," Boston, 1873, pp. 66, 121.

[2] "Recoveries from Mental Disease," *The Alienist and Neurologist*, April, 1880, p. 141.

quainted with the descriptions of it made twenty years previously by Calmeil and others], satisfied himself after the
most thorough examination of the case-books of the McLean
Asylum, that up to that period no instance of it had been
observed in that institution, though since then it has been
common enough."

The development of this uniformly fatal disease within
the time mentioned has, of course, had an influence in rendering the mortality and the incurable cases greater in the
asylums than at former periods.

But, after all, the prognosis of insanity cannot, even under
a system of entirely reliable statistics, be deduced from the
records of lunatic asylums, and this for the reason that the
most curable forms are not sent to asylums. What physician,
for instance, would think of sending to such an institution a
patient who had nothing but a hallucination of sight or hearing under certain circumstances, or one with intellectual subjective morbid impulses, or one with morbid fears (emotional
monomania), or with most of the forms of emotional morbid
impulses, or many of the cases of hypochondria, or of hysterical mania, or of volitional morbid impulses, or of paralysis
of the will, or of puerperal or choreic insanity ?

The subjects of most of these forms are at all times competent to attend to their ordinary business, and they do attend to it. Nevertheless, their minds are deranged. Such
cases are largely of favorable prognosis, and, as they do not
enter asylums, these latter are deprived of the benefit of
counting cases that would legitimately improve their statistics ; whereas they receive a large proportion of the chronic,
the very severe, and the incurable cases.

The prognosis of insanity, as deduced from private practice, is, therefore, taking all these points into consideration, a
very different thing, more reliable and more hopeful than that
of the asylums generally.

CHAPTER XI.

THE DIAGNOSIS OF INSANITY.

THERE is no point connected with the subject of insanity which is of more importance than that of its diagnosis. On the answer which the physician may give to the question, "Is the person insane?" depends often not only the liberty of the individual, his right to his property, his ability to make a will or a contract, but even life itself. Heretofore physicians have frequently allowed legislative bodies and courts to tell them what insanity is. They have confounded insanity with irresponsibility, whereas many of the insane are wholly or in part accountable for their acts, while many who are regarded as sane are not accountable.

Of course it is entirely right and proper that there should be an unyielding line to separate legal sanity from legal insanity, and no better one than that based upon a knowledge of the nature and consequences of an act, and that it is or is not a violation of law, can be devised. Any one possessed of this knowledge is legally sane, and legally responsible for his acts.

But when it comes to the science of the matter the thing is very different. As I have defined insanity in a previous chapter, it consists of "a manifestation of disease of the brain, characterized by a general or partial derangement of one or more faculties of the mind, and in which, while consciousness is not abolished, mental freedom is weakened, perverted, or destroyed." An intellectual subjective morbid impulse, by which a person—as, for instance, the young lady whose case is given on page 383—is compelled to repeat mentally over and over again certain words, or who, like Professor Ball's patient (page 388), could not get rid of a ridiculous idea, is certainly insanity. "One or more faculties of the mind" are deranged, and "mental freedom is weakened, perverted, or destroyed"; but a person the subject of such derangement is not insane according to the legal standard, and ought to be regarded as fully responsible for any crime he or she may commit.

Again, take the instance of the patient whose case is detailed on page 527 as an instance of paralysis of the will. Such a person clearly comes within the definition of insanity, and yet it would be absurd to regard a person as irresponsible for a violation of law, simply because he is unable to determine which shoe to remove first.

In former times the idea of a lunatic was very different among physicians, lawyers, and laymen, from what it is now. There was entire uniformity on the subject, for no one was considered insane who was not a raving maniac, a person who did not know the nature and consequences of his acts. But science has advanced more rapidly than law, and many varieties of insanity are now known to exist which, when Blackstone wrote, were not regarded as departures from the ordinary standard of sound mental health. We know that the smallest deviation from the normal state of any organ of the body impairs to some extent the functions of that organ, and consequently deranges the physical health of the individual. A small fraction of a grain of tartarized antimony taken into the stomach excites nausea, and perceptibly disturbs the system generally. The hundredth of a grain of atropia dropped into the eye destroys for hours the clearness of vision. In both of these instances there is, for the time being, bodily disease. Why, then, should the brain form any exception to the other organs, and why should not slight deviations from its normal mode of action be regarded as instances of mental disease? They are just as much evidences of brain disorder as pus in the urine is evidence of disorder of some portion of the genito-urinary system.

It is from this stand-point—the purely medical one—irrespective of what parliaments and legislatures and courts have decided, that the subject of the diagnosis of insanity will be considered in this work. The medico-legal relations of mental derangement belong entirely to the domain of medical jurisprudence.

In beginning the examination of a person alleged to be insane, the full clinical history should, if possible, be obtained, and no point in his antecedents is altogether unworthy of notice. Inquiry should especially be made relative to the matter of hereditary tendency, the diseases the patient may have had, especially in regard to those of the brain and nervous system generally. The fact of a previous attack of insanity is an important point.

Then the occupation, habits, mode of life, natural character, and disposition should be ascertained, and all possible data in regard to the existing accession, the time of its occurrence, the premonitory symptoms, its mode of development, and present symptoms, especially as to sleep, should be derived from some sensible person who has been in intimate relations with the patient.

Then the subject himself should be carefully examined. Efforts should be made to gain his confidence, and such questions should be put to him—guardedly, if necessary—as the previous information may suggest as most likely to cause him to disclose the present working of his mind. If the patient be an educated person, the physician will require not only a knowledge of medicine, but an acquaintance with the philosophy of the human mind, in order to conduct his examination with skill, and yet at the same time to acquire a proper degree of ascendency over the person whose mental status he proposes to investigate. Many lunatics are shrewd, intelligent, and ready to take advantage of any one whose inferiority to themselves they think they detect. The more extensive and thorough is the general knowledge of the physician, the more readily will he obtain the influence over the patient which is so necessary to a complete examination. It is usually no very difficult task to get a lunatic to speak of his delusions, but sometimes he conceals them with a degree of obstinacy difficult to overcome. Of course, in many cases there is not the slightest difficulty in determining the insanity of a person alleged to be of unsound mind. His restlessness, gestures, play of his countenance, incoherence, mental excitement, extreme loquaciousness, betray him at once, and a lengthened examination is not necessary.

But in more doubtful cases, the perceptions, the emotions, the intellect, and the will, should all be examined into with thoroughness and exactness. The existence or non-existence of illusions or hallucinations ; the sluggishness, hyper-activity, or incongruousness of the feelings ; the degree of intelligence, the power of the judgment, and especially of the memory, should be tested ; the ability to sustain a continuous line of thought should be ascertained ; his appreciation of his surroundings, of his position in life, of his means, his whereabouts, the object of his visit, and the character of the opinions he expresses and of the feelings he reveals, should be the subjects of inquiry. In short, nothing should be omitted which may be necessary to make the physician acquainted with the previous mental organization and present state of mind of the individual he is examining.

By an inspection of the body and its actions a great deal of valuable information can be obtained, and it is all the more useful because it is often of such a character as cannot be concealed or assumed.

First of all comes the *countenance*. Here the expression, as regards joy, or sadness, or stolidity, the play of the facial muscles, the movements of the eyes, the motions of the lips, the stability of the tongue when it is protruded, the presence or absence of fibrillary contractions of its muscles, the condition of the pupils as regards motility to the stimulus of light, their permanent condition of contraction or dilatation, their equality or inequality, the presence or absence of ptosis or diplopia, are all matters of importance.

Then the function of *speech* is capable of affording valuable indications. The character of the articulation, the ability to pronounce words with lingual or labial consonants with ease and accuracy, the degree of effort which it is necessary to make in order to articulate difficult words, the misplacing of words in a sentence, the omission of their final syllables, their clumsy pronunciation, the slurring over of words or syllables, the forgetfulness of words, are points in regard to which the examination cannot be too minute.

The *gestures* and *movements* generally which the patient may make, the degree of mobility, the sluggish condition of the body, the presence or absence of cataleptic phenomena, the actions as regards propriety and decency, the presence or absence of tremor or paralysis of any part of the body, the degree of readiness with which he responds to directions or requests to rise or sit down, to walk or to cease walking, or to put out his tongue, the position in which he holds his head—whether inclined forward in an attitude of weakness, indicating dementia or general paralysis, or thrown back in response to emotions of pride or greatness—are all to be observed.

The gestures which the feelings or passions of the patient may prompt him to make are always indications of great importance as showing the amount of power which he possesses over the expression of his passions. A man who exhibits every passing feeling which he may have, and exhibits it as he may do by an exaggerated or misplaced or incongruous gesture or action, affords some evidence of mental aberration.

The woman with erotomania puts on languishing airs, and makes amorous advances to any man she may meet. The subject of religious monomania falls down on his knees and prays without regard to the fitness of the occasion or the attendant circumstances. The general paralytic, with his delusions of greatness, speaks in a loud tone, struts about the room elevated to his extreme height, strikes his inflated chest to exhibit his strength and endurance, shows his muscular development, etc. The melancholic groans and sobs, wrings his hands, hides his face in order to conceal his tears, refuses to speak, or answers slowly in monosyllables and with evident reluctance.

Relative to the *state of the viscera*, the most important points are connected with the stomach and bowels and bladder. Dyspepsia, want of appetite, constipation, are often present. There may be paralysis of the bladder or its sphincter, or both. In connection with hypochondria, there may be various abnormal sensations in the thoracic, abdominal, or pelvic viscera, to which the attention of the patient is constantly directed, and to which he is anxious to attract the notice of the physician. The condition of the spinal cord and the evidences of its derangement which are supplied by the state of sensibility and motility should be carefully investigated.

The physician may be required to investigate a case in which it is suspected that the individual is feigning insanity. Persons have done this so effectually that they have succeeded in imposing on the superintendents of lunatic asylums, and in being treated as raving maniacs, the object being to observe the system upon which the institutions were managed. A very little intelligence and acquaintance with the phenomena of insanity will enable an impostor to deceive the ordinary average superintendent, who asks a few questions, and, getting incoherent answers and observing an agitated demeanor, jumps at the willing conclusion that he has a lunatic before him. There are superintendents and other medical officers of asylums, however, who, not boasting that they have never made mistakes, are nevertheless difficult persons to deceive by so transparent a fraud as that to which I have alluded, though no one, no matter how skilful an alienist he may be, is beyond the point of being imposed upon for a short time by persons assuming to have certain forms of mental derangement. An individual may tell his physician, for instance, that he has a pain in his great-toe, and will apparently walk with difficulty, and it will be impossible for his medical adviser to determine at the moment whether he has or not. But if he has the opportunity for observation, and he has reasons for suspecting that the patient may have an object in attempting to deceive him, he will probably find out very shortly whether or not he is telling the truth. He will watch him when the man thinks he is not observed, and will ascertain whether or not he walks lame; he will find out whether or not his prescriptions have been used, or his directions not to walk observed. It is almost certain that in a short time any fraud would, under these circumstances, be detected.

So it is with many forms of fraudulent insanity. The existence of illusions and hallucinations may be feigned, as may also all forms of monomania and morbid impulses, all forms of volitional insanity, and several of those of emotional and compound insanities, and the detection of the imposture would be difficult if not impossible at once. If a man says he believes he is the Governor of the State of New York, and acts in accordance with his belief within the limits of his intelligence and power, who can say that he does not believe what he says he does? If opportunity be afforded for watching him, and he is assuming a delusion which he does not entertain, it is quite certain that he will by some incongruous or inconsistent speech or act betray himself. And so of all such fraudulent assumptions, the lack of uniformity and consistency will inevitably be exhibited in time.

If the variety of insanity feigned be of some form characterized by excitement of mind and body, as acute mania, for instance, the performer is almost certain to overact his part. Moreover, a little observation will catch him at times when he does not know that he is watched, and questions put to him suddenly will often take him unawares and receive a rational answer. Waking him suddenly will often so surprise his mind that for an instant he forgets his rôle.

And time here, as in the other instances cited, will leave no doubt as to the real state of the case. No man can consistently play the part of a lunatic for any considerable period; exposure is certain to result. For these reasons, in all cases in which there is some powerful reason which may be an incentive to the assumption of insanity, the physician, if he has any doubt in regard to the matter, after a first examination, should decline to express a definite opinion unless additional opportunities at long intervals be afforded him for making other observations. It often happens that insanity is feigned by persons accused of crime. In such cases there is, of course, the strongest incentive to deceive, but it is believed that no case of the kind can be successfully imposed upon the skilled physician with time and opportunity at his command.[1]

For the purpose of accomplishing certain objects, lunatics sometimes feign another form of insanity from that with which they are affected. This is especially apt to be the case with chronic lunatics, or those who possess original defects of cerebral organization, such as the reasoning maniacs. There is reason for believing that Guiteau, who belonged to this class, feigned a different type of mental aberration from that with which he was born.

In regard to the special varieties of insanity embraced in the classification forming the basis of the present work, it is scarcely possible for errors of diagnosis to be made in the differentiation of one from the other, if the phenomena of such be carefully studied, except as regards a very few of the forms. These I propose now to consider in their diagnostic relations :

It is possible to confound *intellectual monomania of the exalted* form with general paralysis, but a consideration of the facts that the physical symptoms of the latter disease are wanting in the other will prevent any misapprehension. Attention, therefore, should not be concentrated on the mental phenomena, but the pupil, the motility of the face, the articulation, the ophthalmoscopic appearances, the presence or absence of the sense of smell, the gait, should all be the subjects of minute examination.

Intellectual monomania with depression is liable to be confounded with simple melancholia, but the presence of delusions in the first named will suffice to make the diagnosis clear. Moreover, the facts that no matter of how logically

[1] The full consideration of this question belongs more to the department of medical jurisprudence than to a work of the character of the present. The reader is, therefore, referred to the treatises on that branch of science for more complete information on the subject. The works of Wharton and Stillé, Legrand du Saulle, and the " Étude médico-légale sur la simulation de la folie," par Laurent, Paris, 1866, will give all requisite information.

depressing a character the delusions may be, the effect upon the emotions of the patient is not as intense as it should be if they were true, will suffice to distinguish it from all forms of melancholia. The patient seems as though he did not himself fully believe in the truth of his delusions.

In *chronic intellectual mania* there are also delusions, but they are variable to a greater or less extent, and the delirium is usually of a more marked form.

In *reasoning mania* the physician will often require all his acumen and knowledge, as well as time and further opportunities for observation, before he can venture to pronounce a decided opinion. Here the clinical history of the case is of especial advantage.

Hysterical mania presents very few difficulties, if a full clinical history can be obtained. The patients, however, sometimes exercise all their powers of control in order to conceal abnormal manifestations, and again, feign symptoms which they do not possess. They are, nevertheless, easily thrown off their guard.

In the diagnosis of *periodical insanity* and *circular insanity*, time is required to elucidate the character of the mental aberration. Here, again, data in regard to previous accessions will be of great value.

Primary dementia may be mistaken for general paralysis, and in the earliest stages it may for a time be impossible to make the discrimination between the two conditions. But this uncertainty cannot be of long duration, for the symptoms peculiar to either disease are sharp enough to enable a differential diagnosis to be made. It is scarcely possible to confound *general paralysis* with any other form of insanity, but it may be under certain circumstances mistaken for other nervous affections not characterized by mental derangement.

Thus, without very careful inquiry and examination, it might be confounded with certain cases of *cerebral hæmorrhage*, in which there are mental enfeeblement, difficulty of articulation, and inequality of the pupils, as well as more or less paralysis. But the difference in the mental symptoms as well as the mode of onset will enable the physician to diagnosticate the two conditions. There is, however, in old cases of cerebral hæmorrhage sometimes a condition of dementia combined with paralysis very difficult to distinguish from the latter stage of general paralysis.

Chronic alcoholic intoxication, with its tremor, paresis, and mental derangement, presents some features analogous with those of general paralysis; but the prompt disappearance of the phenomena in the former affection as soon as the alcoholic potations are suspended soon indicates the difference.

Progressive muscular atrophy, when it affects the muscles of the face and tongue, presents at first sight phenomena very much like those of general paralysis. Moreover, the troubles of articulation in the two affections are very similar. In an intermission of general paralysis, and in a case without clinical history, and in the early stage, a mistake might readily be made. A little time, however, will serve to rectify the error; and, when general paralysis is in its active state, a failure to diagnosticate the two conditions is scarcely possible. The presence of mental symptoms in the one and their absence in the other, and the oculo-pupillary phenomena of general paralysis, will be sufficient for the purpose.

In *glosso-labio-laryngeal paralysis*, under like circumstances, a mistake may equally readily be made, or general paralysis with a remission or intermission of the mental symptoms may be mistaken for the former disease. In a case which came to my clinique at the New York Post-Graduate Medical School, and which was said to be one of general paralysis, I could detect no mental aberration and no oculo-pupillary symptoms. There were fibrillary movements in the tongue, defective articulation, and the peculiar tremulous movements of the lips met with in both diseases. I hesitated, therefore, to pronounce it one of general paralysis. But two or three days afterward, when the patient returned, there was not only inequality of the pupils in a marked degree but decided mental exaltation. Since then it has several times happened that the pupils were perfectly equal in size, and reacted normally to light.

A few words in conclusion are perhaps necessary in regard to the distinction which sometimes has to be drawn between the condition known as *heat of passion* and certain states known as *transitory mania*, but which have been described in this work under the heads of morbid impulses of various kinds and epileptic insanity.

An act performed in the heat of passion is one prompted by an emotion which for the moment controls the will, the in-

44

tellect being temporarily overpowered by its force. It is an act, therefore, performed without reflection. The passions are, in the normal condition of the individual, more or less under the control of the intellect and the will, and the power of checking their manifestations is capable of being greatly increased by self-discipline. Some persons hold their passions in entire subjugation, others are led away by very slight emotional disturbances. The law recognizes the natural weakness of man in this respect, and wisely discriminates between acts done after due reflection and those committed in the midst of passionate excitement.

The acts performed during heat of passion may in their more obvious aspects, and when viewed isolatedly, resemble those done during the manifestation of some one of the forms of insanity mentioned. But they are so only as regards the acts themselves. Thus, a person entering a room at the very moment when one man was in the act of shooting another, would be unable to tell whether the homicide was done in the heat of passion or under the influence of insanity ; he would be equally unable to say whether it was committed with malice aforethought or in self-defence. The act, therefore, by itself, can teach us nothing. We must look to the attending circumstances and to the antecedents of the perpetrator for the facts which are to enlighten us as to the state of mind of the actor.

In the first place, a crime committed during heat of passion is the direct consequence of a motive, of which the passion is the first result and the act of violence the culmination. It is the direct logical consequence of the motive. Heat of passion, or anger, manifests itself by unmistakable signs with which every one is familiar. Morbid impulses have no such accompaniments, the subjects of them evincing none of the furious excitement of mind and of body characteristic of rage in its most intense form ; and, though in the paroxysms of epileptic insanity there is present a series of phenomena similar to those attendant upon furious anger, the absence of motive and the existence of unconsciousness of the act, as well as the previous history of the patient, will suffice to discriminate between what he may do and what the person previously angry from an obvious cause may do.

It is, therefore, by a study of the attendant circumstances, and by an inquiry into the previous history of the perpetrator of a criminal or violent act, that the distinction between such an act and one committed under the influence of any form of insanity is to be made.

CHAPTER XII.

THE PATHOLOGY AND MORBID ANATOMY OF INSANITY.

As constituting the basis of many of the forms of insanity, and as themselves being one of the classes of mental derangement described in this work, I thought it expedient, for the more thorough elucidation of the subject, to consider the pathology and morbid anatomy of illusions and hallucinations in conjunction with the symptomatology of these affections. It will only, therefore, be necessary in the present connection to prosecute the inquiry so far as concerns the remaining groups.

Although these are five in number, they may properly be reduced to three—the intellectual, the emotional, and the volitional insanities—for the compound and constitutional groups, though necessary in a classification for the study of symptoms, are in reality composed of combinations in varying proportions of the phenomena of the three groups mentioned, with certain peculiarities in some instances which can receive such special considerations as may be required.

The part of the encephalic mass with which we have most to concern ourselves in the study of the pathology and morbid anatomy of insanity is the cerebrum, and the portion of that organ to which our inquiries must especially be directed is the cortex. From their proximity to and intimate anatomical relations with the cortex, the membranes are also of importance, but this importance is quite secondary to that of the structure with which they are in immediate connection.

We have seen, in the earlier chapters of this work, that there is scarcely a doubt that the centres for intellect, emotion, and will, are seated in the cerebral cortex. It is equally certain, therefore, that derangements of either of these categories of mental faculties are the results of lesions perceptible to our means of research, or imperceptible to all the instruments of precision we can bring to bear. But whether visible or invisible, tangible or intangible, is really a matter of very little consequence, so far as the *rationale* of insanity is concerned. For it follows with all possible logical force that, if the intellect, the emotions, and the will result, as we believe they do, from the action of the gray matter of the cortex in its normal condition, the aberrations to which they are subject must be due to the action of the gray matter of the cortex in its abnormal condition.

Further than this we cannot at present go. We cannot say that this or that particular form of insanity is directly associated with lesions of any one portion of the cortex any more than we can say that the intellect is derived from this part, the emotions from that, and the will from some other. Perhaps in time we may acquire this knowledge, but we certainly do not possess it now. It is possible, in view of the researches of Luys[1] and Meynert,[2] that the superior layer of cortical cells is concerned with the intellect and the emotions, and the lowest with volition, but this cannot yet be considered as definitely established.

Beginning with the intellectual insanities, and locating their immediate patho-anatomical cause in the cortex, we have to inquire what are the morbid conditions of this part of the brain to which they can owe their origin? Although the records of morbid anatomy do not teach us as much as we might wish, we are not altogether without information on this point.

In those cases—and they comprise by far the largest proportion—of *intellectual monomania with exaltation* and *intellectual monomania with depression,* in which there are illusions and hallucinations, many instances show, on *post-mortem* examination, the evidences of disease of the optic thalamus of one or both sides, in addition to the lesions of the cortex associated with the intellectual derangement. These latter consist, in recent cases, of dilatation and a tortuous state of the blood-vessels of a greater or less part of the cortex, sometimes of the whole surface of the brain, at others of a single lobe, and again of a portion of a lobe or of even a single convolution. This condition often extends to the membranes, and these may be in patches more or less extensive, adherent to each other, to the cranium, and to the

---

[1] "Recherches sur le système nerveux cérébro-spinal," etc., Paris, 1865.

[2] *Vierteljahrschrift der Psychiatrie,* 1867, Heft i, p. 77 *et seq.*

cortex. In addition, there are often the lacunæ of the peri-vascular canals, made by the distended blood-vessels, and remaining after the contraction of these latter at death. These are found both in the gray and white matter.

These changes, which were noticed by the older writers, Foville,[1] Parchappe,[2] Fischer,[3] Ekker,[4] and others, have been confirmed by later observers, among them Griesinger,[5] Rindfleisch,[6] Tuke,[7] Luys,[8] and Voisin.[9] Sometimes there is a diffused redness extending over portions of the brain, and again there is a swelled or turgid condition of one or more of the convolutions.

Microscopically it is found that the vessels of the cortex are often obstructed by agglomerations of red corpuscles, that the lymphatic sheaths are infiltrated with fatty matter, that the smaller vessels are distended and tortuous, that minute extravasations have taken place, and that there are deformations of various kinds in the nerve-cells. Sometimes these are swollen, at others atrophied; again, they have lost to a greater or less extent their processes; and, again, they are infiltrated with fatty and other granular matter. Sometimes there is pigmentation of certain portions of the cortex.

Voisin[10] reports an instructive case, of which I give the following abstract:

L., a woman forty-one years of age, with some hereditary tendency to neurotic disturbances, and of an impressionable character, became smitten while in church with a missionary. Becoming jealous, she was angry if he spoke to any other woman, and finally accused him of sending men to her apartment to insult her. After the missionary departed to foreign regions, her fury against him increased, and she made many

---

[1] *Dictionnaire méd.-chir. pratique*, art. "Aliéné," Paris, 1829, t. i.

[2] "Recherches sur l'encephale," Paris, 1836–'42, p. 90.

[3] "Pathologisch-anatomisch Befunde im Leichen von Geisteskranken," Lucerne, 1854.

[4] "De cerebri et medullæ spinalis vasorum," Utrecht, 1853.

[5] "Mental Pathology and Therapeutics," *New Sydenham Society Translation*, p. 427.

[6] "A Text-Book of Pathological Histology," American translation, Philadelphia, 1872, p. 644.

[7] *British and Foreign Medico-Chirurgical Review*, April, 1873.

[8] "Traité clinique et pratique des maladies mentales," Paris, 1881, pp. 336, 392.

[9] "Leçons cliniques sur les maladies mentales," etc., Paris, 1883, p. 56.

[10] *Op. cit.*, p. 60.

attacks on persons in the street whom she mistook for him. Then she was arrested and placed in the Salpêtrière. It was found that her memory was good for names, things, and events; articulation normal; often spoke to herself; at times exaltations; hallucinations of sight and hearing; ideas of persecutions. Two years after admission—her mental aberration continuing—she died of typhoid fever.

The encephalon weighed 1,130 grammes. There was no atheroma of the cerebral vessels visible to the naked eye. No thickening or adhesions of the meninges, no sub-arachnoidal effusion. Cranial nerves healthy, except the eighth pair, which were softened. Bulb and protuberance normal. The most internal part of the fissure of Sylvius was covered with a thickened, tough, and opalescent arachnoid, as was also the region in front of the chiasma. The gray olfactive centre of the right sphenoidal lobe presented to the unaided sight many black points and aborizations in large numbers. The left gyrus hippocampi presented also this dotted appearance.

There was a red punctation of the left tubercular quadrigemina. In the space between the corpora geniculata externa and interna there were little lacunæ and slight depressions. A horizontal section of the left hemisphere showed that in front the gray substance was of ordinary color and thickness, but the first frontal convolution (the ascending frontal of Meynert) presented at its most interior part an abnormal appearance characterized by the existence of a general yellow tinge and of a well-defined yellow zone of the breadth of 0 m., .001, which divided the gray substance of this convolution into two very nearly equal parts. This state was found, though to a less extent, in the left second parietal convolution (first parietal of Meynert).

Throughout these altered parts the vessels were found to be larger than was normal, as were also those of the subjacent white substance.

The gray centre of the right optic thalamus was in more than a normally vascular condition, and on antero-posterior section it was seen to be very vascular. In the part immediately subjacent to the olfactive centre there was a little spot the color of lees of wine, and a corresponding depression. There was a lacuna in the middle part.

A portion of the gray substance of one of the parietal convolutions was submitted to microscopical examination, with the following results:

1. There was a large number of vessels of which the lymphatic sheaths were infiltrated with oil-globules.

2. Many vessels were gorged with red corpuscles.

3. Many cells were infiltrated with orange-yellow fat-granules.

4. There were several extravasations.

A part of the olfactive centre of the right sphenoidal lobe, where the black points existed, showed—

1. A large vessel completely gorged with red corpuscles.

2. A mass of orange-yellow hæmatine crystals.

3. A large number of dark-brown extravasations along the course of the vessels.

4. Many fatty cells.

5. Masses of hæmatoidin and hæmatin in the lymphatic wall of some of the vessels, especially at the points of bifurcation.

The examination, therefore, showed the existence of congestion of one optic thalamus and of one sphenoidal lobe, with lesions of the parietal convolutions.

The following case, from my own experience, afforded similar results:

I. L., a man aged forty-five, came to my clinique at the University of New York, in November, 1876, and several times thereafter. He had the delusion that he was about to receive a large fortune, and was in consequence in a mild state of exaltation. At the same time he had hallucinations of persons speaking to him and advising him what to do with his money when he received it. These were supposed to come from both living and dead persons. Among the former were Queen Victoria, General Grant, Victor Hugo, and the King of Sweden, the latter being the chief adviser. His physical symptoms consisted mainly of pain in the head, vertigo, and insomnia. There were no oculo-pupillary symptoms, and his articulation was normal. He talked a good deal, but without much incoherence. I diagnosticated the case as one of intellectual monomania, with exaltation.

In February, 1877, he died of dysentery, and, assisted by Dr. Charles T. Whybrew, my clinical assistant, I made the post-mortem examination. The brain only was examined.

There were no adhesions of the dura mater to the skull,

but the meninges were, at a point beginning at the middle of the right posterior central convolution and extending down to the horizontal branch of the fissure of Sylvius, agglutinated to each other and adherent to the cortex. Over the upper, middle, and lower frontal convolutions of the right frontal lobe, there were opalescent patches and sub-arachnoidal effusions. The membranes in all other regions appeared to be healthy. They were removed as carefully as was practicable, though it was impossible to avoid tearing the cortex a little at the place of adherence. A vertical section was made through both hemispheres immediately in front of the corpus callosum, and including the anterior parts of the upper, middle, and lower frontal convolutions. Numerous *puncta vasculosa* were seen, both in the gray and white substance, in the right frontal lobe, but no abnormal appearance in the left. Another section, carried through both hemispheres, an inch posterior to the first, and passing through the middle of the convolutions mentioned, showed like appearances in the gray and white substances; and a third section, carried through both hemispheres between the optic chiasm and corpora albicantia, and through the part on the right hemisphere at which the adhesions existed, showed an increased state of congestion; the puncta vasculosa were much more numerous, the cribriform state was well marked, and the gray matter of the convolutions was of a decided pink tinge.

The optic thalami were of normal appearance, as were also all other parts of the brain except those specified. Sections through the posterior regions of the parietal lobes and through the occipital lobes showed no evidences of congestion in any part.

Portions of the gray matter of the frontal and central convolutions were taken for microscopical examination.

Inspection of sections of the fresh tissue, made while it was frozen, and then colored with aniline red, showed decided enlargement and increased tortuosity of all the blood-vessels. Most of them were choked with masses of red corpuscles, and in several places the walls of the vessels had given way, and extravasations had taken place. These changes were especially noticeable in sections taken from the anterior central convolution, which appeared to be the centre from which the morbid process radiated. At the bifurcations of many of the vessels deposits of finely granulated, highly refractory matter were found, and along the course of the smaller vessels collections of crystals of hæmatoidin were scattered, and at the bifurcations they were collected in masses. In a section taken from the superior frontal convolution there were several vessels, the calibre of which was entirely filled with masses of red corpuscles.

In all the specimens there were hypertrophied or inflated cells—not in the internal layers, as described by Drs. Batty Tuke, and Rutherford, but in the external layer. These were most numerous in the sections from the central convolutions. The nuclei of these cells were surrounded with granular matter, and had lost in sharpness of outline.

There was decided proliferation of the nuclei of the neuroglia, but no other abnormal feature was observed.

All these conditions were confirmed by the examination of prepared sections, and large numbers of minute extravasations were discovered which were not seen in the fresh specimens.

In *chronic intellectual mania* like changes are detected, and as the affection advances they all become more pronounced. Degeneration of the cells of the gray matter takes place. They lose their processes, and fatty granulations and pigmentary deposits occur in large numbers. Patches of discoloration are found on the surface of the convolutions, and upon microscopical examination these are seen to consist of fragments of the vessels, masses of pigment, and extravasations. Degenerations of the vessels, atheromatous and calcareous, are also often perceived. Miliary aneurisms are not uncommon, and it is from the rupture of some of these that the extravasations are generally produced — though they are sometimes formed by the giving way of the vessels in consequence of the obstruction caused by impacted red corpuscles.

Reasoning mania being the result of congenital conditions, which, although deviating from the normal standard, are not due to existing disease, it is to the structure of the brain and of the cranium that we have to look for the evidences of the mental aberration. Hence, we should not expect to find congestion or abnormalities in the individual cells, but rather variations in the size and direction of the convolutions in the shape of the lobes, and in the development of parts of the brain, or of the organ as a whole.

There are no lesions in reasoning mania, so far as we know. As Campagne [1] says, the morbid anatomy has yet to be discovered. Moreover, as the affection is ·not one which of itself tends to death, the opportunities for making *post-mortem* examinations have been few, and these few have not been improved, mainly for the reason that until quite recently the attention of alienists has not been directed to the subject. Nevertheless, we have some data derived from the study of the crania of living reasoning maniacs, and the results of one *post-mortem* examination, that of Guiteau.

Campagne found from the measurements of the heads of the reasoning maniacs, compared with those of sane persons, lunatics, and idiots, as determined by Panchappe, that the following differences were observed:

1. That the head is smaller than that of persons of sound mind.

2. That it is smaller than that of lunatics in general.

3. That as regards size it is about equal to that of persons of weak minds.

4. That it is larger than that of idiots.

5. That the antero-posterior curve, and particularly the posterior curve of the cranium, are less than those of persons of sound mind, lunatics in general, the weak-minded, and even of idiots. It may be said that reasoning maniacs have a congenital atrophy of the posterior lobes of the brain, and that the cranium has been diminished in size to the detriment of the occipital region.

In the case of Guiteau, disregarding the lesions which indicated that he was passing into the initial stage of general paralysis, we find that he had an unsymmetrical cranium, the right side being smaller than the left, and that there was a marked flattening of the occipital region. The examination of the brain made by Drs. W. J. Morton and C. L. Dana,[2] three quarters of an hour after execution, with all the thoroughness and care of which the circumstances permitted, showed that the organ deviated in many respects from the typical standard.

Thus, it is stated that "the frontal lobes were peculiarly shaped. Looking at them from in front and above, they pre-

[1] "Traité de la manie raisonnante," Paris, 1869, p. 208.
[2] *The Journal of Nervous and Mental Diseases*, New York, July, 1882, p. 613.

sented two protruding points from which the surface sloped away in a concave curve. This pointed apex of the lobes, with the concavity of the orbital and beginning of the frontal surface, was carefully noted by all of us at the first exposure and removal of the brain."

Then, among more or less abnormal features, it is stated that the upper part of the post-central convolution was narrow and shrunken; that the right præcentral lobule was quite small; that the fusiform lobule was smaller on the left than on the right side; and that, to sum up, "the brain was marked by an unusual number of cross and secondary fissures, especially in the frontal lobes, that it was not of the confluent-fissure type, and that the convolutions on the two sides were quite asymmetrical."

It is to be regretted that microscopical examination of the fresh brain was not made, and that facilities were not at hand for accurately weighing the organ, for determining its specific gravity, and for measuring its chords and arcs, its contour and shape. As it is, however, the data obtained are sufficient to show that the brain of this man was of abnormal construction.

In regard to *intellectual subjective and objective morbid impulses*, there are no data on which to found their morbid anatomy, except such as are derived from a consideration of the symptoms observed during life. Here, the vertigo, pain in the head, and insomnia, and morbid dreams which so generally accompany them, and the fact that they frequently result from disturbances of the normal action of the brain in the way of its excessive use or emotional excitement, point to localized hyperæmia as their patho-anatomical basis. If the views of Luys and Meynert be correct, it is mainly in the upper layer of cells of the gray matter of the cortex that we should expect to find the evidences of disease. They have not yet been found, chiefly, in all probability, because they have not been looked for.

In regard to the *emotional insanities*, the remarks just made are applicable to *emotional monomania* and *emotional morbid impulses*, the seat of the lesion of which and its exact character being not definitely known. But here again the probability, from the character of the symptoms, that the latter is hyperæmia, is very great. Doubtless, however, the seat of the lesion is different from that of the intellectual forms specified.

Luys embraces intellectual manias, impulsive manias, and emotional manias in his class of localized hyperæmias of different regions of the brain, according to the phenomena manifested. If the intellect is the result of the action of one part of the brain, it may be taken as an analogous fact that the emotions come from some other part. Like reasoning is applicable to the derangements.[1]

Simple melancholia is regarded by Meynert and others as being the result of exhausted brain-action, conjoined with a deficient supply of arterial blood. Its patho-anatomical basis is from this point of view anæmia, and this state is in uncomplicated cases that which might reasonably be supposed to exist from a study of the phenomena, mental and somatic, which characterize the disease. But in *melancholia with delirium*, while there may be an anæmic condition of some parts of the brain, there is quite certainly a congested state of others. The researches of Voisin[2] abundantly establish this point, and he has been able, in certain cases with impulsions to suicide, to locate the morbid centre with sufficient exactness.

Thus, in the case of a woman, Gris—, who was affected with melancholia, with incessant impulsions to suicide, and who, to accomplish her purpose, not only starved herself but stuffed her mouth with linen, he found that she carried her hand to the cortex, and that there was an elevation of the temperature of that part to the extent of two degrees above that of the axilla. She died of inanition four days after admission to the Salpêtrière, and on *post-mortem* examination the meningeal veins which run to the right and left over the internal part of the ascending frontal convolutions, the first and second parietal, and the most anterior and internal part of the occipital, were found gorged with blood, and the meninges themselves were thickened and in a hyperæmic condition. In addition, there was a serous cyst, the volume of a small apple, which rested on the left parietal convolutions. Besides all this, an antero-posterior and horizontal section of each hemisphere,

---

[1] See the author's " Cerebral Hyperæmia the Result of Mental Strain or Emotional Disturbance," New York, 1879, read before the New York Neurological Society, November 7, 1877 ; also, "On the Effects of Excessive Intellectual Exertion," *Bellevue and Charity Hospital Reports*, New York, 1870 ; also, " A Treatise on Diseases of the Nervous System," New York, 1871, and seventh edition, 1881.

[2] " Leçons cliniques sur les maladies mentales," Paris, 1883, p. 176.

made at the depth of a centimetre, showed the existence of a reddish scarlet tinge in the most internal part of the left ascending frontal and first parietal convolutions, and of the first right parietal.

In another instance, a woman, Chaub., was melancholic, with such persistent impulsions to suicide that it was not safe to leave her alone for an instant. She had tried to hang herself, had then cut her throat, opening the larynx, and had then refused to eat, so that it was necessary to feed her through a tube. She complained of fronto-vertical pains, and the temperature was above the normal standard. She died, and the autopsy showed the existence of a marked degree of meningeal congestion in the fissure between the first frontal and ascending frontal convolutions on the surface of the first parietal, and of the contiguous regions.

These data are important, for they are applicable not only to conditions in which there are impulsions to suicide, but to morbid impulses of all kinds.

In *melancholia with stupor* there is, in the first place, a generalized passive congestion of the brain and its membranes, and this is followed, as Etoc-Demazy pointed out nearly fifty years ago, by an infiltration of serum into the hemispheres, by which the convolutions are subjected to pressure from within, and are, consequently, flattened against the cranium.

Occasionally there is also, as I have seen in several cases, subarachnoidal effusion.

Luys [1] is of the opinion that the condition is often the result of vaso-motor spasm, by which the nervous elements are deprived of their proper supply of blood.

In those cases in which there is at the same time a certain amount of sensorial aberration there is, according to Luys, a hyperæmic state of the optic thalami. Thus, a condition of stupor due to the arrest of intellectual emotional activity and volition can coexist with hallucinations of one or more of the special senses.

In *hypochondriacal mania or melancholia* the condition in the first instance is a passive congestion of some parts with active congestion of others. As this is an affection characterized by the presence of vivid illusions and hallucinations, the optic thalami are in a state of active hyperæmia. As Luys [2]

---

[1] *Op. cit.*, p. 508 *et seq.*   [2] *Op. cit.*, p. 509.

says: "We see in certain cases of hypochondria and melancholia that, while different parts of the cortex are in a state of complete repression, the central regions (the opto-striated bodies) are in a condition of very intense vascularization. This is a very significant fact, and one that demonstrates to us how in the same brain certain regions can be in a state of ischæmia and certain others be very strongly congested. Thus, there are two series of phenomena of quite different natures— one marked by excitation and the other by depression."

But, as the results of the long-continued action of these conditions, permanent alterations of the vessels (even to the extent of their obliteration), sanguineous cysts, adhesions of the meninges, softening, and morbid growths of various kinds, are apt to be produced in different parts of the brain.

Relative to the pathological anatomy of *hysterical mania*, no very definite results are at hand. The probability, however, is that the disease is the result of vaso-motor disturbances in the cerebral circulation, of the nature of both spasm and paralysis of the vessels.

In *epidemic insanity*, there have been no *post-mortem* examinations of the brain made according to the principles of modern research. It is also probably the result of vaso-motor disturbance.

The *volitional insanities* are likewise due to changes in the blood-supply of certain parts of the brain, probably in the lower layers of cortical cells. Although we have no data based upon *post-mortem* examination to support this view, analogy, however, would lead us to the belief that a volitional morbid impulse can be the result of a limited hyperæmia of one portion of the brain, just as intellectual or emotional morbid impulses can result from a like condition existing in other parts. In those cases in which the individual suddenly experiences an impulse to the perpetration of an act not dictated by an idea or an emotion, the excitation is volitional, and it doubtless results from hyperæmia of the volitional centre from vaso-motor paralysis.

In *aboulomania* or *paralysis of the will*, the usual patho-anatomical condition is probably that of vaso-motor spasm, by which the volitional centre is deprived of its due supply of blood, and hence reduced to an anæmic state; but, as the disease is not one which ever terminates fatally, there are no positive data to support this opinion. In some cases the symptoms appear to indicate the existence of cerebral hyperæmia.

As would reasonably be expected, the class of *compound insanities* exhibits great diversities in the character of the patho-anatomical results. In *acute mania* there is a general hyperæmic condition of the brain and its membranes, and the various secondary states which result therefrom. Not only is there intracranial congestion, but the scalp and the bony tissue of the cranium are similarly affected.

On attempting to raise the cranium after it has been entirely sawn through, it is often found that the dura mater has, throughout a greater or less part of its extent, become adherent to the inner surface of the cranium, and that considerable force is required to detach it from its connections. This membrane is seen to be injected, and the sinuses are usually gorged with blood. Sometimes it is adherent to the arachnoid at different places, again it is separated from this membrane by effusions of serum, and again both conditions exist. This exudation may be clear, or red from admixture with blood or its coloring matter. At times the exudation consists entirely of extravasated blood from the rupture of one or more of the over-distended vessels. The arachnoid and pia mater participate in the congested condition. The vessels are seen to be enlarged and tortuous, and there are discolored patches, some red and others opalescent, throughout their extent. Exudations in the meshes of the pia mater of serum, clear or bloody, are common occurrences, and the membranes themselves are thickened. The Pacchionian bodies are almost always enlarged and congested.

On removing the meninges, the cortex is found bathed in serum, or the membranes are adherent to it either in patches or throughout the greater part of its extent. Sometimes there are reddish patches on the surface of the convolutions, and, on section, the evidences of congestion are found in the presence of minute extravasations of blood or *punctæ vasculosæ*, or of a generally diffused reddish tinge. Occasionally certain of the convolutions appear to be swollen or distended.

Section through the white substance shows that the morbid process has extended to this tissue, there are numerous *punctæ vasculosæ*, the cribriform state is well marked, and there are vascular arborizations in different regions.

The basal ganglia and the cerebellum are also involved in

the congestive condition, and the ventricles contain more than the usual amount of fluid.

Sometimes the whole encephalon is softened, or this condition may exist only in the cortex or in other limited portions of the brain, though this may sometimes be a *post-mortem* change.

In the case of a gentleman suffering with acute mania, characterized by hallucinations of sight, hearing, and taste, delusions, high delirium, incoherence, and paroxysms of maniacal fury, during which he attempted to injure those around him, I aspirated the liver for abscess, and evacuated about eight ounces of pus. The maniacal condition, however, continued, and on the ninth day subsequently he became comatose, and on the tenth day death ensued.

The *post-mortem* examination was made by my son, Dr. G. M. Hammond,[1] in my presence, and that of Dr. P. B. Wyckoff, of this city. The dura mater was found to be firmly attached to the cranium throughout the frontal and parietal regions of both sides, and increased in thickness. Under the dura mater, spots of a grayish-white exudation were found scattered over the entire convex surface of the cerebrum. Between the arachnoid and the pia mater a considerable quantity of bluish effusion was observed, and the pia mater was adherent to the brain substance. On microscopical examination of prepared specimens, no deviation from the normal aspect was observed in the size, development, or number of the small or large cells of the gray substance of the cortex. Both the gray and white substance were permeated by great numbers of blood-vessels, all in a state of intense congestion. The duration of the attack was a little over a month.

In *periodical insanity* there are no specially characteristic features of a patho-anatomical character different from those of the form which is repeated. The complete disappearance of the accession is the strongest possible evidence in favor of the view which ascribes the seizure to disturbances in the blood-supply to the brain.

Hebephrenia, depending as it does upon arrest of development, and psychical degeneration supplemented by disturbances of the circulation of blood in the brain, should pre-

---

[1] " A Case of Acute Mania with Abscess of the Liver," by Græme M. Hammond, M. D., *Journal of Nervous and Mental Disease*, April, 1882, p. 300.

sent, on *post-mortem* examination, the characteristics of these conditions. I am not aware, however, that any patho-anatomical examinations of persons dying of the affection have been made.

Circular Insanity.—In the most recent work on the subject of this form of mental derangement, that of Ritti,[1] nothing is said relative to its patho-anatomy. In patients, however, dying during either the period of excitement or that of depression, we should expect to find the evidences of congestion, though probably in different parts of the brain. Or it may be that, in death occurring during the period of excitement, a state of hyperæmia would be found to exist, while in that taking place during the melancholic stage a spasm of the vessels causing anæmia would be discovered.

Katatonia.—*Post-mortem* examinations of the nerve-centres in this disease have been made by Kahlbaum[2] and by Kiernan,[3] assisted by Spitzka. In one case, the details of which are given by Kiernan, the dura mater was adherent to the cranium in patches ; there were firm coagula in the veins and sinuses ; the arachnoid, especially over the fissure of Sylvius, was very opaque ; the pontico-chiasmal lamina were very dense, and a false membrane was formed beneath. Epithelial granulations were present in a rudimentary condition ; the pia mater was nowhere adherent to the cortex except over the frontal lobe. The cortex was pale, and there was a decided sinking of the surface of certain gyri below the neighboring convolutions. There was a fusion of the opposite sides of the anterior cornua of the lateral ventricles. Cysts of the choroid plexus were also present.

In another case, the subarachnoid space was filled with a number of brownish flakes of a gelatinous consistency. Most of these drained away with the cerebro-spinal fluid, but a few were quite firmly adherent to the underlying pia mater. Minute blackish or dark-brown grains were disseminated through them, probably exudative products (?), cerebello-medullary lamina opaque, with whitish dense bands. Sylvian fissure slightly opaque. Along the vessels of the pia mater, minute pale-yellowish, whitish, and reddish bodies were found, which were supposed to be tuberculous. In the Sylvian fissure over

---

[1] " Traité clinique de la folie à double forme," Paris, 1883.

[2] " Die Katatonia," *op. cit.*

[3] " Katatonia," *The Alienist and Neurologist,* October, 1882, p. 558 *et seq.*

45

the island of Reil there was a fusion of the lepto-meninges. The condition of the blood-vessels is minutely described. It may be said of the veins, in general terms, that they presented all the evidences of congestion, being filled with coagula or with thrombi. The white substance generally showed numerous *punctæ vasculosæ*, all of a strikingly venous character. The arteries were in general empty, both in the white matter and in the cortex. The lining membrane of the ventricles was the seat of venous injection, and a mucoid substance covered the floor of these cavities.

The microscopical examination was made by Dr. Spitzka, and is the only one of the kind, so far as I know, on record. It is expedient, therefore, to cite it in full :

"The mucoid matter on the floor of the fourth ventricle was found to consist of an accumulation of round cells, not surpassing a red blood-corpuscle in diameter, some nucleated, others not ; all were perfectly colorless. Interspersed among them were larger elements, identical in every respect with white blood-corpuscles. Isolated bodies of an oblong shape, with a distinct nucleus and pellucid protoplasm, were noticed. All these were embedded in a granular mass, which showed a formation of imperfect fibrils. The arachnoid exudation consisted of the same matters, together with a fair proportion of red corpuscles, large flakes of pigment, and round spheres of a protein nature. The pia mater of the convexity exhibited numerous small nodules, most of which were molecular, others calcareous, and a few contained large and small poly-nucleated cells. These nodules were periadventitial, and hardly visible to the naked eye. The cortical substance of the island of Reil showed a marked increase of the nuclei of the neuroglia. The ganglionic cells, both pyramidal and fusiform, were normally contoured ; processes well developed ; protoplasm healthy, in some cases diffusely pigmented ; and nucleus round and clear. Free lymphoid bodies were accumulated in the peri-cellular spaces in prodigious numbers ; in one instance, no fewer than twenty-three of these cells could be distinguished clustering round one pyramidal nerve-cell of the third layer. Frequently the nerve-cell was altogether hidden from view by such cell-groups. In this respect, the island of Reil presented marked original differences. It was found that areas varying from a line to an inch in diameter were the seat of this appearance, while a similar larger or

smaller adjoining area was either less involved or perfectly
normal in this respect. The transition from the affected to
the healthy areas was sudden.

" The coats of all the vessels were entirely healthy, presenting no deviations from the appearance of cerebral vessels
in some subjects. The arteries were empty; the veins and
many capillary districts filled with blood-corpuscles; these
latter were individually distinct, not compressed or fused by
crowding, as has been described to be the case in the stasis
accompanying general paresis. This engorgement was most
marked in those areas in which the accumulation of lymphoid
bodies was farthest advanced. The periadventitial space was
filled with similar bodies in the case of the vessels referred to.
The same appearances in a less degree were noticed in the
operculum and the convolutions bordering the anterior part
of the great longitudinal fissure. The remainder of the cortex cerebri appeared perfectly healthy. The accumulation of
lymphoid bodies was still more marked in the nucleus len-
ticularis than in the claustrum and island of Reil. The cerebellum, olivary bodies, nuclei of the cranial nerves, corpus
striatum, thalamus, and corpora quadrigemina presented no
deviations from the normal standard."

There was also incipient sclerosis of the antero-lateral and
posterior columns of the spinal cord. From these data, Dr.
Kiernan expresses the opinion that the characteristic pathological condition of katatonia is an inertia of the vaso-motor
centres, whose consecutive injurious effects were concentrated
on the parts lying at the depth of and around the fissure of
Sylvius. Every other lesion is to be considered as secondary
or accidental.

Bearing in mind the readiness with which the cases that
have come under my observation underwent amelioration and
cure, I have no hesitation in entirely concurring in this
opinion.

Primary dementia is doubtless, in the very beginning, the
result of vaso-motor spasms and consequent cerebral anæmia.
The often sudden manner of its appearance as the result of
severe emotional disturbances, and the character of the symptoms point indubitably to this factor as the pathological
cause. But in the late stages of the disease the patho-anatomy does not probably differ essentially from that of *secondary* and *senile dementia*, and hence they can well in this

relation be considered together. Dementia may be regarded as the hopper to which nearly all forms of uncured mental derangement finally come. Hence, there is often a multiplicity of lesions, adherences, extravasations, neoplasms of various kinds, serous exudations, either diffused or encysted softening, induration, etc.

But, notwithstanding the difficulty of determining from this *embarras de richesses* the essential characteristics of dementia, some steps in advance have been taken, so that we are not altogether without definite information on the subject.

Foville [1] was one of the first, if not the very first, to notice that one of the most constant patho-anatomical features of dementia was a diminution of the size of the convolutions, and at the same time a paleness and hardness of their substance. Frequently they were flattened, as if pinched between the fingers. The fissures on the surface of the brain became wider and deeper as the convolutions became smaller, and, as the nervous substance disappeared, serum contained in the commissures of the pia mater took its place.

Marcé [2] found that in senile dementia there were atrophy of the convolutions, alterations of the nerve-cells and fibers, and alterations of the capillaries. The alterations of the nerve-cells and fibres consisted of atheromatous and fatty degenerations ; the former were seen to have lost their processes and to be covered with yellow, fatty granules, while many had entirely disappeared. Sometimes these altered cells were few, at other times there was scarcely a single one that had not undergone change.

The nerve-fibres were deformed and covered with fatty granulations. Later, the contents had disappeared, and they consisted of nothing but a knotted cylinder of an amber-yellow color. At a further stage there was nothing but the sheath, and, still later, the whole fibre had disappeared.

The internal wall of the capillaries was lined with yellow, fatty granulations, which often completely filled the calibre. Sometimes an aggregation of crystals of hæmatin helped to close the vessel.

Dementia, therefore, is characterized by atrophy, which affects both the gray and white matter. With this atrophy

[1] "Dictionnaire de médecine et chirurgie pratiques," t. i, Paris, 1829, art. "Aliénation mentale."

[2] "Recherches sur la démence sénile," *Gazette médicale de Paris*, 1863.

there is sclerosis. In fact, the condition is due to diffuse inflammation of a low form, causing the proliferation of the connective-tissue elements and the deformation and disappearance of the nerve-tissues. To the condition, the term diffused cerebral sclerosis may properly be applied. Cotard[1] has described this condition in other relations, and I[2] have considered it mainly as it occurs in infancy and in connection with other symptoms than those of a mental character.

Among the most thorough observations relative to brain atrophy as the essential patho-anatomical condition associated with dementia are those of Dr. Bucknill.[3]

The general result arrived at was, that:

"In cases of chronic mania, of dementia following mania, and of primary dementia, the amount of cerebral atrophy may generally be calculated upon by the enfeeblement of mental power. In all these forms of disease we have found some amount of atrophy, and have for the most part found this amount to correspond with the amount of mental decadence estimated with its duration. . . .

"It must not be thought that extensive atrophy is only found where the mental symptoms are solely those of impairment or loss of function. It is not inconsistent with much mental excitement or with numerous delusions; but such excitement is powerless, and the delusions are transitory and puerile."

Upon the whole, therefore, it may be considered that the essential patho-anatomical feature of dementia in all its forms—primary, after it has passed the earlier stage, secondary, and senile—is general and interstitial atrophy of the brain substance. Not only is the brain, especially the cerebrum, diminished in size, but the convolutions are changed in form as well as in volume; and it is directly to these changes— just as in progressive muscular atrophy there is a loss of muscular power—that the enfeeblement of the intelligence is due. The flashes of excitement and the childish delusions that sometimes occur are no more in comparison with normal brain-

---

[1] "Étude sur l'atrophie partielle du cerveau," Paris, 1868.

[2] "A Treatise on Diseases of the Nervous System," seventh edition, New York, 1881, chapter xii, "Diffused Cerebral Sclerosis."

[3] "The Pathology of Insanity," *British and Foreign Medico-Chirurgical Review*, January, 1855; also, "A Manual of Psychological Medicine," fourth edition, London, 1879, p. 526.

action than are the fibrillary contractions of the muscular
fibres in progressive muscular atrophy in comparison with
strong voluntary muscular efforts.

General Paralysis.—The morbid anatomy of this disease
has been more thoroughly studied than that of any other form
of insanity, and the results are on a basis of greater certainty
than can be affirmed of any other variety. From the very inception of the discovery of its existence, results of more or
less definiteness have been obtained, until now the essential
nature of the affection is scarcely a matter of any doubt.

Beginning with the naked-eye appearances, and then passing to the consideration of the results of microscopical examination, I shall endeavor to present to the reader a concise view
of what may be considered as established facts relative to the
patho-anatomy of the disease in question. In order to do this,
I shall omit the consideration of many associated conditions
which, however interesting in themselves, are not characteristic of general paralysis, and are mostly to be regarded as accidental complications.

The *scalp* and *cranium* are often found congested. In the
latter, the diploe is injected and of darker color than is normal.

On removing the calvarium the *dura mater* is seen to be
of a dark color, its vessels to be distended ; sometimes there
is an effusion of serum between it and the cranium, but more
generally it is adherent in different places, but especially in
the frontal and vertical regions. False membranes and extravasations of blood, constituting the condition known as
pachymeningitis, are present in about one fourth of the cases.
Besides these, there are occasionally other cystic growths between the dura mater and the arachnoid, and adherent to the
first-named membrane. Generally they contain blood, at
other times serum.

The *arachnoid* is thickened, discolored, congested, and
covered with opalescent or reddish patches, especially on the
frontal and parietal lobes. Sometimes there is an effusion of
serum in large quantity separating this membrane from the
pia mater. Again, they are adherent one to the other.

The *pia mater* is almost invariably thickened, congested,
and its vessels, the veins especially, enlarged and tortuous.
The consistence of the membrane is altered so that it is tough
and resisting and inelastic. Throughout its extent, but nota-

bly over the frontal and parietal lobes, there are extravasations of blood of small size, and consisting for the most part of red corpuscles and hæmatine.

Granulations first described by Boyle are met with mostly in the membrane lining the ventricles, but also on the upper surface over the convex portion of the cerebrum. They are due to a proliferation of the connective tissue of the membrane.

Adhesions of the *pia mater* to the cerebral convolutions are the most common of all the naked-eye patho-anatomical features of general paralysis. I have never seen a case of *post-mortem* examination of the brain of a general paralytic in which they were absent. They are most common over the frontal and parietal lobes, but are met with not only at the convex surface of the cerebrum, but also over the basilar surface. These adhesions exist only between the pia mater and the summits of the convolutions, and, when the membrane is stripped off, a portion of the gray tissue comes with it, leaving the surface of the brain at the points of adhesion torn, rough, and of a reddish appearance. Sometimes the adhesion affects the cortical substances only to the thickness of a sheet of letter-paper, and again nearly the entire depth of the gray matter is involved. It is never the case that the adhesions affect the gray matter of the sulci below the convolutions. The summits only are adherent to the membrane.

Dr. Crichton Browne,[1] on the basis that the six cortical layers of nerve-cells are not developed simultaneously but consecutively, and that the superior layer, perhaps, being developed first, breaks down first, or that, being the seats of a greater and more constant degree of activity, they may be more liable to suffer from irritation and hyperæmia, concludes :

"1st, that the adhesions of the pia mater to the gray matter of the brain are the most frequent and characteristic of the pathological appearances found in general paralysis of the insane ; 2d, that they are caused by a chronic adhesive inflammatory process springing out of excessive functional irritation, and proceeding to disintegration of the cerebral gray matter ; and 3d, that, speaking generally, they represent the cause and distribution of the morbid processes in which the disease essentially consists."

[1] "Notes on the Pathology of General Paralysis of the Insane," *West Riding Lunatic Asylum Medical Reports*, vol. vi, 1876, p. 170 *et seq.*

While agreeing with Dr. Browne relative to the hyper-activity of the superior layer of nerve-cells of the cortex, I think this is to be ascribed to the fact that this layer is, as Meynert and Luys have given us reason to suppose, the seat of ideation ; that during general paralysis, especially in its earlier stages, it is particularly the seat of hyperæmia, as shown by the derangement of the ideas of the patient, and that it is to this localized hyperæmia of the superior layer of cells that the adhesions with the pia mater are to be as-cribed.

Besides being the seat of adhesions, the cortex is often the subject of a *diminution of its consistency,* and of *œdema* from infiltration of serum. Sometimes it is so soft as to be readily washed away by a small stream of water falling on it.

Atrophy of the convolutions is another patho-anatomical feature occasionally met with in general paralysis, especially in those subjects of the disease who have survived its presence many years. In cases in which death occurs after what may be called acute attacks, the white substance presents the *cribri-form* state, and is the seat of numerous *punctæ vasculosæ.*

Section of the gray substance of the cortex shows that it is often the seat of discolored spots, or of a general change of hue from that which is natural to a yellowish gray or brown appearance.

To sum up the data in regard to the naked-eye appear-ances in cases of general paralysis, there are :

1. A congested condition of the scalp and cranium.

2. A similar state of the dura mater and arachnoid.

3. Increased vascularity of the pia mater, with opalescent patches.

4. Adhesions between the pia mater and the summits of certain of the convolutions.

5. Softening of the cerebral tissue.

6. Change of coloration in the cortex.

Microscopical Appearances.—Beginning with the blood-vessels, we find that the most constant lesion is an endarter-itis of the capillaries and arteries, which usually originates in the lymphatic sheath, and then extends to the proper coats of the vessel. Dr. Sankey [1] describes a twisted, or tortuous, condition of the arteries of the cortex, and the presence of a hyaline substance around the capillaries. Both these states

---

[1] "Lectures on Mental Diseases," London, 1866, p. 174.

are normal, and the latter is the peri-vascular sheath described by Robin and His.

Numerous nucleated bodies are found arranged in groups around the vessels, especially at their bifurcations. In addition, there are large quantities of red blood-corpuscles and crystals of hæmatin scattered through the gray tissue, and occasionally there is a development of new capillary blood-vessels.

Sometimes the lumen of the vessels is entirely closed by masses of red globules, and, again, their coats are the seat of dilatations of an aneurismal character. These give way, and minute extravasations of blood are the result.

Mickle[1] found, in regard to the blood-vessels of the cortex, that many contained aggregations of blood-corpuscles, by which they sometimes were completely filled, or were bulged; that there was an increase of the nuclei of the walls of the minute blood-vessels; that sometimes molecular, or pigmentary, deposits were seen in or upon their walls; that there were occasionally appearances of more or less irregular thickening or dilatation of the vascular wall; that now and then some vessels had a soft molecular appearance, and fusiform dilatation was seen; and that, more rarely, there were capillary rupture and extravasation, so that the vessels were surrounded by minute ecchymoses.

On the other hand, Spitzka[2] declares that miliary aneurisms, puriform and dissecting, must be shown to have a definite relation to the symptoms of the disease before they can be considered of any importance, that often they have been produced by faulty methods, and that he has not found a single clear appearance of the kind that would stand all tests.

Cerebral Substance.—The examination of the nerve-tissue relates to the cells, the fibres, and the connective tissue, or neuroglia.

In regard to the cells of the cortex, many undergo fatty degeneration, the nucleus becomes less distinct, and the tissue of the cell is altered by the wasting or entire disappearance of the processes. Finally, the nucleus is no longer seen, it is not even rendered visible by carmine, and the cell appears

[1] "General Paralysis of the Insane," London, 1880, p. 129.

[2] "The Psychological Pathology of Progressive Paresis," *Journal of Nervous and Mental Disease*, April, 1877, p. 277.

as an amorphous body, without any distinctive histological features.

In a communication made to the *Société médico-psychologique*, M. Luys[1] discusses the subject of the patho-anatomy of general paralysis, an affection which he regards as a diffused interstitial sclerosis of the neuroglia of the nervous centres. According to the view he announces, sclerosis acts here exactly as it does when it is the distinguishing characteristic of other affections of the nervous system, or when it involves other tissues—that is, it causes an atrophy and disappearance of the true nerve elements. In a preparation which he submitted, the cells had become bodies of vaguely pyramidal form, without distinctive morphological features.

The *nerve-fibres* of the cortex are deformed and atrophied ; they undergo fatty degeneration, and the nervine escapes into the surrounding tissues.

The *neuroglia* is probably always increased in cases of general paralysis. Rokitansky regarded this as the essential feature of the disease, and Luys, in the communication cited, advances this view with a cogency and amount of evidence that would appear to place the question beyond much doubt. The conclusions he arrives at are :

" That the lesion of general paralysis consists of a generalized hyperplasia of the connective tissue, of which the elements are infinitely developed, and that it constitutes for the nerve-tissue a condition not essentially different from that of cirrhosis of the liver. These lesions appear to have different foci of origin, according to the region invaded. Sometimes they begin in the white substance, sometimes in the gray cortical tissue, at others in the submeningeal regions, and again in some part of the spinal cord, before making their appearance in the brain. It is thus that the existence of general paralysis is sometimes first revealed by disturbances in the motor functions of the spinal cord or medulla oblongata, before there is any manifestation of brain symptoms."

The *white substance* undergoes changes similar in general character to those met with in the cortex — there are like changes in the vessels, there is a proliferation of the connective tissue, but, on account of the comparatively larger quan-

[1] " Anatomie pathologique de la paralysie générale," *Annales médico-psychologiques*, juillet, 1877, p. 106.

tity of this tissue in the white than in the gray tissue, the consistency is increased instead of being diminished.

In regard to the other parts of the brain—the island of Reil, the optic thalamus, the corpus striatum, the medulla oblongata, the pons Varolii, the cerebellum—changes similar to those which occur in the cortex are met with, though not probably to the like extent. Moreover, the nuclei of the cerebral nerves, and the nerves themselves, especially the olfactory, as Voisin has shown, undergo inflammation and softening, or sclerosis. The existence of like lesions in the posterior columns of the spinal cord, and in other anatomical regions of this centre, is also a feature of many cases.

MM. Bonnet and Poincaré[1] regard general paralysis as being primarily a vaso-motor affection, with its origin in the sympathetic system. They deny the existence of any condition of the brain which can in the least degree be assimilated to sclerosis, that the lumen, even of the smallest vessels of the cortex, is ever obscured, or that there is any defect of nutrition due to the impermeability of the vessels. They admit that many cells of the cerebrum, especially of the frontal lobes, contain fatty granulations, and that here and there are reddish-brown patches, probably consisting of extravasations of blood. These changes, however, they regard as secondary to the degenerations existing in the sympathetic ganglia. The nerve-fibres, both of the gray and white substance, they have never found altered, nor have they ever found any evidences of sclerosis in the spinal cord. These views are merely cited in outline in order to show that there is a marked difference of opinion on the subject of the patho-anatomy of general paralysis. It is scarcely necessary to say that they are not entertained by any other pathologists, so far as I am aware. It is, however, quite probable that the very initial point of general paralysis is in the sympathetic system, and that, like many other forms of insanity, it is in the beginning a vaso-motor disorder. Eventually, however, the brain lesions predominate over all others, and constitute the essential characteristics of the disease.

Epileptic Insanity.—In *post-mortem* examinations of persons dying while the subjects of epileptic insanity, the lesions met with are those which are common to simple epilepsy.

[1] "Recherches sur l'anatomie et la nature de la paralysie générale," Paris, 1876.

They may consist of morbid growths of various kinds in the brain or in the cranium, and by their contact with the brain causing irritative adhesions of the membranes to each other and to the cranium, or surface of the brain, diseases of the blood-vessels, fractures of the cranium and consequent injury of the brain, foreign bodies, such as bullets, in the brain, and almost every other possible morbid condition. Very often no lesion is found.

The immediate cause of a paroxysm is a vaso-motor disturbance either of the nature of a spasm or of a paralysis, by which, in the one case, a state of cerebral anæmia is produced, and in the other, one of cerebral hyperæmia. Probably, in those cases in which there are violent fury and excitations to acts of violence, the condition is hyperæmia, while in those characterized by a quiescent state of mind, attended with the tendency to mental automatism, intracranial anæmia exists.

In *puerperal insanity* the patho-anatomical feature is quite surely congestion, in that form which immediately succeeds child-birth, and this view is expressed by Voisin, and is sustained by the data supplied by numerous *post-mortem* examinations. In one case, that of a woman who died during her third attack, there had been religious mania, with intense excitation and incoherence. The autopsy showed the existence of many *punctæ vasculosæ*, and a hyperæmic state of the optic thalami and of all the central portions of the cerebrum. The parietal convolutions exhibited in the perivascular sheaths of their vessels numerous masses of fat-molecules and of pigment. Like aggregations were found in the optic thalami.

In other cases, the meninges of the spinal cord, as well as those of the brain, are in a congested or inflamed condition. In those cases of the disease in question which occur during or soon after the termination of nursing, an anæmic state of the brain is discovered. But, when ensuing on the sudden cessation of lactation, the symptoms indicate cerebral hyperæmia ; and such is the state found on *post-mortem* examination.

The views propounded by Sir James Simpson, and which have already been alluded to, that puerperal mania is the result of uræmic intoxication, and the opinion expressed by others that it is a septic disorder, are not sustained by the experience of those who have seen many cases of the disease. Indeed, the facility with which recovery takes place is of itself a strong argument against the correctness of either hypothesis.

Pellagrous Insanity.—Gintrac[1] says that in cases of persons dying of pellagra the brain is rarely found in a normal condition; it is frequently in a state of congestion on the surface, and often softened. The membranes are the seat of hyperæmia. Billod[2] states that no other lesions different from those found in ordinary cases of insanity are met with than a softening of the white substance of the spinal cord.

Choreic Insanity.—In the insanity which sometimes accompanies chorea, I am led by the attendant phenomena to consider the intracranial condition as one of hyperæmia, affecting mainly the ideational and psycho-motor centres. This, however, is only a hypothesis, as I am not acquainted with the results of any *post-mortem* examinations made with special reference to the state of the brain in the affection in question. Fatal cases of chorea have, however, occurred, and *post-mortem* examinations of them have been made; and in many of these instances the brain was found to be in a state of intense congestion.

Thus, Dr. John W. Ogle,[3] in sixteen fatal cases of chorea, found congestion of the brain and its membranes in some, while in others like conditions existed in the spinal cord.

Fourteen fatal cases were analyzed by Dr. Hughes, and in all but four of these there were intracranial congestion and other structural changes, such as softening opacities and adhesions. And in seven fatal cases collected by Romberg[4] there were softening and degeneration of various parts of the brain and spinal cord.

---

[1] "Nouveau dictionnaire de médecine et de chirurgie pratiques," Paris, 1878, t. xxvi, art. "Pellagre," p. 447.

[2] "Traité de la pellagre," Paris, 1870, p. 192.

[3] "Remarks on Chorea, Sancti Viti, including the History, Course, and Termination of Sixteen Fatal Cases," *British and Foreign Medico-Chirurgical Review*, January, 1868, p. 208.

"Digest of One Hundred Cases of Chorea," *Guy's Hospital Reports*, vol. iv, 1846, p. 360.

[4] "Lehrbuch der Nervenkrankheiten," Band ii.

CHAPTER XIII.

THE TREATMENT OF INSANITY.

BEFORE proceeding to discuss the medical treatment of cases of insanity, there is a point which requires to be first disposed of, for it is one that is suggested both to the physician and the patient's friends at a very early period in the course of the disease, and that is the question:

Shall the insane person be treated at home or in an asylum?

A few years ago there would have been but one answer to such a question, either from the physician or the friends of any patient having the means wherewith to be maintained in a hospital specially set apart for the care and treatment of those so unfortunate as to be the subjects of mental derangement; and for those not having the means, efforts would have been made to procure their admission into a like institution supported at the public expense. But the case is very different now. All are anxious to keep their mentally deranged patients or friends at home so long as this can be done with safety, and matters are fast reaching that point, in some sections of the country, at which no lunatics except those who are dangerous to themselves or others will be sent to asylums so long as they have friends able to take care of them.

But, before proceeding to consider the reasons for this extraordinary change of professional and lay opinion, it is proper, in the first place, to ascertain, as far as practicable, what forms of insanity require asylum treatment, and what forms do not.

All the varieties of insanity given in the table of classification on pages 292 and 293 can, with reference to this point, be arranged into three groups:

1. Those the subjects of which should never, under any circumstances, be forcibly deprived of their liberty by being committed to a lunatic asylum against their will.

2. Those forms a minority of the subjects of which *may* require to be committed to an asylum.

3. Those forms a majority of which *may* require to be so committed.

There is no form of insanity known to alienists all the

subjects of which imperatively require the treatment and restraint of an asylum.

1. The forms embraced in the first group are included in the class of perceptional insanities, comprehending the forms of illusions and hallucinations; the form of intellectual subjective morbid impulses, in the class of intellectual insanities; and the form of aboulomania, or paralysis of the will, in the class of volitional insanities.

There is nothing in pure, uncomplicated cases of any of these forms of mental derangement which requires the treatment of a lunatic asylum, or which would warrant any interference with the full rights and privileges of the individual. On the contrary, forcible confinement in such an institution would tend strongly to cause the disease to pass into some more intense form. The subjects of these varieties of insanity are perfectly aware of their morbid condition, and they generally look forward with horror to a possible termination within the walls of an asylum.

2. The forms embraced in this group are intellectual objective morbid impulses, in the class of intellectual insanities; emotional monomania, emotional morbid impulses, simple melancholia, hysterical mania, and epidemic insanity, of the class of emotional insanities; volitional morbid impulses, of the class of volitional insanities; katatonia, primary dementia, secondary dementia, and senile dementia, of the class of compound insanities; and puerperal insanity and choreic insanity, of the class of constitutional insanities.

Of these groups, it may be that, in the forms of intellectual objective morbid impulses, emotional morbid impulses, and volitional morbid impulses, the tendency is toward the perpetration of some act of violence. If such is ever the case, even in a single instance, the safety of society, as well as the good of the individual, requires that he or she should be placed under restraint of some kind. A few cases of emotional monomania exhibit traits which are prejudicial to the welfare of society, but the majority are harmless, and should not be subjected to any more forcible restraint, if any is necessary, than that which can be imposed by their physician and friends. Simple melancholia is rarely an unmanageable affection, and the subjects of hysterical mania seldom require to be confined in an asylum. Epidemic insanity is generally easily managed at home, as are also katatonia and all the varieties of dementia. Very few cases of puerperal or choreic insanity require the restraint of an asylum.

3. Of the third group, most of the cases of intellectual monomania with exaltation, intellectual monomania with depression, chronic intellectual mania, reasoning mania of the class of intellectual insanities; melancholia with delirium, melancholia with stupor, hypochondriacal mania of the class of emotional insanities; acute mania, periodical insanity, hebephrenia, circular insanity, and general paralysis of the class of compound insanities; and epileptic insanity of the class of constitutional insanities, require to be restrained wholly or in part.

But the opinions here expressed refer to individuals so situated as not to be able to command what they and society require—who either do not have the advantages of a home, friends able and willing to take care of them, or such medical advice and assistance as their cases require. If all these matters can be secured, there is no reason why any lunatic, no matter under what form of insanity he may suffer, should be committed to a public insane asylum. There may be reasons why he should not be kept at home, and then he should be sent to some one of the private institutions, the superintendent of which, finding it to his interest to take care of those committed to his charge, devotes his time and attention and skill to his patients, instead of giving all these to looking after farms and manipulating legislatures. Or, if restraint be required, the law should be so altered as to allow some friend or relative, under bonds and subject to proper inspection, to take the charge of the lunatic, and to place him in such restraint as may be necessary to prevent him committing an act of violence against himself or others, or his own property or that of others. Under such circumstances, public asylums —and by public asylums I mean those supported by the cities, counties, or States in which they are situated—would only be necessary, first, for those who have no money, and, second, for those who have no friends. And even the latter class, if having money, could readily, under the direction of some discreet person appointed by the proper authority, have the advantages of treatment in a private institution or in their own houses. Then the only persons for whom the asylums would still be imperatively required would be those so deplorably situated as have neither money nor friends. Unfortunately there are, and probably always will be, many such. I am aware that there are some excellent public asylums, in which, as I know of my own knowledge, the treatment is skilful and humane, in which the medical officers take a pride in their work, and in which the inmates are as tenderly cared for as though they paid the highest prices for their board, and had the most powerful individuals for their friends. But to-morrow, at the behest of a governor, or legislature, or other political body, they may be ousted from their positions to make way for some medical adventurer who has rendered important services to the "party." Such acts are of common occurrence.

Again, the system of inspection of such institutions, when there is any at all, is so inefficient that the greatest abuses may spring up, and the world be none the wiser, till some day an exposure takes place; and then it is discovered that an asylum which has been the pride of the community is in reality a hot-bed of neglect and cruelty. A legislative inquiry is ordered, a condemnatory report is made, but, through "political influence," it is smothered, and things presumably go on as before. Till the public asylums are organized upon the same general principles as are other hospitals, things are not likely to be better than they are now. As I said[1] several years ago, in a paper read before the Medical Society of the State of New York, "Each should have its corps of visiting physicians and surgeons, and its residents, instead of being placed under the control of one man, whose multitudinous duties with legislatures, visitors, farms, and other non-medical matters, prevent him giving the proper time and attention to his specific obligations. By this plan, to an asylum with six hundred patients there would be a medical board of at least twenty members—and the number could be increased as occasion required—besides a dozen or more of young physicians living in the institution and carrying out the orders of their seniors."

It may be objected against the home treatment of persons the subject of mental aberration that no care which could be exercised could prevent acts of violence. Such an objection would probably be of force in some cases, but are things any better in the public asylums? When we look back over the

[1] "The Non-Asylum Treatment of the Insane," *Transactions of the Medical Society of the State of New York*, 1859.

46

last four or five years only, and bring to mind the long list of the murders, the suicides, the acts of incendiarism, which have been committed, we see what few advantages, even on the score of safety, such institutions offer. Even while these pages are going through the press, we get the account of a poisoning, in a public asylum, by one lunatic of a dozen others, five of whom died in a few minutes. The number of acts of violence committed in public asylums during the last five years is many fold greater than that perpetrated by all the lunatics whose condition has been recognized, and who have been under the care of their friends or in some private institution for the insane.

In conclusion, I have to express the opinion that no insane person who can be properly cared for at home, in the way of medical attendance and nursing, or who can be placed in a private, or what may be called a "family asylum," should be committed to a public institution for lunatics. Several years ago I [1] wrote as follows, and subsequent experience has not only tended to confirm the correctness of the views then communicated, but has caused me to carry them to the point now stated :

"It is not always necessary to confine him (the lunatic) in an asylum, but it is necessary, in the great majority of cases, to place him in such a situation as will secure for him safety, the companionship of sensible people, and the influence and control of some one skilled in the philosophy of the human mind, in the anatomy and physiology of the brain and nervous system, and in medical science generally. The great difficulty with asylums is, that they contain only insane people, and the prevalent idea among the public (and it is often carried out by the officers of the asylums) is, that institutions for the insane are simply places where dangerous or troublesome maniacs are kept in safety. My own idea is, that the best of all places for a lunatic of any kind is the family of a physician—of such a one as I have just mentioned. The association of an insane person day after day, year after year, with others similarly affected, with scarcely the least contact with people of sound minds, is certainly in opposition to the first principles of scientific medicine."

Now, it may be asked, What "companionship with sen-

[1] "A Treatise on the Diseases of the Nervous System," sixth edition, New York, 1876, p. 375.

sible people" has the lunatic immured within the walls of an asylum, without the right to see his friends or even his physician; without even the privilege of writing to them, or to those having authority to correct abuses, if there are any such officials? What "control of some one skilled in the philosophy of the human mind," etc.? Even if the superintendent be such a person—and many of them, I am happy to say, are accomplished and scientific physicians and gentlemen—the other duties which fall to his lot prevent his having any intimate acquaintance with those under his charge.

But, when—as is, I regret to say, sometimes the case—the superintendent, appointed through political influence, not for his medical knowledge, but for the services he has rendered to his party organization, is ignorant of the first principles of the human mind, to whom the anatomy and physiology of the brain is a sealed book, and whose knowledge of insanity has no deeper basis than occasional facetious conversations with the village fool, it is a terrible thing for the poor wretches who have to live under his dominion.

Again, under the system which at present exists in many of the public asylums of this country, the attendants are usually selected from the lowest and most brutal class of the population. They are the henchmen who, having been ever ready to fight for their leader—or "boss," as he is called in the political slang of the day—are also rewarded by being appointed to situations in lunatic asylums. To expect such individuals, whose instincts are not so mild and decent as those of a well-trained dog, to forget their natural and acquired savageism, and to act in a manner approaching that of an average human being, would betray a confidence in the reformatory influence of the American public lunatic asylum, as it sometimes exists, which, I am sorry to say, personal knowledge forbids me to share. It is no matter for surprise, therefore, to learn, as we do every now and then from the reports of legislative committees of inquiry, that the patients "are cruelly gagged, and beaten, and ducked, and ill-fed, and scantily clothed, and 'taken down' and 'spread-eagled' (the technical names for inhuman punishment), and over-worked, and subjected to various needless punishments of revolting severity, and become the victims of inexcusable neglect, and in many cases left in their last moments with no hand to administer to their dying wants"; or to learn that in one insti-

tution a "patient was beaten to death by an attendant"; or
that in another a patient who refused to eat "was caught and
laid on a bench; one attendant held his hands and sat across
his body; another attendant and a patient helped to hold him;
his mouth was plugged to prevent his closing it. The food
(soup) was poured in from a pitcher, his breath was heard to
'gurgle' as it went into his wind-pipe, and in five minutes he
was dead." Or that, in another, one of the keepers carried a
harness-strap with a buckle on the end of it, and that patients
were beaten with the buckle-end, and that the same keeper
knocked patients down with a bunch of keys; and that another knocked a patient down, jumped on him, and kicked
him till he had fits. Such things do not surprise those of us
in this country who have studied the system, and know of
what it is capable. There are lunatic asylums here which are
in all respects as good, and in many respects better, than any
institutions of the kind in the world; there are others worse
than any to be found in a civilized country, and in which
abuses exist to which no other people but the patient and
long-suffering American would for a moment submit.

The means of treatment of the insane, in or out of an asylum, may be advantageously divided into four classes—the
mechanical, the *moral*, the *hygienic*, and the *medicinal*.

The Mechanical Treatment.—The first point under this
head which requires consideration is in regard to the means to
be adopted to prevent a lunatic with tendencies to violence
from inflicting injuries on himself or others, or damaging
property about him. This involves the question of non-restraint, and it is one that deserves more than a mere passing
notice in a work intended mainly for the use of physicians in
a country where the principles of Pinel and Conolly have as
yet only a limited footing.

In 1792, Pinel was appointed chief physician of the Bicêtre, the great lunatic asylum for pauper men in Paris.
He found that all the most violent cases were habitually kept
chained. He struck off their irons, substituted kindness for
blows, improved their diet, and so ameliorated their condition in other respects that many who were regarded as incurable were restored to the world with their mental faculties again to guide them. This was the first grand step
toward treating a lunatic somewhat in accordance with the
methods employed with rational individuals.

But Pinel's[1] methods appear to have sprung more from goodness of heart than from any therapeutical principle ; and, though knocking off the manacles from the maniac's limbs, he still continued to employ in some cases milder methods of mechanical restraint. It was reserved for Dr. Conolly, an Englishman, in 1839, to demonstrate to the world that there was no antagonism between humanity and science in this matter, and that those methods of management which were most kind and gentle were at the same time the most efficacious as curative agents. It is true that for two or three years previously the doctrine of "non-restraint" had been advocated and practiced to some extent at the York Retreat and Asylum, under the charge of the Friends, but it had made little headway till Conolly, at the Hanwell Asylum of London, not only took away every form of apparatus calculated to confine the lunatic's body or limbs, but wrote and spoke so eloquently and logically in support of his views that, before long, they came to be recognized as correct in most parts of the civilized world, the only notable exception being the free and enlightened United States of America. When Dr. Conolly took charge of Hanwell, there were closets full of instruments of restraint, which the attendants were allowed to use at their pleasure. There were strait-waistcoats, "restraint chairs," muffs, leg-locks, various kinds of complicated apparatus, straps of different varieties, and even chains. They do not appear to have had the "crib," that appliance so dear to the hearts of some of our American superintendents. The epileptics, over one hundred in number, were every night fastened by one hand to their bedsteads ; and, in addition, there were over forty patients kept constantly in some form of mechanical bondage night and day. In his first report, Dr. Conolly said, in speaking of the forcible restraint which he found practiced when he took charge of the institution, " that it was in fact creative of many of the outrages and disorders, to repress which, its application was commonly deemed indispensable, and, consequently, directly opposed to the chief design of all treatment—the cure of the disease."

But Dr. Conolly began very cautiously with his measures of reform, and did not at first dispense with every kind of mechanical restraint. For those patients who were continu-

[1] Portions of this sketch are taken from a paper by the author on " The Treatment of the Insane," in the *International Review* for March, 1880.

ally making efforts to take off their clothes, strong dresses were provided, which were secured around the waist by a leathern belt, fastened by a small lock ; and the covering for the feet consisted of warm boots, similarly arranged. For those who were disposed to strike or otherwise injure others, to tear the bedclothes, etc., a dress, of which the sleeves terminated in a stuffed glove without divisions for the fingers and thumb, was provided. "But there was no form of straitjacket, no hand-straps, no leg-locks, nor any contrivance confining the trunk or limbs or any of the muscles," and all the restraint chairs were removed from the wards. During the following year, even these mild forms of restraint were taken away, and then Dr. Conolly enunciated a proposition, the truth of which is entirely established, and which is applicable to any lunatic asylum in any country, that "any contrivance which diminishes the necessity for vigilance proves hurtful to the discipline of an asylum." [1]

This may be considered the starting-point in the theory and practice of non-restraint, as it is carried out in Great Britain, Germany, and other parts of the civilized world.

Now, let us take a brief review of the treatment of lunatics as regards mechanical restraint in this country. While it is certainly true that there are lunatic asylums the superintendents of which are actuated by a desire to keep the number of restraint cases at a minimum, there are only two public institutions—the Kings County Asylum at Flatbush, Long Island, under the charge of Dr. Shaw, and that at Athens, Ohio—in which mechanical restraint in some form or other is not employed ; and in some the proportion equals that at Hanwell before Dr. Conolly instituted his reform measures.

Now, I am not an advocate of absolute non-restraint under all possible circumstances and conditions. There are cases in which it may be indispensably necessary to preserve the life or secure the comfort of the patient. It is never necessary to secure the lives or the comfort of others, and, when used, it should be with all the safeguards against abuse, which sound policy and humanity dictate. Being requested by a recent investigating committee of the Senate of the State of New York to make such suggestions as I might deem proper in regard to the future management of the insane asylums

---

[1] "The Care and Cure of the Insane, being the Reports of the ' Lancet ' Commission on Lunatic Asylums," by J. Mortimer Granville, M. D., London, 1877.

of the State, I stated, among others, the following proposition:

"It should not be allowable for any one but a medical officer of an asylum to order a patient to be placed in mechanical restraint or in seclusion, and even then a record of such instance should be kept in a book provided for the purpose. This book should always be open to the inspection not only of officials in authority, but to the counsel and family physician of the patient, and it should clearly show in detail the reason for the use of such restraint or seclusion. . . .

"At present ignorant and brutal attendants, some of them selected from the very lowest class, can, at their option, from whim, caprice, anger, or any other inadequate cause, order or place a lunatic in the camisole, crib, or other mechanical restraint. There are many instances on record of serious bodily injury and even death having been produced by mechanical restraint improperly applied, to say nothing of the deleterious effect caused on the mind of the patient by such procedure."

These principles appear to be carried out in that excellent institution, the Illinois Eastern Hospital for the Insane at Kankakee, under the superintendence of Dr. Dewey, in which it is stated [1] that:

"The amount of restraint has constantly diminished under the methods employed. The instances in which it has been used on each side, respectively, in the year ending September 30, 1882, could be counted on one's fingers and thumbs—ten times in all on the female side, and six in all in the male division." And this with an average daily population of over three hundred and eight.

There are other insane asylums in the country, notably the one at Athens, Ohio, which could make probably as good a showing as this; but, when we find the superintendents as a body setting themselves against reform in the excessive and indiscriminate use of mechanical restraint, there is little chance of general improvement till many of the present race are weeded out by time, and their places filled by more scientific and progressive men. [2]

[1] "Third Biennial Report," 1882, p. 23.

[2] Thus, at a meeting of the Association of Superintendents, held a few years ago, the president, Dr. Walker, gravely told his fellow-members that he supposed, if anything had been settled to the satisfaction of members of the Association, it is that, in this country, our patients, by original temperament

If restraint be used, the only forms allowable should be leathern mittens, locked to the wrists, to prevent the patient tearing the clothing, and other articles of locked clothing. But, as attendants become more accustomed to the duty of reasoning with the insane, the use even of these measures can be reduced to a minimum—not yet reached in our best asylums—or, perhaps, altogether dispensed with, as at Flatbush, New York,[1] and Athens, Ohio.

Forcible Alimentation.—In those patients who will not eat, means must be taken to secure their nourishment by the compulsory ingestion of food. In some extreme cases, in which there is great physical weakness, this must be done by injections of nutritive substances into the rectum ; in others, the food must be introduced through the œsophagus. Many patients, who at first refuse to swallow food, can be induced to do so by persuasion. At other times, though they may refuse to one nurse, they will readily accede to the request of another, whom they like better ; and, again, it is only some particular kind of food they refuse, or they wish, under the delusion that it is poisoned, to submit it to some test that they have devised. I had a patient once who would never eat or drink anything till he had placed the vessel containing the food or drink in the sunlight, or, if this could not be obtained, near the register by which the heat entered the room. In all such cases it is better to yield to the whim of the patient than to resort to force. If this, however, should be necessary, it should never be left to an attendant, but should be employed by a physician.

The practice, recommended by Guislain,[2] and carried out in some asylums, of forcing open the mouth, closing the nostrils, and pouring liquid food down the throat, is one that should never, in my opinion, be employed. It has resulted

or by some inherent quality of the universal Yankee, will not submit to the control of any person they consider their equal or inferior so readily as to that of mechanical restraint. And another member, Dr. Compton, said: "I think an asylum cannot be found in this country, where the first thing a boy learns to read is the Declaration of Independence, and where every youngster learns that he is in 'the land of the free and the home of the brave,' in which restraint will not be necessary."

[1] "Non-Restraint in the Treatment of the Insane," and "A Second Year's Experience with Non-Restraint in the Treatment of the Insane," *Archives of Medicine,* February, 1881, and April, 1882.

[2] "Leçons orales sur les phrénopathies," Gand, Paris, 1880, t. ii, p. 240.

in death by strangulation, and almost always causes more or less choking.

The better plan is, after having secured the patient so that resistance is impossible, to force the mouth open with a screw wedge, and then, the head of the patient being thrown well back and kept fixed, to introduce the gag, made of smooth wood, with a hole in the centre. Through this hole a large-sized stomach-tube is introduced and carried into the œsophagus. The food, which of course is liquid or semi-liquid, should then be poured into the funnel-shaped upper extremity of the tube, when it readily passes into the stomach. Or the stomach-pump may be used, and the food introduced by its means directly from the vessel in which it is contained. The pump, however, has the objection of requiring the ingesta to be absolutely liquid, to avoid obstruction of the valves.

The introduction of a tube through the nostril has been recommended, but its use is not satisfactory, on account of the smallness of calibre required, and which prevents any but very thin food from being given.

There is nothing in the forcible alimentation of the insane different from the feeding, through tubes, frequently necessary in those cases of disease in which the patient is unable to swallow, except in the one point that force is often required. This should be overwhelming and promptly applied, so as to prevent, as far as possible, the struggles and consequent bruises or other injuries that may be received.

Moral Treatment.—One of the most important means coming under this head is rest. With some patients it is impossible to secure the mental repose required by any efforts they are able to make ; in the cases of others, however, great assistance may be obtained through the intelligent co-operation of the affected individual. Instances in which the reasoning faculties are so far destroyed as to make it a matter of impossibility to be aided by the patients are rare. The difficulty is to discover the way to the light—mere glimmer as it may be—which exists ; and even when this is done, skill in the endeavor to develop it is of almost equal importance. There are no rules which can be laid down in regard to these matters which are of equal applicability in all cases. Some persons have an inborn adaptability by which they readily obtain an influence over all with whom they come in contact. Others, with the best intentions in the world, never succeed in ingratiating themselves with those about them. Patience and tact are probably, in such cases, as indispensable qualities as can be possessed. Without them, all the knowledge that can be acquired in a lifetime will be of but little avail.

Works on insanity written by superintendents of lunatic asylums generally recommend that, for the procurement of the rest which the racked and wearied brain often so imperatively demands, the patient should, at as early a date as possible, be removed to an institution for the insane. As the word asylum is ordinarily understood, I have no hesitation in declaring it to be my deliberate conviction that this is, in most cases, the worst possible thing that can be done. Circumstances may be such that, in cases of persons suffering with some acute form of insanity accompanied with tendencies to violence, some place where the lunatic can be kept in safety is absolutely requisite, and the asylum at once suggests itself. But, if the patient can, even in such a form of the disease, have careful nursing, skilled medical attendance, and isolation in his own house, or, better still, in the house of some physician, who pays special attention to the subject, he will have all the advantages in the way of rest which the best asylum in the land can give him. If these cannot be secured, then send him to the best asylum available.

This subject has already been discussed in other relations, but a few words more in regard to it in this connection appear to be advisable.

It has just been said that in those works on insanity written by medical officers of asylums, the earliest possible deportation of the patient to such an institution is recommended as an indispensable matter. There are some, however, who look at the matter in its true light, and who, hence, make other recommendations.

Thus, Maudsley [1] says :

"The principle which guides the present practice is that an insane person, by the simple warrant of his insanity, shall be shut up in an asylum, the exceptions being made of particular cases. This I hold to be an erroneous principle. The true principle to guide our practice should be this : that no one, sane or insane, should ever be entirely deprived of his liberty unless for his own protection or the protection of society. . . .

[1] "The Physiology and Pathology of the Mind," London, 1867, p. 424.

"Is it not a common thing to hear from an insane person bitter complaints of the associations which he has in the asylum, and of the scenes of which he is an unwilling witness—scenes which cannot fail to occur, notwithstanding the best classification, where all sorts and conditions of madness are congregated together? What, again, can be considered more afflicting to a man, who has any intelligence left, than the vulgar tyranny of an ignorant attendant—a tyranny which the best management cannot altogether prevent in a large asylum? And I might go on to enumerate many more of the unpreventable miseries of life in an asylum which, when superintendent of one, forced themselves painfully on my attention, and often made me sick at heart."

And more recently the same author[1] says:

"The grave and anxious question in a particular case is, whether an asylum is necessary or not. The accepted notions regarding insanity not many years ago were: first, that the best means to promote the recovery of a patient who was laboring under it was to send him to an asylum; and, secondly, that, so long as he was insane, there was no better place for him than an asylum. These opinions had been urged so persistently, and held so long, that they had become a habit of thought which was deemed by some to have the authority of a law of nature. Opinion has now, however, changed so much that the question which first occurs to the mind is, whether it is possible to treat the patient out of an asylum. The decision as to what should be done is often most difficult, since social, pecuniary, and legal considerations come in to complicate the medical question, and most medical men would willingly get rid of the responsibility which it entails."

Dr. Blandford,[2] after mentioning former practices, says:

"Now, from all asylums, patients are sent to the sea-side, the theatre, the picture-galleries. [How much of this is done in the United States?] Each proprietor vies with his fellows in providing recreation and entertainment for his patients—in proving, in fact, how little they need the restraint of an asylum. There will always be a certain number who cannot be allowed so much liberty, who cannot be taken to the sea-side, who cannot even walk beyond the bounds of the asylum grounds, whose life is one incessant struggle to escape by

---

[1] "The Pathology of the Mind," New York, 1880, p. 524.
[2] "Insanity and its Treatment," Edinburgh, 1871, p. 370.

force or fraud, or execute, perchance, some insane project, fraught with danger to themselves or others. Some there will be whose limited means procure for them greater luxury and enjoyment among the numerous boarders of an asylum than could be afforded were they placed alone in a private family. But there are many, with ample means—patients who make the fortunes of asylum proprietors—whose lives would be infinitely happier did they live beyond asylum walls."

Dr. Dickson [1] says :

"As a matter of principle, I should strongly recommend that a patient should never be sent to an asylum if such a course can be avoided. There is no law prohibiting the treatment of a patient at home. The lunatic is not a criminal to be put under locks and bonds, and it is only when he disturbs the public peace, or when by cruel and unusual treatment other people infringe the law as regards him, that authority can interfere in his behalf."

Dr. C. Pinel,[2] while contending for the general principle that lunatics should be sequestered, admits that the exceptions are many. "Every rule," he says, "has its exceptions, and we should, at least in the beginning, when the disease is recent and not of grave character, give the patient the opportunity of remaining in his own house. Thus the subject of maniacal excitement, a restricted monomania, a moderate degree of melancholia, certain kinds of hallucinations and false conceptions not relating to the family, hypochondriacs, of dementia, etc., may properly remain at home."

"In treatment at home," he continues, "if the attentions of the relatives are well received, taken at their first value, accepted with gratitude, eagerly desired, it would be inhuman, indiscreet, and not in accordance with sound medical science, to deprive him of them. Nothing can replace, nothing equal, the tender devotion, the affectionate solicitude of the family. Many times we have been the witness of the inestimable benefit of these moral and physical aids, and it is for us a sacred duty, in the absence of the most imperious necessity, not to separate the lunatic from them."

Dr. Maudsley, Dr. Blandford, Dr. Dickson, and Dr. Pinel

[1] "The Science and Practice of Medicine in Relation to Mind," London, 1874, p. 389.

[2] "De l'isolément des aliénés," *Journal de médecine, mentales,* t. i, Paris, 1861, p. 80.

are, or have been, superintendents of lunatic asylums. The three first are teachers of psychological medicine in prominent London medical schools, and hence their ability to speak intelligently on the subject will not, I presume, be questioned in any quarter.

Hence, in regard to the matter of securing rest for the patient, the physician must take all the circumstances into consideration, and assume the responsibility of so acting in the matter as the facts appear to dictate.

If it be decided to send him to an asylum, or away from his own home to the custody of a physician, nothing can be worse than to inveigle him into going peaceably, by fraud or deceit of any kind. To entice him into a carriage under the pretence that it is for the purpose of giving him a drive, or to take him to see a friend or to a hotel is certainly unjustifiable under any possible circumstances. The deception is one which the patient often keenly remembers, and always with anger; it prejudices him against the superintendent or other person under whom he is to be placed, and puts him into a frame of mind most unpromising for the results of future treatment. If he has to go, and will not go quietly on being told where he is going, and for what purpose, sufficient force should be provided to compel him to go.

In regard to the question of conversing with a lunatic, and humoring or combating his delusions, or morbid fears, or tendencies, some difference of opinion exists among alienists. In former times there was none, and not only arguments and threats were administered to the lunatic for the purpose of coercing him, but measures of supposed still stronger potency were employed. Now these latter are left to the attendants, and by them they are only used surreptitiously.

Less than seventy years ago, a lunatic, named Norris, an officer of the British navy, was confined in the great madhouse Bethlehem. For a threat of violence against the physician, Dr. Haslam, he was subjected to restraint of such a character that we wonder now how the mind of a humane physician, as Dr. Haslam undoubtedly was, could work out the details. An iron collar was put around his neck, another broad and strong band of the same material encircled his body, his arms were confined in the same manner, and the bands around them were united to the one that was fastened around the chest. The ankles were fettered, and then the neck collar was connected by a chain six inches long with an iron ring which slid up and down on a stout bar fixed to the wall at the head of his bed. It was impossible for this unfortunate wretch to lie down, to stand up, or, in fact, to assume any other position than that of sitting on his bed of straw, and yet he lived in this way for nine years in a stone cell.

In Dr. Mead's time, lunatics were beaten as a therapeutical measure to quiet them and rid them of their delusions. Cullen recommends the infliction of corporal punishment as an effectual means of rendering them rational and of impressing them with terror.

Dr. Haslam,[1] while deprecating resort to such harsh measures, nevertheless says:

"In the most violent state of the disease the patient should be kept alone in a dark and quiet room, so that he may not be affected by the stimuli of light and sound—such abstraction more readily disposing to sleep. As in this violent state there is a strong propensity to associate ideas, it is equally important to prevent the accession of such as might be transmitted through the medium of the senses. The hands should be properly secured, and the patient should also be confined by one leg; this will prevent him from committing any violence. The more effectual and convenient mode of confining the hands is by metallic manacles, for, should the patient, as frequently occurs, be constantly endeavoring to liberate himself, the friction of the skin against a polished metallic body may be long sustained without injury, whereon excoriation shortly takes place when the surface is rubbed with linen or cotton."

And this was not all; the mind was worked upon and tortured, and deceptions of various kinds were considered proper and curative.

Thus, Dr. Cox[2] says:

"The conscientious physician, in the execution of his duty, attempting the removal of these deplorable maladies, is under the necessity of occasionally deviating from the accustomed routine of practice, of stepping out of the beaten path, and, in some cases that have resisted the usual methods, is warranted in adopting any others that promise the smallest hope of success. Thus, the employment of what may be termed pious

[1] "Observations on Madness," second edition, London, 1809, p. 289.
[2] "Practical Observations on Insanity," London, 1815, p. 28.

frauds, as when one simple, erroneous idea stamps the character of the disease, depriving the affected party of the common enjoyments of society, though capable of reasoning with propriety, perhaps with ingenuity, on any subject not connected with that of his hallucinations, the connection of which has resisted our very best exertion, and when there is no obvious corporeal disposition, it certainly is allowable to try the effect of certain deceptions contrived to make strong impressions on the senses by means of unexpected, unusual, striking, or apparently supernatural agents; such as often waking the party from sleep, either suddenly or by a gradual process, by imitated thunder or soft music, according to the peculiarity of the case; combating the erroneous deranged notion, either by some pointed sentence, or signs executed in phosphorus upon the walls of his bed-chamber, or by some tale, assertion, or reasoning, by one in the character of an angel, prophet, or devil; but the actor in this drama must possess much skill, and be very perfect in his part."

And by such puerilities, less than seventy years ago, it was attempted to cure insanity! Really, the progress of medicine, as well as the advance in the intelligence of the human race, has not been slight since that time.

But, about forty years ago, Leuret,[1] one of the most eminent mental physiologists the world has produced, proposed and carried out a plan of treatment which he called "moral," and which has been practiced in this country within the last ten or twelve years. It consisted in reasoning with the patient relative to the falsity of his delusions, and, if he persisted in maintaining them, notwithstanding the arguments adduced, of subjecting him to the cold douche on his head and body generally till he announced that he was convinced. Shortly afterward he was asked again whether or not he still held to his false conceptions, and if there was any hesitation to answer in the negative, he got the douche again, and so on till his cure was complete. As an illustration of the method, I quote the following case from Leuret.[2] Speaking of the method, he says:

"The water falling on the head and chest produces in these parts a glacial oppression; the lower parts of the body and the inferior extremities feel almost nothing. It is painful

---

[1] "Du traitement moral de la folie," Paris, 1840.

[2] *Op. cit.*, p. 187 *et seq.*

to receive, but we have tried it for a longer time than any of our patients.''

After having heard a patient, A., speak of his delusions, M. Leuret thus addressed him :

'' 'A., I am going to tell you now what I think of all that you have said. There is not a word of truth in it. All the things that you have related are false, and it is because you are insane that you are here in the Bicêtre.'

''To this, A. replied :

'' 'Monsieur Leuret, I do not think I am insane. I cannot help seeing the light-house, because it is immediately before me, nor the persons who are under my bed, nor the caves, for they are there. You think that all I have said is false, but I know what I see and hear. Now, after what I say, is there no hope that you will let me go out of this place?'

'' 'You can go out, but on one condition. Listen well to what I am about to say. You will go away from here only when you are no longer insane ; and this is what is necessary for you to do to convince me that you are cured : you must not look at the sun or the stars ; you must not believe that there are caves under your bed, for there are none ; you must not believe that you hear voices in these caves, for there are no voices, or that there are persons there who speak to you, for they do not exist ; you are not the saviour of the king, and you must not think that you are watching over his safety. You must cease speaking of all these things, because, if you continue to do so, I shall have still to regard you as insane. And more ; you must never refuse to work, whatever may be the kind of labor you are commanded to perform. If you wish me to be satisfied with you, you must obey, because all that I ask of you is reasonable. Promise me, therefore, that you will not any more think of your delusions ; promise that you will no longer speak of them.'

'' 'If [replied A.] you say they are delusions, and, therefore, you do not wish me to *talk* of them, very well, I will cease *speaking* of them.'

'' 'Will you promise not to *think* of them?'

''The patient hesitated. He was pressed sharply, and finally said :

'' 'No, sir, I will no longer think of them.'

'' 'Will you promise to work every day that you are ordered to work?'

" 'I have an estate of my own. I wish to go out to work on my own land.'

" 'I have told you the conditions on which you will be allowed to work on your estate. Now, I ask you again if you will consent to work?'

" The patient hesitates.

" 'As you have often broken your word to me [continued M. Leuret], and as I cannot depend on your promises, you are going to get the douche, and we will continue to give it to you every day until you come to us of your own accord and ask to be put to work, and until, further, you, without any suggestions from us, confess that all the things you have been talking about are delusions.'

" *Douche!* It is painful to him, and he does not delay long to come out.

" 'You wish me to work. I will. You wish me not to think any more of the things of which I have spoken, because they are only imaginations, as I well know. To all the people who may speak to me of those things I will say that they are not true, but are delusions which I have had in my head.'

" 'Will you go to work to-day?'

" 'Since you compel me, I will.'

" 'Will you go willingly?'

" 'Since you force me, I will.'

" 'You ought to say that you understand that it is for your interest that you should go to work. Do you go willingly, yes or no?'

" Hesitation. *Douche.* After a moment :

" 'Yes, sir. Everything that I have said to you is a delusion. I will go to work.'

" 'You have been a lunatic, then?'

" 'No, I have not been a lunatic.'

" 'You have not been a lunatic?'

" 'I do not think so, at least.'

" *Douche.*

" 'Have you been a lunatic?'

" 'Is a man a lunatic who has imaginations of seeing and hearing?'

" 'Yes.'

" 'Well, sir, and so that is insanity. There have been no women, or men, or companions : all that is insanity.'

47

" 'When you think you hear things of that character, what will you say ? '

" 'I will say it is insanity, and I will give no attention to them.'

" ' And that woman who made court to you ? '

" 'Sir, that is not true ; that is insanity. My head is quieter since I have had the douche. All that I said was insanity, and I no longer think as I did.'

" 'I wish you to come to me to-morrow and thank me for having cured you of your insane ideas.'

" 'I promise to work, and also to thank you for having cured me.'

" 'I want you to work to-day.'

" 'I will go, I promise you.'

" The evening of the same day A. had a douche, which M. Aubanel gave him [M. Aubanel, it may be stated, was one of the medical officers, and is the gentleman to whom we are indebted for that highly "moral instrument of persuasion the ' crib,'" so much liked by certain of our American superintendents] for not having recollected that he had to work that day. He yielded on the second trial. He did not work, he said, because he did not know to whom he was to apply in order to be enrolled with the workers. M. Aubanel, very properly thinking this excuse insufficient, indicated to him the overseer, and A. promised to work on the morrow."

After this a few threats of the douche were sufficient to keep the patient free from delusions, and at the end of about three months he was discharged cured.

All this reads very much like the record of the proceedings in cases of the question being applied to suspected criminals during the middle ages. One method was, that instead of pouring the water on the outside of the body to extort confession, it was poured into the stomach, till the pain caused by the distension became unbearable, and the wretch confessed, either truly or falsely ; or, if endowed with greater powers of endurance than M. Leuret's patient, persisted in silence.

An official record reads as follows : [1]

" Stripped, and placed on the little trestle and bound.

" At the first kettleful, said nothing.

[1] " Les pénalités anciennes. Supplices prisons et grâce en France ; d'après des textes inédits," par Charles Desmaze, conseiller de la cour impériale de Paris, Paris, 1866, p. 422.

"At the second, 'Ah, I know nothing, I am innocent!'"

"At the third, 'I suffer! My God!'"

"At the fourth, 'Enough, enough! Jesus! Mary!'"

"Placed on the large trestle.

"At the fifth, said nothing.

"At the sixth, *idem.*

"At the seventh, 'I can confess nothing.'

"At the eighth, 'Ah, I am dead.'

"Was then placed in bed."

It would be interesting to know the future progress of the case of A. The probability is that, after he got beyond the tender ministrations and persuasive arguments of M. Leuret, he reasserted his delusions with as much vigor as ever. At any rate, it is quite certain that M. Leuret's views and practices of "moral" treatment never made any headway, even in France, where they originated. In fact, intimidation of any kind, while it may make lunatics, as it would many other persons, renounce the expression of beliefs they have held, I do not see how it can change the belief itself. So long as the morbid condition of the brain remains, so long will the morbid condition of the mind continue. Whatever good effects resulted from it were doubtless mainly due to the revulsive effect of the cold water. During the early stages of those forms of insanity in which there are delusions, any attempt, either by mental or physical means, to control them generally results in their being still more tenaciously held. Many lunatics have gone to the scaffold, the stake, and the whipping-post, and have endured all kinds of torture, rather than renounce their opinions, as have also many sane persons. But, while intimidation can be of no permanent service, it should not for a moment be supposed that the lunatic should be humored in his false conceptions, or that any countenance should be given to the delusions of which he may speak.[1] Whether his ideas should be combated by arguments addressed to his reason, is a somewhat different matter. It has been said that it is useless to attempt to convince a lu-

[1] The only possible exception to this rule is in certain cases of hypochondriacal mania, where the delusion is clearly traceable to some circumstance of actual occurrence. In such cases it may be advisable to accept for the moment the statements of the patient in regard to his sensations and beliefs, in order to cure him by some such procedure as that, the details of which are given on page 483.

natic that his erroneous notions are not true. Perhaps this is correct when serious structural lesions exist in the brain. The false intellectual conception is then a fixed result of the altered brain-tissue, and is just as direct a consequence of cerebral action as is a natural thought from a healthy brain. Still, we know that in health it is sometimes possible by argument to counteract the most firmly rooted ideas ; it is, perhaps, yet easier to do this by the aid of certain of the pleasurable emotions. And there appears to be no reason why the like result may not occasionally be produced by arguments addressed to a person with an insane mind, and by bringing into action those feelings which spring from kindness. We know, in fact, that this end is at times accomplished, and that, by never for one instant admitting the truth of an insane delusion, and at suitable times—not obtrusively, but when occasion offers—urging such arguments against it as would be convincing to persons of sound minds, the lunatic comes at last to see the falsity of his ideas, and to laugh at them himself. Little by little he loses faith in his perverted reason, and though he may take up another delusion, the last is held with much less tenacity than the first.

Amusements, especially those which can be taken in the open air, are almost always of service, and a proper system of *rewards* and *punishments* for good and bad conduct is understood by all but the most furious maniacs. Kindness and forbearance, supported by firmness, will not altogether fail in their influence with even the most confirmed and degraded lunatics. Probably the most difficult class of patients to manage by moral means is that of the reasoning maniacs, and next to them those cases of hysterical mania which exhibit marked perversities of character and disposition. But even with such people the principles of justice and fair dealing will not be lost, and eventually an impression will probably be made on subjects incapable of being touched by other measures.

Hygienic Treatment.—The most important point to be considered in this connection is *occupation*. This is naturally of two kinds, *mental* and *physical*.

The system of setting *mental tasks* to lunatics is one which is rarely if ever followed in or out of asylums, and yet it is one from which the best results are likely to flow. Leuret[1]

[1] "Du traitement moral de la folie," Paris, 1840, p. 172.

states that, a school being established at the Bicêtre for the teaching of reading, writing, arithmetic, and orthography to the inmates, he profited by the occasion to make use of its facilities for some of the lunatics under his charge with manifest advantage. If school-teachers—and there are many inmates of asylums who could perform the duty with efficiency—were appointed to every asylum, and the patients whose cases admitted of it were divided into groups according to their form of insanity and intelligence, and systematically caused to exercise their minds in a direction different from that in which they would otherwise flow, the best results would, I am satisfied, be obtained. Reading, language, natural history, and other classes might thus be established, vocal and instrumental music might be properly included in the curriculum, and not only would the lunatic's life be rendered happier, but a powerful curative influence would be brought to bear upon him. I have already given a striking instance (page 438) of the diversion of a gentleman's impulses from stealing to the collection of bottle-corks. Leuret made some of his patients tax the memory with verse, which he required them to learn by heart—and with manifest benefit to their state of mental health. I have on several occasions succeeded by such means in directing the thoughts in such a manner as to abort what there was every reason to believe was an attack of some form of insanity. In one instance, a young lady had incipient delusions of persecution, from which she was entirely freed by means, of which the systematic exercise of her power of attention and of memory were among the chief. She learned to repeat from memory the whole of Campbell's "Pleasures of Hope," besides many other shorter pieces, and took such a degree of interest in her new work that she had little time left for her delusions.

Physical occupation should alternate with that provided for the mind. Where there is a farm or garden, work can be found for many able-bodied lunatics who otherwise would be troublesome people to deal with. Many a time a superfluous amount of nervous energy, which otherwise would have been expended in violent or disorderly conduct, has been gradually expended by manual labor. For women or the more feeble male patients, basket-making and various kinds of ornamental and fancy work might readily be provided.

The good effects of these means cannot be overestimated.

To a great extent they have been neglected in American asylums—though there are several worthy exceptions—to the vast detriment of the patients who day after day pass the time either a prey to their morbid thoughts or in making themselves noisy and troublesome occupants of the wards.

Baths are valuable hygienic adjuncts, besides being indispensable for purposes of cleanliness. In facilities for using water, American asylums are generally far in advance of those of any other part of the world, and yet it is quite true that they rarely make systematic use of the great advantages in this respect which they possess.

Baths should be either warm or cold, according to the indication to be fulfilled. In cases of acute mania and melancholia the *warm bath* at night has a decidedly quieting effect, and will often procure sleep which would not be otherwise obtained but by the use of drugs. It is useful, also, in many cases of hysterical mania and of puerperal insanity. In choreic insanity I have witnessed the most beneficial effects from warm baths at night, the temperature being rather high—from 100° to 105° Fahr.—and continued for not longer than five or six minutes. They should be given just at bed-time. Indeed, there is scarcely a form of insanity in which a warm bath at bed-time is not of service.

Cold baths require to be used with more caution, and are not of such general applicability as those of warm water. In some cases of acute mania they are useful, but the duration should not exceed two or three minutes, and they should only be employed with strong and able-bodied patients.

Employed in the form of the *douche* or *shower bath*, cold water has had a high reputation as a therapeutic agent in the treatment of insanity, and certainly it has an almost immediately quieting effect upon many cases in which there is great mental and motorial excitement. Great care, however, should be exercised in its use, as, if continued for too long a time, alarming prostration may be the result. I have seen strong, healthy men brought to such a state of debility as to be unable to speak or stand from the use of the cold shower bath on the head for three minutes, and I have known of death from its use for seven minutes. I do not think it should ever be continued in the cases of the insane for a longer period than two minutes, and one minute in the vast majority of circumstances would be better.

Brierre de Boismont,[1] basing his memoir on seventy-two cases of insanity, recommended, many years ago, the treatment of insanity by means of prolonged warm baths for the body and irrigation of cold water to the head. Of these cases, thirty-five were of acute mania, ten of maniacal exaltation, eleven of delirium tremens, ten of monomania, and six of chronic intermittent mania. Of the thirty-five cases of mania, thirty-three were cured; of the eleven cases of delirium tremens, all were cured; of the ten cases of maniacal exaltation, six were cured; and of the ten cases of monomania, all were cured. The six cases of chronic intermittent mania resisted treatment.

The duration of the treatment was from one to fifteen days.

The average number of baths used for each patient was six.

The treatment consisted of baths of the temperature of 28° to 30° Cent. (82° to 86° Fahr.), which were allowed to cool slowly, and in which the patients were kept for ten, twelve, or fifteen hours, while a slender stream of cold water of the temperature of 15° Cent. (57° Fahr.) fell on the head from a height of from three to four feet. He arrives at the conclusion, which seems warranted to some extent by the facts, that all kinds of insanity, and especially acute mania, can be cured by this means in from one to two weeks.

Several years subsequently Pinel[2] (nephew) reported that, of one hundred and fifty-seven cases treated after this method, one hundred and twenty-five were cured, and that, of the thirty-two that were not cured, twenty-five were improved.

Other alienists, among them Baillarger and Guislain, speak highly of this form of baths in insanity, and there is no doubt of its efficacy in many cases. It requires care and close watching, in order to avoid extreme weakness or syncope, and should never, therefore, be left entirely to an attendant.

Nothing among general hygienic measures conduces more

---

[1] "De l'emploi des bains prolongés et des irrigations continués dans le traitement des formes aiguès de la folie et en particulier de la manie," *Bulletin de l'académie royale de médecine*, 1846, t. xi, p. 1458; also, *Mémoires de l'académie royale de médecine*, 1848, t. xiii, p. 598.

[2] "Traitement de l'aliénation mentale aiguë par les bains prolonges," *Bull. de l'académie de médecine*, 1852, t. xviii, p. 179.

to the well-being of insane patients of the melancholic types than a full supply of *fresh air* and *sunlight*—and even acute maniacs are benefited by exposure to both these agencies for a portion of the day outside of the building in which they may reside. With the latter, however, too strong a light, long continued, is calculated to increase excitement. The morning sun and air are better than those of the evening. It is scarcely necessary to say that the sensation roused a few years ago relative to the beneficial influence of *blue light* was altogether unwarranted by theory or facts.

Medicinal Treatment.—Looking upon insanity of all kinds as being the direct consequence of morbid conditions of the brain of more or less severity and permanency, it is, of course, a logical inference that the brain is the chief organ to which our remedies are to be addressed. At the same time there may be conditions of other parts of the body which have induced the brain disorder, and there may be various secondary states which require to be treated in order that the patient may be the sooner restored to health.

In the consideration of this division of the treatment of insanity, it appears to be the better plan to continue the system adopted in the other divisions, and to take up in turn the various remedies to which it appears desirable to direct attention; to pursue the other plan of taking up the forms of insanity in their turn, and describing the modes of treatment proper for each, would lead to endless and tiresome repetitions.

The Bromides.—For the purposes of the present inquiry, the bromides of potassium, sodium, ammonium calcium, and lithium may be considered as of similar, and, in fact, almost equal power and efficacy. For general use, I prefer the bromide of sodium, for the reasons that its taste is more pleasant than that of the others, that it appears to be more readily taken into the system, and that it acts more promptly. But it is to be understood that all I shall have to say in regard to the therapeutical effects of the bromide of sodium applies equally to any of the other bromides mentioned.

In another work [1] I have detailed the observations and experiments which brought me to the conclusion that the bromides act upon the vaso-motor system in such a way as to lessen the amount of intracranial blood by diminishing the

[1] "On Sleep and Insomnia," *New York Medical Journal*, June, 1865, p. 203.

calibre of the blood-vessels. For many years I have acted
upon the fact thus established, and have used the bromides
extensively in the treatment of those forms of mental derangement due to a hyperæmic or congested condition of the
brain. In those cases in which there are the somatic phenomena of cerebral hyperæmia, such as pain, a feeling of fulness, distention, or tightness in or around the head, vertigo,
and, above all, wakefulness, the bromides can be relied upon
with almost absolute confidence to restore the healthy state, if
recourse is had to them at a sufficiently early date. Indeed,
there are few cases of *perceptional insanity*, *morbid impulses*, or *morbid fears*, in the early part of their course,
which resist their systematic and intelligent employment.
The uncomfortable feelings in the head disappear, the patient once more sleeps well, and the mind gradually gets rid
of its aberrations and resumes its normal condition.

In such cases the medicine does not require to be given
in large doses. Fifteen grains of the bromide of sodium three
times a day, continued for at least a month, will generally be
sufficient to produce sleep in the course of two or three days.
If not, then larger doses may be administered till this result
ensues, when they may be reduced.

In the management of *intellectual monomania with exaltation*, or *intellectual monomania with depression*, somewhat
larger doses are required, twenty grains of the bromide of
sodium three times a day being about an average dose. It is
also necessary to give it for a longer continuous period, until,
in fact, decided evidences of bromism are induced. I have
persevered with it in cases of either of these forms for six
months without intermission, the condition of the patient
gradually improving through the whole period, and an ultimate cure being effected.

In *emotional monomania* other than those varieties embraced under the designation of morbid fears, its influence in
eradicating the mental disease is not so well marked, though
I have succeeded with it in several striking instances of this
form of insanity.

In *simple melancholia* it is sometimes beneficial, especially in those cases in which there are the somatic evidences
of cerebral congestion, and which have not been of very long
duration. Relapses, however, are apt to ensue, and in such
cases it can rarely be got to act favorably again.

In *melancholia with delirium* and *melancholia with stupor* it has no very decided influence.

I have succeeded in several recent cases of *hypochondriacal mania* in entirely arresting the course of the disease and restoring the patient to his normal condition. In one case which had lasted over a year, and which was a few weeks since before my class at the New York Post-Graduate Medical School, the delusions entirely disappeared in about two months under the use of the bromide of sodium and aloetic purges.

Few cases of uncomplicated *hysterical mania* resist the continued use of the bromides in sufficiently large doses. If there is much mental and physical excitement, I usually give a hundred grains at a dose, and repeat it in twelve hours, or even less, if occasion seems to require. Then the medicine is continued in doses of from fifteen to twenty grains three times a day for as long as may seem necessary. Relapses are not uncommon, however, and then, unless a considerable interval has elapsed, the bromide does not act so well as in the first instance. They are also useful in some cases of *aboulomania*, in which there are marked symptoms of cerebral hyperæmia. In the fourth case of my own, described under that head, the bromide of sodium always controlled the trouble so long as the patient took it.

In *acute mania*, as well as in *periodical* and *circular insanity*, large doses of the bromides are important adjuncts in the treatment, and they may be continued in addition to other measures of more rapid action. They certainly exercise a beneficial effect in allaying excitement and in facilitating a favorable result.

In *katatonia* they are even still more advantageous. Here, also, large doses—from fifty to a hundred grains—should be given at first—for two or three days—and then when the force of the disease is broken, doses of fifteen or twenty grains three times a day will be sufficient.

In the early stages of *general paralysis*, and during any paroxysm of excitement or convulsion occurring in the course of the disease, the bromides are useful in quieting the patient and giving sleep.

In *epileptic insanity* they are indispensable, but they may have to be given for several years, or even during the lifetime of the patient. Indeed, many patients have paroxysms of the disease if the administration be stopped for only a few days. They should be given in large doses at first, and then subsequently in smaller ones, in cases in which the accessions are frequent and very severe. In milder cases the doses need not exceed fifteen grains three times a day for the first six months, with an increase of five grains every six months for two or three years.

In a patient recently under my charge, and in whom there were monthly attacks of epileptic insanity corresponding with the menstrual period, the attacks could always be prevented by a dose of a hundred grains of bromide of sodium, taken with the appearance of the menstrual discharge.

In *puerperal insanity* the bromides are almost invariably useful, especially in the beginning of the attack. The doses should at first be about thirty grains three times a day, which, as the patient passes under the influence of the medicine, may be reduced to fifteen grains.

In *choreic insanity* they are occasionally useful, though often more rapidly acting remedies are required. A large dose, taken just before bedtime, will, however, generally prove serviceable in stopping the hallucinations of sight to which patients with this form of insanity are subject.

It must not be forgotten, however, as previously stated, that the bromides sometimes themselves cause mental derangement. An analogous fact has been noted by Dr. H. M. Bannister,[1] who found that in certain insane epileptics—not cases of epileptic insanity—an increase of excitement was caused by the bromides. He is, however, inclined to regard this result as rather due to the suppression of the convulsive seizures than to any direct effect of the medicine.

Opium and its Preparations.—The preferable form in which to administer an opiate in cases of insanity is undoubtedly some one of the salts of morphia. In this country the sulphate is the one generally in use.

Morphia, systematically administered, is of undoubted efficacy in many forms of insanity as a curative agent, in addition to the immense benefit to be derived from its employment in cases in which an immediate calming effect is desired.

Morphia is especially beneficial in the treatment of those forms of *insanity which are characterized by mental depres-*

[1] "Note on a Peculiar Effect of the Bromides on certain Insane Epileptics," *The Journal of Nervous and Mental Disease,* July, 1881, p. 560.

sion. Although it had been previously used with success in other cases, Clerici[1] appears to have been the first to use it with a clear conception of its method of action in a case of melancholia, and shortly afterward Marcé[2] employed opium in a similar case with a successful result.

If melancholia is, as Meynert asserts, the result of exhausted brain action conjoined with a deficient supply of arterial blood, the indications would, of course, be to secure rest for the over-excited organ, and to increase the flow of blood to its arteries.

In a valuable memoir, Dr. Courtenay,[3] of the Derby County Lunatic Asylum, England, insists upon the use of opium as a remedy calculated to fulfil the objects in view, and he relates the details of a number of cases in which the most favorable results followed. Indeed, he regards opium in small doses as the most valuable of all medicines in the treatment of the condition in question. He appears, however, to be unaware of some experiments of my own (already described in this work, p. 156), performed several years ago, which tend to enforce very decidedly the correctness of the conclusions which he has reached by independent observations. The inference from these experiments, as well as from those of Dr. Courtenay, is that opium should be administered with discrimination, and that, when the object is to stimulate an exhausted and anæmic brain, the doses should be small. In my own practice in the class of cases under consideration, I have always derived very great benefit from doses rarely exceeding half a grain, repeated three or four times a day, and continued systematically for several weeks. Or from the eighth to the sixth of a grain of the sulphate of morphia may be given as often by the mouth, or twice daily as a hypodermic injection, if the patient will not take the medicine otherwise.

Voisin[4] is also an advocate for the continued use of morphia in all forms of insanity in which there is reason to suspect the existence of cerebral anæmia.

In larger doses I have found, in accordance with the ex-

[1] *Gazzetta medica de Lombardia*, Novembre, 1856.

[2] *Annales médico-psychologiques*, 1859.

[3] "The Use of Opium in the Treatment of Melancholia," *West Riding Lunatic Asylum Medical Reports*, vol. ii, 1872, p. 254.

[4] "Leçons cliniques sur les maladies mentales," Paris, 1883, p. 687.

periments referred to, that morphia is an efficient adjunct to
the bromides in the treatment of all the forms of mental derangement in which they are useful. As a small dose produces cerebral hyperæmia, a moderate dose causes cerebral
anæmia. It should, therefore, when used, in hyperæmic
forms of insanity, in conjunction with the bromides, be given
in doses of a quarter of a grain once or twice a day, or a grain
of opium may be administered in like manner. I have frequently obtained the most happy results by the employment
of the drugs in their combined form.

In cases of *acute mania*, or of *melancholia with delirium*,
or of any other variety in which there is a state of high mental and physical excitement, hypodermic injections of from
half a grain to a grain of sulphate of morphia will often quiet
the patient and induce a sound sleep of several hours' duration. Such a quantity as my experiments show, given to a
healthy man, would cause stupor, and perhaps death.

Chloral Hydrate.—As a means of securing sleep, chloral is
sometimes of service, though I very seldom employ it, owing
to the uncertainty of its action so far as the life of the patient
is concerned. It is used extensively in lunatic asylums, however, not as a curative agent, but solely as a hypnotic. I have,
however, known a person to take doses with impunity which
afterward resulted in her death.[1] It is not so much a hypnotic as it is a soporific.

Hyosciamus, or rather *hyosciamine*, is a valuable adjunct
in the treatment of conditions of mental excitement, especially when conjoined with great motorial activity. I have
given as much as the twentieth of a grain of the crystallized
hyosciamine by hypodermic injection with excellent effect in
a case of *acute mania*, and a like dose in a case of *general
paralysis* in which there was an exacerbation of mania. In
an instance of *melancholia with stupor* four drops of a solution of a grain of Merck's crystallized hyosciamine to one
ounce of water, equal to about the one hundred and twentieth
of a grain, were given three times a day with good results.
The quantity was gradually increased up to fifteen drops—
nearly the thirtieth of a grain—three times a day, some six
weeks being taken to reach this dose, the patient gradually

[1] "Fatal Cerebral Congestion following the Administration of Hydrate of
Chloral," by George G. Needham, M. D. *The Journal of Psychological Medicine*, January, 1871, p. 93.

improving and ultimately going on to recovery, even after the administration was stopped.

Digitalis.—I have used digitalin in *simple melancholia* and in *melancholia with stupor.* In the latter affection its action is sometimes particularly good. In the case of a young lady from New London, suffering from this form of mental derangement, the doses were carried up to the twentieth of a grain three times a day, beginning with the sixtieth. In this case the bromides had been given, before I saw the patient, with a decidedly deleterious effect. The digitalin acted well. The force of the heart was increased, her general circulation became more active, and complete recovery was the result. In another similar case, however, it produced no effect upon the mental condition, though given in doses of the tenth of a grain.

Conium.—The fluid extract of the seeds is the most eligible preparation of this drug to employ, and, as Dr. Seguin has shown, it may be given in much larger doses than are ordinarily thought admissible. There is, however, in my opinion, no form of insanity in which it is particularly indicated, though it may be useful in those cases in which there is mental and motorial excitement—choreic insanity, for instance.

Ergot, especially in combination with the bromides, is an exceedingly useful remedy in the hyperæmic forms of insanity. I usually give the fluid extract as the solvent instead of water for the bromide of sodium. It is indicated in all those varieties in which the bromides are useful.

Amyl Nitrite.—Inhalations of the nitrite of amyl are often of especial value in the treatment of the paroxysms of *hysterical mania* of the variety known as *hystero-epilepsy.* Ten drops may be poured on a handkerchief, and held over the nose and mouth. Similar treatment is frequently efficacious in the accessions of *epileptic mania.* In either case the administration may be made immediately before an expected seizure or during its action.

It is also useful in cases of *melancholia* generally. In the instance of a lady suffering from simple melancholia, who had several times attempted to commit suicide, and who had been for six months in a lunatic asylum, no other medicine was given, and the result was a complete recovery in about five weeks. In this instance ten drops of the remedy were administered by inhalation six times a day.

I have used the drug internally in doses of a drop or more up to ten drops, with the idea of preventing the paroxsyms of both these affections, but without any notable result.

Nitro-glycerine, or *glonoine*, as an internal remedy for certain forms of insanity, is of unquestionable value. A solution of one per cent in alcohol is a safe preparation to employ, and in the beginning the dose should not exceed a drop, which, however, may be taken if necessary every hour or two. I have used it in this way in the treatment of *simple melancholia*, in *melancholia with stupor*, in *hysterical mania*, in *primary dementia*, and in *epileptic insanity*, and have found it a valuable remedy. It is especially indicated in those forms of mental derangement in which cerebral anæmia is the chief intracranial morbid condition, such as the groups of melancholias and dementias.

I have also used it with entirely satisfactory results in three of the cases of *aboulomania* referred to when the symptomatology of the disease was under consideration. Whether this affection be due to a state of passive congestion or of anæmia of a portion of the brain, nitro-glycerine would appear to be indicated, and the results have been, in my experience, in accordance with the views I have expressed relative to its pathology. I gave a drop every hour for sixteen hours a day in the three cases first described, and continued this treatment for twenty days. After the second day in one case— the second—and the third day in the others, the power of the will began to augment, and gradually reached its normal degree of force, so that by the twentieth day no difficulty was experienced in causing it to act. The medicine was continued in the doses of two drops three times a day for a month longer, and then its administration was entirely stopped. In none of the cases has there been, so far as I know, any recurrence of the trouble. In the fourth case, which was one of long standing, the condition was aggravated by the nitro-glycerine.

Nitro-glycerine can be also given in the form of pills,[1] each one of which contains the one hundredth of a drop of the substance, but I prefer the solution, as acting more rapidly.

Sulphuric ether is of very limited application in the treatment of insanity. I have used it only in a few cases of *hysterical mania, epileptic insanity*, and *choreic insanity*. Its

[1] As prepared by Metcalf, of Boston, whose solution I have also found eminently satisfactory in its action.

effects are temporary only so far as the first two named are concerned, but in choreic insanity it has exercised a tranquillizing influence which did not altogether cease with the return of the patient to consciousness.

Bromide of Ethyl.—This substance was recommended two years ago by MM. Bourneville and d'Olier,[1] who used it with success in several cases of hysterical mania, hystero-epilepsy, and epilepsy. Recently Roux [2] has employed it in two cases of acute mania, of which one was cured.

My personal experience with this agent in the treatment of insanity is limited to a single case of *intellectual monomania with depression.* In this case there were hallucinations of voices uttering abuse and threats of violence, with delusions of persecution. After each inhalation the patient was decidedly better, both the hallucinations and delusions being of less intensity, and occasionally disappearing altogether, but they soon returned ; and, as after two weeks' treatment there was no improvement, the use was discontinued.

I gave it twice daily in doses of from a drachm to a drachm and a half dropped on a handkerchief two or three times, and held to the mouth. I continued the anæsthetic condition for fifteen or twenty minutes each time. No ill effects attended the administration. In view of the experience gained by Roux, it would appear that the remedy is worthy of further trial, and especially in cases of acute mania.

Iodide of Potassium.—The iodide of potassium has been used with benefit in some cases of *general paralysis,* and I have myself employed it with advantage in this affection. Apparently, under its influence the delusions have ceased to exist, many of the somatic symptoms have disappeared, and the patient has resumed his ordinary business. Eventually, however, in all but two cases they have reappeared. In these two instances, the intermissions have been thus far respectively eighteen months and six months, and both patients are free from all signs of mental aberration, except, perhaps, a slight degree of emotional impressionability, and from all physical symptoms except inequality of the pupils. In both cases the disease was of syphilitic origin, or, at least, the patients

---

[1] " Recherches sur l'action physiologique et thérapeutique de homme d'ethyle dans l'épilepsie et de l'hystérié," *Gazette médicale de Paris,* 26 mars, 1881, p. 173.

[2] *Thèse de Paris,* 1882.

had had primary disease. The doses in both cases were carried up to one hundred and twenty grains three times a day, and at intervals the medicine is still taken. Of course, these results may be mere coincidences, as remissions lasting as long as these are occasionally met with.

The iodide of potassium is of great service in all forms of *insanity which are of syphilitic origin*. It should be given in gradually increasing doses, up to one, two, or even three or four hundred grains at a dose if the diagnosis as to the cause is clear, and amendment does not result from smaller quantities.

Mercury is useful as an adjunct to the iodide of potassium. I usually give, in the cases in which the latter drug is indicated, from the thirtieth to the sixteenth of a grain of the bichloride with each dose of the potassium salt.

Mercury is sometimes useful as a purgative, but the occasions for its employment for this object are not many.

Strychnia and *phosphorus* are of advantage as tonics in all cases in which the vital powers are low, and which are such as may be supposed to result from an anæmic condition of the brain. These are included in the groups of melancholias and dementias. The former substance can almost always be relied upon in doses of from the sixtieth to the thirtieth of a grain three times a day, to increase the activity of the cerebral circulation.

Quinine and *iron* have a like applicability. In *melancholia with stupor* quinine in conjunction with strychnia is often of striking efficacy.

Arsenic is a very valuable remedy in all forms of the hyperæmic or congestive type. It is certainly a powerful agent in diminishing the amount of intracranial blood, as Lisle [1] pointed out several years ago. I generally give it in the form of the pills of arsenious acid which are now found ready-made at the pharmacists. The dose at first may be the twenty-fifth of a grain three times a day after eating, and the number of pills should be gradually increased for several weeks up to four or five at a dose—that is, to about half a grain daily. It is indicated in all those forms in which the bromides are useful, and may be given with advantage in conjunction with them. Fowler's solution may be administered instead of the

---

[1] "Du traitement de la congestion cérébrale et de la folie avec congestion et hallucinations par l'acide arsénieux," Paris, 1871.

48

arsenious acid in its solid form in corresponding quantities, though it has appeared to me that the latter preparation is preferable.

Besides its own specific effect upon the brain, arsenic is an excellent tonic, and tends to prevent the excessive debility which sometimes accompanies the use of the bromides in large doses.

There are other medicines which are also of great service in the treatment of insanity, to obviate certain pre-existing, accompanying, or secondary conditions. Thus, *emmenagogues* are indispensable when there is a functional arrest of the menstrual flow; *diuretics*, when the kidneys are inactive; *purgatives*, when the bowels are constipated; and so on with other classes of remedial agents. The latter are very generally required at some time or other in nearly every case of mental derangement.

Schroeder van der Kolk[1] has pointed out the efficacy of aloetic purges in certain cases of mental derangement with depression, accompanied with accumulations in the colon. I have frequently had occasion to be gratified with the success obtained by following the plan of treatment in question. I often give a grain of the watery extract of aloes in pill three times a day for a month, or even more if necessary, and again one pill at bedtime only, consisting of two grains of the watery extract of aloes, three of inspissated ox-gall, and from a quarter to half a grain of podophyllin. Under this plan of treatment I have repeatedly seen the most intense melancholia disappear in a few days. The treatment is also of service in all forms of insanity except the dementias and certain of the constitutional types, unless specially contraindicated.

Electricity.—In the chapter on insanity in the earlier editions of my work on "Diseases of the Mind and Nervous System," I stated that "electricity had not in my hands been productive of any marked benefit, though I have used it in all its various forms and methods." Since those lines were written, the great improvements which have been made in the construction of statical or Franklinic electrical machines have enabled us to employ statical or Franklinic electricity to

---

[1] "Die Pathologie und Therapie des Geisteskranken auf anatomisch-physiologischer Grundläge," Braunsweig, 1863, p. 185 *et seq.*; also, translation by Dr. James T. Rudall, London, 1870, p. 134.

much better effect than was then possible. I now very generally employ it as a counter-irritant, capable of making a very rapid and decided impression on the system. In cases of mental derangement coming under the class of *emotional insanities*, and in *primary* and *secondary dementia*, it is of decided benefit. I place the patients on the insulated stool and draw long sparks from the whole length of the spine. They very generally express themselves as feeling better, and they are perfectly willing to have the operation repeated. Whether or not the action is anything more than that of a counter-irritant I do not pretend to know. The *seance* may be repeated daily, or every alternate day, for as long as benefit appears to be derived. No single application should last longer than ten minutes.

Dr. Clifford Allbutt[1] has called attention to the good results derivable from the use of the continuous or galvanic current in certain forms of insanity. In cases of acute primary dementia decided improvement took place ; in mania and atonic melancholia—melancholia with stupor—the benefit was less decided ; in chronic dementia and in some cases of melancholia, no effect was produced ; while in hypochondriacal melancholia and, perhaps, in brain wasting, the result was unfavorable.

General bloodletting, once so much in vogue, can scarcely ever be required at the present day. There may be cases of acute mania in which it might be useful, and perhaps also certain instances of *epileptic insanity*, but certainly no others. On the other hand, *local bloodletting* by cups or leeches is often a useful measure, especially in those cases in which there are pain and heat in the head accompanied with insomnia and excitement. A half dozen or so of cups to the nape of the neck, or as many leeches to the temples, are often of marked and immediate advantage. A couple of leeches to the inside of the nostrils are remarkably efficacious in relieving cerebral hyperæmia and mitigating the violence of the physical and mental symptoms resulting from it.

In milder cases, *dry cups* may be applied to the nape of the neck and upper part of the spine every day with good results.

As to *counter-irritants*, such as *blisters, croton oil, tar-*

[1] " The Electric Treatment of the Insane," West Riding Lunatic Asylum Medical Reports, vol. ii, 1872, p. 203.

tarized antimony, and the *actual cautery*, cases every now and then appear in which they seem to be of service. I have, however, several times aggravated the mental and physical symptoms of insanity by their use. I suppose the most generally advantageous agent of the kind is the actual cautery very lightly applied to the nucha, but then the action in such a case can scarcely be called counter-irritant.

In a few cases of *chronic intellectual mania* I have derived slight benefit from the use of croton oil to the scalp, but it is scarcely worth while to go through so much to get so little.

The application of *cold* to the head or nape of the neck is useful in all cases of insanity belonging to the hyperæmic type, unless there is some special reason why it should not be employed. In mild cases it is sufficient to apply a lump of ice to the nape of the neck for two or three minutes just before going to bed. It generally aids effectually in producing sleep. In more severe cases the ice may be applied in a special ice-bag to the upper part of the spine and the occiput, and in others to the cortex.

In those cases due to cerebral anæmia embraced in the groups of melancholias and dementias, heat immediately applied is of great service, not only in quieting agitation when it exists, but in rousing the mind to something like its original degree of activity. I suppose one reason why good results have not more generally been derived from its employment is that it has not been used to a sufficiently high degree, and another is that it has not been continued long enough. The bags used for ice may be also used for hot water, and the application may be made in a manner like that employed for ice. Water heated up to 120° or even 130° is not generally of too elevated a temperature.

INDEX.

THE END.

MENTAL ILLNESS AND SOCIAL POLICY
THE AMERICAN EXPERIENCE

AN ARNO PRESS COLLECTION

Barr, Martin W. Mental Defectives: Their History, Treatment and Training. 1904.

The Beginnings of American Psychiatric Thought and Practice: Five Accounts, 1811-1830. 1973

The Beginnings of Mental Hygiene in America: Three Selected Essays, 1833-1850. 1973

Briggs, L. Vernon, et al. History of the Psychopathic Hospital, Boston, Massachusetts. 1922

Briggs, L. Vernon. Occupation as a Substitute for Restraint in the Treatment of the Mentally Ill. 1923

Brigham, Amariah. An Inquiry Concerning the Diseases and Functions of the Brain, the Spinal Cord, and the Nerves. 1840

Brigham, Amariah. Observations on the Influence of Religion upon the Health and Physical Welfare of Mankind. 1835

Brill, A. A. Fundamental Conceptions of Psychoanalysis. 1921

Bucknill, John Charles. Notes on Asylums for the Insane in America. 1876

Conolly, John. The Treatment of the Insane Without Mechanical Restraints. 1856

Coriat, Isador H. What is Psychoanalysis? 1917

Deutsch, Albert. The Shame of the States. 1948

Dewey, Richard. Recollections of Richard Dewey: Pioneer in American Psychiatry. 1936

Earle, Pliny. Memoirs of Pliny Earle, M. D. with Extracts from his Diary and Letters (1830-1892) and Selections from his Professional Writings (1839-1891). 1898

Galt, John M. The Treatment of Insanity. 1846

Goddard, Henry Herbert. Feeble-mindedness: Its Causes and Consequences. 1926

Hammond, William A. A Treatise on Insanity in Its Medical Relations. 1883

Hazard, Thomas R. Report on the Poor and Insane in Rhode-Island. 1851

Hurd, Henry M., editor. The Institutional Care of the Insane in the United States and Canada. 1916/1917. Four volumes.

Kirkbride, Thomas S. On the Construction, Organization, and General Arrangements of Hospitals for the Insane. 1880

Meyer, Adolf. The Commonsense Psychiatry of Dr. Adolf Meyer: Fifty-two Selected Papers. 1948

Mitchell, S. Weir. Wear and Tear, or Hints for the Overworked. 1887

Morton, Thomas G. The History of the Pennsylvania Hospital, 1751-1895. 1895

Ordronaux, John. Jurisprudence in Medicine in Relation to the Law. 1869

The Origins of the State Mental Hospital in America: Six Documentary Studies, 1837-1856. 1973

Packard, Mrs. E. P. W. Modern Persecution, or Insane Asylums Unveiled, As Demonstrated by the Report of the Investigating Committee of the Legislature of Illinois. 1875. Two volumes in one

Prichard, James C. A Treatise on Insanity and Other Disorders Affecting the Mind. 1837

Prince, Morton. The Unconscious: The Fundamentals of Human Personality Normal and Abnormal. 1921

Putnam, James Jackson. Human Motives. 1915

Russell, William Logie. The New York Hospital: A History of the Psychiatric Service, 1771-1936. 1945

Sidis, Boris. The Psychology of Suggestion: A Research into the Subconscious Nature of Man and Society. 1899

Southard, Elmer E. Shell-Shock and Other Neuropsychiatric Problems Presented in Five Hundred and Eighty-Nine Case Histories from the War Literature, 1914-1918. 1919

Southard, E[lmer] E. and Mary C. Jarrett. The Kingdom of Evils. 1922

Southard, E[lmer] E. and H[arry] C. Solomon. Neurosyphilis: Modern Systematic Diagnosis and Treatment Presented in One Hundred and Thirty-seven Case Histories. 1917

Spitzka, E[dward] C. Insanity: Its Classification, Diagnosis and Treatment. 1887

Supreme Court Holding a Criminal Term, No. 14056. The United States vs. Charles J. Guiteau. 1881/1882. Two volumes

Trezevant, Daniel H. Letters to his Excellency Governor Manning on the Lunatic Asylum. 1854

Tuke, D[aniel] Hack. The Insane in the United States and Canada. 1885

Upham, Thomas C. Outlines of Imperfect and Disordered Mental Action. 1868

White, William A[lanson]. Twentieth Century Psychiatry: Its Contribution to Man's Knowledge of Himself. 1936

Willard, Sylvester D. Report on the Condition of the Insane Poor in the County Poor Houses of New York. 1865